Health assessment

Health assessment

■ **LOIS MALASANOS, R.N., Ph.D.**

Professor, Department of General Nursing, College of Nursing,
University of Illinois at the Medical Center,
Chicago, Illinois

■ **VIOLET BARKAUSKAS, R.N., C.N.M., M.P.H.**

Assistant Professor, Department of Public Health Nursing,
College of Nursing, University of Illinois at the Medical Center,
Chicago, Illinois

■ **MURIEL MOSS, R.N., M.A.**

Assistant Professor, Department of Public Health Nursing,
College of Nursing, University of Illinois at the Medical Center,
Chicago, Illinois

■ **KATHRYN STOLTENBERG-ALLEN, R.N., M.S.N.**

Former Assistant Professor, Department of Public Health Nursing,
College of Nursing, University of Illinois at the Medical Center,
Chicago, Illinois

with 769 illustrations

The C. V. Mosby Company

Saint Louis   1977

The C. V. Mosby Company
11830 Westline Industrial Drive, St. Louis, Missouri 63141

Library of Congress Cataloging in Publication Data

Main entry under title:

Health assessment.

    Includes bibliographies and index.
    1. Nursing. 2. Medical history taking.
3. Physical diagnosis. I. Malasanos, Lois, 1928-
[DNLM: 1. Physical examination. 2. Medical
history taking. WB205 H434]
RT48.H4   616.07'5   77-2179
ISBN 0-8016-0478-8

GW/CB/B 9 8 7 6 5 4 3 2

To family, friends, and colleagues
who were our clients, counselors, and sustainers.

For those students who gave us the need to write
by their persistent efforts to find the information
that would enable them to provide better health care.

Preface

This text is designed for beginning practitioners who are learning skills that will enable them to assess the health status of the client by obtaining a health history and performing a physical examination. The acquisition of clinical skills is best accomplished when learning experiences are organized and the learner is provided with opportunities to acquire knowledge and to practice with experienced preceptors in settings that enhance learning (for example, a laboratory where learners can practice their new skills with each other or a clinical setting where the clients have been informed of the learner's purpose and have agreed to participate). Therefore, this text is intended for use in conjunction with a course of study that provides structured learning experiences enabling the learner to acquire the theory and skills of health assessment.

Health assessment skills are useful to the practitioner in any clinical setting. However, this text is especially aimed at helping the practitioner who is preparing for a role in primary care, where the health maintenance of the client is a priority. The focus is on wellness, and the parameters of normal health are incorporated into the process of obtaining a health history and performing a physical examination. The discussion of selected problems is also included in the text as a way of demonstrating differences or deviations from the parameters of normal health. Within the framework of health maintenance, emphasis is placed on the early detection of changes in the health status of the client for the purpose of preventing a more serious problem or disability. This is compatible with the plan to assist the learner in defining the parameters of wellness and the subtle or gross deviations that occur in the presence of illness.

The consumer of health care is referred to as the *client* in this text because it is a term that implies the ability of a person to contract for health care, whether well or sick, as a responsible participant with the providers of health care. The label *patient* has been avoided because it can only be used to describe someone who is ill and therefore more apt to be a dependent receiver of care. Health providers can no longer expect consumers of care to accept health advice or treatment plans unless they have been included in the decision-making process. Thus, the use of the term *client* is more appropriate in today's world.

The text is intended as a guide to assist the learner in conceptualizing the assessment of the whole person, taking into account the parameters of good health practices and the factors that impinge on health. The assessment that incorporates these components provides a basis for the development of an optimal plan for health care and health teaching that is reasonable in terms of the individual client's life situation.

The components of the assessment, including the history and physical examination, are organized to allow the learner to proceed from an assessment of the overall function of the client to the more specific function of each body system. A discussion of the purposes and techniques of interviewing precedes the chapter on the health history in order that the learner may become more sensitive to the process of obtaining information within the framework of a beginning or continuing relationship with the client. The chapters that discuss aspects of daily health care—nutrition and sleep—and the developmental assessment are placed in the beginning portion of the text to help the practitioner gain an appreciation of the whole person and some aspects of individual life-styles before proceeding to the more specific assessment of the body systems.

Finally, the learner is encouraged to consider specific ways of organizing the assessment and the recording of the data obtained. There is little value in obtaining information that is lost to the practitioner or other members of the health team at a future time when it may be of critical importance as part of an overall data base from which problems are identified and actions planned.

Regarding the techniques utilized to assess the health of the client, we have described the standard techniques of history taking and the use of inspection, both direct and via instrumentation (for example, the otoscope and ophthalmoscope), palpation, percussion, and auscultation. In addition, we have made an effort to expand on the techniques and to describe the instruments. For example, the client's history not only includes the chief complaint, present illness, review of systems, and so on, but also focuses on the daily patterns of activity and sleep and on the developmental stage or level of the individual. In those sections where the use of examination techniques (including instrumentation) pertains, those techniques and instruments are described; for example, the techniques of percussion are discussed in the chapter on the respiratory tract ex-amination, a description of the ophthalmoscope is found in the chapter on the eye examination, a description on the otoscope accompanies the chapter on the ear examination, and material on the stethoscope accompanies the chapter on the cardiovascular examination. Thus, a discussion of the various techniques utilized in health assessment is presented with the system relevant to that technique.

Many people have contributed to the development of this text. Without their support and assistance it would not have been possible. Carrie Schopf, M.D., has been our reviewer, supporter, and teacher. Patricia Urbanus, R.N., M.S.N., our photographer, has been consistently interested and creative in helping us despite the enormous demands made on her time. And our thanks is extended to Scott Thorn Barrows, William R. Schwarz, Robert Parshall, and Christo Popoff for their outstanding artwork.

Lois Malasanos
Violet Barkauskas
Muriel Moss
Kathryn Stoltenberg-Allen

Contents

CONTENTS

Health assessment

1 Introduction

RECOGNITION OF THE NEED FOR HEALTH ASSESSMENT AND UNIVERSAL HEALTH CARE

As long ago as the beginning of the Civil War an article was published recommending periodic health examinations in the interest of the early detection of disease (Dobell, 1861). This concept was adopted by the American Medical Association in 1922 in the form of a resolution advocating periodic health assessment. In 1925 the procedure was formalized in a manual published by this organization.

In 1956 the declaration that health care is a basic human right was made at a White House Conference on Aging. The general public has expressed with increasing frequency the expectation that preventive health care constitutes a fundamental part of this care. Leavell and Clark have defined preventive health care in three categories: primary, secondary, and tertiary prevention. Primary prevention involves those aspects of health care that are aimed at avoiding the contraction of a disease. Secondary prevention is aimed at stopping or attenuating the process of disease, and tertiary prevention deals with rehabilitative processes. The objective of tertiary prevention is the restoration of optimal function to a person after the disease process has been arrested.

Each level of prevention is based on a thorough assessment of the client's health status. Preventive health care can be planned only from a complete data base of both the client and his family.

Government leaders emphasize the need for provision of adequate and accessible health care for all Americans regardless of their ability to pay and regardless of where they live. The two words that frequently appear in discussions relevant to this issue are equity and access.

The need to establish facilities for health care in the communities where people live is receiving more attention among legislators. The negative aspects of asking the client to travel long distances for preventive care are increasingly clear. In many cases the distance to the physician or hospital is the major determinant of whether a client seeks care. The famous anecdote among the people of Watts makes the point well. In this community the cost of a taxi to the hospital is ten dollars. These people often have to be quite sick before they seek medical help. When they do go to the hospital, they refer to themselves as being "ten dollars sick."

One way that the government of the United States has recognized the universal need for comprehensive health care has been through the establishment of health maintenance organizations. These institutions are designed to provide preventive health care that is community based.

On the other side of the coin, physicians control health care in the United States as a result of both legislative action and tradition. Although the number of physicians has increased to 170 per 100,000 population, a number greater than at any other time in the history of this country, there are wide gaps between the consumer, the health care demands, and the capabilities of the available physicians to meet them. The major deficit is in the number of primary care physicians prepared to provide the degree of preventive health care known to be needed. Several British writers have taken the position that it is the primary care practitioner who can give preventive care most effectively.

The process of specialization in medical practice makes it increasingly more difficult for physi-

1

cians to obtain salient family and community information. At this time the majority of preventive care is performed in physicians' offices and in emergency rooms. Care essentially involves providing prescriptions and treatment for symptomatic clients.

Thus, most health care treatment in this country is oriented toward dealing with crisis situations. Health maintenance efforts are directed toward large industrial groups, antenatal women, well babies, school children, and military groups but remains on the whole a matter of individual responsibility.

ADVANTAGES OF ASSESSMENT

The value of periodic health examinations has been attested to in several studies. As early as 1921 the Metropolitan Life Insurance Company reported a 28% reduction in mortality due to early disease detection incurred through periodic health examinations. Studies related to disability reported in the 1960s showed a savings in employee disability payments that amounted to four times more than the cost of the examinations; the studies also showed that as much as 13% of the disease that produces disability in executives could be detected in the periodic health examination before the disability was incurred. Although later studies have failed to substantiate the wide margins suggested in these early studies, there is little doubt that the general public would benefit not only from the early detection of disease but also from the provision of a constantly updated baseline of relevant data. This information would benefit the individual by allowing a comparison of parameters obtained during a well visit with those observed during a suspected illness; this comparison would potentially afford a more accurate diagnosis. Furthermore, significant epidemiological data obtained during these examinations would be a secondary gain.

INCREASING ACCESSIBILITY TO ASSESSMENT

The health examination is frequently the mechanism of entry into the health care system. Since accessibility has been shown to be an important factor in determining whether a client will seek health care, alternate modes of providing health care to greater numbers of people have been explored.

Recent studies have indicated that although periodic health examinations have proved ben-

efits, they may not necessarily need to be performed by a physician. Controlled studies comparing physicians' and nurses' problem lists after they have examined the same client show no appreciable differences. The examinations are certainly less costly to the client when they are done by health care workers other than physicians. At least one author has suggested that as many as three fourths of the clients who visit a primary care physician for health care could be safely monitored by an allied health professional and at a considerable financial saving. It is reasonably clear that making health services available to the entire population in an effective manner will include both medical and nurse practitioners.

That there is a need to develop a core of individuals skilled in assessing the health status of persons seeking such care has been attested to by the Russians' use of Feldsher and by the utilization of public health nurses, nurse practitioners, and physicians' assistants in the United States. These paramedical practitioners have helped to make preventive care an actuality by increasing accessibility to the system, both through increasing the number of people able to give this care and by providing care in communities that had previously been underserved. The provision of these services is evidence of sensitivity to the public's need and an effort to make health care more convenient.

These groups of health care workers have entered into situations involving varying degrees of responsibility for patient care. In all cases they are involved in the assessment of health status; there are some differences in expectations of their abilities to identify normal versus abnormal traits. In many cases standardized treatment schedules or protocols allow these individuals to render treatment and follow-up care. This can be a workable reality in those cases where the medical community has achieved consensus as to appropriate care for specific problems.

OBJECTIVES AND TYPES OF ASSESSMENT

The purposes of health assessment include surveillance of health status, the identification of latent or occult disease, screening for a specific type of disease (called case finding), and follow-up care.

The public has been educated and often required to seek certain health examinations, such as well baby, preschool, premarital, precollege, prenatal, preemployment, and preinsurance examinations. Both men and women in their middle years have been educated to their increased vulnerability to disease and thus seek care at this time.

Many words have developed to describe the act of health assessment. Some of these are *physical examination, health appraisal, checkup,* and *screening examination*. These types of assessment generally include a history, a physical examination, and a routine battery of clinical laboratory tests. Such appraisals are often thought of as isolated incidents. The *periodic health examination,* on the other hand, is regarded as occurring at regular intervals. A return or follow-up visit is one that is scheduled to assess the progress or abatement of diagnosed dysfunction.

Examinations performed for the purpose of case finding are directed at significant diseases for which there is a recognized treatment. Furthermore, definitive tests or examinations should be recognized as being specific to the condition and the population tested. In addition, there should be an early symptomatic or latent stage of the disease, so that intervention will prevent progress of the disease.

FREQUENCY OF ASSESSMENT

There is considerable controversy surrounding the issue of how often the periodic health examination should be performed on the ostensibly healthy client. Early recommendations suggested that the health examination should be done each year. More recent evaluation of the findings of examinations by age groups suggests that younger individuals need not be assessed as frequently as older people. One recommendation is that persons under 35 years of age be assessed every 4 to 5 years, that persons 35 to 45 years of age be assessed every 2 to 3 years, and that only persons over 45 years of age undergo a thorough health assessment every year.

INCREASING CLIENT PARTICIPATION IN HEALTH CARE

The health assessment should accurately define the health and sick care needs for the individual at that specific point in time.

The information obtained in the interview and physical examination is used to formulate the exchanges of responsibility in defining the contract. The client should be apprised of the services available that will be useful in dealing with his problems.

Table 1-1. Recommendation for the frequency of health assessment

Client's age	Frequency of health assessment
<35	Every 4 to 5 years
35 to 45	Every 2 to 3 years
>45	Every year

The findings of the health assessment are shared with the client in a clearly understandable manner. In many cases this may mean educating him to the anatomy and physiology of his diseased tissues so that he can fully understand the meaning and level of his dysfunction.

Only with a clear definition of his problem is the client capable of assuming active involvement in decision making for his own care.

The World Health Organization (WHO) has defined health education as the active mechanism of facilitating an optimal state of social, emotional, and physical functioning that should be available to all people. Patient education is implicit in preventive care.

Primary prevention may be facilitated through teaching the client the general tenets of a healthful life-style. Some of the topics that may be explained are the optimal nutritional habits, sleep-activity patterns, exercise regimens, and recreational patterns. The client may also be warned against such potentially dangerous health patterns as smoking and diets typified by high sugar content.

The adolescent may particularly benefit by educational efforts concerning alcohol, drugs, and sexuality.

Genetic counseling may be considered one form of primary prevention, the need for which may become apparent during the course of the health assessment.

Several authors contend that individuals should be educated to the most common problems experienced by the general public in their particular geographical locale in order to take care of themselves more effectively. Moreover, the public needs sufficient information to make responsible use of the health services available to them.

In many situations clients may be taught to monitor their own disease process. More common examples are the hypertensive client who follows his own blood pressure and the diabetic client who tests for the presence of sugar and acetone in his urine. Many assessment techniques may be easily taught to clients, particularly those involving inspection and palpation.

Another form of increasing the participation of the client in the management of his health problems is one of teaching him the untoward side effects that commonly occur with medications that are prescribed for him and the steps he should take in the event these side effects happen to him.

An exploration with the client should be planned that will allow the practitioner to understand the attitudes and feelings of the client toward the health care system. Questions may be formulated that will reveal the nature of the client's earlier experiences with physicians, nurses, and allied personnel and health care agencies. This discussion may also bring out an appreciation of the kind of problems the client feels would warrant a visit to a health care agency. This information may be utilized in planning the mechanisms that will help the individual to continue in the system.

Several studies have been done that contribute to the knowledge of the client's attitudes and values toward health care. Some of the findings are useful. The client imparts to the health professional a faith in the fact that technical competence is a given, that the professional's educational preparation has guaranteed this aspect. The client further expects that all the equipment necessary for his examination is available and in working order and that all the tests necessary to explore his problems will be ordered, performed, and interpreted correctly. The health professional is expected by the client to show a genuine interest in his general welfare, that the client is worth the time required to evaluate and intervene in the disease processes the professional may find. The client frequently correlates the competence of the health professional with the amount of time the professional is willing to spend with the client, the professional's demonstrated willingness to allow the client to fully discuss his problems, and the degree to which the professional answers questions lucidly and honestly. The client is not loath to visit several health professionals if the opinion of specialists is needed in reaching a diagnosis. He is, however, better satisfied if the health professional he visits actively intervenes in his disease process.

The prospect of an individual seeking health care in relation to a specific illness corresponds directly with his perception of (1) the dangers of the disease (disability, death), (2) his own susceptibility to the disease, and (3) the possibility that the illness can be cured by the intervention of health professionals.

The levels of income and education are positively correlated with those populations who seek health care. Furthermore, those with education regarding hygiene are more prone to ensure their well-being by attaining health surveillance. They are also more likely to secure verification of symptoms that they feel may connote disease.

The aged, the poorly educated, and the socioeconomically disadvantaged are less likely to feel that health care is meeting their needs. It has been shown that women, poorly educated individuals, and elderly individuals are less likely to demonstrate compliance in health care. Thus, these groups are less likely to seek a health examination, to follow the therapeutic regimen established for them, and to return for further help.

Studies have shown that women with family responsibilities only are less likely to seek health care than those with family responsibilities who have career commitments as well.

Conditions for which health care is needed include self-destructive behavior leading to early death, sickness, and debility. Such conditions may be drug dependency, alcoholism, venereal disease, unwanted pregnancy, and obesity. Because of the stigma attached to many of these states, the affected individuals may not seek health care. Frequently, inadequate services are available for those who do. The individual feels devalued in his own estimation and is hesitant to reveal what he considers a weakness, an aberration, over which he feels he "should" have control. It has been shown that return visits of such individuals are increased by encouraging them to assume responsibility for planning.

ASSESSMENT TECHNIQUES

Although the major emphasis of this volume is health assessment, there are certain physiological functions and perceptions that are considered to be integral to examination of the client; these are the skills that contribute to the art of physical diagnosis. The four major procedures of physical diagnosis are inspection, palpation, percussion, and auscultation. These procedures are described here and are further developed in chapters dealing with their application for specific organs and systems.

■ Inspection

Inspection (L. *inspectio*, the act of beholding) is the act of concentrating attention to the thorough and unhurried visualization of the client. Inspection also involves listening to any sounds emanating from the client as well as being attuned to any odors that may be present.

Lighting must be adequate. Daylight or artificial light is suitable. The specific cues to which the examiner alerts himself are discussed in Chapter 7 on General inspection.

■ Palpation

By palpation (L. *palpatio,* the act of touching), the examiner's hands may be used to augment the data gathered through inspection. The skilled examiner will use the most sensitive parts of the hand for each type of palpation. The pads of the fingers are thought to be most effective in those tasks requiring discrimination through touch. Rough measures of temperature are best determined with the dorsum of the hand. Vibration is detected most effectively with the palmar surface of the metacarpal phalangeal joints. The position and consistency of a structure may best be determined by employing the grasping fingers. The examiner may utilize touch to seek out and determine the extent of tenderness and tremor or spasm of muscle tissues or to elicit crepitus in bones and joints. Individual structures within body cavities, particularly the abdomen, may be palpated for position, size, shape, consistency, and mobility. The examining hand may be used to detect masses or to evaluate abnormal collections of fluid. The skin and hair are examined for moisture and texture through the use of touch.

■ Percussion

Percussion (L. *percussio,* the act of striking) involves a cause-and-effect relationship. This summary term includes the act of striking or otherwise producing the impact of one object against another—this is the cause. The result of this rapping is the production of a shock wave that in some cases results in vibration. The vibration may produce sound waves that may reach the ear to be interpreted as sound. In the process of physical diagnosis, percussion means the striking or tapping of a body surface such as the back or the abdomen while listening with the unassisted ear or with the stethoscope.

Auenbrugger, the originator of the technique, described what has been termed *immediate percussion.* Immediate percussion means the striking of a finger or hand directly against the body. The term *mediate percussion* is used to describe the refinement in technique that was developed some time in the 19th century. Instruments called the pleximeter and plexor were devised. The plexor was a small rubber hammer, much like the reflex hammers used today. This plexor was used to strike a blow against the pleximeter, a small, flat, solid object, often made of ivory, that was held firmly in place against the client's body.

Mediate percussion using the middle finger of one hand as the plexor that strikes against the middle finger (pleximeter) of the other hand is the method in use in current clinical practice.

The passive hand is placed gently against the body surface. The finger is dealt a blow at or immediately proximal to the distal interphalangeal joint with the middle finger of the other hand. The blow must be delivered crisply, sharply, and with the plexor perpendicular to the pleximeter.

The speed and force of a blow by the plexor is made possible by wrist action. The hand is flexed back on the forearm and brought forward with a clean, snapping motion that allows a fast strike and rapid removal of the plexor (Fig. 13-13).

Fatty tissue overlying the tissue to be percussed may dampen the blow. In order to overcome this, it has been suggested that more force can be brought to bear on the body surface by striking the lateral aspect of the thumb. Rapid pronation of the forearm is used to provide the quick, striking movement.

The vibration produced through percussion involves only the tissue closely adjacent to the pleximeter. The most resonant tissues may vibrate up to 5 cm from the pleximeter. Percussion over bones is affected by lateral transmission of vibration.

The change from resonance to dullness is more easily perceived than the dull-to-resonant transition. Thus, the examiner organizes his percussion protocol to progress from more resonant regions to lesser ones.

Fist percussion is, as the name implies, striking with the hand in a fisted position. The blow is delivered to the dorsum of the other hand. The purpose of this type of percussion is to elicit sensation by the vibration of the tissue. The most common applications are to stimulate pain or tenderness due to hepatitis, cholecystitis, or kidney disease.

The sound waves that result from percussion are evaluated with reference to intensity, pitch, quality, and duration.

Sound is produced by vibrating structures. The vibrations generate a series of compression waves in the medium that is capable of sound transmission. Solids, liquids, and gases that are sufficiently elastic to convert energy to motion may

Table 1-2. Sounds produced by percussion

Characteristics of sounds produced	Record of finding	Anatomical regions where sounds may be encountered
Musical note, higher pitch than resonance; sustained longest time	Tympany	Air in closed structure vibrates in concert with tissues surrounding it: the stomach, intestines
Moderate to high pitch; sustained longer than resonance	Hyper-reso-nant	Air-filled lungs
Moderate pitch; sustained moderate time	Resonant	Lung tissue
High pitch; short sound	Dull	Relatively airless, solid tissue: liver, spleen
High pitch; short sound	Flat	Solid tissue, least amount of trapped air: muscles of arm, leg

transmit sound. The compression waves initiate vibrations of the tympanic membrane, which moves in and out with the frequency of the sound waves. The mechanical energy of the compression waves is transduced into neural signals by receptor structures of the middle ear. These neural signals are transmitted to the temporal cortex and perceived as sound.

Intensity, loudness. The physical property of sound called intensity produces the effect of loudness in the human auditory apparatus. As a sound wave travels through a point in the air, the air molecules are compressed and then expanded in the wake of the compression wave. The difference between maximum pressure and minimum pressure is the amplitude of the sound wave. The greater the displacement of air, the more movement during vibration of the tympanic membrane and the louder the perception of sound. Loudness is a psychological variable as well. The individual listener may be attentive to or selectively unaware of the many sounds in his milieu.

Pitch, frequency. The frequency of sound is a physical property that corresponds to the number of vibrations of the sound source per second. Pitch is related to the frequency of sound.

The waveform of a sound of single frequency is sinusoidal, ⌇⌇ with perfectly matched

hills (peaks) and valleys (troughs). The distance from 1 peak to the next is 1 cycle. The recording of frequency is in cycles per second (cps), or hertz (Hz). The human ear is capable of detecting sounds in the frequency range of 15 to 30 cps, to 20,000 cps. With advancing age, the human ear becomes progressively less sensitive to the higher sound frequencies. The sounds of speech and music (250 to 2,048 cps) are most frequently lost. However, most sounds of importance in physical diagnosis are in the frequency range below 1,000 cps and more particularly in the range of 40 to 500 cps.

Quality, harmonics. Harmonic, or overtone, refers to the physical property of sound that causes the psychological effect called quality or timbre. A sound of single frequency produces a pure tone. The lowest frequency at which a piano wire vibrates is called the fundamental. Most objects vibrate at more than one frequency. The piano wire may vibrate as a single unit or in halves or thirds that oscillate at their own frequency. These frequencies will be whole number multiples of the single frequency. The fundamental and the multiples of the single frequency are the harmonics. Sound quality is produced by the sum of the harmonics present and their intensities. The quality is recorded in descriptive terms such as *humming*, *buzzing*, or *roaring*. The fundamental is the first harmonic. A musical sound is one wherein the mix of intensity and pitch is pleasing to the ear, whereas *noise* is the term given an unpleasant sensation. Most sounds heard in the course of the physical examination are perceived as noise.

An axiom of the physical examination is that, like the drum, the more air tissue contains (the less dense the tissue), the deeper, louder, and longer the sound will be. The corollary is that the more compact the tissue, the higher, fainter, and shorter the sound will be. The sounds elicited in percussion are recorded in relation to the density of the tissue being vibrated. The least dense tissues produce tympany, whereas successively more dense tissue results in hyperresonance, resonance, impaired resonance, dullness, and flatness.

■ Auscultation

Auscultation (L. *auscultate*, to listen to) is the process of listening for the sounds produced by the human body. The sounds of particular importance are those produced by (1) the thoracic or abdominal viscera and (2) the movement of blood in the cardiovascular system. *Direct*, or *imme-*

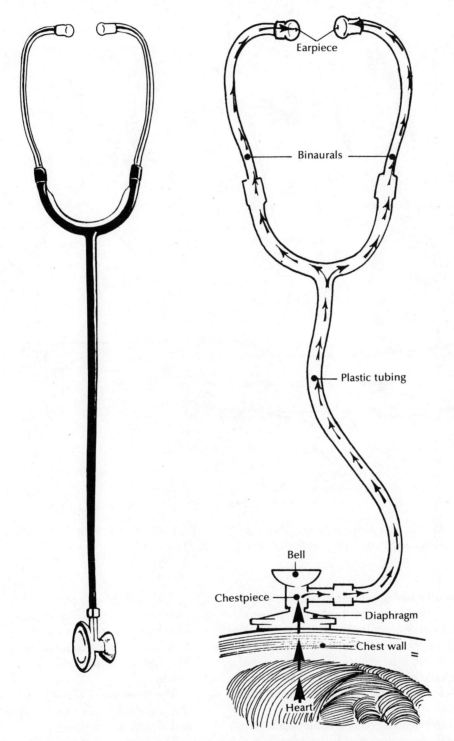

Fig. 1-1. Acoustical stethoscope. (From Patient Care, March 15, 1974. © Copyright 1974, Miller and Fink Corp., Darien, Conn. All rights reserved.)

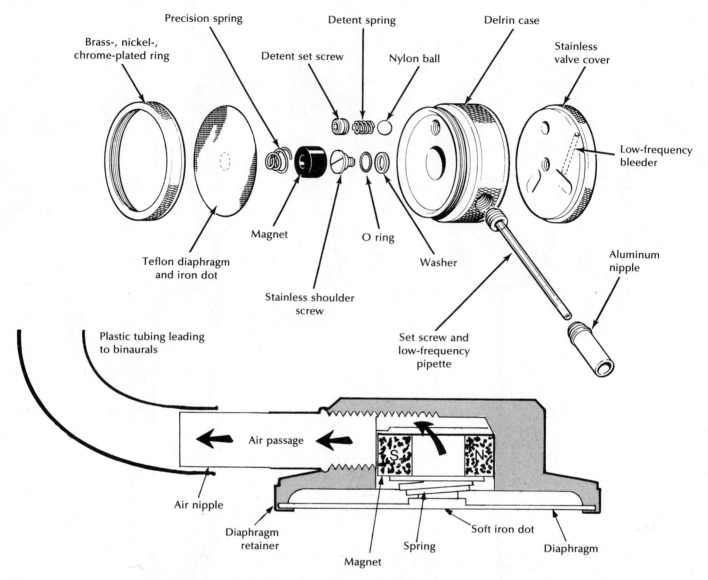

Fig. 1-2. Magnetic stethoscope. (From Patient Care, March, 15, 1974. © Copyright 1974, Miller and Fink Corp., Darien, Conn. All rights reserved.)

diate, auscultation is accomplished by the unassisted ear, that is, without any amplifying device. This form of auscultation often involves the application of the ear directly to a body surface where the sound is most prominent. The use of a sound augmentation device such as a stethoscope in the detection of body sounds is called *mediate auscultation.*

Hippocrates described chest sounds in his writings, and Harvey mentioned heart sounds in the early 1600s. Direct, or immediate, auscultation was practiced until 1816, when Laennec devised the first stethoscope, which consisted of a series of rolled up papers held in place with gummed paper. Laennec continued to improve the device

and ultimately utilized a wooden tubing with an earpiece. Later, flexible ear trumpets were modified for use in auscultation. This monaural form of mediate auscultation was succeeded by a binaural instrument in the middle of the 19th century.

The three types of stethoscopes that enjoy clinical popularity today are the acoustical, magnetic, and electronic stethoscopes.

The *acoustical stethoscope* (Fig. 1-1) is essentially a closed cylinder, which serves to inhibit the dissipation of the compression waves produced by the sound source in the column. The diaphragm of the acoustical stethoscope screens out low-frequency sounds and is therefore most

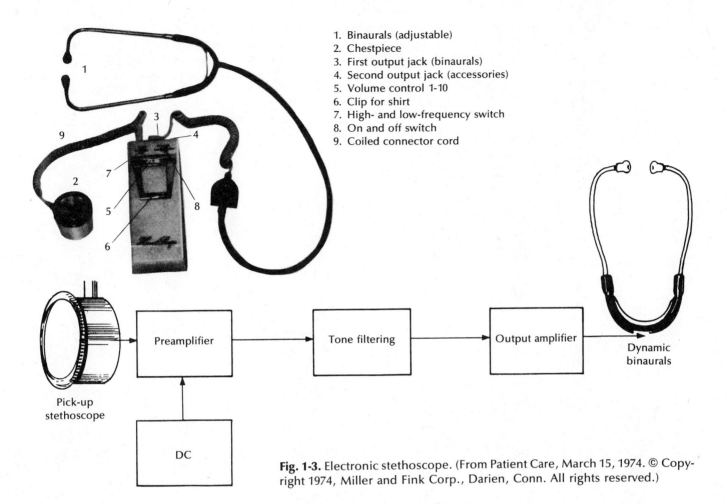

1. Binaurals (adjustable)
2. Chestpiece
3. First output jack (binaurals)
4. Second output jack (accessories)
5. Volume control 1-10
6. Clip for shirt
7. High- and low-frequency switch
8. On and off switch
9. Coiled connector cord

Fig. 1-3. Electronic stethoscope. (From Patient Care, March 15, 1974. © Copyright 1974, Miller and Fink Corp., Darien, Conn. All rights reserved.)

effective in assessing high-frequency sounds. The diaphragm is applied firmly to the skin so that it moves synchronously with the body wall. The bell-type head is most effective in detecting low-frequency sounds. Care is taken not to flatten the skin by pressing the bell too firmly, since the vibrations of the surface tissues in response to visceral vibration are the source of sound; stretching these tissues inhibits vibration, actually converting the tissue to a diaphragm.

The Harvey stethoscope, a variation of the acoustical type, has three heads: a bell for low frequencies, a corrugated diaphragm for midrange, and a flat diaphragm for high frequencies. This stethoscope also has separate tubes leading to each head.

The *magnetic stethoscope* (Fig. 1-2) has a single head that is a diaphragm. Magnetic attraction is established between an iron disk on the interior surface of the diaphragm and a permanent magnet installed behind it in the head. A strong spring keeps the diaphragm bowed outward when not compressed against a body surface. Ap-

plication of the diaphragm with the appropriate amount of pressure allows activation of the air column. A dial allows the user to adjust for high-, low-, and full-frequency sounds.

The *electronic stethoscope* (Fig. 1-3) operates as a result of vibration of a diaphragm or microphone occurring as a result of the body surface vibrations. These vibrations are transduced into electrical pulses, which are amplified and converted back to sound at a low speaker.

The use of the stethoscope is described in Chapter 13 on Assessment of the Respiratory System and in Chapter 14 on Cardiovascular assessment: the heart and the neck vessels.

BIBLIOGRAPHY

Andreopoulos, S., editor: Primary care; where medicine fails, New York, 1974, John Wiley & Sons, Inc.

Collen, M. F.: Periodic health examinations, Primary Care 3:197, 1976.

Garfield, S. R., Collen, M. F., Richart, P. H., and others: Evaluation of new ambulatory medical care delivery system, N. Engl. J. Med. **294**:426, 1976.

Hart, C. R.: Screening in general practice, Edinburgh, 1975, Churchill Livingstone.

Javits, J.: National health care policy for the future, J. Politics Policy Law 1:5, 1976.

Leavell, H. R., and Clark, E. G.: Preventive medicine for the doctor in his community, ed. 3, New York, 1965, McGraw-Hill Book Co.

Mushkin, S. J., editor: Consumer incentives for health care, New York, 1974, Prodist.

Spitzer, W. O., Sackett, D. L., Sibley, J. C., and others: The Burlington randomized trial of the nurse practitioner, N. Engl. J. Med. 290:251, 1974.

2 The interview

The major purpose of the interview conducted prior to the physical examination is to obtain a health history and to elicit symptoms and the time course of their development. The goal of an effective interview is a complete and accurate data base. However, although assessment may be the main emphasis of a given exchange, the primary care practitioner must bring to bear skillful communication techniques in order to establish the rapport necessary for a full sharing of the client's relevant life experiences. A climate of trust must be established that will allow a full expression of the client's needs. Furthermore, an analysis of the reactions of the client during the interview will allow the examiner to predict the ability and willingness of the client to comprehend and carry out the directions given him as part of the therapeutic plan.

The communication skills and sensitivity of the practitioner during the interview process may well be the most important examiner skills making up the assessment armamentarium. To this end, the practitioner must develop a flexible framework for obtaining the information or behavior needed in the assessment that will also facilitate the interaction necessary for a therapeutic relationship.

The most effective place to learn how to interview is at the bedside and in the clinic while dealing with actual clients. Initial interviews should be supervised by a skilled professional who will provide approbation or suggestions for modification immediately after leaving the client.

The use of a written record of the interview, called a process recording, may be helpful in identifying communication problems. However, a tape recording of a verbal interchange between the client and the practitioner may serve the same ends.

One frequently observed error is the monopoly of the interview by the practitioner. Particularly at the first interview, the client should be allowed to talk freely, to ramble on in his description of his health condition. Frequently clients report that they did not mention symptoms, because they did not have an opportunity or were not encouraged to do so. When one of the participants does most of the talking during the interview, in essence delivers a monologue, the other may be silent for long periods or repeat certain phrases again and again. Thus, "uh huh" or "okay" said repeatedly by one person in the interview is characteristic of stifled communication. The practitioner should bear in mind that the perception of what is being said in conversation is often decreased when one is listening to a long presentation. The most effective communication exists when the client takes an active role in the interview.

THE CONTRACT

The interview is a verbal and nonverbal exchange that provides for the beginning and development of a relationship. Initially, the participants are strangers, each presenting his own style of relating and adapting. Defining the terms of the relationship early in the interview obviates unnecessary stressors and provides goals for the participants. Common symbols must be achieved, since the quality of the communication will determine the value of the relationship. Unlike many others, the association between health professional and client has a mutual concern, the well-being of the client. This commonality of interest will facilitate progress toward the sharing of information, ideas, and emotions. A mutually understandable language, as well as an understanding of the significance of body language, such as gestures and facial expressions, will increase the exchange of information between the client and the practitioner and enrich the data obtained.

The contract, or basic operating agreement between the client and the practitioner should include:

1. Time and place the interview and subsequent examinations will occur
2. Duration of time involved in the present and future examinations
3. Number of sessions required
4. Expectations for participation by the client in the assessment process
5. Confidentiality of shared information and findings—responsibilities of each member
6. Rules regarding the presence of other professionals or of the client's relatives or other advocates
7. Cost to the client where applicable

The advantage of the contract to the practitioner is that the client is relieved of misconceptions, fears, or fantasies he may have had concerning what might happen during the interview and examination. Thus, the contract establishes norms and role behavior. A social system with definable, interdependent parts, so that a change in one part effects changes in other parts, has been identified. The practitioner and the client have expectations of each other. Abrogation of responsibility threatens the relationship.

The expectation that there will be shared decision making in the management of his health care should be made very clear to the client. To this end, the client is encouraged to learn more about himself in order to identify health needs and to recognize that he has an option in determining if and how his health needs may be met.

In traditional health care relationships there is an inequity in that the health professional is in the authority role whereas the client is, at least to some degree, dependent. The client has initiated the interview by seeking help for his problems. In his efforts to obtain aid from the professional, the client must determine the kind of information and behavior he must give. The professional is obligated to analyze the client's communication pattern in order to explain to the client what is needed for the professional to give the help that is needed. The interaction provides a kind of negotiation for the terms on which the relationship can continue, that is, a contract defining the roles of the participants. The verbal and nonverbal dialogue that occurs in the first few minutes of this social exchange may well determine not only the reliability and amount of information the client will furnish to the interviewer but also the character of the relationship that follows.

SETTING

To promote the most effective attention to communication and therefore to build rapport, the practitioner should carefully construct the interview environment to avoid interruption, distraction, or discomfort. Although geographical privacy may not be a luxury that can be obtained in large clinics or in multiple bed units in the hospital, psychological protection may be provided. Some of the assurances important to the client are that (1) the client is not being heard by other clients or personnel not concerned in his care, (2) the practitioner is giving his highest level of attention to the client, and (3) the information the client is sharing will be regarded as confidential.

In the more ideal setting the privacy of the client's thoughts and his comfort can be guaranteed by conducting the interview in a private room where optimum temperature and lighting can be controlled.

The physical position of the practitioner as related to the client can have implications in the control process. For a mutual sharing of the control of the interview or to suggest that the client has some option for control, the chairs or other furniture should be arranged so that a face-to-face alignment is possible. The commonly used position of standing over the client (looking down at) suggests that the practitioner has assumed leadership for the interchange.

Excessively long interviews are tiring to the client. There may be a need to schedule more than one session to complete the data base, particularly if the health history is complex or the client is critically ill or debilitated.

COMMUNICATION PROCESS

Anxiety is an anticipated element in an initial interview for both the health professional and the client. Some of the indications of acute anxiety include a furrowed brow, squinting, dilated pupils, tensed facial muscles, distended neck vessels, rapid talk, a dry mouth, frequent hand gestures, a tense posture, an increased heart rate and blood pressure, sweaty palms and axillae, and a sweaty pubic area. The client's anxieties may be associated with the symptoms of his illness, with the practitioner's reaction to him, with fees, or with expectations of future appointments. The practitioner is concerned with the client's response to the interview, with his (the practitioner's) ability to get appropriate information, and with his ability to synthesize the data provided so that the problems can be correctly defined. The practitioner is further concerned that problem management is appropriate and that referral is properly instituted. Clues that interview items are anxiety producing are long pauses, nervous laughter, dry coughing, and sighing.

To facilitate the development of rapport, the health professional must use his communication skills to project to the client that he is interested and concerned with providing the support needed by the client. The practitioner might convey support by assuring the client, "I'll do all I can to find out what is making you feel this way." To demonstrate interest and the willingness to listen, the practitioner must also be aware of the message conveyed nonverbally.

The practitioner must deal with both the information needed and given by the client and with the process of the interview. This process is the developing relationship and will include not only what is said but those elements that are implied by words and gesture, that is, the manner in which data is supplied and withheld as well as the client's efforts to control the interview.

Particular attention is given the remarks made as the client is entering the room or as he is leaving, since these comments frequently have special significance. The client may reveal his chief complaint at these times and avoid mentioning it during the formal interview.

The amount of structure that is brought to bear in the interview is dependent on the level of organization of ego functioning exhibited by the client. In general, the client with the lesser degree of organization needs more structure in the interview in order to increase the amount of data obtained in a given period of time and to decrease anxiety.

The communication process involves feedback in that each message sent involves a response. This response affects the next message sent and its reaction. The skilled practitioner readily settles in the communication mode that is most effective for the individual client. This is particularly important in the choice of the type of questions used to obtain the health history.

A common communication error that occurs in this society is that of thinking of the next remark, thereby not fully perceiving what is being said. This is a particular hazard for the student who is not yet fully comfortable with the interview pattern. Such an individual may perceive little of valuable data being given him by the client since he must concentrate on the format of questioning as well as on how best to word the next query.

Types of questions

Open-ended questions or suggestions. Although the interview is aimed at getting more or less specific answers concerning the events surrounding the client's signs and symptoms, each point should be developed by the client in his own words. An open-ended question or suggestion is one aimed at eliciting a response that is more than one or two words in length. This type of question is effective in stimulating descriptive or comparative responses. Observation of the client as he describes a symptom may give valuable information concerning his attitudes and beliefs. In addition, it allows the client to provide information when he is ready to disclose it; he is not forced to divulge information when sharing it may trouble him. This free description may also provide clues to the alertness, or level of mental abilities, of the client and to the organization of his ego functioning, revealed through the organization of his thoughts and through his vocabulary. Furthermore, rapport is strengthened through the demonstration that the practitioner wants to invest time in hearing the thoughts of the client.

Examples of open ended questions or suggestions are "How have you been feeling lately?" and "Tell me about your problem."

The disadvantage of this type of question is that it may result in responses that are not relevant to a specific point being assessed. The client may use the opportunity provided by an open-ended question to digress in order to avoid discussing relevant data because it is distressing to him. Although this technique might yield important information, there are times when the examiner needs data quickly and must sacrifice to get it. This is particularly true in emergency care. When the drug overdose victim rouses, the only piece of data of importance may be elicited by a closed question ("What did you take?").

Closed questions. The closed question is a type of inquiry that requires no more than a one- or two-word answer. This might be agreement or disagreement. The response may be a yes or no and may be answered nonverbally by a nod of the head. This is the kind of question most appropriate for eliciting age, sex, marital status, and other forced-choice responses.

Examples of closed questions are "What did you eat for dinner last night?" and "What medication did you take?"

The educationally impoverished or those who lack culturally enriching experiences are often more comfortable with this type of question since they know what is expected. The open-ended question may pose anxiety to the client with poor articulation, since he may be afraid that the display of his lack of verbal skill will disadvantage him with the practitioner. On the other hand, the closed question by its nature limits the amount of information that is obtained in the health history and may convey to the client that the practitioner is too busy or disinterested to listen to him. It has been observed that practitioners use more closed questions in initial interviews and when the process is stressful, as well as when time constraints are marked.

Biased or leading questions. Questions that carry a suggestion of the kind of information that should be included in the response are called leading or biased. The client is presented with an expectation by the practitioner. This kind of question may seriously limit the value of the health history. For example, the question "You haven't ever had venereal disease, have you?" implies that the possibility that the client *has had* venereal disease would be outside the limits of reality for the practitioner. The client who has experienced the disease may not say so since to do so might mean disappointing the questioner.

The presence of emotionally charged words in a given question may make the question a biased one. This is one in such questions as "You haven't been masturbating, have you?" Since the Judeo-Christian ethic defines masturbating as "bad," bias has been inflicted. In this case the practitioner has suggested that the answer should be no. The client may well avoid all matters dealing with sexuality in order to avoid the possible loss of the approval of the practitioner.

Use of silence

Periods of silence during the interview are helpful in making observations, such as is the client comfortable? Angry? Confused? Silence provides an opportunity to assess the level of anxiety in both the practitioner and the client. Second, the client is provided with sufficient time to carefully organize his thoughts for a coherent explanation in response to questions. The rapid presentation of questions may not allow time for sufficient thought or reflection by the client. Silence is also useful as an indicator of the amount of anxiety the client is experiencing. Silence may indicate absorbing thought, boredom, deep affection, or grief.

Methods for assuring understanding

The practitioner must use validation maneuvers to determine if both participants understand what has been said. A clear understanding of what the client is trying to say is essential to the establishment of an accurate data base. The health history should not contain assumptions of what the client meant but a clear accounting of exactly what he said. There are many techniques that provide for encouragement of the client to expand on a description or to clarify the explanation that has been given. A workable example might be "Tell me more about it."

Use of a common language. The practitioner must carefully plan questions and give particular care in selecting the vocabulary to be used in order that the client perceives the question in the same sense that it is intended by the practitioner. The practitioner is aided in processing the language and behavior of the client for what is usual or "normal" by having an understanding of cultural and ethnic differences. Medical terminology or jargon should not be used excessively. When medical diagnoses are employed, the meaning should be explained to client when the words are first used.

Frequently, the professional uses these terms to avoid communication altogether or to terminate conversations with clients. Should the client use a medical diagnosis, the practitioner should ascertain that the client's understanding of the word matches his own. For example, many lay people believe that *neoplasm* is synonymous with *cancer*.

Planning the questions. In order for the client to give the information needed for the health history, the questions must be phrased in such a way that the client knows what kind of answers are expected. When the client's response is not appropriate, a reordering of the sentence or a more explicit choice of vocabulary may be indicated. It may be helpful to emphasize the key words in the question. In designing questions, one should avoid the use of ambiguous terms, medical language, or words with more than one meaning.

Use of an example. Comparison with a common experience, that is, a concrete happening, may help to clarify an abstract concept or hazy terminology. The practitioner may use an example as part of the questioning process when the meaning is not clear. For example, the practitioner may ask the client, "Was it as large as a cherry?"

Restatement. Restatement is the formulation of what the client has said in words that are more specific; it provides an opportunity for validation of the practitioner's conception. The client is cued that he is expected to give attention to the thought by phrases such as "Do you mean . . ." "In other words . . ." or "If I understand you correctly . . ."

Reflection or echoing. Reflection, or echoing, means repeating a phrase or a sentence the client has just said. The suggestion to the client that the practitioner is still involved in that part of the communication may focus further attention or rumination on that thought. The strategy is aimed toward further elaboration in the form of the recall of facts or feeling states that surrounded the circumstance. The technique should allow clarification or expansion of the information just given by the client. Examples are "You say your mother is an alcoholic?" and "Painful?"

Encapsulation or summary. Encapsulation, or summary, is a technique that allows for the condensation of facts into a well-ordered review. It is particularly useful following a rambling, detailed description. The summary further signals the client that this particular segment of the interview is terminating and suggests to him that he should give further input immediately, since closure is imminent.

Filling in omitted data

Clinical impressions reached by the practitioner must be regarded as fluid in the sense that in further conversation with the client new information may be provided. The client may withhold information if he fears that sensitive information may be shared indiscriminately or if he has not been able to trust the practitioner. Furthermore, he may regard certain facts as unimportant or irrelevant to the focus of the interview. There are many instances when the client is so eager to comply with questions that he gives a hurried accounting and leaves out significant data. In ordering the data the practitioner may note that information is missing or that there are inconsistencies. Further interviews may be scheduled. The client may simply need to be given a summary of his previous conversation in order for him to detect the areas where he needs to interject information. These gaps may be filled by direct questioning. Another method of asking for the missing facts may be to suggest to the client that the practitioner is confused and needs to be told again a particular sequence of events. A remark such as the following would invite this input: "Now, tell me again all that you remember from the time you first vomited until you came here."

In addition, the possibility of past evaluation and treatment of symptoms should be investigated. The important facts are those obtained by asking when, where, and by whom. Were laboratory or other diagnostic tests performed? Are results available? What diagnosis was made? Was a treatment instituted? Was the treatment helpful?

Obtaining data from people other than the client

The client who is critically ill, confused, or intellectually impaired may be unable to give the information necessary to an adequate history. A close relative or a person who knows the client well may be able to provide the information necessary to understand the presence or nature of problems of the individual being examined. If an ineffective attempt has been made to obtain the history from the client, it may be psychologically prudent to ask permission to go over the details again with the second person. Such comments as "I want to be sure that I have what has happened to you correctly in my mind," or "I'd like to go over this one more time to make sure I've got the facts right and in the correct order," may help to gain the client's permission to interview relatives or friends. The parents may be the only reliable source of information for the young child.

Nonverbal communication

Nonverbal communication is that which takes place in the form of behavior patterns that are expressive in the use of (1) body movements, (2) space or territoriality, (3) voice tone, (4) time, and (5) appearance. The behaviors can convey emotional or feeling state messages or can be used to impart instruction or direction.

Communication through body movement

Some of the gestures to be observed are movements of the body, limbs, hands, or feet; facial expressions, particularly smiling and frowning; and eye behavior such as blinking, the direction of gaze, and the length of time of gaze. Posture is particularly expressive.

Extension of large muscles is associated with relaxation, whereas contraction of large muscles is associated with anxiety and fear. The individual who sits stretched out and gestures away from the body gives an aura of assurance.

Kinesis is the communication provided through body movement. The posture or movement of the client's body may provide valuable clues to his health status. The messages given by the client through his body language may provide additional and sometimes more reliable information than his words, since many persons employ less conscious control over this aspect of behavior. Thus, by his actions the client may convey thoughts that he cannot or refuses to commit to words. Interpretation of the full meaning of the gestures and action of the client must be performed against a comparison of their sociocultural meanings. For instance, the downcast eyes of the Muhammadan woman could only be interpreted as the usual or normal response to the practitioner, whereas in the United States one might become alert to other indications of fear, withdrawal or depression, or lack of attentiveness. The use of eye contact assumes a good deal of meaning among Greek and Indian cultures, whereas torso messages are common in Africa.

Oculesics. Oculesics is the communication that occurs through glances and eye movements. The practitioner may detect signals of disagreement, aversion, or disgust in the client through subtle eye movements. Dilation of the pupils of the eyes generally accompanies pleasurable experiences, whereas innocuous or unpleasant circumstances generally result in contracted pupils.

Touch. The act of touching is one of the most intimate forms of nonverbal communication. Cultural traditions prescribe the ritual of touch or define the taboos. Touch is regulated by social-distancing techniques and is apparent in all living groups. Touch has special meaning among health professionals. Many professionals conceive of themselves reaching out in support of their clients. Touch when used judiciously conveys a message of closeness, encouragement, and caring and plays a prominent part in the health practitioner–client interaction.

Although in our culture a pat on the back, the handshake, a gentle squeeze of the hand, or a slap on the cheek may be well understood, the practitioner must bear in mind that this community of understanding does not exist for many touching processes. The physical contact of palpation may be misperceived as it is translated from stimulus received to perception. Touch as a form of communication precedes speech in the individual's life. Manners and mores involving touch are given to the developing child through the actions of his significant others. In America there is a taboo against touching without permission to do so. So, we talk about the reassuring pat of the hand and the warm handshake and define who is permitted to do these acts. There is often confu-

sion when the client opts to touch the health professional.

Effect of space or territoriality on communication

A good deal of symbolism has been attributed to one's position in a group. Definition of a cultural group's concern or rejection is provided by distancing. The distance between the practitioner and the client may determine the relationships developed.

The size of space allowed the client may be related to status or to the differential importance accorded him.

Hall has coined the word "proxemics" to describe the use of space by people in this country as zones that he calls intimate, personal, social, and public.

Intimate distance. Intimate distance is the distance used for physical lovemaking and intense verbal exchange and is defined as a distance of zero to 18 inches. This is the distance from which most of the clinical examination is performed. Body contact is expected during the physical examination and the practitioner must use the intimate space of the client and must be concerned with sensory overload. Thus, sensation may frequently be distorted. The presence of another body at this close distance intrudes on the senses and is sometimes overwhelming to the client.

At this close distance the odors of each body are prominent in the senses. The examiner is aware of diagnostic body odors and of the patient's general hygiene. The examiner should also be aware of his own body smells; the use of pungent toiletries is often offensive to the client. Even the heat extruded by the bodies of participants may be a part of the interchange.

This close phase is also the distance used by the client for touch and intimate skin manipulation. This may be pleasurable and reassuring, or threatening to the client. Muscular tension is heightened as though in preparation for movement.

Visual detail is sharpened. The eyes are pulled inward in accommodation, and the individual may appear to squint. Vocalization may be involuntary at the near point but become low and more frequent as the periphery of this zone is approached.

Since it would appear that it is a natural instinct to maintain and protect the space immediately around us, the intrusion on the client's intimate zone should be carefully planned. The client may be carefully assessing the practitioner's use of space. His perceptions may be largely determined by what he assesses of the practitioner in the visual domain.

Frequently the use of social measures that allow the acceptance of a shortened distance for communications may be helpful; these include introductions, an explanation of the roles of the practitioner and the client, and an explanation of the benefits to be achieved by allowing the closer contact. The client should have each procedure communicated to him before its actualization with the full knowledge that he has the option to refuse. The practitioner should use simple sentences and a carefully chosen, nonthreatening vocabulary.

The hospital room or clinic office visit seriously threatens the control of space by the client. He is told where and how he must cooperate in order that his body may be invaded by tactile, visual, auditory, and olfactory probing. The culture may permit this invasion of privacy by physicians and nurses since they are given special status by the professional roles. The endowment of the role with technical skill, authority, and confidentiality protects the client from the shame that has been cultivated in him for exposure of the body to a stranger. It has been shown that when more evidence is given of the roles of health professionals and these roles are well understood, it is easier for the client to submit to the encroachment of privacy. To this end, the professional uniform of white coat, and so on, is effective, as is the health professional's careful adherence to the behaviors recognized to be part of that role.

The client needs time to adjust to the levels of the space provided for the physical examination. The interview allows a reordering of the perimeters defining the client's space bubble. The client should be allowed as much decision making as possible. He should be allowed to order the disposition of his personal belongings. Questions regarding the use of space should be seriously attended.

Personal distance. Personal distance limits physical contact and is defined as a distance of 1½ to 4 feet. Although holding and grasping are possible at the near point, touching is the form of physical contact most frequently used. Visual perception is less distorted, and there is a three-dimensional impression of the person involved. As the distance between participants lengthens, the gaze may encompass the entire face rather than a single part of it, such as the eye or the chin. Vocal volume is moderate, and body odors and heat are less intruding.

This is the ideal distance for viewing nonverbal behaviors and is the distance most frequently utilized for the interview. Trust is best developed from this distance.

Social distance. Social distance provides protection from others without one's having to declare or demand it and is defined as a distance of 4 to 12 feet. The visual image includes more of the total person, and the fine detail of the body is lost. Eye contact becomes more important. Body heat and odor are lost. Vocalization is louder and loses its aura of privacy because it can be overheard. Interaction becomes more ritualized or formal. The threat of domination is less from this distance. This distance allows a limited view of the physical aspects of the client, and his revelation of attitudes and feelings in general is censored from this distance.

Vocalics

Vocalics is the information that is transmitted through the delivery of speech. The individual who screeches "I'm not afraid of the operation" reveals that he is terrified.

Chronemics

Chronemics is the term used to describe the information that is transmitted through the use of time. The health practitioner is generally perceived by the client to be the one of superior status in the health care visit. Thus, the client deems it appropriate to wait past the appointment time. On the other hand, the client may be revealing some of his opposing feelings by a pattern of lateness in meeting appointments.

Similarly, the person with perceived superior status is allowed to talk longer. Interruption of the practitioner by the client with an unrelated thought while the practitioner is explaining treatment requirements may signal that the client holds the advice at low value.

Effect of appearance on communication

Both clothing and cosmetics may be used to create an impression. In general, adults aim to reflect the current mode of "handsome" or "beautiful" and, in most cases, "young." Furthermore, financial status may be revealed by the cut of the garments or the label of the manufacturer.

Persons in the health professions, as well as the bulk of American society, are more generous and outgoing in their feelings toward the physically attractive individual. This is true of practitioners working with all age levels. The practitioner must frequently work through his attitudes and emo-

Guideline	Interview items to elicit symptom description
1. Anatomical location Radiation of the symptom	"Tell me where it hurts." "Show me where it hurts."
2. Quality or character	"What does it feel like?" "Can you compare this to something you have felt in the past?"
3. Quantity	"How bad [intense] is the pain?" "How much does the pain immobilize you?" "What effect does the pain have on normal daily activities?"
4. Time sequence	"When did you first notice the pain? "How long does it last?" "How often have you had it since that time?"
5. Geographical or environmental factors	"Where were you when the pain occurred?"
6. Precipitating conditions	"Do you find that the pain occurs at a certain time of day?" "Does heat or cold seem to affect the pain?" "What causes the pain?"
Conditions making the symptom more severe	"Have you noticed anything that makes the pain worse?"
7. Alleviating condition	"What seems to help you when you have the pain?"
8. Concomitant symptoms	"Have you noticed any other changes that are present when you have the pain?"

tions in order to touch the diseased individual without visible indications of restraint or repugnance, such as tensed musculature, frowns, or touching only with the fingertips.

Supportive remarks and actions should be a part of the interview process. Although it is not credible to attest to supportiveness, the practitioner should try to convey interest and understanding of the client's problem as well as the desire to help the client meet and work through his problems.

Gestures that say "I like you; you're acceptable" include smiling and moving closer. The basic projection is pleasant, and the words that are chosen say nice things.

■ Encouraging a complete description of the symptom

The descriptions by the client of the changes he has perceived in the structure of his body or its

functions are called symptoms. The interview should provide the most accurate and constructive picture of the symptom that can be obtained, since this is the base from which the client's problems can be defined.

The practitioner carefully avoids devaluing the client's symptoms by such remarks as "You have nothing to be nervous about," or "That's nothing; now, last week we had a really bad case."

There are eight criteria that can be used to provide this delineation: anatomical location, quality of the symptom, quantity of the symptom, time sequence of the symptom, geographical or environmental locale in which the symptom occurs, precipitating conditions that cause the symptom to be more severe, circumstances that alleviate the symptom, and other symptoms that occur in conjunction with the symptom.

To clarify the use of these guidelines in the interview setting, consider a client who comes for treatment with a chief complaint of pain (see upper left column).

The accuracy of the diagnostic process is dependent on exploring the ramification of these eight areas for data collection.

BIBLIOGRAPHY

Bernstein, L., Bernstein, R. S., and Dana, R. H.: Interviewing: a guide for health professionals, New York, 1974, Appleton-Century Crofts.

Bernstein, L., and Dana, R. S.: Interviewing and the health professions, New York, 1970, Appleton-Century-Crofts.

Engel, G. L., and Morgan, W. L., Jr.: Interviewing the patient, Philadelphia, 1973, W. B. Saunders Co.

Fast, J.: Body language, New York, 1970, M. Evans & Co., Inc.

Gill, M., Newman, R., and Redlich, F.: The initial interview in psychiatric practice, New York, 1954, International Universities Press.

Gordon, R.: Interviewing; strategy, techniques and tactics, Homewood, Ill., 1969, Dorsey Press.

Hall, E.: The silent language, Greenwich, Conn., 1959, Fawcett.

Hall, E.: The hidden dimension, Garden City, N.Y., 1969, Doubleday & Co., Inc.

MacKinnon, R. A., and Michels, R.: The psychiatric interview in clinical practice, Philadelphia, 1971, W. B. Saunders Co.

Morgan, W. L., Jr., and Engel, G. L.: The clinical approach to the patient, Philadelphia, 1969, W. B. Saunders Co.

Richardson, S., Dohrenwend, B. S., and Klein, D.: Interviewing, its forms and functions, New York, 1965, Basic Books, Inc., Publishers.

Sullivan, H.: The psychiatric interview, New York, 1954, W. W. Norton & Co., Inc.

3 The health history

The health history is an extremely important part of the health assessment. Its performance is the primary vehicle by which rapport is established between the practitioner and the client. The information derived from the history-taking interview assists the practitioner in assessing and diagnosing the client's health problems and in obtaining knowledge of the client's problems and needs within the context of that particular client's life. The health history not only records the problems of the client but also describes the client as a whole and in relation to his social and physical environment. Thus, it records not only weaknesses and abnormalities but also the strengths that will support therapy and care.

Other important components of the history data base are the perceptions of the client regarding his health, his illness, and his past experiences with health delivery systems. These perceptions must be known if future care is to be relevant and, consequently, effective.

In practice, the taking of the health history is implemented in two phases: (1) the client interview phase, which elicits the information, and (2) the recording of data. The information as presented in this chapter is organized according to a systematic method for recording the history. The client interview may or may not proceed in the same sequence. Each portion of the health history discussed contains descriptions of processes for both eliciting and summarizing data. Examples of two recorded health histories are included at the end of this chapter.

Certain principles of the history-taking procedure should be emphasized. The importance of privacy seems obvious, but this principle is too often violated in actual practice. Another apparent principle is the maintenance of eye contact, but what does one do about recording? The practitioner must immediately note specific information, such as dates, age, and so on, or he may forget. Also, the client expects the practitioner to consider his information important enough to have it recorded. It is a temptation to attempt to complete one's recorded history during the interview, but it not possible to do this and simultaneously observe the client and his responses.

FORMAT

The health history, as described in this chapter, is an extremely complete one. In many actual client care situations, it may not be possible, or even appropriate, to obtain the complete history. For clients receiving continuous care, the history can be obtained in portions during several encounters.

For clients requiring episodic care, decisions regarding the data essential for immediate therapy guide the content of the history.

However, the beginning historian should practice obtaining the complete health history in order to develop skill in interviewing and in recording data. During this practice process the learner will develop an appreciation for the client management implications of each portion of the health history.

The format used in this text for the complete health history is as follows:

A. Biographical information
B. Chief complaint or client's request for care
C. Present illness or present health status
D. Past history
E. Family history
F. Review of systems
　1. Physical
　2. Sociological
　3. Psychological
G. Developmental data
H. Nutritional data

▪ Biographical information

At the beginning of any health record, there should be a place to record commonly used and sometimes critically important biographical information. This information should be obtained early during the client's first visit or admission; otherwise, it may be omitted, only to be needed in an emergency or at a time when the client is unavailable or unable to respond.

The following information is to be recorded in the introductory and biographical section of the health history:

A. Full name
B. Address and telephone numbers
   1. Client's permanent
   2. Contact of client
C. Birthdate
D. Sex
E. Race
F. Religion
G. Marital status
H. Social Security number
I. Occupation
   1. Usual
   2. Present
J. Birthplace
K. Source of referral
L. Usual source of health care
M. Source and reliability of information
N. Date of interview

First, the client's name is recorded. Persons in an ethnically homogenous geographical area often have similar names. Precise identification, using first, middle, and last names, assists in assuring accurate information retrieval and coordination.

Next, the client's full mailing address and telephone number are recorded. Also recorded are the name, address, and telephone number of one of the client's friends or relatives, someone with whom he is in frequent contact and who would be willing and able to relay a message to the client in an emergency or if the client could not be located.

Birthplace, sex, race, marital status and religion information are self-explanatory. Many health problems and needs are age, sex, race, or social situation related. This information might be correlated with problems discovered later in the history.

There are justifiable reasons for the notation of the client's Social Security number, including the precise identification of each client and a potential access to a large pool of health-related information. Potential violations of confidentiality are a disadvantage.

A significant difference may exist between the client's current and usual occupations. The nature of the difference may be indicative of the severity of the client's health problems and the level of disability resulting from them. In addition, knowledge of past occupations might provide clues to past or present environmental hazards contributing to the present illness. A mine worker with a respiratory system complaint is an example.

Knowledge of the client's birthplace provides geographical implications for the origin of problems and cultural implications for therapy and health maintenance.

If the current care giver is not the usual and primary source of the client's care, the name and address of the individual or institution so identified should be recorded. In addition, the practitioner should record the reason for the client's entering a new health care system. The client may be in crisis, he may be dissatisfied with past care, or he may be "shopping." If the past source of care possesses significant data about the client's health and if the client intends to continue in the current health care system, the client should be asked to sign a permission for the transfer of information. Later in the health history, the practitioner will have the opportunity to record, in some detail, past patterns of health care.

Next, the practitioner makes a statement about the source of the information to follow. In most cases the source is the client, but this can not be assumed unless the informant is specifically identified. If the information is given by someone other than the client, the degree of the informant's contact with the client should be described. For example, in the case of a child, the practitioner would utilize the history given by a grandmother who resides with the child differently from one given by a grandmother who visits the child once a week.

Along with the statement of the informant, an evaluation of his reliability is made. For example, one of the following may be stated: "inconsistent," "unclear about recent events," "evasive," or "cooperative and reliable." These statements serve as simple criteria by which the remainder of the information in the history is judged by other health care providers and may indicate a need to retake or supplement the history at a future date or to consult with other informants to determine the accuracy of the data.

The history is dated. In a situation where the client's condition changes rapidly, events can be correlated only if their temporal relationships are known.

Chief complaint or client's request for care

The chief complaint (CC) statement is a short statement, preferably in the client's own words and recorded in quotation marks, that indicates the client's purpose for requesting health care at this time. In the case of a client who is ill, the CC statement is of the acute or chronic problem (or problems) that is the client's priority for treatment. The CC statement, whenever relevant, includes a notation of the problem's duration. The duration, as stated by the client, may not be the actual duration of the symptoms. However, it is an indication of the time during which the complaint has become intolerable enough to motivate the client to seek help.

In the case of a well client, the CC statement may be a statement of the client's request for a health examination for health screening, health promotion, or disease case-finding purposes.

The CC statement is not a diagnostic statement. Actually, it is very hazardous to state a chief complaint in diagnostic terms. For example, a client who has frequent asthmatic attacks appears for treatment with respiratory system complaints and states that he is having an "asthmatic attack." This may or may not be the case. In this early portion of the history, client and interviewer bias must be avoided; otherwise the interview and the problem solving may be set in one, and potentially a wrong, direction.

The following are examples of adequately stated chief complaints:

"Chest pain for 3 days."
"Swollen ankles for 2 weeks."
"Fever and headache for 24 hours."
"Pap smear needed. Last pap 9/8/73."
"Physical examination needed for camp."

The following are examples of inadequately stated chief complaints:

"Thinks she might be pregnant."
"Sick."
"Nausea and vomiting."
"Hypertension."

The CC statement may seem superfluous, especially since the next section on the present illness describes the symptoms in detail. However, this is one of the few places in the recorded history of a client's encounter with the health care system where he has the opportunity to have recorded, in his own words, his needs. Too often

the practitioner loses sight of the client's priorities for care. The consistent recording of a chief complaint or reason for the visit will assist in keeping the system responsive to the client's perceived needs.

In some instances the client may present several complaints. No more than three should be stated in this portion of the history and the client's stated priorities should be noted first.

Present illness or present health status

The present illness (PI) section describes the information relevant to the chief complaint. In the case of a client with a health problem, this portion of the health history challenges the interviewing, clinical knowledge, and written communication skills of the practitioner. The practitioner needs to learn the minute details of the chief complaint and its associated phenomena. Information must be comprehensive, it must be recorded concisely and comprehensively, and it must provide the practitioner with enough information to initiate additional assessment and the intervention measures.

In the case of a well client, the interviewer usually describes the client's usual health and briefly summarizes his health maintenance needs and activities.

The following are the components of the PI section:

I. Introduction
  A. Client's summary
  B. Usual health
II. Investigation of symptoms: chronological story
  A. Onset
  B. Date
  C. Manner (gradual or sudden)
  D. Duration
  E. Precipitating factors
  F. Course since onset
    1. Incidence (frequency)
    2. Manner
    3. Duration (longest, shortest, and average times)
    4. Patterns of remissions and exacerbations
  G. Location
  H. Quality
  I. Quantity
  J. Setting
  K. Associated phenomena
  L. Alleviating or aggravating factors
III. Negative information
IV. Relevant family information
V. Disability assessment

Introduction. The introduction to the PI section should be succinct; its major purpose is to provide the reader with a general orientation to the client.

The introduction indicates which admission or visit this particular one is for this client to the institution or service. Next, there is a short summary of the client's biographical data. Age, race, marital status, employment status, and occupation are the items of information usually recorded. If the client is being hospitalized and has been hospitalized in the past, the client's total number of hospitalizations and the number of hospitalizations for complaints related to the current illness are noted.

The practitioner next describes the client's usual health and records any significant past diagnoses or past or current health problems that might have caused the client to enjoy anything other than good health.

Investigation of symptoms: chronological story. The practitioner usually initiates the PI description by asking the client: "Tell me about it [the problem mentioned in the CC statement]," or "How did it start and what has happened since it started?" The client will usually respond to this inquiry with a long but usually diagnostically incomplete discourse about his health problems and needs. The practitioner exercises skill in determining when to interrupt the client and more specifically direct his responses by asking additional, clarifying questions and when to allow the client to continue the narration of those events significant to him.

The practitioner needs a mental or actual list of the areas of symptom investigation as an aid in attaining comprehensive information. Regardless of the nature of a problem, each of the areas of investigation is relevant, and any health problem analysis would be incomplete without the description of all areas.

The practitioner also attempts to determine the chronological sequence of the client's problem. The client is apt to best remember his most recent episode of illness and in the case of a prolonged illness will need direction in tracing the problem back to its first symptomatic event. Once this first event is identified, it is investigated in detail and its date, manner of onset, duration, and precipitating factors are described in the recording.

Each symptom's course since onset is described. Frequency in a specific time interval is determined. Clients may state vaguely that they have a symptom "all the time." This may mean once a month to one client or ten times a day to another. To obtain specific information, the practitioner might ask, "How many times a day (or a week, or a month) does it occur?" Although the practitioner avoids suggesting answers with his questions, occasionally it may be necessary to pursue frequency with leading questions, for example, "Does it occur more often than five times a day?"

The practitioner determines the usual manner of onset for the illness episodes. Any change in onset is specifically mentioned. In the case of many episodes, the longest, shortest, and average durations of the episodes are noted. If there have been only several episodes, the length of each is identified.

In prolonged illnesses, the patterns of remission and exacerbation are described according to their duration and frequency. The practitioner needs to be watchful for environmental or other clues that might be precipitating factors for the illness events.

In recording, there are several suggested methods that can be used in assisting readers to easily identify temporal relationships. The practitioner describes the initial event first and then the subsequent events. The chronological story may be indexed in the left-hand column of the history sheet, using the reference base *prior to admission* (PTA). For example, the index might be listed as follows: "6 years PTA," "3 years PTA," "6 months PTA," "1 day PTA," and so on, with the corresponding narrative along side of and below the temporal index heading.

A method of demonstrating the progression of illness is accomplished by the use of a diagram illustrating the disease process (Fig. 3-1). A diagram is especially helpful in the case of multisymptomatic illnesses.

As the chronological story evolves, the other areas of symptom investigation are integrated into the text of the narrative. Whenever appropriate, the sign's or symptom's location, quality, quantity, setting, associated phenomena, and alleviating and aggravating factors are described, especially whenever there is a change in any of them.

Location. The exact site of the sign or symptom is determined. Subjective events, such as pain, pose some problem. Having a client point to the exact point of pain and trace its radiation with his finger assists in location. In recording location, one uses body hemispheres and landmarks.

Quality. Quality refers to the unique properties of the complaint. Signs, such as discharge, are described according to their color, texture, composition, appearance, and odor. Sound and

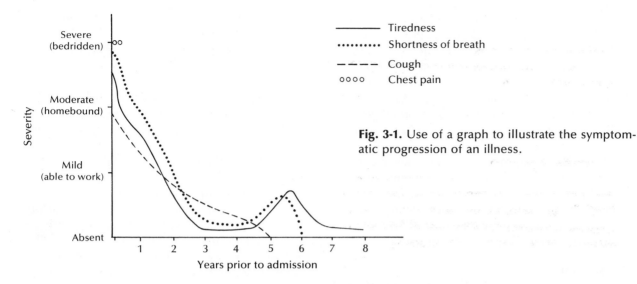

Fig. 3-1. Use of a graph to illustrate the symptomatic progression of an illness.

temperature may be descriptive attributes of other phenomena.

Subjective events, such as pain, challenge the creativity of the practitioner. The quality of pain is frequently characterized as dull, aching, sharp, nagging, throbbing, stabbing, or squeezing.

Whenever appropriate, the client's descriptions are used with quotation marks.

Quantity. Quantity refers to the size, extent, number, or amount, for example, of the pain, rash, discharge, or lesion. With objective signs, the practitioner can use commonly understood measures, such as centimeters, cups, or tablespoons. In describing subjective events, pain, for example, one should note that evaluations such as "a little" or "a lot" have different meanings among persons. The quality of such phenomena can be more accurately understood by describing the client's response to the symptom. For example, does he have to stop and sit or does he continue on with what he is doing?

Setting. Whenever something occurs, the client is somewhere and is either with someone or alone. Physically or psychologically the setting may have an effect on the client, and knowledge of this information may provide the practitioner with clues of the cause of the problem and implications for treatment.

Associated phenomena. Associated phenomena are those symptoms that occur with the chief complaint. They may be related to the chief complaint or may be a part of a totally different syndrome. Often the client will spontaneously identify these events. In addition, the practitioner may ask if there is anything else occurring with the chief complaint or ask about the presence or absence of certain specific events. A complete review of the implicated problem system or systems is indicated. Positive responses are recorded with a complete description of all reported symptoms. Negative responses are recorded in the negative information section.

Alleviating or aggravating factors. When an illness occurs, a person often accommodates to it or treats himself. He may decrease activity, eat more or less, wait, or actively medicate and treat himself. The practitioner should nonpunitively probe into the client's actions in response to the problem and into the effect of these actions. If there has been professional intervention, the nature, source, and effect of each intervention are recorded. The client, through treatment or through accommodation, may have discovered something that alleviates the symptom. The client is asked what makes his problem better. The nature of the client's solution may provide valuable therapeutic data and may reflect the nature of his adaptation to illness.

The client is asked about that which makes the chief complaint worse. Usually clients have noticed aggravating factors, but may need assistance in recalling them. The practitioner may ask about the effect of movement, positioning, or eating, for example. Again, valuable therapeutic data may be obtained.

Negative information. In analyzing a problem, one may find negative information as significant as positive information in determining the diagnosis.

Each system implicated in the PI section is thoroughly reviewed. All of the client's positive replies are recorded in the text of the chronological story. All of the negative information is recorded in this separate category of the PI section.

Relevant family history. The client is queried about any problem similar to the chief complaint in his blood relatives. Positive replies are recorded, identifying specifically the relative and his problem. A negative reply is recorded generally, for example, "None of the client's blood relatives have diabetes."

Disability assessment. The practitioner determines the extent to which the symptoms identified in the PI section have affected the client's total life. Not only are the physiological effects determined, but also the sociological, psychological, and financial impacts of the problem.

■ **Past history**

The purpose of the past history (PH) section of the health history is to identify all major past health problems of the client.

The following indicates the information to be obtained and recorded in the PH section of the health history:

  A. Past illnesses
    1. Childhood illnesses
    2. Injuries
    3. Hospitalizations
    4. Operations
    5. Other major illnesses
  B. Allergies
    1. Environmental
    2. Ingestion
    3. Drug
    4. Other
  C. Immunizations
  D. Habits
    1. Alcohol
    2. Tobacco
    3. Drugs
    4. Coffee, tea
  E. Medications taken regularly
    1. By practitioner prescription
    2. By self-prescription

The recording of childhood illnesses is probably more relevant to and more easily obtained for a child's history than for an adult's history. However, all adults should be asked minimally if they have had rheumatic fever. Whenever there is a positive reply, the age of the client at occurrence, the fact or absence of a medical diagnosis, and the sequelae of the disease are determined.

The client is asked to recall accidents and disabling injuries, regardless of whether he was hospitalized for them or was treated on an outpatient basis. The precipitating event, the extent of injury, the fact or absence of medical care, the

names of the practitioner and institution, and sequelae are determined and recorded. The practitioner investigates for patterns of injuries or for the presence of consistent environmental hazards.

Descriptions of hospitalizations include all the times the client was admitted to an inpatient unit. Dates of stay, the primary practitioner, the name and address of the hospital, the admitting complaint, the discharge diagnosis, and the follow-up care and sequelae should all be recorded.

Obstetrical hospitalizations are recorded in the review of systems portion of the health history under the review of the female genital system.

Operations are recorded together, under this specific category. The history should include as complete a description of the nature of the repair or removal as is possible. However, clients are generally and unnecessarily unaware of the nature of their operations. Past records may need to be consulted for accurate and complete information.

Clients may have had major, acute illnesses or chronic illnesses that have not required hospitalization. The course of treatment, the person making the diagnosis, and the follow-up care and sequelae are noted.

Information under the categories of hospitalizations, operations, and other major illnesses may, in some cases, be redundant. Information is not recorded more than once, but the presence of a past problem is stated, and the reader is referred to the section where the original notation was made.

The practitioner specifically asks about allergies to food, environmental factors, animals, and drugs. (The practitioner should particularly ask about past administrations of penicillin; the number of administrations and reactions are noted in the record.) If the client admits to an allergy, specific information is obtained about the causative factor, the reaction, the diagnosis of causative factor, the therapy, and the sequelae. Caution must be exercised in assessing drug allergies. A drug reaction may not always be an allergic response; it may be an interaction with a concurrently administered drug, a misdose, or a side effect.

Habits that may have relevance to the health of an individual are excessive alcohol, coffee, or tea ingestion; smoking; and the addictive use of legal or illegal mood-altering substances. In the case of habits, the number of cigarettes, ounces, tablets, and so on, per day are noted along with the duration of the habit.

If therapy is to be logically planned by informed practitioners, it is critical that all medications that are currently being used by the client are known and recorded. Clients usually admit to vague patterns, such as "a white pill once a day for water," but forget to tell the practitioner about the aspirin or antacid they take several times a day unless they are specifically asked about nonprescription items. Here, the health practitioner has the opportunity to educate clients about the names, doses, and uses of their medications and about the necessity of knowing such information.

■ Family history

The purpose of the family history (FH) section is to learn about the general health of the client's blood relatives, spouse, and children and to identify any illnesses of environmental, genetic, or familial nature that might have implications for the client's current or future health problems and needs.

The practitioner inquires about the health of the client's family members, including maternal and paternal grandparents, parents, siblings, aunts, uncles, spouse, and children. Information is obtained about the current health status, presence of disease, and current age or age at death of each family member. If a member is deceased, the cause of death is recorded.

If the nature of the client's established or possible illnesses have known or suspected familial tendencies, the client is again questioned about similar problems of family members.

Inquiries about the presence of the following diseases are made because of their genetic, familial, or environmental tendencies: epilepsy, diabetes, blood dyscrasias, Huntington's chorea, cancer, hypertension, arteriosclerosis, gout, obesity, allergic disorders, coronary artery disease, tuberculosis, and kidney disease.

The information in the FH section may be outlined in the record or put in the form of a family tree chart. Fig. 3-2 is an example of such a chart.

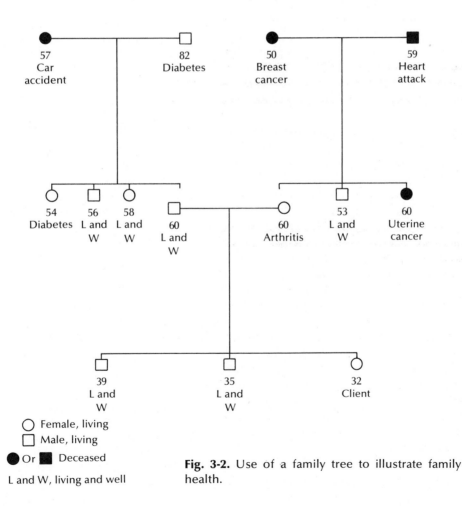

Fig. 3-2. Use of a family tree to illustrate family health.

○ Female, living
□ Male, living
● Or ■ Deceased
L and W, living and well

■ Review of systems

The review of systems (ROS) portion of the history includes a collection of data regarding the past and present health of each of the client's systems. This review of the client's physical, sociological, and psychological health status may identify problems not uncovered previously in the history and provides an opportunity to indicate client strengths as well as liabilities.

Generally, the ROS portion of the history is organized from cephalad to caudad, from physical to psychosocial. Clients are instructed that they will be asked a number of questions. Both beginning and experienced interviewers usually need a check list or written reminder of the questions usually asked each client.

Physical systems

In the review of physical systems section, the practitioner asks about symptoms or asks a specific question and then pauses, allowing the client to think and respond. If the client responds positively, the examiner analyzes the symptoms according to the characteristics of symptoms discussed in the PI section of the history. The practitioner asks questions quickly enough to be efficient, yet slowly enough to allow the client time to think. Questions generally emphasize the presence of past or current common anatomical or functional problems of the system and the health functioning and maintenance of the system.

Obviously, the signs and symptoms need to be creatively translated into questions and terms that can be understood by the client. For example, questions concerning a symptom such as intermittent claudication would need to be presented in lay, descriptive terms.

The presence or absence of all signs or symptoms regarding which inquiry has been made is stated in the record. The general term "negative" for a total system is meaningless; the reader, if he is not the recorder, does not know which questions were asked and consequently does not know the context of "negative"; if the reader is also the recorder, he probably will not, after time, remember which specific questions were asked. An exception might exist in a health care system where the review of physical systems section is routinized and where "negative" indicates an inquiry into and a negative response to predetermined, universally known, and always-reviewed items of exploration.

In the PI section the practitioner has already reviewed the problem system thoroughly. The practitioner can, under that system in the review of physical systems section, advise the reader to refer to the PI section for information about that system.

Systems and body regions for review and exploration of health status, functional and anatomical problems, and health maintenance in the review of physical systems section are:

General

Usual state of health
Episodes of chills
Episodes of weakness or malaise
Fatigue
Fever
Recent and significant gain or loss of weight (if present, amount, time interval, and possible causes are recorded)
Sweats
Usual, maximum, and minimum weight

Skin

Usual state of health	Masses
Previously diagnosed and treated disease	Odors
	Petechiae
Color changes	Pruritus
Dryness	Temperature changes
Ecchymoses	Texture changes
Lesions	Care habits

Hair

Alopecia	Use of dyes
Texture changes	

Nails

Changes in appearance
Texture changes
Health maintenance (usually not recorded unless there is a positive response to a symptom; if positive, pattern of bathing and use of soaps, creams, and so on, are recorded)

Head and face

Usual state of health	Past trauma
Dizziness	Syncope
Pain	Unusual or frequent headache

Eyes

Use of corrective or prosthetic devices
Current vision, with corrective lenses if applicable
Cataracts
Changes in visual fields or vision
Diplopia
Excessive tearing
Glaucoma

Eyes—cont'd

Infections
Pain
Pattern of eye examinations
Photophobia
Pruritus
Unusual discharge or sensations

Ears

Usual state of health	Tinnitus
Use of prosthetic devices	Otalgia
Discharge	Vertigo (subjective or
Hearing	objective)
Infections	Care habits, especially
Presence of excessive	ear cleaning
environmental noise	

Nose and sinuses

Usual state of health	Pain in infraorbital or
Olfactory ability	sinus areas
Discharge (seasonal asso-	Postnasal drip
ciations)	Sinus infection
Epistaxis	Sneezing (frequent or
Frequency of colds	prolonged)
Obstruction	

Mouth and throat

Usual state of health	Hoarseness
Use of prosthetic devices	Lesions
Abscesses	Odors
Bleeding or swelling of	Sore throats
gums	Voice changes
Dryness	Pattern of dental care
Excessive salivation	Pattern of dental hygiene

Neck and nodes

Masses	Swelling
Node enlargement	Tenderness
Pain with movement or palpation	

Breasts

Discharge	Tenderness
Masses	Self-examination pattern
Pain	

Respiratory and cardiovascular systems

Usual state of health
Past diagnosis of respiratory or cardiovascular system
disease
Cough
Cyanosis
Dyspnea (if present, amount of exertion precipitating
it is recorded)
Edema
Hemoptysis
High blood pressure

Respiratory and cardiovascular systems—cont'd

Orthopnea (number of pillows needed to sleep com-
fortably is recorded)
Pain (exact location and radiation, effect of respiration
are recorded)
Palpitations
Sputum
Stridor
Wheezing
Paroxysmal nocturnal dyspnea
Date of last roentgenogram or electrocardiogram

Gastrointestinal system

Usual state of health	Hematemesis
Appetite	Hemorrhoids
Bowel habits	Hernia
Previously diagnosed	Indigestion
problems	Infections
Abdominal pain	Jaundice
Ascites	Nausea
Change in stool color	Pyrosis
Constipation	Rectal bleeding
Diarrhea	Rectal discomfort
Dyschezia	Recent changes in habits
Dysphagia	Thirst
Flatulence	Vomiting
Food idiosyncracies	Previous roentgenograms

Urinary system

Usual state of health	Incontinence
Past diagnosed problems	Nocturia
Usual patterns of urination	Oliguria
Anuria	Polyuria
Change in stream	Pyuria
Dysuria	Retention
Enuresis	Stress incontinence
Flank pain	Suprapubic pain
Frequency	Urgency
Hematuria	Urine color change
Hesitancy of stream	

Genital system

Male

Usual health	Pain
Lesions	Prostate problems
Impotence	Swelling
Masses	

Female

Diagnosed problems	Obstetrical history (for
Lesions	each pregnancy)
Pruritus	Prenatal course
Vaginal discharge	Complications of
Frequency of pap	pregnancy
smear	Duration of pregnancy
Menstrual history	Description of labor
Age at menarche	Date of delivery

Genital system—cont'd

Female–cont'd

Frequency of menses	Type of delivery
Duration of flow	(vaginal, caesarean
Amount of flow	section)
Date of last menstrual	Condition, sex, and
period (LMP)	weight of baby
Dysmenorrhea	Postpartum course
Menorrhagia	Place of prenatal
Metrorrhagia	care and hospital-
Polymenorrhea	ization
Amenorrhea	
Dyspareunia	

Both sexes

Ability to perform and	Infertility
enjoy satisfactory	Sterility
sexual intercourse	Venereal disease

Extremities and musculoskeletal system

Usual state of health	Muscles
Past diagnosis of disease	Cramping
Extremities	Pain
Coldness	Weakness
Deformities	Bones and joints
Discoloration	Stiffness
Edema	Swelling
Intermittent claudica-	Redness
tion	Heat
Pain	Limitation of move-
Thrombophlebitis	ment
	Fractures
	Back pain

Central nervous system

Usual state of health	Motor
Past diagnosis of disease	Ataxia
Anxiety	Imbalance
General behavior change	Paralysis
Loss of consciousness	Paresis
Mood change	Tic
Nervousness	Tremor
Seizures	Spasm
Speech	Sensory
Aphasia	Pain
Dysarthria	Paresthesia (hyperes-
Cognitive ability	thesia, anesthesia)
Changes in memory	
Disorientation	
Hallucinations	

Endocrine system

History of physical growth and development
Adult changes in size of head, hands, or feet
Diagnosis of diabetes or thyroid disease
Presence of secondary sex characteristics
Dryness of skin or hair

Endocrine system—cont'd

Exophthalmos
Goiter
Hair distribution
Hormone therapy
Hypoglycemia
Intolerance to heat or cold
Polydipsia
Polyuria
Polyphagia
Postural hypotension
Weakness

Hematopoietic system

Past diagnosis of disease	Blood type
Anemia	Bruising
Bleeding tendencies	Exposure to radiation
Blood transfusion	Lymphadenopathy

Sociological system

The practitioner cannot effectively diagnose a disorder or treat a client by knowing the client's physical status only. The client is a unique and whole person. In order for therapy to be effective, the problem must be assessed and treated within the context of that person. The practitioner should, in some organized way, gather information about the sociological status of the client, as well as his psychological, developmental, and nutritional status.

The following is a suggested organization of sociological data:

A. Relationships with family and significant others
1. Client's position in the family
2. Persons with whom client lives
3. Persons with whom client relates
4. Recent family crises or changes
B. Environment
1. Home
2. Community
3. Work
4. Recent changes in environment
C. Occupational history
1. Jobs held
2. Satisfaction with present and past employment
3. Current place of employment
D. Economic status and resources
1. Source of income
2. Perception of adequacy or inadequacy of income
3. Effect of illness on economic status
E. Educational level
1. Highest degree or grade attained
2. Judgment of intellect relative to age
F. Daily profile
1. Rest-activity patterns

  2. Social activities
  3. Special weekend activities
G. Patterns of health care
  1. Private and public primary care agencies
  2. Dental care
  3. Preventive care
  4. Emergency care

This outline is recommended for gathering the sociological data of the majority of adult clients; obviously, adaptations will need to be made for other individuals. Many clients may be unaccustomed to extensive questioning about nonphysical matters during the taking of a health history. The practitioner may need to explain the use of such data by stating to the client, for example, "In order to treat you most effectively, it is important that I know something about you as a person."

First, the practitioner asks about the client's role or roles in the family and household. A member may have a societally assigned role, relating to birth, for example, that of son, father, or grandfather, as well as a circumstantially defined role, for example, that of provider, "black sheep," child, and so on. Both should be identified.

Next, the practitioner inquires about the people with whom the client lives and relates on a regular basis. Information can be used to hypothesize, for example, the effect on the family of a long illness of the provider. Also, the practitioner could identify strengths in the presence of strong family or friend relationships. The client should also be asked about the closeness and compatibility of the relationships. Sometimes unsatisfactory social relationships produce stress, which can be a factor in the exacerbation or causation of illness.

It has been epidemiologically demonstrated that there is a higher than expected incidence of morbidity in those who have undergone recent important life crises or changes. Each client should be asked if any recent event has had a significant impact on his life. Resultant positive data might provide clues of causation or implications for prevention of illness.

Physical as well as psychological environments can have a profound effect on the health status and potential of an individual. The practitioner asks about the client's satisfaction with the appearance and general comfort of his house, his community, and his work situation. The practitioner might ask if the client considers his environment healthy or unhealthy. The pursuit of "why" in the case of negative responses will provide the practitioner some insight into the client's value system as well as possible informa-

tion regarding significant health hazards and clues to the etiology of the present illness. Again, the practitioner asks about recent change or loss. Positive responses are recorded.

Occupational history information can be used to identify past environmental hazards, to determine the fit between personal ability and productivity, and to plan rehabilitation. The practitioner asks about jobs held, satisfaction with those jobs, and the place of current employment.

The practitioner does not, in many cases, need to know the exact annual income; however, he should know the source of income and the client's assessment of its adequacy. Clients whose resources are too insufficient to enable them to follow therapy must be identified early, and appropriate referral for financial assistance made. In the case of probable prolonged illness, financial reserves are discussed and recorded. If the client is covered by any health insurance, the type of insurance, the name of the insurer, and the policy number are recorded.

The educational level of the client is determined. The highest degree or grade completed is recorded. The practitioner may also wish to make a judgment regarding intellectual ability relative to age. Interviewing up to this point in the history has provided the opportunity for extensive observation of the client's understanding, response, and judgment.

Knowledge of the client's daily pattern helps the practitioner know the client as a person, with habits that encourage or impede health. The practitioner asks the client to describe a typical 24-hour day and to indicate weekend differences. Work, activity, sleep, rest, and recreational pursuits are specifically identified in the recording.

Part of the client's past social interaction has been with the health care system, and past responses may be predictive of future patterns. The client is asked about the health agencies that he has used in the past for acute, preventive, and maintenance health care. It can be determined whether the client is a health facility "shopper" or whether care has had continuity.

Psychological system

The following is an outline of the information obtained and recorded in the psychological assessment of the client.

A. Cognitive abilities
  1. Comprehension
  2. Learning patterns

B. Response to illness and health
  1. Reaction to illness
  2. Coping patterns
  3. Value of health
C. Response to care
  1. Perceptions of the care givers
  2. Compliance
D. Cultural implications for care
  1. Patterns of therapy
  2. Patterns of illness response

In the assessment of cognitive abilities, the practitioner determines the comprehension ability of the client. Usually this assessment is accomplished more indirectly than directly. Prior to this point in the history-taking process, the client has demonstrated his ability to respond to some rather complex questions. The recording is the judgment summary of the practitioner regarding the client's general comprehension ability.

Since education should be an essential component of all therapy, it is useful to determine the client's health-learning patterns. Some clients need personal instructions; others learn best through reading or group discussion. Knowledge of the client's preference can enable efficient use of provider effort and also involve the client in decision making concerning the process of his therapy.

A discussion of the client's behavior in past illnesses and in health will probably be predictive of future responses. The practitioner asks: "What does health mean to you, and what do you do to keep yourself healthy?" "How do you feel, and what do you do when you become slightly ill? When you become very ill?" "Who do you go to for help if you are ill?" Most clients will be able to answer these questions easily. A summary of the client's responses is recorded concisely. Information can alert the practitioner about strengths, weaknesses, and possible problems in therapy.

Skill may be required in learning the client's real responses to care, since he is often placed in a position of subjugation by the health care system. The practitioner might ask the client how comfortable he feels in asking questions of his health care providers and if he has considered himself a partner in care with them. Answers may be recorded verbatim or summarized.

The practitioner asks about the client's amount of compliance to past courses of therapy. If compliance has been minimal, reasons should be determined for noncompliance. Problems resulting from lack of understanding and financial constraints are more easily solved than problems relating to distrust, indifference, or denial.

If the client is of a cultural group different from that of the practitioner and the majority of the care providers, it would be useful to ask the client what he expects of care and therapy, what general things are done in his culture for persons with needs similar to his. If the chief complaint is of an illness, the practitioner asks about the feelings and responses of the client and his significant others to the fact of the illness. Responses may guide the care provider into more efficient and fewer unacceptable routes of intervention.

■ Developmental data

A detailed description of the developmental assessment is presented in Chapter 4 (Developmental assessment).

The recording of this data minimally includes a summary of the client's development to date; a judgment of its normalcy, abnormality, or questionable retardation or fixation; and a statement of current developmental functioning.

■ Nutritional data

A detailed description of nutritional assessment is presented in Chapter 5 (Nutritional assessment).

The recording of data minimally includes a description of an average day's food intake, an assessment of adequacy, inadequacy, or excess of the components of the Basic Four food groups and the presence of any past nutritional problems.

WRITTEN RECORD OF THE HEALTH HISTORY

The written record is the permanent, legal, and working documentation of what was seen, heard, and felt during the examination. It will serve as the baseline by which subsequent changes will be evaluated and therapy advised. It is very often utilized by a reader who does not have access to the recorder and is consequently subject to interpretation.

It is important that the record be objective, concise, and specific. The history is not the place for the recorder to bias the reader with opinions of diagnoses. Other portions of a client's record allow for the recorder to elaborate on hypotheses and plans.

The record should be specific enough for the reader to clearly determine what was asked and examined, and the result of the interview and examination. An entry such as "Eyes—negative" or "Eyes—normal" does not supply information regarding procedures done, areas of the eyes examined, or information regarding the condition of the eyes. The range of "normal" is wide. Change in condition, even within the range of "normal" may be significant for an individual client.

The record, however, should be concise. Regional entries should be easily located and read. An extremely verbose and disorganized record may be less effective than an incomplete one because its appearance may frustrate the busy reader, who simply will not read it.

Two examples of recorded health histories are presented. One is an example of a history taken on an ill client who is being admitted to a hospital. The other is an example of a history taken on a well client. An example of a recorded physical examination is included in Chapter 23 on Integration of the physical assessment.

EXAMPLE OF A RECORDED HEALTH HISTORY: ILL CLIENT

Client: John Donald Doe
Address: 9037 N. Sheridan St.
      St. Louis, Mo. 63125
Telephone: 735-1946
Contact: Mrs. Clara Doe (mother)
Address: Same address as above; client will move in with mother after discharge from hospital
Telephone: Same telephone number as above
Birthdate: March 3, 1945   Sex: Male   Race: White
Religion: Presbyterian (inactive)   Marital status: Separated
Social Security number: 097-32-7259
Usual occupation: Offset printer
Present occupation: None; on disability for 1 year
Birthplace: New York, N.Y.
Source of referral: Self
Usual source of health care: Dr. Ryan
              1346 W. North Ave.
              St. Louis, Missouri 63122
Source and reliability of information: Client; attempted to be cooperative; however, was frequently vague about the nature and time of events
Date of interview: Jan. 9, 1975

Chief complaint
"Pain in the left side of stomach for 2 days."

Present illness
Usual health

This is the fifth Healer's Hospital admission for this 29-year-old white, separated, unemployed male who has been drinking an average of 2 to 3 fifths of hard liquor daily. Total past admissions number 8; none of these have been for abdominal complaints. Client is presently on disability income due to a diagnosis of tuberculosis (11/73). Also has a history of drug abuse and gastric ulcer.

Chronological story

14 years PTA	Began drinking heavily and regularly.
7 years PTA	Diagnosed as having a gastric ulcer by Dr. Ryan. Treated by him on an outpatient basis with Maalox and Valium prn. Had x-rays at that time. Has complained of slight to moderate gastric discomfort and food intolerance intermittently since then. Unable to relate the specific frequency or specific characteristics of episodes of illness. States that they are usually accompanied by "hangovers." Generally experiences left upper quadrant (LUQ) discomfort, feelings of hunger, nausea, and vomiting of mucous material 6 to 8 hours after drinking heavily. Drinks heavily 3 to 4 days a week and states symptoms occur approximately 2 times a week. Appetite generally has been good. Meal patterns are erratic. Takes Valium for sleep each night. Drinks 2 to 3 8-oz bottles of Maalox per week. No pattern of follow-up care with Dr. Ryan. Symptoms relieved somewhat with Maalox. Bowel movements have been regular, formed, and brown.
1 day PTA	Had not been drinking the night before. Awoke at approximately 7:00 AM and took several alcoholic drinks (amount approximately 1 cup). After an hour experienced nausea and vomiting after an attempt to drink orange juice.

Continued.

EXAMPLE OF A RECORDED HEALTH HISTORY: ILL CLIENT—cont'd

Present illness—cont'd
Chronological story—cont'd
1 day PTA—cont'd

At 10:00 AM walked to his mother's home (2 blocks). On arriving, experienced a sharp, continuous, nonradiating pain in his upper left abdominal area. Indicates LUQ. The intensity required him to lie down. Position changes provided no relief. A whole bottle of Maalox did not affect the pain, which built in intensity over the next 2 hours. After 2 hours the pain remained constant but was more nagging than sharp. Tried to take some soup and orange juice but immediately vomited it. At 2:00 PM vomited again, and this time there were red streaks in the vomitus, which was a green, thick material. (Exact amount of vomitus or blood streaks unknown.)

Throughout the remainder of the afternoon and early evening, took 5 mg Valium for a total of 4 times. Obtained no relief; pain remained nagging and continuous. Was able to walk with no increase in discomfort but felt most comfortable lying down.

At bedtime took a sleeping pill but states it did not really help him sleep. Spent a fitful night, and the pain persisted with increased intensity. States he took his temperature at midnight and had a fever of 102° F.

Date of admission
Rose at 9:00 AM and was driven to Dr. Ryan's office but found it closed. Then came directly to Healer's outpatient clinic, where he was seen and admitted.

Negative information

Denies unusual weakness, chills, or fever prior to the onset of symptoms. Denies injury to the abdomen, unusual activity or exercise, pain in other locations, diarrhea, constipation, change in stools, jaundice, ascites, flatulence, hemorrhoids, rectal bleeding, or dysphagia.

Relevant family history

The only significant family history (hx) for a serious, persistent gastrointestinal disorder was a maternal uncle who was a heavy drinker and who died of stomach cancer at age 40.

Disability assessment

Client states that he has not felt really well in the past 7 years. Has not spent a great deal of time in bed but has not worked regularly and has been either drinking or "hung over" most of the time. Was diagnosed as having tuberculosis, 11/73, and was placed on a disability income plan at that time. This insurance will cover medical expenses.

Past history
Childhood illnesses

Exact illnesses or dates unknown. Assumes he had all childhood illnesses, for example, measles, mumps, chicken pox; denies hx of rheumatic fever.

Injuries

Client unable to provide exact dates for any of the following:
1. Age 9 (1954). Hit in the eye by rock. States has had a permanent decrease in vision in that eye. No medical care.
2. Age 14 (1959). In an automobile accident. Was hospitalized in Lakeside Hospital, Chicago, for 1 week. Physician unknown. Discharged from hospital with no follow-up required.
3. Age 15 or 16 (1960 or 1961). Fractured right ankle while playing football. Cast applied at Johnson Hospital, Chicago, and was followed in their orthopedic clinic. Apparently healed.
4. Age 18 (1963). Head injury from blow with blunt object, which was thrown. Was unconscious for approximately 30 minutes. Head sutured in emergency room (ER) of Healer's Hospital, St. Louis. No follow-up except for removal of sutures. No sequelae.
5. Age 21 (1966). Stab wound in left shoulder; was attacked and robbed. Sutured in ER of Lakeside Hospital, Chicago. No follow-up except for removal of sutures. No sequelae.

Hospitalizations

1. Age 10 (1955). Hernia repair at Lakeside Hospital, Chicago. Dates and events of hospitalization unclear.
2. Age 14 (1959). Automobile accident. See item 2 under Injuries.
3. Age 20 (1965). Pneumonia. Under the care of Dr. Warner at St. Peter's Hospital, Chicago. Hospitalized for 2 weeks during December. No follow-up.
4. Age 23 (1968). Surgery for priapism at Lakeside Hospital. Under the care of Dr. Meyer. Follow-up for 1 year after surgery because was unable to obtain an erection. No other complications or current disability.

EXAMPLE OF A RECORDED HEALTH HISTORY: ILL CLIENT—cont'd

5. Age 24 (1969). Drug overdose. Under the care of Dr. Ryan, Healer's Hospital, St. Louis. Hospitalized for 2 weeks; was to start methadone maintenance; did not. Dates of stay not known.
6. Age 26 (1971). Drug overdose. Under the care of Dr. Ryan, Healer's Hospital. In the hospital for 1 week. Discharged against medical advice (AMA).
7. Age 28 (1973). Drug overdose. Under the care of Dr. Ryan. Hospitalized at Healer's Hospital for 2 weeks (1/73). Discharged on methadone maintenance.
8. Age 28 (1973). Hemorrhoidectomy. Under the care of Dr. Ryan and Dr. Jones, Healer's Hospital. Hospitalized 1 week. No complications; 1 follow-up visit.

Operations
See Hospitalizations for details.
1. Age 10 (1955). Hernia repair.
2. Age 23 (1968). Correction of priapism.
3. Age 28 (1973). Hemorrhoidectomy.

Other major illnesses
1. Age 23 (1968). Diagnosed as having a gastric ulcer by Dr. Ryan after an outpatient evaluation including x-rays. See PI section for follow-up and sequelae.
2. Age 28 (1973). Tuberculosis diagnosed and treated by staff of the St. Louis Health Department as an outpatient. Medications for 1 year. Off medications for the past 3 months. Followed with yearly x-rays and evaluation.

Allergies
None known. Denies allergies to penicillin, other drugs, foods, or environmental components; has had at least 3 courses of penicillin.

Immunizations
Unknown.

Habits
Cigarettes—smokes 1 pack a day. Habit regular since age 12.
Hard drugs—all types, including heroin. 1969-1973 had a "$90.00 a day habit."
Alcohol—started to drink heavily at age 16. Drinking decreased during period of drug addiction. Has been drinking 2 to 3 fifths of hard liquor a day for the past 2 years.
Coffee—drinks 6 to 7 cups a day.

Medications
Maalox—for ulcer prn with varied dosage since 1968. Prescribed by Dr. T. Ryan. Client states he uses 2 to 3 8-oz bottles a week.
Valium—10 mg prn for ulcer and nervousness since 1968. Client states he uses at least 1 to 2 tablets a day.
Methadone—40 mg daily for 6 months, 1973. Given through drug abuse program.
Streptomycin—IM daily, dose? For TB, 11/73 to 9/74.
INH—tid for TB, 11/73 to 9/74.
Salve—name unknown, a nonprescription drug; topically every day for scaling skin on soles of feet; since approximately 8/74.
Magnesium citrate—for constipation approximately once ($\times$1) monthly or less frequently; prescribed by self. Uses 1 tbsp prn.
Sleeping pill—prn. Name and dose unknown. Prescribed by Dr. Ryan; 1 every night.

Family history
Maternal and paternal grandparents deceased. Ages at death and causes of death unknown. Denies family hx of diabetes, blood disorders, arteriosclerosis, gout, obesity, coronary artery disease, tuberculosis, cancer, hypertension, epilepsy, kidney disease, or allergic disorders. Uncertain about health history of aunts and uncles.
    Mother—age 52; alive and well.
    Father—deceased, age 50, 1960; cause unknown.
    Siblings—no maternal miscarriages.
        1. ♀ Age 27; alive and well.
        2. ♂ Age 20; deceased 1973; drug overdose.
        3. ♀ Age 21; alive and well.

Continued.

EXAMPLE OF A RECORDED HEALTH HISTORY: ILL CLIENT—cont'd

Family history—cont'd
    4. ♂ Age 18; deceased 1970; gunshot wound.
    5. ♀ Age 19; alive and well.
  Children
    1. ♂ Age 10; alive and well.
    2. ♂ Age 7; alive and well.
  Wife—age 31; obese, otherwise well.

Review of physical systems
General

Chronically ill, white male adult; usual wt about 176 lb. Reports approximately 10-lb wt loss over the past 3- to 4-month period. Feels this is due to not eating when drinking heavily. States he has felt a generalized fatigue and malaise for over 1 year, since onset of TB, but denies requiring daily naps or extra sleep. States he cannot exercise due to fatigue. Denies chills (other than those associated with PI), sweats, and seizures.

Skin, hair, and nails

Denies lesions, color changes, ecchymoses, petechiae, texture changes, unusual odors, or infections. Pruritus; soles of feet dry and scaling for 6 months; condition stable (using nonprescription salve, name unknown). States he has had small cracks at corners of mouth for 1 month. Denies cold sores. States hair breaks off and falls out but denies patchy alopecia. Denies brittle, cracking, or peeling nails. States bites nails. Has 1 birthmark on upper back but is not aware of any change in size or color.

Head and face

Denies pain, headache, dizziness, or vertigo. Hx of injury with blow to forehead. Reports frequent losses of consciousness after drinking; duration unknown, probably 1 to 8 hours.

Eyes

Has worn corrective lenses since 1955, age 10. States rt eye 20/20, lt eye 20/50. Hx of 1 eye injury, age 9. States visual acuity decreased after injury. Denies pain, infection, watery or itching eyes, diplopia, blurred vision, glaucoma, cataracts, decreased peripheral vision. Last ophthalmological examination 2 years ago.

Ears

Denies hearing loss. Denies discharge, pain, irritation, or ringing in ears. States he was "cut in a fight" on rt auricle. Cleans ears with a toothpick.

Nose and sinuses

Denies sinus pain, postnasal drip, discharge, epistaxis, soreness, excessive sneezing, or obstructed breathing. Denies injuries. States he has approximately 2 colds a year. Olfaction not good; attributes this to smoking.

Oral cavity

Complains of frequent dryness in mouth and cracking of lips and tongue. No false teeth. Gums bleed frequently. Denies hoarseness, pain, odor, frequent sore throats, voice change. Dental care infrequent. Brushes teeth "occasionally."

Neck

Denies pain, stiffness, or limitation of range of motion (ROM). Denies masses.

Nodes

Denies enlarged or tender nodes in neck, axillary, or inguinal area.

Breasts

Denies surgery, pain, masses, or discharge.

Chest and respiratory system

Denies pain, wheezing, asthma, or bronchitis. Hx of pneumonia, age 20 (see Hospitalizations). Denies shortness of breath or dyspnea. Sleeps on 2 pillows but is not dependent on them for breathing. Hx of TB, 1973-1974 (see Major illnesses). Last chest x-ray on present admission, negative. States he had 1 episode of hemoptysis, 1968, associated

EXAMPLE OF A RECORDED HEALTH HISTORY: ILL CLIENT—cont'd

with his ulcer. Details of this unclear. States he has "smoker's cough" (dry cough in the morning) but denies sputum.

Cardiovascular system
Denies chest pain, coronary artery disease, rheumatic fever, or heart murmur. Denies hypertension, palpitations, cyanosis, or diagnosis of cardiac disorder. States he has occasional slight edema in rt ankle.

Gastrointestinal system
See PI. Also see Hospitalizations re hemorrhoidectomy. Appetite good. Denies dysphagia, belching, or hematemesis. Hx of ulcer (see PI) and hernia repair (see Hospitalizations). Denies melena, clay-colored stools, or diarrhea. Takes laxative, citric magnesium, approximately ×1 monthly or less for constipation. Denies jaundice. Reports decreased appetite with alcohol intake but denies specific intolerance to any food.

Genitourinary system
Denies bladder or kidney infections, urgency, frequency, hesitancy, painful micturation, incontinence, nocturia, or polyuria, hx of VD. Denies testicular pain. Hx of surgery for priapism with inability to have erection for 1 year following (p̄) surgery. No dysfunction at present. States sex life is "fair." Alcohol decreases "urge." Fertile; states he has fathered 7 children.

Extremities
Hx of fractured rt ankle, age 15 or 16. Reports swelling of ankle without pain. Denies varicose veins, thrombophlebitis, joint paint, stiffness, swelling, gout, arthritis, limitation of ROM, or color changes.

Back
Denies pain, stiffness, limitation of movement, or disc disease.

Central nervous system
Reports loss of consciousness (1963) following blow to head; duration approximately 30 minutes. Denies clumsiness of movement, weakness, paralysis, tremor, neuralgia, or paresthesia. States he is a "nervous" person but denies hx of nervous breakdown. Hx of drug and alcohol abuse. States he will periodically (every 2 to 3 weeks) have spontaneous jerky movement of legs during rest. There are 4 to 5 movements in each episode. This has never occurred while legs were wt bearing. Denies disorientation or memory disorders. Denies seizures or epilepsy. "Passes out" frequently after heavy alcohol ingestion and sleeps for 5 to 6 hours. Wakes with headache and nausea.

Hematopoietic system
Denies bleeding, bruising, blood transfusion, or exposure to x-rays or toxic agents.

Endocrine system
Denies diabetes, thyroid disease, or intolerance to heat or cold. Growth has been within normal range.

Review of sociological system
Family relationships
Has been separated from wife for 6 to 7 months and is in the process of being divorced. States his marital problems do not interfere with seeing his children. Plans to move to his mother's home when discharged from hospital. States relationships with his family are good.

Occupational history
Offset printer since 1971. Presently unemployed. Was advised not to work for 6 months when tuberculosis was diagnosed and has not been "able to get back to work." States he liked that occupation but expresses no urgency to return to work.

Economic status
On disability income, because of tuberculosis and need to rest. States he does not have trouble making ends meet on present income.

Daily profile
Lives alone in a room. States he spends time during the day at home or with friends, drinking. Has no special hobbies or activities to occupy time. Has habit of heavy daily drinking. States "I just hang around all day." Does do some

Continued.

EXAMPLE OF A RECORDED HEALTH HISTORY: ILL CLIENT—cont'd

Review of sociological system—cont'd

Daily profile—cont'd

spur-of-the-moment traveling. Weekdays are no different from weekends. States he dropped out of college because of disinterest. Meal patterns are erratic; sleeps 8 to 10 hours every day, usually 1 AM until 9 to 11 AM.

Educational level

States he is "smart enough." Dropped out of college after 2 years because of disinterest. States he has no aspiration except to "get by in life."

Patterns of health care

Has maintained relationship with same physician for episodic care for the last 10 years. Does return for periodic examinations and follow-up when symptoms "scare him."

Environmental data

Birthplace—New York, N.Y.

Home—plans to move to his mother's home. Will share the 5-bedroom residence with his mother and 2 siblings. Neighborhood is residential; describes it as "beautiful."

Review of psychological system

Cognitive abilities

Oriented to present events. Has fairly adequate vocabulary. Has a fair to poor memory. Cannot recall details of some important events. No history of psychiatric treatment.

Response to illness

States he "quit" drinking when he entered the hospital and plans to abstain in the future. Verbalizes that his health problems are his own fault and that he will die soon if he does not resolve them. States illness does not bother him except when "it gets out of control." Definition of health entails being able to play baseball again.

Response to care

States he has sometimes not followed medical advice, because of fear or because drug or alcohol did not allow him to think "straight." "People have been nice to me." States all care has been "OK."

Cultural implications

Inactive Presbyterian at present but is concerned about conflict with religious beliefs and life-style. Fourth-generation American.

Developmental data

Adult male who has had problems with interpersonal relationships in his marriage. Has demonstrated drug and alcohol abuse since entering adulthood. Present lifestyle seems to lack motivation. Does not express concern regarding his inability to work; has abandoned his college attendance. Immediate plans for the future involve moving in with his mother and trying to stop drinking. Speaks of his children as playmates; expresses few fathering needs or activities.

Nutritional data

States he does not eat when drinking heavily and must build his tolerance to food by taking liquids such as soup or juices after drinking. States he does eat 3 complete meals daily when not drinking. Includes foods from the four basic food groups.

EXAMPLE OF A RECORDED HEALTH HISTORY: WELL CLIENT

Client: Mary Rose Doe
Address: 1056 N. East St.
      St. Louis, Mo. 60347
Telephone: 278-9274
Contact: Mrs. Elsa Smith (mother)
Address: 3496 Oak St.
      St. Louis, Mo. 63047
Telephone: 926-8711
Birthdate: Feb. 6, 1945   Sex: Female   Race: Black
Religion: Methodist (active)   Marital status: Married
Social Security number: 396-47-8911
Usual occupation: Grade school teacher
Present occupation: Same—Greenwich School
Birthplace: St. Louis, Mo.
Source of referral: Self
Usual source of health care: St. Louis Health Maintenance Organization
                              4693 C. Division St.
                              St. Louis, Mo. 63044
Source and reliability of information: Client; cooperative, apparently reliable
Date of interview: Dec. 12, 1975.

Reason for visit

Annual physical examination; last exam, 1/74.

Present health status

Usual health

This is the third St. Louis Health Maintenance Organization (HMO) visit for this 30-year-old black, married female school teacher who has been in good health for all of her life. Client has been hospitalized twice for the purposes of normal childbirth only. Has no major chronic diseases.

Summary

Client is presently well and requests a physical examination for health maintenance and screening purposes. Is concerned about a strong family history of hypertension and believes that monitoring of her blood pressure status is important.

   Also requests a pap smear and evaluation for continuance of oral contraceptives. Has been taking Ortho-Novum 1+50 since the birth of her last child in 1969. Client enrolled in the health plan a year ago.

Past history

Childhood illnesses

Had rubella, chicken pox—not diagnosed by a physician. Has not had rheumatic fever.

Injuries

None.

Hospitalizations

See obstetrical data in Review of physical systems.
1. Age 20 (1965). Childbirth.
2. Age 24 (1969). Childbirth.

Operations

None.

Major illnesses

None.

Allergies

None known. Denies allergy to penicillin, other drugs, foods, or environmental components. Has had a course of penicillin (10 d, oral).

Continued.

EXAMPLE OF A RECORDED HEALTH HISTORY: WELL CLIENT—cont'd

Past history—cont'd

Immunizations

Had full series of diphtheria-pertussis-tetanus (DPT) when a preschooler. Had oral polio when an adolescent.

Habits

Cigarettes—smoked 15 cigarettes a day for 5 years (age 20-25).
Hard drugs—none.
Alcohol—drinks 3 to 4 mixed drinks during a weekend.
Coffee, tea—drinks approximately 10 cups of coffee a day. Drinks tea rarely.

Medications

Ortho-Novum 1+50 oral contraceptives since 1969.
Aspirin (ASA) for headache—takes approximately ×10 gr twice a month.
Milk of magnesia for constipation—takes 1 tablespoon about once a month.
One-a-Day multiple vitamins—takes 1 a day.

Family history

Denies family history of diabetes, blood disorder, gout, obesity, tuberculosis, epilepsy, kidney disease, or gastrointestinal disease.

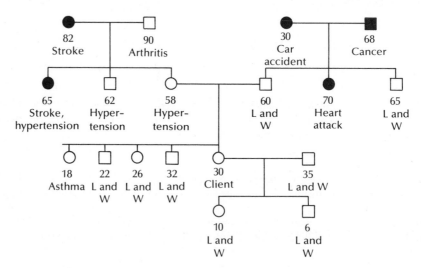

Review of physical systems

General

Usually well. Usual-minimum-maximum weight: 135-125-160 lb. No increase or decrease in weight. Denies fatigue, malaise, chills, sweats, fever, seizures, or fainting.

Skin, hair, and nails

Denies lesions, color change, ecchymoses, masses, petechiae, texture changes, pruritus, sweating, or unusual odors. No alopecia or brittle hair. Denies brittle, cracking, or peeling nails. No birthmarks. Washes hair once a week; does not use dyes.

Head and face

Denies pain, dizziness, vertigo, or history of injury or loss of consciousness.

Eyes

Has worn corrective lenses since age 7; currently wears contact lenses all day. Denies recent change in visual acuity, pain, infection, watery or itching eyes, diplopia, blurred vision, glaucoma, cataracts, or decreased peripheral vision. Last ophthalmoscopic examination 2 years ago.

Ears

Denies hearing loss, discharge, pain, irritation, or ringing in the ears. Cleans ears with cotton-tipped applicator.

EXAMPLE OF A RECORDED HEALTH HISTORY: WELL CLIENT—cont'd

Nose and sinuses

States she has sinus pain, congestion, and subsequent nasal discharge several times each winter. Takes Contact prn (approximately 1 q 12 hours × 3d) for each episode of rhinitis; gets relief. Denies epistaxis, soreness, excessive sneezing, obstructed breathing, or injuries. States olfaction is good.

Oral cavity

Visits a dentist every 6 months for cleaning and examination. Brushes teeth twice a day. Denies toothache, lesions, soreness, bleeding of gums, coated tongue, disturbance of taste, hoarseness, or frequent sore throat.

Neck

Denies pain, stiffness, limitation of ROM, or masses.

Nodes

Denies enlarged or tender nodes in neck, axillary, or inguinal area.

Breasts

Denies masses, pain, tenderness, or discharge. Examines breasts monthly, right after menses.

Chest and respiratory system

Denies pain, wheezing, shortness of breath, dyspnea, hemoptysis, or cough. Denies hx of asthma, pneumonia, or bronchitis. Has yearly chest x-ray, required for work in the schools.

Cardiovascular system

Denies precordial pain, palpitations, cyanosis, edema, or intermittent claudication. Frequently bicycles in summer and downhill skis in winter. Walks 2 miles a day. Denies diagnosis of heart murmur, hypertension, coronary artery disease, or rheumatic fever.

Gastrointestinal system

Denies history of gastrointestinal disease. Appetite good. Bowels active daily, stools are always brown. Denies pain, constipation, diarrhea, flatulence, vomiting, hemorrhoids, hernias, jaundice, pyrosis, or bleeding. Has never had GI x-rays.

Genitourinary system

Denies hx of bladder or kidney infections, hematuria, urgency, frequency, dysuria, incontinence, nocturia, polyuria, or VD. Menses—onset 13 years; frequency, every 26 to 30 days; duration, 5 days; flow, heavy for 3 days, light for 2 days; last menstrual period (LMP), 12/1/75. Denies dysmenorrhea, menorrhagia, metrorrhagic discharge, or pruritus. Last pap smear, 12/74.

Obstetrical history

1. Sept. 12, 1965. Girl, 6 lb, 8 oz. Vaginal delivery at St. Francis Hospital, St. Louis. Prenatal, intrapartum, and postpartum course normal for mother and baby.
2. Oct. 9, 1969. Boy, 7 lb, 2 oz. Vaginal delivery at St. Francis Hospital, St. Louis. Prenatal, intrapartum, and postpartum course normal for mother and baby.

Sexual history

Age at first intercourse was 17 years. Enjoys intercourse with husband—no dyspareunia and able to achieve satisfactory orgasm most of the time. Using oral birth control medication. Not sure yet if she will have another child. Will consider sterilization when family is complete.

Extremities

No past problems. Denies deformities, varicose veins, thrombophlebitis, joint pain, stiffness, swelling, gout, arthritis, limitation of ROM, color changes, or temperature changes.

Back

No past problems. Denies pain, stiffness, or limitation of movement; no history of disc disease.

Central nervous system

No past problems. Denies loss of consciousness, clumsiness of movement, difficulty with balance, weakness, paralysis,

Continued.

EXAMPLE OF A RECORDED HEALTH HISTORY: WELL CLIENT—cont'd

Review of physical systems—cont'd
Central nervous system—cont'd

tremor, neuralgia, paresthesia, history of emotional disorders, drug or alcohol dependency, disorientation, memory lapses, or seizures. Speech articulate.

Hematopoietic system

No past problems. Denies excessive bleeding and bruising, blood transfusions, or excessive exposure to x-rays or toxic agents. Blood type A, Rh positive.

Endocrine system

Denies history of diabetes or thyroid disease, polyuria, polydipsia, polydysplasia, intolerance to heat or cold, or hirsutism.

Review of sociological system
Family relationships

Lives in own home with husband and 2 children. Husband is a school teacher also; couple shares finances, childrearing, and housekeeping responsibilities. Client's parents live ½ mile away, and relationships are described as "good." Couple has several close friends; also, siblings are in frequent contact. No recent family crisis or change.

Occupational history

Has been a grade school teacher for 5 years. Holds BS and MA degrees and feels secure that she can retain her job as long as she wants it. Enjoys children and states job is very satisfying.

Economic status

Client and husband achieve a combined gross income of over $30,000 a year. Feels this is very adequate. Has hospitalization insurance.

Daily profile

During the week, works 8 AM to 3 PM. Returns home around 3:30 and works until 5 PM on school work. Then cooks dinner and interacts with family. Has meetings 1 or 2 evenings a week. Weekends, client and husband usually have 1 evening out with friends, to movie or concert. Family attends church each Sunday. Client is involved with photography as a hobby. Sleeps 7 to 8 hours every night (approximately 11 PM to 7 AM).

Educational level

Highest degree attained is the master's degree. Obtains most of health knowledge by reading.

Patterns of health care

Has always had a primary care provider. Cared for by Dr. Richard Smith, a family practitioner until first pregnancy. Then seen regularly by Dr. Janice Lawson, for obstetrical and gynecological care. Family enrolled in HMO a year ago; all family members are being seen here. Dental care regular and at the HMO.

Environmental data

Birthplace—Greenwood, Miss. Grew up in Trenton, N.J.

Home—family lives in their own 8-room home in a residential St. Louis neighborhood. Client describes home as comfortable. Has lived there for 10 years.

Community—community is middle income, integrated, consisting primarily of young professional families.

Work—teaches fourth grade in a community grade school. States that the work situation is fairly good. School is in good condition, and classes are small. A recent stress is a new assistant principal with whom client does not get along. May consider transfer to another school.

Review of psychological system
Cognitive abilities

Oriented to time, place, and person (×3). Is articulate, asks questions, has a good memory. Able to understand directions.

Response to illness

States she has never been seriously ill, so does not know what personal response would be. Feels she is "too busy" to be ill for any length of time. Uses the resources of HMO for preventive and therapeutic needs of self and family.

EXAMPLE OF A RECORDED HEALTH HISTORY: WELL CLIENT—cont'd

Response to care

States she enjoys encounters with health care providers. States she usually follows through on the advice that is given. Feels that the services of the HMO are adequate to meet her family care needs and has been very satisfied with the care to date.

Cultural implications

Client states she and her family are involved in a racially integrated community. She grew up in a predominantly black northern community. Cannot identify any way in which her black culture would especially affect her response to illness or therapy in the case of illness. Active Methodist; believes that religious concerns would influence her response to illness and treatment.

Developmental data

Adult female; wife, mother, and career teacher. Is able to manage the tasks of all these roles effectively. Development to date has proceeded normally in the physical, social, and psychological areas.

Nutritional data

Diet adequate; high in fats and carbohydrates. Has no food intolerances.
Usual breakfast—toast with butter, fried egg, orange juice, and coffee with cream.
Usual lunch—eats with school children; consists of meat, 1 vegetable, 1 carbohydrate, dessert, and beverage.
Dinner—meat (beef, chicken, or pork), salad, 1 vegetable, potato or bread, dessert, and coffee with cream.
Snacks—may have cheese and crackers, or peanuts in the evening.

BIBLIOGRAPHY

Berg, R. L.: Health status indexes, Chicago, 1973, Hospital Research and Educational Trust.

Bernstein, L., Bernstein, R. S., and Dana, R. H.: Interviewing; a guide for health professionals, ed. 2, New York, 1974, Appleton-Century-Crofts.

Bird, B.: Talking with patients, ed. 2, Philadelphia, 1973, J. B. Lippincott Co.

Blum, L. H.: Reading between the lines; doctor-patient communication, New York, 1972, International Universities Press, Inc.

Bowder, C. L., and Burnstein, A. G.: Psychosocial basis of medical practice, Baltimore, 1974, The Williams & Wilkins Co.

Froelich, R. E., and Bishop, F. M.: Medical interviewing; a programmed manual, ed. 2, St. Louis, 1972, The C. V. Mosby Co.

Mitchell, P. H.: Concepts basic to nursing, New York, 1973, McGraw-Hill Book Co.

Small, I. F., editor: Introduction to the clinical history, Flushing, N.Y., 1971, Medical Examination Publishing Co.

Tumulty, P. A.: The effective clinician, Philadelphia, 1973, W. B. Saunders Co.

Yarnall, S. R., and Wakefield, J. S.: Acquisition of the history database, ed. 2, Seattle, 1972, Medical Computer Services Assoc.

4 Developmental assessment

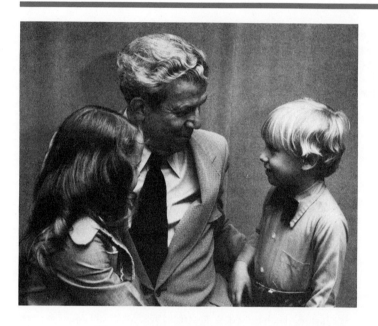

The purpose of this chapter is to provide the student of health assessment with some guidelines and ideas on the developmental assessment of individuals throughout the lifespan. It is hoped that this type of assessment will enhance the scope of "whole person" assessment and provide a broadened perspective on what total health assessment includes.

The chapter does not include a detailed delineation of the many theories and extensive research related to development and the continuous aging process; for a guide to that type of information, the reader is referred to the bibliography at the end of the chapter.

THE CHILD

The assessment of a child's development is carried out formally or informally by the practitioner during each examination. The opportunity to observe the development of many children enhances the ability to define the parameters of normal development, and the experienced examiner often responds to subtle behavioral cues with an intuitive hunch that all is not well with the child. However, it is usually difficult to verify this initial impression and make a determination of the presence or absence of a developmental deficit while examining a child in a busy clinical setting. The practitioner may need to plan additional time in order to focus attention on the assessment of the child's development or may need to seek the assistance of experts in child development.

The information obtained from the developmental assessment has many uses. It will aid the practitioner in providing assistance to the parents when they have questions about their child's behavior. Most parents will be interested in learning that their child is developing normally, and with anticipatory guidance they can gain a greater appreciation of ways to support the normal development of their child. The developmental assessment also provides information that can be useful at a future time. For instance, the child who has been developing in a normal fashion and then demonstrates a developmental lag presents a different problem than the child who has been consistently slower in development. Finally, the developmental assessment is helpful in screening for some of the more obvious deficits in development that deserve further investigation.

It is most important to keep in mind that the developmental assessment is not a test of the child's intelligence and does not allow the practitioner to make a diagnosis. It does allow the practitioner to collect data that indicates whether the development of the individual child is within the normal range.

The appraisal of the child's development is somewhat easier to accomplish during infancy and early childhood, because the nature and stages of development have been documented and the data incorporated into various developmental screening tests. In contrast, the development of the school age child and adolescent occurs at a slower rate and is not as easily observed; few screening tests for these children have been devised.

Although there are many theories of development that can provide a framework for observing and assessing the development of children, the discussion in this chapter is limited. However, it is reasonable to expect that each practitioner with an interest in children will be challenged to increase his understanding of the behavior presented by children of different ages.

The discussion in this section includes a conceptual framework for organizing the developmental assessment; approaches to the developmental assessment of the child, which can be incorporated into the plan for the health history and examination; and a brief discussion of selected screening tests that can be helpful to the practitioner.

■ Conceptual framework

A systematic appraisal of the child's development can be organized in different ways. Although each behavior of the child is part of an indivisible whole, it is clinically useful to separate behaviors into several categories whether the assessment is carried out as a part of the health examination or is done according to a more formal procedure. Different categories of behavior are used, but many of the screening tests commonly focus on three categories: fine and gross motor development, language and communication, and personal-social behavior. These categories are especially useful in the assessment of the infant and preschool child, when observable changes occur most rapidly. When the development of the older child is being assessed, it is important to include questions about the child's adjustment to school and the grade level achieved and about his relationships with peers, siblings, and significant adults.

The stages of motor development have been documented and are well-known, as is the relationship of motor skills to neuromotor organization. The practitioner will find information about the expected norms for achieving specific motor skills in most standard textbooks of pediatrics or child development. What is not usually discussed in regard to developing motor abilities is the way the child uses these skills. Is the child active and using his skills in a variety of ways? Or is the child quiet, showing little apparent interest or pleasure in walking, running, and climbing? Information as to the amount of activity may lead to questions about the environment. Does it offer too much stimulation or too little? Differences in the use of skills may also be related to organic problems, which are sometimes demonstrated by the hyperactive, impulse-ridden child.

The normal age range for the sequential development of language and communication skills is also well documented, as well as the relationship of speech development to intellectual functioning. The assessment of the child's language and communication skills should provide information about the size of the child's vocabulary, his understanding of language, his clarity of articulation, and his use of phrases and sentences. The speech of the young child is easily disturbed when there are physical problems or problems with the people in the environment. Speech disturbances may be transitory, may indicate an impairment of the hearing or speech apparatus, or may indicate the presence of a mental disability. Although a delay in speech development may be a temporary problem, it is a concern that deserves further investigation even when the child is very young.

The appraisal of the personal-social behavior of the child provides information about the child's developing awareness of himself as a person, his ability to interact with people, and his adaptive behaviors. These abilities can also be described as the intellectual, emotional, and social skills of the child. Erik Erikson's "conceptual itinerary" of the psychosocial stages of life provides a plan, or a guided overview, of the changes and adaptive behaviors of the child in each of the sequential stages of childhood. Each stage is identified with a core problem or crisis that allows the child to increase his sense of self and his capacity to act in an organized fashion in his social and physical environment if a satisfactory solution is reached. However, the core problems are never totally resolved; and even though the child is successful, he will be left with the negative as well as the positive aspects of the conflict in the continuing, dynamic condition of human life. Erikson's core problems of childhood are presented in the following paragraphs.

"Trust *versus* mistrust" is the core problem of

the infant. Successful growth during this period means that the child comes to trust the people in his environment and himself. As he becomes attached to the people who care for him, especially his mother, be begins to demonstrate trust when he rewards them with spontaneous smiles and playfulness by 2 or 3 months of age. He demonstrates increasing trust during the fourth and fifth months by his ability to wait a short while before having his needs met. He becomes increasingly aware of the environment as separate from himself during the last half of the first year and becomes more demanding of his mother's attention. He will protest if she leaves his view. Also, he no longer accepts attention passively from other people and may show anxiety with strangers. When his behavior is understood and he continues to receive loving attention, his trust in himself and others can be maintained and strengthened.

The toddler experiences a sense of "autonomy *versus* shame and doubt." He enjoys his newly acquired skills, such as walking and climbing. He is eager to explore and manipulate objects in the environment. If there are opportunities for him to make successful choices, his feelings of autonomy will grow. However, if his choices result in disaster, the negative feelings of shame arise. The child of this age is happiest when he is free to move and explore without unnecessary restraints, but he has little inner control. He needs a safe environment that allows him to use his wonderful new skills.

The preschool child from 3 to 6 years of age is developing a sense of "initiative versus guilt." The child of this age is developing a sense of himself as a social person in relation to other people. He is also learning about the physical world. This is the early period of socialization, when the child identifies with the parent of the same sex. Play is creative and provides the child with the opportunity to "try out" different experiences and roles perceived in his daily life. His conscience is developing, and he is eager to please. He is able to cooperate and enjoy other children. He is also more responsible for his own actions and enjoys doing some things independently, such as dressing himself. He is vulnerable to criticism and punishment because of the initiative he takes in learning and seeking new experiences that may bring him into conflict with his social environment. When he is successful, his feelings of well-being increase; but when he fails, he feels guilty.

The core problem of the child from 6 to 12 years of age is "industry versus inferiority." The child is able to be a serious worker at this age and wants to participate well. However, he is now concerned about gaining the approval of his peers, teachers, and other significant adults, as well as that of his family. If he fails to meet the standards that are set for him, he will feel inferior and inadequate. He works hard to achieve and needs to be successful.

The adolescent from 13 to 18 years of age is involved in the developmental crisis of "identity versus role confusion." The adolescent struggles to reorganize and integrate his past roles and the roles he hopes to play in the future. He is uncertain about himself as a person. His tasks include emancipation from his parents, acceptance of a sexual role, and a plan for a career or vocation.

■ Approaches to assessment

The practitioner with limited time would be well served to find ways to incorporate aspects of the developmental assessment into the routine health examination of every child. A good deal of information can be gained by including questions about the child's development in the history. Also, since it is traditional to include observations of the child's behavior as part of the general inspection of the physical examination, it is relatively easy to pay special attention to particular aspects of behavior in order to obtain data about the child's level of functioning. However, it is well to keep in mind when observing the child in a clinical setting that the behavior demonstrated may not be typical, because of the stress that may result from the unfamiliar environment or from particular problems of illness that the child is experiencing.

A "Schedule for Preventive Health Care," developed by the American Academy of Pediatrics, and published in the second edition of *Standards of Child Health Care*, includes suggestions and recommendations for the examination of the child during each visit for health care during the first 6 years of life. Items from the Denver Developmental Screening Test that are appropriate for the chronological age of the child at the time of each visit have been incorporated. This schedule offers an excellent example of a plan for the continuing appraisal of specific developmental milestones at the time the child is seen for health care.

Because there are limited opportunities to observe the child's behavior in the clinical setting, the history becomes the major tool for obtaining information about the child's development.

First, the history allows the practitioner to obtain data about the factors that will increase the chances of the child's being at risk for problems that may interfere with his development. Una Haynes outlines many of the factors that contribute to the "at risk" status of the child. This information can be elicited from the past history of the child in the prenatal, natal, and postnatal period of life; from the family history; from the sociological assessment; from the developmental data; and from the history of illnesses and injuries. The history that reveals problems such as prematurity, precipitate delivery, or hyperbilirubinemia in the first 48 hours of life will alert the practitioner that the child is at greater risk than most children for developmental problems. However, this information should not bias the practitioner's perception of the child's development but should encourage a sense of "benign suspicion," a term used by Sally Provence (1968a) to describe the attitude of the examiner.

The pediatric history as outlined in Chapter 21 on Assessment of the pediatric client includes a developmental history that provides information about the age at which the child achieved certain developmental milestones. This information can be used to determine whether the early development was within average or normal limits. The history of the present health or present illness should include a description of the child's current level of functioning. The practitioner can review the achievements expected of the child at a specific chronological age as outlined in many texts on child development. Table 4-1 provides such an outline. Questions about these expected achievements will provide information about the

Table 4-1. Child development from 1 month to 5 years*

1 month

Motor
1. Moro reflex present.
2. Vigorous sucking reflex present.
3. Lying prone (face down): lifts head briefly so chin is off table.
4. Lying prone: makes crawling movements with legs.
5. Held in sitting position: back is rounded, head held up momentarily only.
6. Hands tightly fisted.
7. Reflex grasp of object with palm.

Language
8. Startled by sound; quieted by voice.
9. Small throaty noises or vocalizations.

Personal-social-adaptive
10. Ringing bell produces decrease of activity.
11. May follow dangling object with eyes to midline.
12. Lying on back: will briefly look at examiner or change his activity.
13. Reacts with generalized body movements when tissue paper is placed on face.

2 months

Motor
1. Kicks vigorously.
2. Energetic arm movements.
3. Vigorous head turning.
4. Held in ventral suspension (prone): no head droop.
5. Lying prone: lifts head so face makes an approximate 45° angle with table.
6. Held in sitting position: head erect but bobs.
7. Hand goes to mouth.
8. Hands often open (not clenched).

Language
9. Is cooing.
10. Vocalizes single vowel sounds, such as: ah-eh-uh.

Personal-social-adaptive
11. Head and eyes search for sound.
12. Listens to bell ringing.
13. Follows dangling object past midline.
14. Alert expression.
15. Follows moving person with eyes.
16. Smiles back when talked to.

3 months

Motor
1. Lying prone: lifts head to 90° angle.
2. Lifts head when lying on back (supine).
3. Moro reflex begins to disappear.
4. Grasp reflex nearly gone.
5. Rolls side to back (3-4 months).

Language
6. Chuckling, squealing, grunting, especially when talked to.
7. Listens to music.
8. Vocalizes with two different syllables, such as: a-a, la-la (not distinct), oo-oo.

*Reprinted by permission of Walter M. Block, M.D., Child Evaluation Clinic of Cedar Rapids, Iowa. © Copyright 1972.

Continued.

Table 4-1. Child development from 1 month to 5 years—cont'd

3 months—cont'd

Personal-social-adaptive
9. Reaches for but misses objects.
10. Holds toy with active grasp when put into hand.
11. Sucks and inspects fingers.
12. Pulls at clothes.

Personal-social-adaptive—cont'd
13. Follows object (toy) side to side (and 180°).
14. Looks predominately at examiner.
15. Glances at toy when put into hand.
16. Recognizes mother and bottle.
17. Smiles spontaneously.

4 months

Motor
1. Sits when well supported.
2. No head lag when pulled to sitting position.
3. Turns head at sound of voice.
4. Lifts head (in supine position) in effort to sit.
5. Lifts head and chest when prone, using hands and forearms.
6. Held erect: pushes feet against table.

Language
7. Laughs aloud (4-5 months).
8. Uses sounds, such as: m-p-b.
9. Repeats series of same sounds.

Personal-social-adaptive
10. Grasps rattle.
11. Plays with own fingers.
12. Reaches for object in front of him with both hands.
13. Transfers object from hand to hand.
14. Pulls dress over face.
15. Smiles spontaneously at people.
16. Regards raisin (or pellet).

5 months

Motor
1. Moro reflex gone.
2. Rolls side to side.
3. Rolls back to front.
4. Full head control when pulled to or held in sitting position.
5. Briefly supports most of his weight on his legs.
6. Scratches on table top.

Language
7. Squeals with high voice.
8. Recognizes familiar voices.
9. Coos and/or stops crying on hearing music.

Personal-social-adaptive
10. Grasps dangling object.
11. Reaches for toy with both hands.
12. Smiles at mirror image.
13. Turns head deliberately to bell.
14. Obviously enjoys being played with.

6 months

Motor
1. Supine: lifts head spontaneously.
2. Bounces on feet when held standing.
3. Sits briefly (tri-pod fashion).
4. Rolls front to back (6-7 months).
5. Grasps foot and plays with toes.
6. Grasps cube with palm.

Language
7. Vocalizes at mirror image.
8. Makes four or more different sounds.
9. Localizes source of sound (bell, voice).
10. Vague, formless babble (especially with family members).

Personal-social-adaptive
11. Holds one cube in each hand.
12. Puts cube into mouth.
13. Re-secures dropped cube.
14. Transfers cube from hand to hand.
15. Conscious of strange sights and persons.
16. Consistent regard of object or person (6-7 months).
17. Uses raking movement to secure raisin or pellet.
18. Resists having toy taken away from him.
19. Stretches out arms to be taken up (6-8 months).

8 months

Motor
1. Sits alone (6-8 months).
2. Early stepping movements.
3. Tries to crawl.
4. Stands few seconds, holding on to object.
5. Leans forward to get an object.

Language
6. Two-syllable babble, such as: a-la, ba-ba, oo-goo, a-ma, mama, dada (8-10 months).
7. Listens to conversation (8-10 months).
8. "Shouts" for attention (8-10 months).

Table 4-1. Child development from 1 month to 5 years—cont'd

8 months—cont'd

Personal-social-adaptive

9. Works to get toy out of reach.
10. Scoops pellet.
11. Rings bell purposely (8-10 months).
12. Drinks from cup.
13. Plays peek-a-boo.
14. Looks for dropped object.

10 months

Motor

1. Gets self into sitting position.
2. Sits steadily (long time).
3. Pulls self to standing position (on bed railing).
4. Crawls on hands and knees.
5. Walks when held or around furniture.
6. Turns around when left on floor.

Language

7. Imitates speech sounds.
8. Shakes head for "no."
9. Waves "bye-bye."
10. Responds to name.
11. Vocalizes in varied jargon-patterns (10-12 months).

1 year

Motor

1. Walks with one hand held.
2. Stands alone (or with support).
3. Secures small object with good pincer grasp.
4. Pivots in sitting position.
5. Grasps two cubes in one hand.

Language

6. Uses "mama" or "dada" with specific meaning.
7. "Talks" to toys and people, using fairly long verbal patterns.
8. Has vocabulary of two words besides "mama" and "dada."
9. Babbles to self when alone.
10. Obeys simple requests, such as: "Give me the cup."
11. Reacts to music.

15 months

Motor

1. Stands alone.
2. Creeps upstairs.
3. Kneels on floor or chair.
4. Gets off floor and walks alone with good balance.
5. Bends over to pick up toy without holding on to furniture.

Language

6. May speak four to six words (15-18 months).
7. Uses jargon.
8. Indicates wants by vocalizing.
9. Knows own name.

Personal-social-adaptive—cont'd

15. Bites and chews toys.
16. Pats mirror image.
17. Bangs spoon on table.
18. Manipulates paper or string.
19. Secures ring by pulling on the string.
20. Feeds self crackers.

Personal-social-adaptive

12. Plays "pat-a-cake."
13. Picks up pellet with finger and thumb.
14. Bangs toys together.
15. Extends toy to a person.
16. Holds own bottle.
17. Removes cube from cup.
18. Drops one cube to get another.
19. Uses handle to lift cup.
20. Initially shy with strangers.

Personal-social-adaptive

12. Cooperates with dressing.
13. Plays with cup, spoon, saucer.
14. Points with index finger.
15. Pokes finger (into stethoscope) to explore.
16. Releases toy into your hand.
17. Tries to take cube out of box.
18. Unwraps a cube.
19. Holds cup to drink.
20. Holds crayon.
21. Tries to imitate scribble.
22. Imitates beating two cubes together.
23. Gives affection.

Language—cont'd

10. Enjoys rhymes or jingles.

Personal-social-adaptive

11. Tilts cup to drink.
12. Uses spoon but spills.
13. Builds tower of two cubes.
14. Drops cubes into cup.
15. Helps turn page in book, pats picture.
16. Shows or offers toy.
17. Helps pull off clothes.
18. Puts pellet into bottle without demonstration.
19. Opens lid of box.
20. Likes to push wheeled toys.

Continued.

Table 4-1. Child development from 1 month to 5 years—cont'd

18 months

Motor

1. Runs (stiffly).
2. Walks upstairs—one hand held.
3. Walks backwards.
4. Climbs into chair.
5. Hurls ball.

Language

6. May say six to 10 words (18-21 months).
7. Points to at least one body part.
8. Can say "hello" and "thank you."
9. Carries out two directions (one at a time), for instance: "Get ball from table."—"Give ball to mother."
10. Identifies two objects by pointing (or picking up) such as: cup, spoon, dog, car, chair.

Personal-social-adaptive

11. Turns pages.
12. Builds tower of three to four cubes.
13. Puts 10 cubes into cup.
14. Carries or hugs a doll.
15. Takes off shoes and socks.
16. Pulls string toy.
17. Scribbles spontaneously.
18. Dumps raisin from bottle after demonstration.
19. Uses spoon with little spilling.

21 months

Motor

1. Runs well.
2. Walks downstairs—one hand held.
3. Walks upstairs alone or holding on to rail.
4. Kicks large ball (when demonstrated).

Language

5. May speak 15-20 words (21-24 months).
6. May combine two to three words.
7. Asks for food, drink.
8. Echoes two or more words.
9. Takes three directions (one at a time), for instance: "Take ball from table." "Give ball to Mommy."—"Put ball on floor."
10. Points to three or more body parts.

Personal-social-adaptive

11. Builds tower of five to six cubes.
12. Folds paper once when shown.
13. Helps with simple household tasks (21-24 months).
14. Removes some clothing purposefully (besides hat or socks).
15. Pulls person to show something.

2 years

Motor

1. Runs without falling.
2. Walks up and down stairs.
3. Kicks large ball (without demonstration).
4. Throws ball overhand.
5. Claps hands.
6. Opens door.
7. Turns pages in book, singly.

Language

8. Says simple phrases.
9. Says at least one sentence or phrase of four or more syllables.
10. Can repeat four to five syllables.
11. May reproduce about 5-6 consonant sounds. (Typically: m-p-b-h-w).

Language—cont'd

12. Points to four parts of body on command.
13. Asks for things at table by name.
14. Refers to self by name.
15. May use personal pronouns, such as: I-me-you (2-2½ years).

Personal-social-adaptive

16. Builds five to seven cube tower.
17. May cut with scissors.
18. Spontaneously dumps raisin from bottle (without demonstration).
19. Throws ball into box.
20. Imitates drawing vertical line from demonstration.
21. Parallel play predominant.

2½ years

Motor

1. Jumps in place with both feet.
2. Tries standing on one foot (may not be successful).
3. Holds crayon by fingers.
4. Imitates walking on tiptoe.

Language

5. Refers to self by pronoun (rather than name).
6. Names common objects when asked (key, penny, shoe, box, book).
7. Repeats two digits (one of three trials).
8. Answers simple questions, such as: "What is this?"—"What does the kitty say?"

Table 4-1. Child development from 1 month to 5 years—cont'd

2½ years—cont'd

Personal-social-adaptive

9. Builds tower of eight cubes.
10. Pushes toy with good steering.
11. Helps put things away.
12. Can carry breakable objects.
13. Puts on clothing.
14. Washes and dries hands.

3 years

Motor

1. Stands on one foot for at least one second.
2. Jumps from bottom stair.
3. Alternates feet going upstairs.
4. Pours from a pitcher.
5. Can undo two buttons.
6. Pedals a tricycle.

Language

7. Repeats six syllables, for instance: "I have a little dog."
8. Names three or more objects in a picture.
9. Gives sex. ("Are you a boy or a girl?")
10. Gives full name.
11. Repeats three digits (one of three trials).
12. Knows a few rhymes.
13. Gives appropriate answers to: "What: swims-flies-shoots-boils-bites-melts?"
14. Uses plurals.
15. Knows at least one color.
16. Can reply to questions in at least three word sentences.
17. May have vocabulary of 750 to 1,000 words (3-3½ years).

4 years

Motor

1. Stands on one foot for at least five seconds (two of three trials).
2. Hops at least twice on one foot.
3. Can walk heel-to-toe for four or more steps (with heel one inch or less in front of toe).
4. Can button coat or dress; may lace shoes.

Language

5. Repeats ten-word sentences without errors.
6. Counts three objects, pointing correctly.
7. Repeats three to four digits (4-5 years).
8. Comprehends: "What do you do if: you are hungry, sleepy, cold?"
9. Spontaneous sentences, four to five words long.
10. Likes to ask questions.
11. Understands prepositions, such as: on-under-behind, etc. ("Put the block *on* the table.")
12. Can point to three out of four colors (red, blue, green, yellow).
13. Speech is now an effective communicative tool.

Personal-social-adaptive–cont'd

15. Eats with fork.
16. Imitates drawing a horizontal line from demonstration.
17. May imitate drawing a circle from demonstration.

Personal-social-adaptive

18. Understands taking turns.
19. Copies a circle (from model, without demonstration).
20. Builds three-block pyramid (⌂).
21. Dresses with supervision.
22. Puts 10 pellets into bottle in 30 seconds.
23. Separates easily from mother.
24. Feeds self well.
25. Plays interactive games, such as "tag."

Personal-social-adaptive

14. Copies cross (+) without demonstration.
15. Imitates oblique cross (×).
16. Draws a man with four parts.
17. Cooperates with other children in play.
18. Dresses and undresses self (mostly without supervision).
19. Brushes teeth, washes face.
20. Compares lines: "Which is longer?"
21. Folds paper two to three times.
22. Can select heavier from lighter object.
23. Cares for self at toilet.

Continued.

Table 4-1. Child development from 1 month to 5 years—cont'd

5 years

Motor

1. Balances on one foot for eight to ten seconds.
2. Skips, using feet alternately.
3. May be able to tie a knot.
4. Catches bounced ball with hands (not arms) in two of three trials.

Language

5. Knows age ("How old are you?").
6. Performs three tasks (with one command), for instance: "Put pen on table—close door—bring me the ball."
7. Knows four colors.
8. Defines use for: fork-horse-key-pencil, etc.
9. Identifies by name: nickel-dime-penny.
10. Asks meaning of words.
11. Asks many "why" questions.
12. Relatively few speech errors remain—90% of consonant sounds are made correctly.
13. Counts number of fingers correctly.
14. Counts by rote to 10.
15. Comments on pictures (descriptions and interpretations).

Personal-social-adaptive

16. Copies a square.
17. Copies oblique cross (×) without demonstration.
18. May print a few letters (5-5½ years).
19. Draws man with at least six identifiable parts.
20. Builds a six-block pyramid from demonstration.
21. Transports things in a wagon.
22. Plays with coloring set, construction toys, puzzles.
23. Participates well in group play.

child's current level of development; this information can then be included in the description of the child's present health.

Provence (1968a) mentions two questions that are helpful for the examiner to keep in mind when making judgments about the development of a child: (1) What has the child achieved in the various sectors of development that one can observe, describe, or measure? (2) How does the child make use of the skills and functions available to him? The first question requires the practitioner to find out about the developmental progress of the infant or child from helplessness at birth to his current level of development. The second question requires the practitioner to find out about the adaptation the child is making to his life. The second question is usually more difficult to answer, because it is not based on standardized developmental schedules. However, information about the child's adaptation can be obtained by asking the parent to describe the child. This description can be broadened by asking whether the child is quiet or active, happy or sad, and mischievous or very good.

Ronald Illingworth (1975) stresses that purely objective tests result in obtaining information about scorable items in the area of sensorimotor skills and that it is of great importance to also determine the child's alertness, responsiveness, and interest in surroundings, which cannot be scored.

Arnold Gessell calls these latter behaviors "insurance factors." If the child demonstrates these behaviors but has delays in some of the sensorimotor behaviors, an opinion should be reserved and the child followed over a longer period of time before a judgment is made about the developmental skills of the child.

If there are questions or concerns about a child's development that are identified as the result of the routine appraisal, it would be well to set aside time so that a complete developmental assessment could be done that would include a careful review of the history of the developmental milestones and an appraisal of the child's current level of function. It would be appropriate to use one of the more structured screening tests.

■ **Developmental screening tests**

There are several screening tests that the practitioner may find useful in carrying out the developmental assessment of a child.

The Washington Guide to Promoting Development in the Young Child (outlined by Barnard and Powell) was designed for assessing the development of the child from birth to 5 years; it asists the practitioner in determining the child's level of function and in providing parental counseling in terms of anticipatory guidance and suggestions for activities to promote the child's development.

The Denver Developmental Screening Test is widely used for children up to 6 years of age. Items were selected from 12 developmental and preschool intelligence tests on the basis of (1) ease of administration and interpretation and (2) a relatively short time span from the point at which a few children could perform an item to the point at which most children could perform the item.

The Developmental Screening Inventory, developed by Knoblock and Pasamanick, screens children from 1 month to 18 months. It can be used for serial observations over a period of time for purposes of monitoring the development of a normal child or for continued observation of the child who may have a developmental problem.

In *Standards of Child Health Care,* The American Academy of Pediatrics has adapted a communication chart from an unpublished report of a Special Ad Hoc Committee of the Children's Bureau, 1965; this chart is for assessing the normal developmental expectancies regarding responses to acoustic stimuli, the learning of language, and speech output for children from birth to 3 years.

THE ADULT

Development is an ongoing life process occurring continually throughout the life span. Although in the past much attention on the assessment of developmental processes has focused on the child, the phenomenon of human development does not end with adolescence. In adulthood, development is less along the lines of the rapid acquisition of physical and cognitive skills of childhood and adolescence; rather, it is more along the lines of growth in relationships and responsibilities, in coping with the situational demands and changes that life imparts, and in acquiring experience and, hopefully, some quantity of wisdom in relation to all of these. Changing, growing, and learning are not the perogatives only of youth; at all times in one's life, one is dealing with some task of development.

Assessment of the developmental level, including the appropriateness of tasks pursued and the handling of maturational and situational crises, is as important in whole-person assessment as is the physical examination, though the former may not necessarily be performed as quickly or at the same visit as the latter. In addition to providing a more complete picture and understanding of the client, developmental assessment provides the health care provider with data for appropriate counseling and preparatory guidance of the client; the health care provider's goal is to assist the client in contemplating his current developmental status and those developments and changes that are likely to be ahead. This can enhance the development of a functional and versatile attitude toward a life perspective that makes constructive use of past and present experiences in creative preparation for the near and distant future.

Furthermore, as the life expectancy increases for a greater portion of the population and as a larger proportion of the total population is composed of persons in their adult years, it will become increasingly important to understand and deal with the experiences of the adult years. An understanding of human patterns and potentials is also important because changes in technology affecting the work world will likely yield greater amounts of time for persons in the adult years to spend on self and social development.

There are several vantage points from which to assess human development. The types of tools described earlier in this chapter for the developmental assessment of children are not generally available or in use for adults. Also, it is noteworthy that the developmental assessment of adult individuals is a process covering tremendous diversity. As individuals age, each becomes increasingly more like himself and less like any other. Each person is a reflection of all he has done with his days and years, and of all that his days and years have done to him. In this section, Erikson's delineation of adult developmental stages and a number of the now commonly unacknowledged tasks of adulthood are discussed. Also, some of the maturational and situational crises involved in task accomplishment during late adulthood are pursued.

■ Erikson's stages of ego development

Erikson's formulations on the stages of ego development provide a useful organizing principle around which to examine adult development; of his eight stages of ego development, three relate to the adult experience.

In young adulthood, the development of affiliation or intimacy expressed as mutuality with a loved partner of the opposite sex with whom one is willing and able to regulate the cycles of work, procreation, and recreation is a central task. This involves the capacity to commit oneself "to concrete affiliations and partnerships and to develop the ethical strength to abide by such commitments, even though they may call for significant sacrifices and compromises" (Erickson, 1963, p. 263). Isolation threatens this experience.

In middle adulthood, the development of a sense of generativity expressed through care and concern in establishing and guiding the following generation occurs. Stagnation endangers this experience.

In late adulthood, there is the development of ego integrity, a ripening of what has occurred during a lifetime. This involves (1) the sense that one "has taken care of things and people and has adapted himself to the triumphs and disappointments adherent to being" (Erikson, 1963, p. 268) and (2) a basic acceptance of one's life as appropriate and meaningful. A sense of despair including the fear of death threatens this level of ego development.

Although these stages may predominate during one phase of the life span, the issues of each may also be present at earlier and at later periods in life. Although the stages are presented as separate entries, they may be mutually existent; and one stage need not necessarily be completely and finally resolved before the next one is experienced to some extent.

■ Developmental tasks of adulthood

The three stages of early, middle, and late adulthood also provide a perspective for looking at a series of tasks. According to Robert Havighurst, developmental tasks are defined as follows: The tasks the individual must learn—the developmental tasks of life—are those things that constitute healthy and satisfactory growth in our society. They are the things a person must learn if he is to be judged and to judge himself as a reasonably happy and successful person. A developmental task is a task that arises at or about a certain period in the life of the individual, successful achievement of which leads to his happiness and to success with later tasks, whereas failure leads to unhappiness in the individual, disapproval by society, and difficulty with later tasks (Havighurst, 1952, p. 2).

Havighurst describes the following tasks for the three stages of adulthood:

A. Early adulthood (ages 18-30)
1. Selecting a mate
2. Learning to live with a marriage partner
3. Starting a family
4. Rearing children
5. Managing a home
6. Getting started in an occupation
7. Taking on civic responsibility
8. Finding a congenial social group
B. Middle age (ages 30-55)
1. Achieving adult civic and social responsibility
2. Establishing and maintaining an economic standard of living
3. Assisting teenage children to become responsible and happy adults
4. Developing adult leisure-time activities
5. Relating to one's spouse as a person
6. Accepting and adjusting to the physiological changes of middle age
7. Adjusting to aging parents
C. Later maturity (ages 55 and over)
1. Adjusting to decreasing physical strength and health
2. Adjusting to retirement and reduced income
3. Adjusting to the death of one's spouse
4. Establishing an explicit affiliation with one's age group
5. Meeting civic and social obligations

Not every individual can or desires to fulfill all tasks presented for each age category; for example, those who do not marry will not become involved in the marital or parental roles but will nevertheless develop home management, occupational, civic, and social roles.

The student of health assessment may use a categorization such as this to investigate the type and appropriateness of tasks that a client is currently pursuing. In addition to discovering which tasks are salient, the student should assess the individual's reactions to, feelings about, and coping mechanisms involved in the realization of the tasks or the barriers to their accomplishment. For the purpose of example, several tasks of adulthood and potential crisis and resolutions are discussed.

At each level there is an exchange of energy between the individual and his social system. During the years of early adulthood, much time and energy is expended on the beginning of long-term involvements, that is, the process of beginning a family, a work-occupational role, social and civic interactions, and leisure-time activities. The individual is faced with a need to develop in response to these new and growing roles in several areas.

During the middle years, some of the roles continue to develop and expand whereas others begin to diminish in their intensity and energy demands. An example of the latter is the completion of some of the child-rearing tasks. As the children reach first adolescence and then early adulthood and leave the family, beginning their own adult development, the parents are in the position, once again, of relating more directly with each other. For many, this is an opportunity for stimulating rediscovery of a partner, since the demands of offspring on a daily or hourly basis are no longer present. It can also be a time of stress if the parents have, in the intervening years, expended most of their available energy on child rearing and the struggle for economic security and stability rather than on continuing to develop their relationship with one another. During these middle years, individuals also may develop roles of status in their work or civic area.

The years of late adulthood are accompanied by a number of difficult developmental tasks. Adapting to advancing age is, however "an active, energy requiring process, not merely the passive submission to the passage of time" (Pfeiffer, 1973, p. 2). The multiple aspects of the aging process affect people differently at various times in their lives, and there are those who seem always to have been old and those who seem to stay young in heart, attitude, and appearance. Although much of the awareness of aging is concerned with multiple losses—of job, income, friends, spouse, and so on—it should not be forgotten that the later years may also be characterized by gains in experience, opportunities for personal growth, and opportunities to focus on things of greatest interest to the individual, leading to a seasoned, historical perspective and a sort of active wisdom.

Whereas some tasks of the later years involve the continuation of earlier-developed activities and processes, others necessitate the relinquishment of certain of these long-standing roles and activities. Major changes may occur in the areas of work, income, health, and social relationships. The changes may be sudden, as in the area of retirement, or subtle and gradually accruing, as in the area of health.

Changes in the physical organism occur as a result of progressive changes in body structure and function. There may be degrees of loss in the sensory organs and slowing of the neuromuscular system. Although chronic disease does not necessarily accompany aging, it is not uncommonly present to some degrees with mild to severe discomfort or disability.

In addition to these internal changes, other changes occur in relation to the position of the individual as a member of a family and community. Retirement from work often results in a sense of uselessness and purposelessness to the person who has not prepared for retirement by developing other interests and activities. This causes a stress on the internal psychological and physiological systems and also on the interpersonal relationships of the individual. Loss of a job is usually associated with a reduced income necessitating changes in certain areas of the life-style. Retirement may also result in a considerable increase in uncommitted time. Adjusting to the use of that time in productive and satisfying ways is important. At this time in human history, couples are likely to have a number of years together after their children have left home to establish their own life-styles. Because the life expectancy is longer for women than for men, there is a high likelihood that a woman's last years will be spent in widowhood. For either sex, adjustment to being alone and often lonely and to taking on responsibilities previously shared requires considerable energy. For persons who have remained single, the death of a close friend or family member with whom they have lived or shared many experiences can have similar effects.

As an individual grows older, the process of a life review, of looking back over the years and accepting the events that occurred and the responses that were made as acceptable, appropriate, and the best that could have been done within the circumstances is an important activity. This process of review may be repeated over and over during many periods of reminiscence and conversation in order to arrive at a personal understanding and acceptance of all that has transpired.

Another developmental task is that of coming to terms with the reality of one's own death. Preparation for death really evolves over many years as part of an attitude toward life and its meaning; yet in the later years, as the propinquity of death is increased, coping with it takes on a greater personal meaning.

In summary, individuals who arrive near the latter end of life's continuum must learn to find personal fulfillment and satisfaction in new modes of activity and leisure rather than in the activities of the working world; they must review life, its meanings and its satisfactions; they must adapt to and cope with changing, and often diminishing, body functions; and while continuing to live in the present, they must look both backward and forward, accepting the passing of the days and the inevitable fact of death.

Individuals approach the developmental tasks of adulthood in a great variety of ways and move through them with varying satisfaction. Some adjust satisfactorily to the tasks, demands, and changes of adulthood with energy and vitality. A level of satisfaction does not necessarily depend on a high degree of activity, (though maintenance of numerous activities often does provide continuing satisfaction) but may also be derived from a gradual withdrawal from some of one's previous activities. Other adults find less satisfaction in life and its tasks because of difficulties in the physical or emotional area that prevent them from making the adaptations they perceive as optimal. Some attempt to deny the changing needs and tasks of the years by clinging to earlier patterns and life-styles, whereas others adapt more readily to changes within and around themselves.

The changes that occur throughout life may become crises if adequate coping mechanisms are frustrated or unavailable. Some assessment of an individual's adjustments to developmental tasks can be made by examining crises incidents. By inquiring into crises recently or currently faced, the degree of distress related to them, and alternative ways of dealing with them, one can gain appreciation for the individual's style of dealing with adversity. All individuals are from time to time faced with confusion, uncertainty, depression, hopelessness, frustration, and anger. Learning to live through crises and to cope with the difficult feelings they often engender is in itself another task of human development.

The student of health assessment should be sensitive to inquiries and observations about the developmental tasks of clients throughout the life span. The growth and development of the elderly client can be as interesting as that of the infant, though it is of a very different nature. Every individual, whether near the beginning, in the middle, or approaching the end of life is marked by potential, growth patterns, and limitations. Each carries within and about himself a growing sum of skills and experiences and a sense of success or failure, of satisfaction or some lack thereof. The variability and complexity of human development provides a wealth of client and human understanding if it is sought.

BIBLIOGRAPHY

Barnard, K. E., and Powell, L.: Teaching the mentally retarded child; a family care approach, St. Louis, 1972, The C. V. Mosby Co.

Bier, W. C.: Aging; its challenge to the individual and to society, New York, 1974, Fordham University Press.

Birchenall, J., and Streight, M. E.: Care of the older adult, Philadelphia, 1973, J. B. Lippincott Co.

Brantl, V. M., and Brown, M. L., editors: Readings in gerontology, St. Louis, 1973, The C. V. Mosby Co.

Burnside, E. M., editor: Nursing and the aged, New York, 1976, McGraw-Hill Book Co.

Busse, E. W., and Pfeiffer, E., editors: Behavior and adaptation in late life, Boston, 1969, Little, Brown and Co.

Butler, R. N., and Lewis, M. I.: Aging and mental health; positive psychosocial approaches, St. Louis, 1973, The C. V. Mosby Co.

Cook, R. E., editor: The biological bases of clinical pediatrics, New York, 1968, McGraw-Hill Book Co.

DeAngelis, C.: Basic pediatrics for the primary care providers, Boston, 1976, Little, Brown and Co.

Erickson, M. L.: Assessment and management of developmental changes in children, St. Louis, 1976, The C. V. Mosby Co.

Erikson, E. H.: Childhood and society, ed. 2, New York, 1963, W. W. Norton & Co., Inc.

Frankenburg, W. K., and Dobbs, J. B.: The Denver Developmental Screening Test, J. Pediatr. 71(2): 1967.

Gesell, A., and Amatruda, C.: Developmental diagnosis, ed. 2, New York, 1947, Paul B. Hoeber, Inc.

Green, M., and Haggerty, R. J., editors: Ambulatory pediatrics, Philadelphia, 1968, W. B. Saunders Co.

Havighurst, R.: Developmental task and education, New York, 1952, David McKay Co., Inc.

Havighurst, R.: Human development and education, St. Louis, 1953, Warren H. Green, Inc.

Haynes, U.: A developmental approach to casefinding with special reference to cerebral palsy, mental retardation and related disorders, 1969, Washington, D.C., U.S. Department of Health, Education, and Welfare, Bureau of Community Health Serivce.

Illingworth, R. S.: The normal child, ed. 5, Baltimore, 1972, The Williams & Wilkins Co.

Illingworth, R. S.: The development of the infant and young child, normal and abnormal, ed. 6, Edinburgh, 1975, Churchill Livingstone.

Knoblock, H., and Pasamanick, B.: Predicting intellectual potential in infancy, Am. J. Dis. Child. 43: 106, 1963.

Neugarten, B. L., and others: Personality in middle and late life, New York, 1964, Atherton Press.

Pfeiffer, E.: Successful aging; a conference report, Durham, N.C., 1973, Duke University Press.

Provence, S.: Developmental assessment. In Green, M., and Haggerty, R. J., editors: Ambulatory pediatrics, Philadelphia, 1968, W. B. Saunders Co. (a)

Provence, S.: Developmental history. In Cooke, R., editor: Biological basis of pediatric practice, New York, 1968, McGraw-Hill Book Co. (b)

Riley, M. W., and Foner, A.: Aging and society, vol. 1, An inventory of research findings, New York, 1968, Russel Sage Foundation.

Riley, M. W., Johnson, M., and Foner, A.: Aging and society, vol. 3, A sociology of age stratification, New York, 1972, Russell Sage Foundation.

Riley, M. W., Riley, J. W., and Johnson, M.: Aging and society, vol. 2, Aging and the professions, New York, 1969, Russell Sage Foundation.

Smart, M. S., and Smart, R. C.: Children; development and relationships, ed. 2, New York, 1972, MacMillan, Inc.

Spencer, M. G., and Dorr, C. J., editors: Understanding aging; a multidisciplinary approach, New York, 1975, Appleton-Century-Crofts.

Standards of child health care, ed. 2, Evanston, Ill., 1972, American Academy of Pediatrics.

Williams, R. H., and Wirths, C. G.: Lives through the years, New York, 1965, Atherton Press.

Working with older people; a guide to practice, U.S. Department of Health, Education, and Welfare, Pub. No. HSM 72-6005, vols. 1-4, 1969-1972; vol. 1, The practitioner and the elderly; vol. 2, Biological, psychological and sociological aspects of aging; vol. 3, The aging person—needs and services; vol. 4, Clinical aspects of aging.

5 Nutritional assessment

Savitri Kamath, Ph.D.

Although the widespread occurrence of malnutrition has been recognized in developing countries for more than a quarter of a century, its occurrence in the "affluent" United States has been publicized only recently. Following the publication of *Hunger U.S.A.* by the Citizens Board of Inquiry into Hunger and Malnutrition in 1968 and the CBS television program *Hunger in America,* there was a great deal of concern about the nutritional problems in this country. Senate Hearings on Nutrition and Human Needs from 1968 to 1974 and the White House Conference on Food, Nutrition, and Health in 1969 are the outcome of this revelation. Many nutrition intervention programs have been planned and implemented at the national and local levels to combat hunger and malnutrition in the United States. Examples of such programs are the School Lunch Program, The Special Milk Program, the School Breakfast Program, and the Commodity Distribution Program.

How were the needs for these programs identified? How will the efficacy of these programs be evaluated? The best way is to assess the nutritional status of the population periodically, before and following the implementation. A recent comprehensive attempt to assess the nutritional status of the American people resulted in the National Nutrition Survey. A detailed discussion of the results of this survey is found in the Health, Education, and Welfare (HEW) publication *Ten-State Survey, 1968-1970.* The results do indicate the existence of severe primary nutritional disorders, such as kwashiorkor; however, the incidence is very, very low when compared to that of developing countries. But more rampant are the subclinical deficiencies of certain nutrients such as iron and vitamin A, as judged by biochemical parameters. How these chronic sub-

clinical deficiencies affect one's health in the long run is not known at this time. It is important to control the deficiency at early stages; otherwise, severe deficiency may occur in a situation of stress, such as surgery or infection. Therefore, nutritionists are concerned with developing sensitive techniques to identify marginal deficiencies so that preventive measures can be undertaken to avoid further aggravation of the conditions.

A great deal of concern has recently been expressed regarding evidences of malnutrition in hospitalized clients. Several concerned researchers have brought to attention the occurrence of poor nutritional care of hospitalized clients and the resulting malnutrition in this population. This is particularly unnecessary, since many products and techniques are available through which nutritional support can be given to clients who are unable, for a variety of reasons, to consume adequate amounts of the usual foods served. Some of these nutritional problems are of a secondary nature, such as maldigestion or malabsorption; increased requirements, as in fever or infection; or inadequate intake due to trauma or alcoholism. As a result, adult kwashiorkorlike or marasmuslike syndromes develop.

Currently, drug-induced malnutrition is another cause of concern. Subacute deficiencies of nutrients as a result of drug interference in the bioavailability of the nutrient to the cell are sometimes encountered in clients receiving prolonged drug therapy.

In consideration of these factors, it would appear very desirable to make every health professional aware of the existing and potential nutritional problems in their communities and institutions. Every individual in this country has a right to receive adequate health care, and an integral part of health care is nutritional care.

Nutritional care is a problem-solving process involving assessment before implementation of the care plan and during the period that the plan is carried out. So that nutritional care may be provided to each individual, as many health professionals as possible should be trained to evaluate the nutritional status of individuals or populations. This assessment is one of the techniques necessary to the implementation of the preventive aspects of health care.

Nutritional status may be defined as the state of health enjoyed as a result of nutrition. The World Health Organization (WHO) has defined health as a state of "complete physical, mental and social well being and not merely the absence of disease or infirmity."

Nutritional assessment aids in (1) the identification of malnutrition in an individual or in a population, of current nutritionally high-risk groups in the community, and of factors related to the cause of malnutrition; (2) providing information on resources available in planning efforts to overcome malnutrition; and (3) evaluating the efficacy of the nutritional care provided to the individual or the efficacy of the nutritional programs implemented in the community.

DEVELOPMENT AND NATURE OF MALNUTRITION

Malnutrition results from faulty or imperfect nutrition. At its fundamental level, it represents an inadequate supply of nutrients to the cell. A series of factors may be responsible for cellular malnutrition. Psychosocial, economic, personal likes and dislikes of foods, and political factors may contribute to inadequate intake of food or nutrients, resulting in *primary malnutrition*. On the other hand, factors such as inadequate digestion, improper absorption, faulty utilization, and increased requirement or excretion of nutrients may lead to decreased bioavailability of the nutrient to the cell, causing *secondary malnutrition*. Fig. 5-1 should be helpful in determining factors related to the bioavailability of nutrients.

Although both primary and secondary malnutrition ultimately result in similar manifestations, the cause needs to be identified in order to treat the condition. For instance, the vitamin A deficiency resulting in individuals due to a lack of intake could be overcome by administering this nutrient through foods or supplements. However, the secondary deficiency of this vitamin ob-

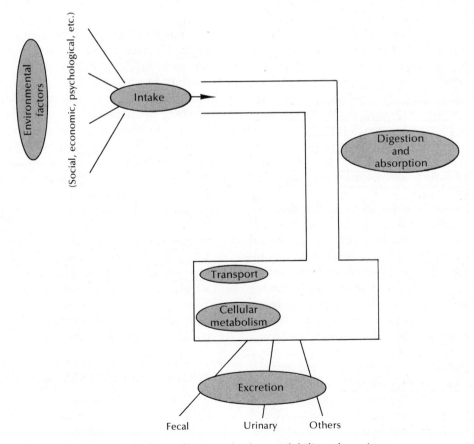

Fig. 5-1. Factors affecting the bioavailability of nutrients.

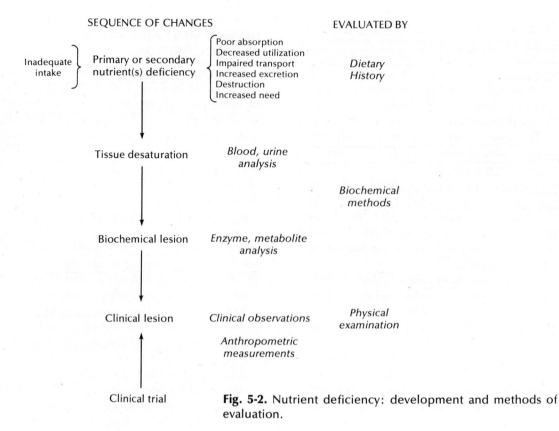

SEQUENCE OF CHANGES

EVALUATED BY

Inadequate intake

Primary or secondary nutrient(s) deficiency

Poor absorption
Decreased utilization
Impaired transport
Increased excretion
Destruction
Increased need

Dietary History

Tissue desaturation

Blood, urine analysis

Biochemical methods

Biochemical lesion

Enzyme, metabolite analysis

Clinical lesion

Clinical observations

Physical examination

Anthropometric measurements

Clinical trial

Fig. 5-2. Nutrient deficiency: development and methods of evaluation.

served in severe protein deficiency can be alleviated only by instituting protein therapy. Malnutrition may be *acute*, that is, the result of temporary adverse conditions that can be rapidly overcome, leaving no long-standing effects. Malnutrition may also be *chronic*, that is, the result of adverse conditions continued without relief over a period of time. Chronic malnutrition may lead to irreparable losses, such as blindness and growth retardation, and occasionally may even lead to death.

Fig. 5-2 describes the steps in the development of a nutrient deficiency. As to how fast and to what degree the deficiency of a nutrient would proceed is determined by the level of dietary intake and by the previous nutritional status, reflecting the extent of body stores and the body's ability to adapt to lower levels of the nutrient intake. Irrespective of the rate of progression, the general pattern in which the disease develops is similar to the one shown.

In the gradual development of a nutrient deficiency, tissue reserves are first mobilized in an effort to maintain the necessary supply of the nutrient to the cells. This is reflected in a reduced concentration of the nutrient in the blood or tissues as well as in decreased urinary excretion of

the nutrient. As the deficiency progresses, the tissue reserves are depleted, resulting in an inadequate supply of the nutrient to the cell. This leads to biochemical lesions such as changes in enzymes, coenzymes, and metabolites, the levels of which would be altered in the blood and in the tissues. Further progression of the deficiency is manifested in the anatomical lesions and clinical symptoms detectable in a thorough physical examination by an alert practitioner. Clinical manifestation of vitamin deficiencies such as beriberi, pellagra, and scurvy are easily recognized.

In summary, it is possible to identify the development of a nutrient deficiency at the intake level, at the blood and tissue level, and during a physical examination. This is the principle on which the major methods of nutritional assessment, namely food intake studies, biochemical parameters, anthropometric measurements, and clinical examinations, are based.

PROCEDURES FOR ASSESSMENT

Whether the assessment is of a single individual or of a group of people in a population, the procedures are basically the same. However, when individual cases are considered, a more thorough nutritional assessment can be made, including an accurate nutritional history and sophisticated laboratory studies. When population groups are assessed, general methods, simple and fast, perhaps with less accuracy and precision, may have to be resorted to because of limitations of time, personnel, and facilities.

The nutritional profile of a community can be determined from various sources, such as food balance sheets, vital statistics, and agricultural data. Although food balance sheets provide information on the per capita availability of food and nutrients to the population, it does not consider individual food consumption and the variation in intakes due to age, sex, socioeconomic condition, personal preference, or other factors affecting the food intake. Likewise, vital statistics may be helpful in the identification of morbidity and mortality but may not be reliable in terms of tracing the mortality and morbidity to the nutritional status.

Four major methods are important in the assessment of nutritional status:

1. Dietary surveys
2. Clinical appraisal
3. Anthropometry
4. Biochemical appraisal

In all these methods, data obtained from various techniques have to be evaluated in relation to "norms" or standard guidelines. Uses and limitations of individual guidelines are discussed under each method. However, one point worth stressing is that the norms used here are statistical norms obtained from a sample of the "healthy" population. Whether these are identical with the biological norms compatible with good health is a matter of debate.

■ Dietary surveys

Dietary surveys, or food intake studies, deal with collecting information on the dietary practices of people, including intakes of specific foods or nutrients over a known period of time. Populations subsisting on marginal intakes may not show physical signs of deficiency, or lesions. For these "subclinical" states, food intake studies have advantages since biochemical methods are extensive in comparison. In addition, this method serves as a check on the validity of the biochemical and clinical observations and vice versa.

Dietary surveys, if carried out appropriately, provide information on (1) the food or nutrient intake of the individual or population group, (2) the nutritional practices of the individual or population group, (3) ration allowances in emergency situations, (4) menu preparation and food procurement, and (5) the nutritional quality of foods available and of those foods actually consumed.

In communities, dietary surveys also help in identifying resources that can be utilized in programs for improving the nutritional status of the population. Information gathered is also applied when plans are developed for modifying existing economic, agricultural, and food management policies and programs.

It must be remembered that dietary surveys yield information of the situation during a limited time, whereas much of the clinical and biochemical evidence reflects the long-term nutrition of the individual. A recently improved diet would not immediately relieve the biochemical and clinical lesions; thus, a discrepancy between dietary and other findings can be expected and explained.

Dietary surveys are carried out in a number of ways. Each has merits and limitations. The method of choice depends on several factors, such as the size of the sample; the background of the individual or population group surveyed; the availability of personnel; and the provisions for data collection, analysis, and interpretation.

Two types of food intake studies are mainly in vogue: the family or group method, and the individual food intake method.

Family or group method. The family or group method is useful in obtaining information on the intake of a homogenous population, such as persons in the same institution or in a family sharing a common kitchen. Common methods of gathering information include the food record method and the food list method. In both methods, full cooperation from the individual in charge of the food service is essential. One of the drawbacks is in the need for estimating the food wastage occurring during the period of the study. Approximately 10% of the energy value of the diet has been estimated as this loss, though it varies from study to study.

Food record method. The food record or inventory method consists of keeping a record of all the foods in the kitchen at the beginning of the survey, of all foods obtained during the period of the survey (2 to 4 weeks), and of all the foods remaining at the end of the survey. Food waste occurring during the study and foods eaten away from home also are recorded. From these lists, amounts of foods consumed over the period are determined.

Food list method. In the food list method, an estimate of the quantities of foods used during a given period of time is obtained through an interview with the person responsible for the food service.

Individual food intake method. Individual food intake studies generally consider both qualitative and quantitative aspects. Three approaches have usually been in practice. These include the food intake record, the 24-hour recall method, and the dietary history method.

Food intake record. Food intake at each of the meals is recorded concurrently over a known period of time by means of weights, household measures, or estimates of quantities of specific foods. As to how many days this survey should last and which of the weekdays is to be included are debatable points. In view of the fact that the day-to-day diet varies in this country, a 1-day intake is not representative of the usual intake. It is desirable to include more than 1 day. The longer the duration, the better the reliability; however, since subjects tend to lose interest in keeping records after a while, it is advantageous to limit the record keeping to short periods.

A 3-day food intake record appears to be quite satisfactory, both in terms of the subject's cooperation and in terms of obtaining reliable information. Since a person's eating pattern tends to change during the weekend, inclusion of a weekend day may be advocated. Some researchers have found that inclusion of a weekend day along with 3 weekdays provides a satisfactory record.

Weighed-food records are a modified version of the food intake method and involve weighing all the foods consumed by the subject. The subject may be trained to weigh the foods accurately, or an investigator may be assigned to do this. This version is expensive and is mainly used in metabolic research studies.

In general, the food intake record has the disadvantage of making the subject conscious of his eating pattern, and this consciousness might make him modify his intake. When the subject is asked to estimate his intake, discrepancies related to the concept of serving size might also occur.

Twenty-four hour recall method. The 24-hour recall method is very practical and useful in nutrition clinics. Intake of specific foods is recalled in terms of either estimates or quantities determined by means of weights or household measures. From the memory point of view, the best recall period appears to be the immediate past 24 hours. A trained interviewer, generally a dietitian, usually carries out this method. To improve the reliability of the informant's memory, cross-check methods have been devised. The same questions are asked in different ways at different times in the interview. However, this procedure is time consuming and expensive and may be used only when the interviewer's time is not a limiting factor.

The accuracy of this method will vary. Women appear to be more accurate than men, and younger people more than elderly people, in giving data. Intake determined by the 24-hour method tends to be higher than that reported in a 7-day record. The day-to-day variation in meal pattern and in food intake make the 24-hour recall method not entirely representative of the individual's usual intake. Validity of the data obtained from the recall method has also been questioned. However, for all practical purposes, this method seems to provide sufficient information. It has been shown that for group comparisons, 24-hour recall records on a larger number of people provide better criteria than long-term studies on a limited population.

Dietary history method. The dietary history method yields qualitative information on long-standing food habits. This information is useful in interpreting the biochemical and clinical findings since the latter are indicative of long-standing food habits. The individual is asked to report his current or past intake in terms of frequency of occurrence of food items, changes in meal pattern, methods of food preparation, food likes and dislikes, shopping practices, and any other pertinent information. The history not only reflects the individual's food behavior but also is informative in terms of identifying the cause of nutritional problems. The dietary history also is a check for the validity of the intake reported in the 24-hour recall method. Dietary histories in conjunction with a 24-hour recall enhance the accuracy of the information.

Tactics for eliciting data. Since individuals' food habits are of a very intimate nature, much of the success in eliciting suitable information on food habits depends on the interview. All the tactics described for an effective interview would be helpful here, also. Rapport between the interviewer and the informant is of utmost importance. A positive environment enhances the interaction between the interviewer and the interviewee. On an individual basis, a 30 to 45 minute interview using a suitable questionnaire or nutrition history form will yield useful information. Highly trained personnel can obtain very reliable information if the proper interview techniques are used.

To facilitate communication, the interviewer may use various-size glasses, spoons, bowls, and food models to help the subject estimate food quantities more accurately. Repetition may be necessary to cross-check information. Data on meal patterns over weekends and holidays helps in deciding the days to be included for the food intake study. In addition to likes and dislikes, accessibility and availability of foods, and meal patterns, it may be necessary to gather information on such data as age; sex; occupation; educational background; economic level; cultural heritage; use of dietary supplements, fortified foods, and recipes; cooking facilities; and shopping practices. To overcome the problem of reliability, socioeconomic data can also be used as a check. The combined problems of reliability and accuracy make it apparent that the quality of data obtained is determined by the skill, personality, and sensitivity of the interviewer as well as the honesty of the informant.

Analysis and evaluation of data. Food intake data are evaluated in terms of either the foods in the diets or the nutrients, or both. Tools used for analysis and evaluation include the Basic Four food guide, food composition tables, and chemical analysis.

Basic Four food guide. The Basic Four food guide, though not perfect, serves as a practical tool for rapid analysis and evaluation of diets. The guide was recommended by the United States Department of Agriculture (USDA), based on the essentials of an adequate diet. Table 5-1 describes the Basic Four food guide. The intake of the recommended number of servings of determined amounts from each of the food groups is assumed to provide an optimal diet. A discussion of the uses and limitations of the Basic Four food guide may be found in any textbook on nutrition.

Food composition tables. It is possible to calculate the amount of nutrients provided by a diet from food composition tables if the food is described in the table. The standard food composition table is the *Agriculture Handbook No. 456* (Adams). Data compiled from various laboratories sometimes consider the variety of foods, the method of preparation, and other factors that affect the nutritive value of foods.

With the influx of convenience foods in the market, it is rather hard to analyze diets with these tables, since so many of the foods are not listed. Sometimes it may be necessary to obtain the information from the manufacturer.

A short method of dietary analysis could be resorted to if one uses tables in which similar foods are grouped in broad categories and an average value for the nutrient represents the whole group.

With the limitations of food composition tables, nutritive values should not be considered as accurate figures but as estimates of intakes.

Also, with food composition tables, as well as with the Basic Four food guide, the inaccuracy generated in the description of the food consumed is reflected in the analysis.

Chemical analysis. Chemical analysis of food eaten is sometimes carried out to accurately determine the nutrient intake. This is an elaborate and expensive method and, as such, is employed only for research purposes. The food intake is weighed accurately, excluding the plate waste. A representative sample is then analyzed for nutrients in the laboratory.

Standards for evaluating the nutrient intake. Once the diet is analyzed for nutrients, the next step is to judge the intake for adequacy. Guidelines used for this in the United States are the Recommended Dietary Allowances (RDA) set up by the Food and Nutrition Board of the National Research Council of the National Academy of Sciences. The values for various ages are presented in Table 5-2. The RDA do not represent minimal requirements. Intakes lower than the RDA do not necessarily mean nutrient deficiency. In fact, intakes of two thirds or more of the RDA have been interpreted as adequate in nutritional surveys. An intake of less than this amount is considered suboptimal intake. Because of individual variations in nutrient needs, care should be taken to interpret the individual intake on the basis of the RDA.

Table 5-1. Basic Four food guide (1956)

Food group	Essentials of an adequate diet
Milk and milk products	Children, 3 to 4 cups Adults, 2 or more cups
Fruits and vegetables	4 servings
Green and yellow vegetables	1 serving
Citrus fruits or raw cabbage	1 serving
Potatoes, other vegetables, and fruits	
Meat, poultry, fish, and eggs	2 or more servings
Bread, flour, and cereal (enriched or whole grain)	4 or more servings

Table 5-2. Recommended daily dietary allowances,[a] revised 1974*

Designed for the maintenance of good nutrition of practically all healthy people in the U.S.A.

	Age (years)	Weight		Height		Energy (kcal)[b]	Protein (gm)	Fat-soluble vitamins			
								Vitamin A activity		Vitamin D (IU)	Vitamin E activity[e] (IU)
		kg	lb	cm	in			RE[c]	IU		
Infants	0.0-0.5	6	14	60	24	kg × 117	kg × 2.2	420[d]	1,400	400	4
	0.5-1.0	9	20	71	28	kg × 108	kg × 2.0	400	2,000	400	5
Children	1-3	13	28	86	34	1,300	23	400	2,000	400	7
	4-6	20	44	110	44	1,800	30	500	2,500	400	9
	7-10	30	66	135	54	2,400	36	700	3,300	400	10
Males	11-14	44	97	158	63	2,800	44	1,000	5,000	400	12
	15-18	61	134	172	69	3,000	54	1,000	5,000	400	15
	19-22	67	147	172	69	3,000	54	1,000	5,000	400	15
	23-50	70	154	172	69	2,700	56	1,000	5,000		15
	51+	70	154	172	69	2,400	56	1,000	5,000		15
Females	11-14	44	97	155	62	2,400	44	800	4,000	400	12
	15-18	54	119	162	65	2,100	48	800	4,000	400	12
	19-22	58	128	162	65	2,100	46	800	4,000	400	12
	23-50	58	128	162	65	2,000	46	800	4,000		12
	51+	58	128	162	65	1,800	46	800	4,000		12
Pregnant						+300	+30	1,000	5,000	400	15
Lactating						+500	+20	1,200	6,000	400	15

*From The Food and Nutrition Board, National Academy of Sciences–National Research Council, 1974.

[a]The allowances are intended to provide for individual variations among most normal persons as they live in the United States under usual environmental stresses. Diets should be based on a variety of common foods in order to provide other nutrients for which human requirements have been less well defined

[b]Kilojoules (kJ) = 4.2 × kcal.

[c]Retinol equivalents.

[d]Assumed to be all as retinol in milk during the first 6 months of life. All subsequent intakes are assumed to be half as retinol and half as β-carotene when calculated from international units. As retinol equivalents, three fourths are as retinol and one fourth as β-carotene.

Table 5-3. Suggested guide to interpretation of nutrient intake data*

	Deficient	Low	Acceptable	High
Protein (gm/kg)	<0.5	0.5-0.9	1.0-1.4	>1.5
Iron (mg/day)	<6.0	6-8	9-11	>12
Calcium (gm/day)	<0.3	0.30-0.39	0.4-0.7	>0.8
Vitamin A (IU/day)	<2,000	2,000-3,499	3,500-4,999	>5,000
Ascorbic acid (mg/day)	<10	10-29	30-49	>50
Thiamine (mg/100 kcal)	<0.2	0.20-0.29	0.3-0.4	>0.5
Riboflavin (mg/day)	<0.7	0.7-1.1	1.2-1.4	>1.5
Niacin (mg/day)	<5	5-9	10-14	>15

*From Manual for nutrition surveys, ed. 2, Washington, D.C., 1963, Interdepartmental Committee on Nutrition for National Defense.

Water-soluble vitamins							Minerals					
Ascorbic acid (mg)	Folacin[f] (µg)	Niacin[g] (mg)	Riboflavin (mg)	Thiamin (mg)	Vitamin B$_6$ (mg)	Vitamin B$_{12}$ (µg)	Calcium (mg)	Phosphorus (mg)	Iodine (µg)	Iron (mg)	Magnesium (mg)	Zinc (mg)
35	50	5	0.4	0.3	0.3	0.3	360	240	35	10	60	3
35	50	8	0.6	0.5	0.4	0.3	540	400	45	15	70	5
40	100	9	0.8	0.7	0.6	1.0	800	800	60	15	150	10
40	200	12	1.1	0.9	0.9	1.5	800	800	80	10	200	10
40	300	16	1.2	1.2	1.2	2.0	800	800	110	10	250	10
45	400	18	1.5	1.4	1.6	3.0	1,200	1,200	130	18	350	15
45	400	20	1.8	1.5	2.0	3.0	1,200	1,200	150	18	400	15
45	400	20	1.8	1.5	2.0	3.0	800	800	140	10	350	15
45	400	18	1.6	1.4	2.0	3.0	800	800	130	10	350	15
45	400	16	1.5	1.2	2.0	3.0	800	800	110	10	350	15
45	400	16	1.3	1.2	1.6	3.0	1,200	1,200	115	18	300	15
45	400	14	1.4	1.1	2.0	3.0	1,200	1,200	115	18	300	15
45	400	14	1.4	1.1	2.0	3.0	800	800	100	18	300	15
45	400	13	1.2	1.0	2.0	3.0	800	800	100	18	300	15
45	400	12	1.1	1.0	2.0	3.0	800	800	80	10	300	15
60	800	+2	+0.3	+0.3	2.5	4.0	1,200	1,200	125	18+[h]	450	20
80	600	+4	+0.5	+0.3	2.5	4.0	1,200	1,200	150	18	450	25

[e]Total vitamin E activity, estimated to be 80% as α-tocopherol and 20% other tocopherols.

[f]The folacin allowances refer to dietary sources as determined by *Lactobacillus casei* assay. Pure forms of folacin may be effective in doses less than one fourth of the recommended dietary allowance.

[g]Although allowances are expressed as niacin, it is recognized that on the average 1 mg of niacin is derived from each 60 mg of dietary tryptophan.

[h]This increased requirement cannot be met by ordinary diets; therefore, the use of supplemental iron is recommended.

Table 5-4. Dietary standards used by the U.S. Public Health Service in evaluating dietary intake in the National Nutritional Survey, 1970*

Age	Energy (kcal/kg)	Protein (gm/kg)	Calcium (mg)	Iron (mg)	Thiamine	Riboflavin	Vitamin A (IU)	Ascorbic acid (mg)
6-7 years	82	1.3	450	10	0.4 mg/1,000 kcal	0.55 mg/1,000 kcal	2,500	30
10-12 years								
Male	68	1.2	650	10	0.4 mg/1,000 kcal	0.55 mg/1,000 kcal	2,500	30
Female	64	1.2	650	18	0.4 mg/1,000 kcal	0.55 mg/1,000 kcal	2,500	30
17-19 years								
Male	44	1.1	550	18	0.4 mg/1,000 kcal	0.55 mg/1,000 kcal	3,500	30
Female	35	1.1	550	18	0.4 mg/1,000 kcal	0.55 mg/1,000 kcal	3,500	30
Adults								
Male	38	1.0	400	10	0.4 mg/1,000 kcal	0.55 mg/1,000 kcal	3,500	30
Female	38	1.0		18	0.4 mg/1,000 kcal	0.55 mg/1,000 kcal		
Pregnant	+200	+20	800	18	0.4 mg/1,000 kcal	0.55 mg/1,000 kcal	3,500	30
Lactating	+1,000	+25	900	18	0.4 mg/1,000 kcal	0.55 mg/1,000 kcal	4,500	30

*From Guthrie, H. A.: Introductory nutrition, ed. 3, St. Louis, 1975, The C. V. Mosby Co.

A second standard, used mostly in the International Survey, is the Suggested Guide to Interpretation of Nutrient Intake Data, developed by the Interdepartmental Committee on Nutrition for National Defense (ICNND) (Table 5-3). This guide applies only to the 25-year-old, 67-inch tall, physically active man who weighs 143 lb. In order to overcome this problem of age and sex, yet another standard has been developed for the National Nutrition Survey. This new standard is derived from the ICNND guidelines and the RDA and is outlined in Table 5-4.

Because of the limitations of these standards, interpretation of dietary data is not diagnostic but only indicative of a deficiency.

■ Clinical appraisal

Clinical appraisal is concerned with the physical examination of certain parts of the body, such as the eyes, hair, mucous membranes, skin, and oral cavity (lips, teeth, gums, and tongue), in order to detect the symptoms of nutritional deficiency. Generally, this examination is carried out by a physician. However, auxiliary health workers may be trained in nutritional diagnosis based on clinical appraisal. The auxiliary health worker would then alert the physician to the presence or absence of clinical symptoms.

Clinical appraisal is the least sensitive technique among the methods used in the nutritional assessment. Some reasons for this are:

1. Subjectivity of the examiner or examiner bias is involved in the judgment. Different evaluators differ regarding the identification and degree of malnutrition of the same lesion. The more nonspecific a lesion is, the more differing are the opinions. An example of this is seen in the examiner variability observed in the recordings of three examiners in an area included in the recent Ten-State Nutrition Survey (Table 5-5). Another example is that of the examiner who judges the leanness of a male subject's body in relation to his own and that of the female subject's in relation to the contour of his wife. Therefore, standardization of examiners' parameters must be carried out often. Color slides would be very useful in the identification and standardization of signs of deficiency.

2. Because of the nature of the development of nutrient deficiencies, clinical assessment may or may not correlate well with the food intake data or with the biochemical parameters.

Table 5-5. Percentage of adult clinical findings by three examiners in a selected area of the Ten-State Nutrition Survey*

	Examiners		
	1	2	3
Number of examinations	1,123	1,127	589
Filiform papillary atrophy	4.1	1.1	11.2
Follicular hyperkeratosis	4.0	0.6	6.8
Swollen red gums	2.8	3.7	4.1
Angular lesions	0.4	0.4	1.2
Glossitis	0.6	0.4	0.5
Goiter	3.6	6.6	3.6

*From Laboratory tests for assessment of nutritional status, Sauberlich, H. E., Dowdy, R. P., and Skala, J. H., CRC Crit. Rev. Clin. Lab. Sci. 4:215, 1973. © CRC Press, Inc., 1973. Used by permission of CRC Press, Inc.

3. The nonspecific nature of clinical lesions encountered may complicate the diagnosis. The same lesion could be traced to a deficiency of one or more nutrients. The lesion could also be due to some other reason, such as allergy or trauma.

In spite of its drawbacks, clinical appraisal does have a definite role in the total assessment procedure:

1. It provides information to supplement that obtained in anthropometric, dietary, and biochemical methods.
2. As seen in Fig. 5-2, anatomical lesions do not appear until the deficiency is far advanced. The presence of clinical symptoms in some individuals of a community would indicate the possibility of a subclinical deficiency in others. This identification could lead to correction at earlier stages.
3. Clinical assessment may reveal a host of other diseases not diagnosed earlier but which merit diagnosis and treatment.
4. A physical examination may detect nutritional deficiency not detected by dietary or biochemical methods.

Table 5-6 summarizes certain of the symptoms associated with specific nutrient deficiencies in man. Some of the observations made on specific tissues that are useful in the assessment procedure are briefly discussed below. One should note, however, that although prolonged and severe deficiencies of nutrients are manifested in anatomical lesions, not all the changes observed can be traced to nutritional origin.

Sometimes complaints from patients who have

Table 5-6. Clinical syndromes associated with deficiencies of specific nutrients*

Calories: Underweight, underheight, weight loss, lethargy, anemia, edema, marasmus

Protein: As above, fatty liver, kwashiorkor

Fat: Dermatoses in infants (essential fatty acid deficiency), deficiencies of the fat soluble vitamins A, D, E, and K

Vitamin A: Growth failure, follicular hyperkeratosis, night blindness, xerophthalmia, keratomalacia

Vitamin D: Rickets, tetany, osteomalacia

Vitamin E: Unknown, macrocytic anemia

Vitamin K: Decreased plasma prothrombin activity with prolonged coagulation time and hemorrhages

Thiamine: Anorexia, beriberi, polyneuropathy, toxic amblyopia, heart disease, the ophthalmoplegia of Wernicke's syndrome

Riboflavin: Photophobia, corneal vascularization, angular stomatitis, glossitis, dermatitis

Niacin: Pellagra, dermatitis, glossitis, diarrhea, mental confusion and deterioration, encephalopathy

Pyridoxine: Anemia, convulsions (infants), polyneuropathy, seborrheic eczema

Pantothenic acid: Nutritional melalgia (burning feet syndrome)

Folic acid: Glossitis, archrestic anemia, megaloblastic anemia of infancy, megaloblastic anemia of pregnancy, nutritional macrocytic anemia, sprue

Vitamin B$_{12}$: Glossitis, macrocytic anemia, pheripheral neuropathy, combined system disease (posterolateral column degeneration), mental changes and deterioration

Biotin: Seborrheic dermatitis

Choline, inositol, and carnitine: Unknown

Ascorbic acid: Scurvy, scorbutic gums, subperiosteal hemorrhages, petechial hemorrhages, anemia, impaired wound healing

Iron: Anemia, achlorhydria, glossitis

Iodine: Simple goiter

Fluorine: Dental caries

Calcium: Osteomalacia, a role in the production of senile osteoporosis has been suggested but not proven

Magnesium: Neuromuscular irritability, tetany

Potassium: Alkalosis, muscle weakness and paralysis, cardiac disturbances

Salt (NaCl): Anorexia, nausea, vomiting, lassitude, asthenia, muscle cramps, circulatory collapse

Water: Thirts, dehydration, oliguria, mental changes progressing to coma

*From Goodheart, R. S., and Wohl, M. G.: Manual of clinical nutrition, Philadelphia, Lea & Febiger, 1964.

deficiencies of specific nutrients aid in diagnosing the symptoms faster. Examples of these complaints are general weakness, chronic fatigue, loss of appetite, loss of weight, bleeding gums, and soreness of the eyes and mouth.

Eyes. Dryness of the cornea and conjunctiva and corneal opacity (xerophthalmia) are usually associated with vitamin A deficiency. Infiltration of the cornea by blood vessels is associated with vitamin B$_2$, or riboflavin, deficiency.

Skin. Some of the dermatitides are associated with certain vitamin deficiencies. In niacin deficiency, dermatitis of skin exposed to sunlight is observed. In vitamin A deficiency, xerosis or roughness of skin due to the hardness of papillae at the base of the hair follicle is seen. Nasolabial dermatitis is often considered a pyridoxine deficiency. Essential fatty acid deficiency results in eczematic skin, particularly in infants. Ascorbic acid deficiency resulting in capillary fragility is the cause of perifollicular petechiae.

Oral cavity. Riboflavin deficiency is considered to be the cause of cheilosis or angular stomatitis, that is, cracks and fissures in the lips, particularly at the corners of the mouth. Often this is followed by redness, swelling, and ulceration of the lips. Riboflavin deficiency sometimes causes the tongue to have a magenta hue, which could also be due to folic acid or vitamin B$_2$ deficiencies. A scarlet, raw appearance of the tongue with a loss of papillae is a sign of niacin deficiency. Bleeding gums are associated with ascorbic acid deficiency; and mottled teeth, with excessive intakes of fluorides. Dental caries may be a result of fluoride deficiency or faulty nutritional practices after tooth eruption.

Hair. Lack of luster, depigmentation, and decreased hair diameter are often the outcomes of protein deficiency.

Glands. Enlargement of the thyroid gland, goiter, is a manifestation of a lack of iodine availability to the thyroid cells.

■ Anthropometry

Anthropometry deals with the measurements of a part or whole of the body. Because nutrition is one of the determinants of growth and development, it is not surprising that over the decades researchers have attempted to establish this criterion as a measure of nutritional adequacy. Anthropometry is of particular interest in the nutritional assessment during the growing years.

However, the nonspecificity of this method should be kept in mind in light of present findings that the ultimate growth and development of an individual is the result of a complex web of factors, such as genetic tendencies, maternal and childhood nutrition, infections and diseases influencing the growth process from the time of conception to maturity, and environmental factors.

The most commonly used parameters in anthropometry are height; weight; skinfold thicknesses; and the circumference of the arm, chest, and head.

Height and weight

Data collection. Exact height and weight data depend on the accuracy of instruments used, as well as on correct techniques. Weighing machines are convenient. Regular checking and recalibration of the scales may be necessary. Lever balances are more reliable than spring balances. In practice, however, many modifications to accuracy need to be made, depending on the situation. Ideally, the nude weight of the individual should be considered, but this is often impractical. An indirect and practical method of determining the nude weight is to recommend that similar amounts of clothing be worn by the individual each time he is weighed. The deduction of this weight from the total weight would yield an estimate of the nude weight.

Standing height should be measured on a standard scale. The individual should stand erect, and a sliding headpiece may be helpful in judging accuracy. With infants, recumbent length is considered. Here again, innovative methods are often employed when measuring is carried out in developing countries.

Norms. Efforts to correlate height and weight in relation to age and sex with nutritional status have been met with limited success, mainly because of the norms used for comparison. If the standards for height and weight consider body builds without defining the builds—small, medium, or large frame—as was done in the 1959 Build and Blood Pressure Study by the Society of Actuaries, a great deal of subjectivity enters the evaluatory mechanism. On the other hand, if stature is not considered, too high a degree of homogeneity may be assumed, which would also contribute to errors in assessment. The lateral bony chest measurement by roentgenographic determination may be used as a stature reference, but the procedure is expensive and may not be practical in population studies.

The most commonly used standard height and weight tables for age 25 and over were published in 1960 (Tables 5-7 and 5-8). These were derived from the Build and Blood Pressure Study and give ideal or desirable weights in relation to heights for different statures (frames). The ranges of weight given in the tables are those that were associated with lowest mortality. It should be remembered that these tables are based on people who buy insurance and may not be a representative example of the population.

Smoothed average weights for adult men and women by age and height are given in Table 5-9. Published by the National Center for Health Statistics, U.S. Public Health Service, these data on height, weight, and selected body dimensions were collected in 1960-1962 and were based on a nationwide probability sample. They are, therefore, more representative of the adult civilian, noninstitutionalized population in the United States than are data from the Build and Blood Pressure Study, which represents an insured population.

Height and weight standards used for children are the Harvard growth charts and the Iowa growth charts, which mainly reflect the growth rate of middle-class white children. The more recent standards by Falkner (Table 5-10) include the fifth, fiftieth, and ninety-fifth percentile heights and weights for white North American children from birth to 18 years. Falkner suggests that children falling outside the fifth and ninety-fifth range may have to be further assessed for nutritional imbalances.

Many factors, such as secular trends and healthier mothers with better nutrition giving birth to larger babies, have contributed to significant increases in average heights and weights of the present generation. In view of this, height and weight norms developed a decade or more ago would tend to become obsolete.

Again, growth charts developed for a specific population may or may not be applicable for another population. However, unavailability of reliable standards have often made these charts useful for practical purposes in nutritional surveys.

Skinfold thickness. The rising incidence of obesity has necessitated the screening of obese individuals from those that are of above-average weight. Obesity is the excessive accumulation of fat in the adipose tissue as a result of caloric surplus in the system. Therefore, efforts are directed toward evolving methods to measure body fat. Fatness can be determined from such variables as body density, lean body mass, and soft

Table 5-7. Desirable weights for men 25 years of age and over*†

Height with shoes on (1-inch heels)		Small frame	Medium frame	Large frame
Feet	Inches			
5	2	112-120	118-129	126-141
5	3	115-123	121-133	129-144
5	4	118-126	124-126	132-148
5	5	121-129	127-139	135-152
5	6	124-133	130-143	138-156
5	7	128-137	134-147	142-161
5	8	132-141	138-152	147-166
5	9	136-145	142-156	151-170
5	10	140-150	146-160	155-174
5	11	144-154	150-165	159-179
6	0	148-158	154-170	164-184
6	1	152-162	158-175	168-189
6	2	156-167	162-180	173-194
6	3	160-171	167-185	178-199
6	4	164-175	172-190	182-204

*Courtesy Metropolitan Life Insurance Co: How to control your weight, New York, 1960 supplement. Based on 1959 Build and Blood Pressure Study.
†Weight in pounds, according to frame (in indoor clothing).

Table 5-8. Desirable weights for women 25 years of age and over*†

Height with shoes on (2-inch heels)		Small frame	Medium frame	Large frame
Feet	Inches			
4	10	92-98	96-107	104-119
4	11	94-101	98-110	106-122
5	0	96-104	101-113	109-125
5	1	99-107	104-116	112-128
5	2	102-110	107-119	115-131
5	3	105-113	110-122	118-134
5	4	108-116	113-126	121-138
5	5	111-119	116-130	125-142
5	6	114-123	120-135	129-146
5	7	118-127	124-139	133-150
5	8	122-131	128-143	137-154
5	9	126-135	132-147	141-158
5	10	130-140	136-151	145-163
5	11	134-144	140-155	149-168
6	0	138-148	144-159	153-173

*Courtesy Metropolitan Life Insurance Co.: How to control your weight, New York, 1960 supplement. Based on 1959 Build and Blood Pressure Study.
†Weight in pounds, according to frame (in indoor clothing).

Table 5-9. Smoothed average weights[1] for men and women (by age and height: United States 1960-1962)*

Height	Weight (in pounds)						
	18-24 years	25-34 years	35-44 years	45-54 years	55-64 years	65-74 years	75-79 years
Men							
62 inches	137	141	149	148	148	144	133
63 inches	140	145	152	152	151	148	138
64 inches	144	150	156	156	155	151	143
65 inches	147	154	160	160	158	154	148
66 inches	151	159	164	164	162	158	154
67 inches	154	163	168	168	166	161	159
68 inches	158	168	171	173	169	165	164
69 inches	161	172	175	177	173	168	169
70 inches	165	177	179	181	176	171	174
71 inches	168	181	182	185	180	175	179
72 inches	172	186	186	189	184	178	184
73 inches	175	190	190	193	187	182	189
74 inches	179	194	194	197	191	185	194
Women							
57 inches	116	112	131	129	138	132	125
58 inches	118	116	134	132	141	135	129
59 inches	120	120	136	136	144	138	132
60 inches	122	124	138	140	149	142	136
61 inches	125	128	140	143	150	145	139
62 inches	127	132	143	147	152	149	143
63 inches	129	136	145	150	155	152	146
64 inches	131	140	147	154	158	156	150
65 inches	134	144	149	158	161	159	153
66 inches	136	148	152	161	164	163	157
67 inches	138	152	154	165	167	166	160
68 inches	140	156	156	168	170	170	164

*From Obesity and health; a source book for professional health personnel, U.S. Department of Health, Education, and Welfare, U.S. Public Health Service. Adapted from National Center for Health Statistics: Weight by height and age of adults, United States, 1960-1962, *Vital Health Statistics*. PHS Pub. No. 1000—Series 11, No. 14. May 1966.
[1]Estimated values from regression equations of weights for specified age groups.

Table 5-10. Height and weight of children 4-18 years of age*

Ages (years)	Height (inches)			Weight (pounds)		
	5th P†	50th P	95th P	5th P	50th P	95th P
			Boys			
4	38.3	40.8	43.3	30.0	36.1	42.2
5	40.3	43.4	46.4	33.0	40.3	47.6
6	42.8	45.9	49.0	36.0	44.7	53.4
7	44.8	48.1	51.4	40.3	50.9	61.5
8	46.9	50.5	54.1	44.4	57.4	70.4
9	48.8	52.8	56.8	48.0	64.4	80.4
10	50.6	54.9	59.2	51.4	71.4	91.4
11	51.9	56.4	60.9	53.3	78.9	102.5
12	53.5	58.6	63.7	60.0	86.0	113.5
13	55.2	61.3	67.4	65.3	98.6	131.9
14	57.5	64.1	70.7	75.5	111.8	148.1
15	61.0	66.9	72.8	88.0	124.3	160.6
16	63.8	68.9	74.0	97.8	133.8	169.8
17	65.2	69.8	74.4	106.5	139.8	174.0
18	65.9	70.2	74.5	110.3	144.8	179.3
			Girls			
4	38.1	40.7	43.3	28.8	36.1	43.4
5	40.6	43.4	46.2	32.2	40.9	49.6
6	42.8	45.9	49.0	35.5	45.7	55.9
7	44.5	47.8	51.1	38.3	51.0	63.7
8	46.4	50.0	53.6	42.0	57.2	72.4
9	48.2	52.2	56.2	45.1	63.6	82.1
10	49.9	54.5	59.1	48.2	71.0	95.0
11	51.9	57.0	62.1	55.4	82.0	108.6
12	54.1	59.5	64.9	63.9	94.4	124.9
13	57.1	62.2	66.8	72.8	105.5	138.2
14	58.5	63.1	67.7	83.0	113.0	144.0
15	59.5	63.8	68.1	89.5	120.0	150.5
16	59.8	64.1	68.4	95.1	123.0	150.1
17	60.1	64.2	68.3	97.9	125.8	153.7
18	60.1	64.4	68.7	96.0	126.2	156.4

*From Falkner, F.: Some physical growth standards for white North American children, Pediatrics **29**:448, 1962.
†P, percentile.

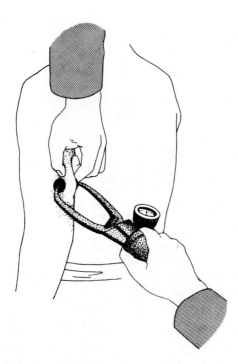

Fig. 5-3. Measuring triceps skinfold with calipers. From Guthrie, H. A.: Introductory nutrition, ed. 3, St. Louis, 1975, The C. V. Mosby Co.

Table 5-11. Obesity standards for Caucasian Americans* (minimum triceps skinfold thickness in millimeters indicating obesity†)

Age (years)	Skinfold measurements	
	Males	**Females**
5	12	14
6	12	15
7	13	16
8	14	17
9	15	18
10	16	20
11	17	21
12	18	22
13	18	23
14	17	23
15	16	24
16	15	25
17	14	26
18	15	27
19	15	27
20	16	28
21	17	28
22	18	28
23	18	28
24	19	28
25	20	29
26	20	29
27	21	29
28	22	29
29	23	29
30-50	23	30

*From Obesity and health; a source book for professional health personnel, U.S. Department of Health, Education, and Welfare, U.S. Public Health Service. Adapted from Seltzer, C. C., and Mayer, J.: A simple criterion of obesity, Postgrad. Med. **38:**101, 1965.
†Figures represent the logarithmic means of the frequency distributions plus one standard deviation.

tissue roentgenograms; but the most inexpensive and simple, and therefore practical, method of assessing body fat is to measure the skinfold thickness. Skinfold measurements are indicative of subcutaneous fat and of the caloric status. However, this variable appears to be more useful in assessing normal and moderately fat people rather than really obese people.

Data collection. Calibrated calipers are used in measuring skinfold thickness. Langes calipers are an example. The calipers allow most of the assessors to obtain reasonably reliable numerical values, provided the inter- and intrapersonnel variabilities in measurement are overcome. Standardization with the instrument and with the assessor are needed. The skinfold is pinched up to the point where the sides are parallel. Care should be taken not to touch the muscle or the bone. The thickness is then measured by means of standard calipers (Fig. 5-3), using constant pressure. Selection of the site for measurement is critical, since not all the sites are practical or reliable as indicators of fatness. The lower thoracic site appears to be ideal but impractical. The most commonly selected sites are the deltoid triceps, the subscapular region, and the upper abdomen. According to some researchers, a single skinfold measurement of the triceps is useful in diagnosing obesity.

Norms. Normal values for this variable are presented in Table 5-11. These norms are derived for the American white population and is more applicable to this specific group. If used for other groups, discretion is indicated. However, these norms are invariably used for all groups because of the unavailability of any other standard.

Measurement of circumferences (head, arm, and abdomen). With the present concern, though controversial, over the relationship between nutrition and mental development, the need for methods to assess brain growth is being recognized. Measurement of head circumference is being utilized as a tool for this purpose.

This parameter is of importance in infancy since it is an indicator of brain development, most of which is complete in the first year of life. Head circumference is more satisfactory if taken with the infant lying on his back. The measuring tape is passed around the head. The largest circumference is measured by placing the tape anteriorly over the lower forehead just above the supraorbital ridges and by passing it posteriorly over the most prominent part of the occiput. Values ranging from 31 cm to 37 cm at birth have been considered normal. Lower values should be a matter of concern.

Arm circumference measurement is a useful criterion for the musculature and therefore in determining the extent of protein-caloric malnutrition. A soft tape measure calibrated in centimeters is placed around the arm, usually the left arm, at its midpoint. The tape should be firmly wrapped around but without compressing the underlying muscle. A value of 29.3 cm for male subjects and 28.5 cm for female subjects is considered normal. For further discussion on this, refer to Jelliffe (1966).

Invariably, anthropometrists have attempted to construct formulas based on various anthropometric measurements to provide an index of nutritional status. In some cases they have proved useful in the nutritional diagnosis; however, in others they have been less satisfactory. Therefore, height and weight are still the choice criteria in community assessment. Depending on the resources and enthusiasm of the assessor, other criteria could be included.

■ Biochemical appraisal

The biochemical method—or laboratory assessment, as it is sometimes called—measures levels of nutrients; their metabolites; and enzymes associated with or even compounds clearly related to the nutrient under consideration in blood or other body fluids, urine, or tissues such as liver and bone. Since tissue biopsies are hazardous and difficult techniques are involved, tissues are rarely used for analysis; rather, blood or urine is used.

Biochemical assessment is more objective than clinical and dietary methods. In addition, this method detects marginal or subclinical deficiencies before overt clinical lesions appear. It can also indicate metabolic alterations caused by a deficiency of the detected nutrient. Generally, two types of tests are used: (1) measurement of

the circulating nutrient in blood or urine and (2) a functional test to evaluate biochemical functions that are dependent on an adequate supply of nutrients. Whereas the former aids in detecting the presence of the problem in earlier stages, the latter indicates the severity.

Specimen collection, handling, and storage are of critical importance, as is the standardization of various laboratory methods in order to overcome the interpersonal and interlaboratory variabilities. A detailed discussion of this can be found in the manual by the ICNND. Recent changes in the quantity and quality of the diet may result in variations in blood and urine composition. The composition of nutrients in blood and urine has also been noted to vary during the day. Therefore, blood samples are usually collected for analysis from a fasting subject.

Parameters. Although nutritional status cannot be completely assessed by the biochemical method, different parameters may be used to assess the status of specific nutrients. The parame-

Table 5-12. Nutritional assessment data obtained from clinical laboratory parameters

Nutrient	Blood	Urine*
Protein	Protein (P)† Albumin (P) Amino acids (P)	Total nitrogen Urea Creatinine OH—proline
Iron	Hemoglobin Hematocrit Transferrin (S) Iron (S)	
Vitamin A	Vitamin A (P) Carotene (P)	
Vitamin C	Vitamin C (S) Vitamin C (WBC)	Vitamin C
Thiamine	Transketolase (E)	Thiamin
Riboflavin	Glutathione reductase (E)	Riboflavin
Niacin		N. methyl nicotinamide
Vitamin B_6	GOT (E)‡ GPT (E)‡	Xanthurenic acid Pyridoxine
Folic acid	Folic acid (S)	FIGLU (Formiminoglutamic acid)
Iodine		Iodine
Vitamin B_{12}	Vitamin B_{12} (S)	

*Urinary values are often considered per unit weight of creatinine excreted.
† P, plasma; S, serum; WBC, white blood cell; E, erythrocyte.
‡Glutamic-oxalacetic transaminase; glutamic-pyruvic transaminase.

ter to be chosen for a specific nutrient depends on the physiological significance of the test and also on the facilities and resources available, including the cost. Some test methods are still in the experimental stages. Some are utilized only in research or in individual assessments. However, the parameter should be sensitive enough to assess the status of the particular nutrient. Table 5-12 describes some of the parameters used to assess the status of certain specific nutrients.

Biochemical parameters have also been used to identify and screen certain diseases. For instance, elevated levels of serum cholesterol and triglycerides have been implicated in heart disease. Efforts are being continued to evolve more sensitive parameters and newer and more accurate techniques. Hair biopsy sample analysis for certain trace minerals and protein status are being considered. Urinary hydroxyproline as an index for detecting protein-calorie malnutrition is another more recent parameter being used. However, the need for large numbers of parameters is being questioned. Whether fewer variables could be utilized for screening population groups is also being debated. Much more experimentation and study is necessary before a decision can be made.

Methods. The biochemical methods utilized vary in cost, reliability, and the degree of techni-

cal expertise. They are also constantly being revised and improved. Analytical techniques for evaluating constituents of blood have been adopted for use on very small samples. These microtechniques have enabled the determination of 15 to 20 biochemical constituents on as small a sample as 1 ml of blood. Microtechniques have not only added to the convenience of the individual being tested but have also facilitated the usage of more biochemical parameters in the nutritional assessment. The selection of a test and method and the interpretation of results depends on resources available and on the preference of the researcher.

Norms. Norms for biochemical parameters that are frequently used have been developed by the ICNND. These standards refer to the adult male only. Therefore, in the recent National Nutrition Survey, standards referring to all age groups are derived on the basis of research findings and the ICNND standards (Table 5-13).

The norms used are often criticized. The arbitrarily chosen cut-off points, indicative of some degree of risk (deficient, marginal, and acceptable), are a matter of controversy. This is not surprising in view of the fact that the specificity of laboratory evaluation of nutrients and the physiological significance of the tests used are still not conclusive in nature.

Table 5-13. Criteria for evaluating some frequently used biochemical measures of nutritional status (levels indicative of a deficiency state)*

	Adult males	Children	
		2-5 years	6-12 years
Blood data			
Hemoglobin (gm/100 ml)	<12	<10	<10
Hematocrit (% packed cell volume)	<37	<30	<30
Serum albumin (gm/100 ml)	<2.8	†	†
Serum ascorbic acid (mg/100 ml)	<0.1	<0.1	<0.1
Plasma vitamin A (μg/100 ml)	<10	<10	<10
Serum iron (μg/100 ml)	<60	<40	<50
Transferrin saturation (%)	<20	<20	<20
Serum folacin (mg/ml)	<2	<2	<2
Serum vitamin B_{12}	<100	<100	<100
Plasma vitamin E (mg/100 ml)	<0.2	<0.2	<0.2
Urinary data			
Thiamine (μg/gm creatinine)	<27	<85	<70
Riboflavin (μg/gm creatinine)	<27	<100	<85
Tryptophan load (100 mg/kg) (mg xanthurenic acid/24 hr)	>75	>75	>75

*From Guthrie, H. A.: Introductory nutrition, ed. 3, St. Louis, 1975, The C. V. Mosby Co. Adapted from Christakis, G., editor: Nutritional assessment in health programs, Am. J. Public Health **63** Supplement, Nov. 1973.
†No values available.

Interpretation. Biochemical data indicate the deviation from the norm but not always the cause of the deviation. Further difficulty in interpretation is encountered when the body's homeostatic mechanisms, which could cause a nutrient deficiency, are considered. Only when the body's homeostatic mechanisms fail, do deficiencies in specific nutrients become apparent.

The interpretation of biochemical findings is difficult and therefore should be left to expert hands.

Conclusion

More positive correlation between biochemical parameters and dietary intake data have been found in nutrition surveys than between laboratory and clinical findings. This is not surprising in consideration of the nonspecific nature of clinical lesions and the development of biochemical variations before physical abnormalities are apparent.

This does not mean that the clinical method is not of importance or that one method of assessment is better than the other. The data from all the methods should be collected, integrated, and then interpreted to be assured of a reasonable degree of diagnostic accuracy and sensitivity.

Nutritional assessment is an expensive procedure. Presently, the need for large numbers of variables is being questioned. Efforts are being made to reduce the number of tests necessary to identify nutritionally vulnerable individuals and groups without reducing the diagnostic potential. Statistical analysis (factor analysis) of the data collected on more than 25 variables in the Ten-State Survey indicated that perhaps as few as 8 to 10 of these parameters would provide as much information as that provided by all the variables together.

BIBLIOGRAPHY

Adams, C. F.: Nutritive value of American foods in common units, Agriculture Handbook No. 456, Washington, D.C., 1976, Agriculture Research Service, U.S. Department of Agriculture.

Arroyave, G.: Biochemical evaluation of nutritional status of Man, Fed. Proc. 20:39, 1960.

Beal, V. A.: The nutritional history in longitudinal research, Am. J. Diet Assoc. 51:426, 1967.

Bollet, A. J., and Owens, S.: Evaluation and nutritional status of selected hospitalized patients, Am. J. Clin. Nutr. 26:931, 1973.

Butterworth, G., and Blackburn, G.: Hospital malnutrition, Nutr. Today 10:8, 1975.

Christakis, G. M., editor: Nutritional assessment in health programs, Am. J. Pub. Health (suppl.) 63:1, November 1973.

Food and Nutrition Board: Recommended dietary allowances, ed. 8, Washington, D.C., 1974, National Academy of Sciences, National Research Council.

Garn, S. M.: The applicability of North American growth standards in developing countries, Grad. Med. Assoc. J. 93:914, 1965.

Gueney, M. J., and Jellife, D. B.: Arm anthropometry in nutritional assessment; monogram for rapid calculation of muscle circumference and cross sectional muscle and fat areas, Am. J. Clin. Nutr. 26:912, 1973.

Guthrie, H. A., and Guthrie, G. M.: Factor analysis of nutritional status data from Ten-State Survey, Am. J. Clin. Nutr. 29:1238, 1976.

Guthrie, H. A., Owens, G. M., and Guthrie, G. M.: Factor analysis of measures of nutritional status of preschool children, Am. J. Clin. Nutr. 26:497, 1973.

Hillman, R. W.: Concordance among clinical signs suggestive of malnutrition, Am. J. Clin. Nutr. 20:1118, 1967.

Hollingsworth, D.: Dietary determination of nutritional status, Fed. Proc. 20:50, 1960.

Howells, G. R., Wharlon, B. A., and McCance, R. A.: Value of hydroxyproline indices in malnutrition, Lancet 1:1082, 1967.

Interdepartmental Committee on Nutrition for National Defense (ICNND): Manual for nutrition surveys, Bethesda, Md., 1963, ICNND.

Jellife, D. B.: The assessment of the nutritional status of the community, WHO Monogr. Ser. 53, 1966.

Kelsey, J. L.: A compendium of nutritional status studies and dietary evaluation studies conducted in the United States, 1957-1967, J. Nutr. (suppl. 1, part II) 99:123, 1969.

Klevay, L. M.: Hair as a biopsy material; assessment of zinc nutriture, Am. J. Clin. Nutr. 23:284, 1970.

Krehl, W. A., and Hodges, R. E.: The interpretation of nutrition survey data, Am. J. Clin. Nutr. 17:191, 1965.

Leevy, C. M., Cardi, L., Frank, O., and others: Incidence and significance of hypovitaminemia in a randomly selected municipal hospital population, Am. J. Clin. Nutr. 19:259, 1965.

Medical assessment of nutritional status; report of the Joint FAO/WHO Expert Committee, WHO Techn. Rep. Ser. 258, 1963.

Pearson, W. N.: Biochemical appraisal of the vitamin nutritional status in man, J.A.M.A. 180:49, 1962.

Pekkarinen, M.: Methodology in the collection of food consumption data, World Rev. Nutr. Diet 12:145, 1970.

Plough, I. C., and Bridforth, E. B.: Relations of clinical and dietary findings in nutritional surveys, Public Health Rep. 75:699, 1960.

Selzer, C. C., Goldman, R. F., and Mayer, J.: The triceps skinfold as a predictive measure of body density and body fat in obese adolescent girls, Pediatrics 36:212, 1965.

Standard, K. L., Lovell, H. G., and Garrow, J. S.: The validity of certain physical signs as indices of generalized malnutrition in young children, J. Trop. Pediatr. 11:100, 1966.

Suaberlich, H. E., Dowdy, R. P., and Skala, J. H.: Laboratory tests for the assessment of nutritional status, CRC Crit. Rev. Clin. Lab. Sci. September, 1973, p. 215.

U.S. Department of Health, Education, and Welfare: Ten-state nutritional survey, 1968-1970, vols. 1-5, Atlanta, Ga., Health Services and Mental Health Administration.

Wilson, C. S., and others: A Review of methods used in nutrition surveys conducted by the Interdepartmental Committee on Nutrition for National Defense (ICNND), Am. J. Clin. Nutr. 15:29, 1964.

6 Assessment of sleep-activity patterns

BIOLOGICAL RHYTHMS IN MAN

Normal man is characterized as an organism that adapts its functions in such a way as to have a different physiochemical and psychological makeup for each hour of the day. Yet each of these changes is carefully regulated for the given hour. This ability to maintain a relative internal constancy has been termed *homeostasis* or, more precisely, *homeokinesis*. Thus, the healthy individual represents the integration of a myriad of cyclical alterations of psychophysiological functions.

Since the cyclical nature of human function has been defined, a good deal of experimentation has been focused on determining whether one or more factors in the environment are the cause of the rhythms. Further work has been devoted to locating receptors in man that sense these external factors and are responsible for the establishment of the rhythms.

Man adapts to environmental cues of an immediate nature as well as to external sequences or cycles of regularly changing conditions. Examples of regular external periodicities that are known to be incorporated into organisms' adaptive behavior are the tides, the light-dark cycle, the lunar cycle, and the seasons. This adaptive process involves the establishment of an endogenous rhythm that approximately corresponds to the environmental stimulus. These rhythms are known as the biological clocks that allow the organism to adjust to the changes occurring outside. Once the internal rhythm is established, the environmental cue that caused the change becomes a synchronizing stimulus and is called a *Zeitgeber* (Ger. *Zeit*, time; and *Geber*, giver).

Biological rhythms have been described for all levels of biological functions. It has been shown that cells may be influenced directly by gravity and electrostatic and magnetic fields. The nervous system seems important to the control of rhythms in higher organisms, particularly as related to photoperiodicity. At least one researcher has hypothesized different levels of rhythm organization: neural, endocrine, and cellular. In this system, the neural system is thought to be entrained by dominant synchronizers and the cellular elements by weaker synchronizers. In man it is necessary to include a fourth level, psychosocial organization, which may serve to modify rhythmic trends.

The influence most frequently observed in plants and animals is the day-night, or light-dark, cycle. Such circadian (L. *circa*, about; and *dies*, day) rhythms have been identified for all cells and functions of the human body from enzyme levels to complex neural events. Since most human rhythms are 23 to 25 hours in length, they are termed circadian. However, although most human functions are entrained by a period approximating 24 hours, the peaks (high-function point) and troughs (low-function point) of daily rhythms for various functions can occur at different times; and although these functional records show phase relationships to each other, it is not known if all the rhythms for the various functions are entrained by *Zeitgeber* stimuli or by other rhythms internal to the person.

It has been hypothesized that functions such as the sleep-wakefulness cycle are weakly entrained whereas functions such as urinary output, body temperature, cortical secretion, enzyme production, and cellular division are more strongly incorporated. Data to support this hypothesis are those from experiments wherein subjects are placed in light- and soundproof enclosures for weeks to months. As many stimuli as possible are removed, and this is termed the free-running condition, which means that cyclical events occur in the absence of their respective *Zeitgeber*. The sleep-wakefulness cycle becomes desynchronized to 30 to 33 hours. The more deeply entrained cycles, the vegetative functions, retain a 25-hour cycle. Thus, many endogenous cycles may be in new phase relationships.

The 24-hour temperature rhythm was defined soon after the development of the clinical thermometer in the eighteenth century. However, a refined experimental approach to the study of biological rhythms in human physiology had its origin in the 1920s when it was shown that rhythms occur even in metabolism. Table 6-1 reflects some of the data useful to the health care professional in this still relatively unknown field.

Table 6-1. Time of maximum amplitude of physiological rhythms in a person whose sleep cycle is 11 PM to 7 AM

	Peak of cycle*
Vital signs	
Temperature (rectal)	4-6 PM
Heart rate	4 PM
Respiratory rate	2-3 PM
Blood pressure	7-10 PM
Cardiac output	Midnight
Venous pressure	Midnight
Oxygen consumption	Midnight
Physical vigor	3-4 PM
Optical reaction time	3 AM
Grip strength	2-8 PM
Blood	
Sodium	4-5 PM
Calcium	9-10 PM
17-hydroxycorticosteroid	7-8 AM
Hematocrit	9-10 PM
Polymorphonuclear cells	12-1 PM
Lymphocytes and monocytes	11-3 AM
Urine	
Sodium	12-1 PM
Potassium	12-1 PM
Calcium	3-4 PM
Magnesium	1 AM
Dopamine	3 PM
Catecholamines	5-7 PM
Vanillylmandelic acid	5-7 PM
17-hydroxycorticosteroids	9-10 AM
Rate of excretion	8-9 AM
Mitosis-epidermal	11-12 PM
Body weight	6-7 PM

*The valley or low period for these values occurs approximately 12 hours later.

It has been shown that the sensitivity to many pharmacological agents, such as morphine and ethanol, to bacteria, and to carcinogens varies over the 24-hour period. Thus, the time the client takes a given medication may influence the effectiveness of the drug.

Some cycles appear to be significantly related to one another; for instance, the pulse rate and respiratory rate in the normal adult demonstrate a 4:1 ratio, and any long-term deviation from this ratio may be the diagnostic feature of abnormal function.

Nocturnal diuresis has been given as an example of a phase change (180°) in a biological rhythm; the change in time for this function was recognized as abnormal and given diagnostic significance long before circadian rhythms were well defined.

Periodic mood changes are described in both normal mental states and in emotional illnesses. Dramatic changes in affect occur in manic-depressive illness. One group has reported that some hormonal functions may free run whereas other rhythms adhere to the 24-hour cycle and has correlated depression with the times when hormonal functions are out of phase.

A good deal of work has been devoted to determining whether interference with circadian rhythms results in disorders in the affected individual. Two particularly fruitful areas for this study have been work situations requiring a change in the sleep-wakefulness pattern and rapid travel across time zones.

Industrial shift workers demonstrate changes in accuracy and accident proneness. Workers who change shifts given an indication of some imbalance in rhythms through a higher incidence of ulcers and nervousness. Temperature fluctuations in the individual who works at night are reduced in amplitude.

Translongitudinal passage or long-distance travel across time zones results in a derangement of rhythms, so that several days are required to adapt to local time. A 5-hour flight westward results in a readjustment period of 2 days for the sleep-wakefulness cycle, 5 days for body temperature, and 8 days for cortisol secretion.

The health professional is faced with the responsibility for establishing exact limits of normal values for man. Experimental data have allowed the establishment of separate sets of norms for men and women, accounting for individual differences in size, various age groups, and various levels of activity. More precise diagnosis will be possible when data are also available for all the body functions, particularly those that will allow the limits of normal to be established for changes that occur throughout the day, seasons, and year. The changing resistance of the body to disease phenomena must be defined, as well as the changing susceptibility to pharmaceutical agents. What is needed is a 24-hour tolerance test for the circadian range of values for each bodily parameter.

SLEEP-WAKEFULNESS PATTERNS

During sleep, the individual shows a greatly increased threshold for external stimuli. Thus, sleep is a normal, physiological condition that can be regarded as an altered state of consciousness from which the subject can be aroused by stimuli of sufficient magnitude. Although the precise function of sleep has not been made clear, most persons agree that the act of sleep is refreshing, that it is a time of physiological and psychosocial reintegration.

It has been shown that sleep disorders are due for the most part to situational stresses or crises, to medical pathophysiology, to psychosocial illness, to drug-related disorders (particularly withdrawal), and to the effects of the aging process. Furthermore, it has been recorded that one third to one half of clients who seek health care complain of a difficulty related to sleep and will want a prescription to help them obtain a sleep pattern they would consider more desirable. Clients may complain of disordered sleep as a primary problem or as a concomitant of another condition. Often the client complains that lack of sleep is making him so "nervous and irritable" that his job is in jeopardy and his friends are deserting him. Thus, the magnitude of sleep problems can be appreciated in both the numbers of individuals involved and in the degree to which a client may be incapacitated. The primary care practitioner must assess the client's sleep pattern in order to determine if a problem related to sleep exists.

Sleep habits vary markedly from one individual to another. However, any one person's sleep period may demonstrate consistency.

Factors identified as those which influence the length of time an individual will spend sleeping and the quality of that sleep are (1) anxiety related to the need to meet a task, such as finishing a paper or going to work; (2) the promise of pleasurable activity, such as starting a vacation; (3) the conditioned patterns of sleeping; (4) physiological makeup, such as the metabolic level; (5)

age; and (6) physiological alteration, such as disease or alcoholism.

The affective response to sleep, that is, whether the individual feels he had a "good night's sleep," has been found to be dependent on the number of times he was awakened as well as on the total number of hours of sleep.

The practitioner needs to be aware of the unique rest and sleep needs of the individual client.

■ Sleep research

Sleep research has been systematically conducted for only the past 20 years. The reported findings of this research have shown the diagnostic value of having the client report his sleep-wakefulness pattern as part of the history. This data will indicate the need for further intervention. The electroencephalographic (EEG) tracings of subjects who are asleep have been analyzed by many researchers. Their findings have been correlated with physiological alterations that accompany various EEG sleep patterns as well as with affective phenomena reported by the subjects when they awaken naturally or are awakened by the observers. These studies have indicated that clients' complaints of inability to sleep well may have their basis in organic diseases.

Furthermore, observation for signs of sleep disturbance may yield valuable data for the ongoing assessment and management of the hospitalized client. It has been shown that sleep consists of cyclic patterns of physiological signs that recur periodically throughout the night.

The physiological measurements most valuable to defining the sleep pattern are (1) the recordings of electrical potential made from electrodes placed on the surface of the head (EEG), (2) the tracing made from sensors (electro-oculogram [EOG]) of ocular movement made from both eyes, and (3) the record derived from sensors for skeletal muscle tone (electromyogram [EMG]); these sensors are generally placed beneath the client's jaw.

The differentiation of sleep stages from the EEG tracing is based on alterations in the frequency and amplitude of the brain wave tracings recorded from subjects who are asleep (Fig. 6-1). Waves of 8 to 12 cycles per second (cps) are called alpha activity. Sleep spindles are defined as waves of 12 to 16 cps, and those greater than 16 cps are called beta activity. Slower waves of 4 to 7 cps are called theta activity, and those of 1 to 3 cps are described as delta activity.

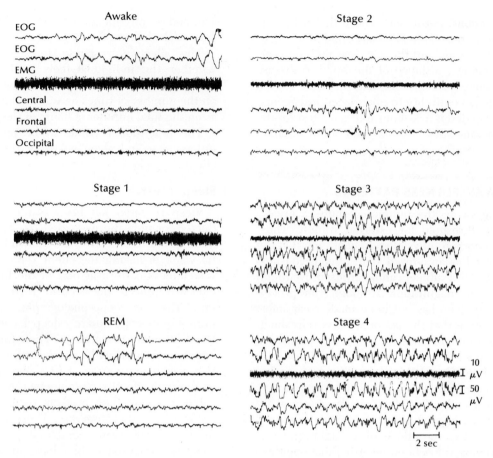

Fig. 6-1. Sleep stages. The same six channels are used throughout, as labeled in the *awake* record. EOG: eye movements; EMG: muscle tonus from beneath the chin. Note the high EMG and eye movements in the awake state, the absence of REMs in stage 1 (NREM), and REMs with decreased muscle tonus during REM sleep. Stages 2, 3, and 4 show progressive slowing of frequency and an increase in amplitude of the EEG. (From Kales, A.: Ann. Int. Med. **68,** 1078, 1968.)

The normal adult has low-amplitude, fast-frequency activity in the waking state. Alpha activity is the most frequent type of activity recorded during what the subject felt was a period of rest.

Some authorities refer to the awake and resting states as stage zero of the sleep cycle. During sleep, five characteristic tracings can be isolated; these make up the stages of sleep called 1, 2, 3, 4, and rapid eye movement (REM). These five stages constitute the sleep cycle.

■ The sleep cycle

In the critical stage of falling asleep, alpha waves decrease in the EEG record. Sleep spindle waveforms appear within 1 to 2 minutes and herald the beginning of stage 2. As noted, these spindle forms occur at 12- to 16-second intervals,

superimposed on a base of low-amplitude, fast-frequency activity. The duration of stage 2 sleep is 5 to 10 minutes, and its termination marks the end of light sleep. Stage 3 is identified on the EEG record as the appearance of delta activity. These slow waves make up 20% to 50% of the EEG sleep record. This is the transition stage between light and deep sleep and may last about 10 minutes. As stage 4 sleep is entered, sleep spindles disappear and high-voltage slow waves occupy 50% or more of the EEG record. This stage lasts from 5 to 15 minutes.

During these four stages of sleep, eye movements are not observed and skeletal muscle tone is only slightly less in amplitude than during the waking state. Calling these four stages non-REM (NREM) allows for categorization of sleep into two categories: NREM and REM.

During a normal sleeping period, the client experiences stage 1 sleep followed by stages 2, 3, and 4 sleep. Then there is a reverse from stage 4 sleep to stages 3 and 2. After about 60 to 90 minutes of this pattern of sleep, the first period of REM sleep occurs. The EEG is characterized by lower voltage and by the absence of big, slow waves and sleep spindles.

Gross eye movements can be seen and can be recorded (EOG). The first REM period of sleep lasts approximately 10 minutes and is demonstrated by body movement. This period is thought to be the time that most dreaming occurs. The client may only recall the dream if awakened during the REM stage. The remembered ideation occurring in NREM sleep seems more like the thinking that surrounds daily life activities.

At the end of the initial REM period, the sleeper returns to stages 2, 3, and sometimes 4, returning again to stage 3 and then to stage 2. This second period of NREM sleep lasts about 60 to 90 minutes. This is followed by another, slightly longer REM period (10 to 12 minutes). The transition from stage to stage is accompanied by body movement. A healthy adult probably experiences 30 to 40 turns during a night's sleep. The mobility of sleep protects the sleeper from the hazards of remaining motionless, that is, pressure changes in the microcirculation, thrombus formation, or diminished respiration, possibly leading to pneumonia.

As the sleep period continues, the length of the NREM sleep periods decrease and the REM periods increase. In addition, the depth of sleep usually that of stages 2 and 3, decreases. Thus, the client achieves the greatest amount of stages 3 and 4 sleep early in the sleep period, whereas most of the REM sleep occurs in the later cycles of the sleep period (Fig. 6-1).

The total number of cycles in a normal sleep period range from four to six, depending on the total length of the sleep period.

REM sleep. Phasic activity that occurs during REM sleep may be considered that of an arousal state generated by bursts of central nervous system (CNS) activity resulting in muscle twitches, eye movements, phasic changes in pupil size, and cardiopulmonary irregularities.

REM sleep has been described as a physiologically active period. The forebrain appears to be aroused. Animal studies have demonstrated that there is an increase in cerebral blood flow as well as in brain temperature. Lability of cardiopulmonary parameters is the rule with REM sleep. That is, there is a marked variation in heart and respiratory rate as well as in blood pressure. Tonic inhibition of skeletal muscles occurs during REM sleep. The absence of EMG activity, particularly as recorded from the digastric or neck muscles, has been cited in the support of the statement that there is generalized, skeletal motor inhibition. On the other hand, some muscles are not suppressed. These are the diaphragm, extraocular, middle ear, intercostal muscles, some facial muscles, and the muscles of the pharynx and larynx. Tendon reflexes are suppressed.

This stage is also referred to as paradoxical rhombencephalic, emergent, dream, or desynchronized sleep. Although data show that most REM sleep occurs during the last half of the sleep period, REM can occur during naps if the sleep period has sufficient duration. For the night sleeper, morning naps contain largely REM sleep, whereas afternoon naps are largely made up of stage 4 sleep. Several investigators have posited that REM sleep serves to reprogram the brain, particularly through the assimilation of new experiences into the existing personality structure. Some theorists contend that the function of REM sleep is to keep disturbing or threatening information from reaching the waking consciousness. Another theory is that the REM arousal periods are the mechanism for vigilance during the rest period that may have contributed to our distant ancestors' survival.

NREM, or slow-wave, sleep. An afternoon nap can be regarded as the beginning of NREM sleep, which represents 80% of the total sleeping time and is also called slow-wave sleep. NREM sleep is characterized by a decrease in tempo of the body's physiological processes. The basal metabolism rate (BMR) is decreased 10% to 15%, resulting in a decrease in body temperature of approximately 1° F. The pulse rate is decreased 10 to 30 beats, and the respiratory rate shows compensatory slowing. The blood pressure is slightly decreased. Muscle tone is minimal. Knee jerks are abolished. All of these characteristics represent an acute inhibitory process. Reflexes are weaker and slower to appear. The pupils of the eye are constricted in sleep and, with relaxation of the extraocular muscles, appear to "roll," that is, are not aligned.

Significance of the sleep stages. The clinical significance of the presence or absence of the sleep stages in man is still not clearly understood. Furthermore, it is difficult to make a judgment from the client's explanations of his sleep patterns whether he is more REM or NREM sleep de-

Table 6-2. The initial sleep cycle*

Stages of sleep	EEG brainwaves	Time span	Approximate percentage of total night's sleep	Affective aspects	Physiological alterations
NREM sleep					
Stage 1	Alpha activity	1-2 min	5%-10%	Fleeting thoughts; may be un-aware of being asleep	Light sleep, easily awakened; pulse rate decreased 10-30 beats per min; BMR decreased 10%-15%; temperature and respiration decreased; muscle tone minimal; knee jerks abolished; slight decrease in blood pressure
Stage 2	Sleep spindles	5-10 min	50%		
Stage 3	Delta activity appears	10 min	10%-20%		Transition sleep
Stage 4	Delta activity predominates	5-15 min			Deep sleep; difficult to awaken
REM sleep	Desynchronized pattern of low-voltage beta activity—similar to waking EEG	10 min, first cycle; 10-12 min, second cycle; 20-30 min as length of total sleep increases	20%-25%	Dreams believed to occur	Physiologically active; paradoxical muscle movements, that is, rapid eye movements; increase in cerebral blood flow, brain temperature, and body oxygen consumption (most skeletal muscle tone depressed; tendon reflexes depressed)

*The sleeper, on falling asleep, goes through stages 1 through 4 and then returns to stage 3 and then to stage 2, followed by a period of REM sleep. Further sleep involves stages 2, 3, and sometimes 4, returning to stage 3 and then to stage 2 with another slightly longer REM period.

prived. Some investigators have reported, however, that loss of REM sleep is more likely to cause agitation and irritability, or in some persons, apathy and depression. Most clients report malaise or tiredness when the REM sleep period is shortened.

The EEG pattern may provide support to other data in differentiating such conditions as depression, narcolepsy, endocrine abnormality, or drug dependency.

■ Sleep patterns throughout the life cycle

Over the life cycle decrements are noted in the time spent in total sleep, in stage 4 sleep, and in REM sleep.

Sleep patterns in the young adult. The young, physically active and healthy adult spends 20% to 25% of sleep time in REM sleep, 50% in stage 2 sleep, and 5% to 10% in stage 1 sleep. The re-

maining 10% to 20% of sleep time is spent in a combination of stages 3 and 4 sleep (Fig. 6-2). Although most adults sleep 7 to 8 hours a day, many normal individuals sleep more than 9 hours, and another group of normal individuals sleep 6 hours or less in a 24-hour period. One study showed that the long sleepers had a high incidence of mild to moderate anxiety, depression, and social introversion, whereas the short sleepers were predominantly healthy, efficient, and energetic persons who tended to work hard or otherwise keep busy and who were satisfied with themselves and their lives.

Sleep patterns in the infant and child. The newborn infant spends 50% of his sleep time in REM sleep. By the age of 1 year, this is reduced to 20% to 30%, which is the adult value. Stage 4 sleep is greater in amount during childhood. Sleep cycles in the neonate are 45 to 60 minutes

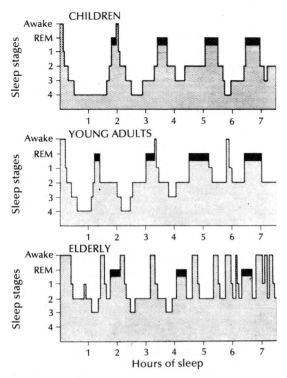

Fig. 6-2. Sleep cycles of normal subjects. The sleep of children and young adults shows early preponderance of stages 3 and 4, progressive lengthening of the first three REM periods, and infrequent awakenings. In elderly adults there is little or no stage 4 sleep, REM periods are fairly uniform in length, and awakenings are frequent and often lengthy. (From Kales, A.: Ann. Int. Med. **68,** 1078, 1968.)

in length and increase as the individual approaches maturity. The total sleep time for the normal newborn may be 14 to 18 hours a day.

Sleep patterns in the aged. "Nap most of the day; can't sleep at night," is a frequent description of the sleep of the elderly client. Stage 4 sleep is markedly decreased and sometimes absent in the aged adult. The total sleeping time is diminished as a result of frequent and prolonged waking periods.

Although REM sleep continues to occupy 20% to 25% of the total sleep time, REM latency at every period (the time from the onset of sleep to the first REM activity) is decreased, and the first REM period is longer. The EEG record may show poorly formed spindles that occur at a lower frequency. Insomniacs who are less than 50 years of age generally have difficulty in falling asleep; those over 50 complain of difficulty in staying asleep or of awakening early in the morning.

The sleep-deprived elderly client shows def-icits in both stage 4 and REM activity. A question to elicit a description of sleep pattern changes relevant to the aging process might be "Is your sleep the same as it has always been?"

BEHAVIORS AND/OR DISORDERS RELATED TO SLEEP
■ Effects of sleep deprivation

The affective description associated with sleep loss includes tiredness or fatigue, the sensation of a tight band around the head, and eye problems such as burning or heaviness of the eyelids.

Neurological changes associated with sleep loss have included muscle tremor, particularly of the hands; skeletal muscle weakness, such as neck flexion; lack of coordination of motor movements; dysarthria and decreased facial expressive movement; and decreased attention span. Prolonged sleep deprivation has been accompanied by visual distortion; the individual may see halos around light sources or cobwebs on the floor. The sleep-deprived individual may appear apathetic. The individual functions more poorly during the time that he would normally be asleep. The poorest performance of the sleep-deprived individual occurs in monotonous and prolonged tasks. Accurate assessment of functioning on short-term tasks is difficult, since these individuals appear capable of concentrating effectively for short periods of time.

Laboratory tests performed on sleep-deprived individuals show an increase in creatinine phosphokinase (CPK), glucose, and cortisol, whereas a decrease is seen in plasma iron and cholesterol.

The individual has an increased total sleep time following total sleep deprivation, with the increment reflected to stages 3 and 4. Although total REM sleep is increased in the first recovery night, the percentage of REM activity shows little actual change.

Most sleeping pills decrease REM sleep and, therefore, dreaming. Withdrawal of the medication is followed by an increase in REM sleep and dreaming.

Psychotropic drugs—or those which alter the function of the CNS—sedatives or tranquilizers, hypnotic antidepressants, and stimulants, have been observed to alter the course of sleep.

■ Night terrors and dream anxiety attacks

Two types of frightening dreams have been described as night terrors and dream anxiety attacks. Night terrors occur during slow-wave sleep and are accompanied by autonomic anxiety symptoms. Children who experience night terrors generally do not display daytime anxiety, whereas adults are likely to have anxiety symptoms. Dream anxiety attacks are the most common and are considered to be milder than night terrors. Autonomic anxiety signs may or may not accompany these episodes. Mental confusion frequently occurs, particularly if the sleeper is awakened suddenly.

■ **Primary sleep disorders**

Primary sleep disorders are those in which disordered sleep is the only symptom or sign of a problem. These disorders include sleeping periods in excess of and less than what is considered a normal sleeping period. Insomnia is the general term for a shortened sleeping period. Hypersomnia and narcolepsy are examples of conditions wherein the client sleeps longer than the normal individual.

Insomnia. The term insomnia includes the inability to fall asleep, frequent or prolonged awakening, or shortened sleep periods (early morning awakening).

EEG studies of insomniacs have shown the affected individuals to have longer sleep latencies, shorter sleep periods, and less efficient sleep. These individuals are believed to have greater levels of REM sleep than other persons.

Several subgroups of insomniacs have been cited based on the pattern of sleep loss. They are described as follows:

1. *Initial insomnia:* Inability to fall asleep, usually due to either rumination on situational stress, sleep phobia, or anxiety. Autonomic activity is higher during sleep in these persons as compared to the normal sleeper.

   The cause of sleep latency may be apparent from the history. Examples of questions that might reveal situational stress or anxiety as the cause of initial insomnia include: "How are things going at work?" "Have you had a lot of worries lately?" or "How are you getting on with your wife?" Initial insomnia is the most common type of sleep loss in young adults.

2. *Maintenance or intermittent insomnia:* Disruption of sleep occurring during midcycle due to a startle reaction from internal or external stimuli.

3. *Terminal insomnia:* Early awakening; may be due to aging or may be an important sign of depression; could also mean the person is napping during the day or retiring early.

4. *Imaginary insomnia:* Subjective insomnia; the person appears to have slept but claims he has not.

Insomniacs often show an improved sleeping pattern following a judicious increase in activity and exercise during the waking period. However, activity just before bedtime has an excitatory effect in most instances. A thorough assessment of a client who reports insomnia includes a description of his activities of daily living. It is important, particularly, to determine the amount and vigorousness of exercise subscribed to by the client who has difficulty sleeping.

Some investigators have suggested that most insomniacs have problems in sexual adjustment or functioning. The client's description of sexual activity is therefore assessed.

Hypersomnia. Hypersomnia is the term used to describe the condition wherein an individual has a tendency to sleep for excessive periods. In some clients the sleep period may be extended to 16 to 18 hours a day. The episodes of hypersomnia may be acute or chronic. The EEG sleep patterning is normal. Victims of hypersomnia are found to have higher pulse and respiratory rates than normal individuals both during sleep and wakefulness.

Perihypersomnia is a condition that is described as an increased need for sleep (18 to 20 hours a day) that lasts for only a few days, following which the client is fine.

Hypersomnia has been correlated with uremia, increased intracranial pressure, and diabetic acidosis. The hypothyroid client may report longer hours spent in sleep and sleepiness when awake.

In some cases hypersomnia may be a conversion symptom. The severely anxious client may be escaping discomfort in sleep. The hysterical personality and the depressed individual are predisposed to conversion symptoms. This mechanism should be looked for particularly when the need to sleep occurs repeatedly in conjunction with potentially troublesome experiences, such as "Whenever my mother-in-law comes for a visit."

Narcolepsy. Narcolepsy ("sleep attacks") is the term used to describe the uncontrolled onset of sleep. Although the pathophysiology of narcolepsy is not clearly understood, it is safe to say that the condition is a disorder in the sleep regulatory mechanism. The episode of sleep occurs when the client is engaged in what are considered to be work-time activities. Some 10% of diagnosed narcoleptics have described situations of falling asleep while driving and causing accidents. Others have fallen asleep in such unusual activities as standing at attention while in the military service or while eating. It is particularly important to be alert to the evidence that will establish the diagnosis so that treatment may be instituted, since the untreated narcoleptic is dangerous to himself and to others.

The episodes of involuntary sleep may begin just before puberty, that is, at approximately 12 years of age in girls and 14 years of age in boys. The range of age for the first attack may occur any time between 10 and 40, however. The familial involvement should be explored, since family members show an incidence of narcolepsy 20 times that of the general population.

Clinical records indicate that affected individuals may have the condition for as long as 15 years before it is diagnosed. This is particularly reprehensible since the attacks can be eliminated by amphetamines or methylphenidate (Ritalin) hydrochloride.

Because most normal people feel sleepy from time to time during the day, particularly at quiet times, such as during a dull lecture or television broadcast, a careful history is necessary to differentiate this dozing phenomenon from narcolepsy.

Automatism is sometimes reported by the narcoleptic victim's relatives. He appears to be awake but may act irrationally. The client does not remember the episode.

Diagnosed narcoleptics are observed to sleep fewer hours than their normal counterparts, and the sleep they do obtain is interrupted and restless. They fall asleep remarkably quickly, sometimes with 15 seconds after lying down and complain of difficulty in waking up.

Narcolepsy has been described as a tetrad of four symptoms: sleep attacks, cataplexy, hypnagogic hallucinations, and sleep paralysis. The final two symptoms occur in the transition period between sleep and wakefulness and are only indicative of narcolepsy when accompanied by the preceding symptoms.

Sleep attacks. The uncontrolled sleep in the early stages of the disorder occurs infrequently and under conditions that are described by normal people as sleep inducing. The episodes increase in number and occur in increasingly bizarre circumstances. Eventually the episodes occur 3 to 5 times a day, lasting 5 to 15 minutes. Some of these victims fall asleep without warning, whereas others feel sleepy for minutes or hours before succumbing to sleep.

Cataplexy. Approximately 4 to 5 years after the disorder is initiated, cataplexy may be experienced by the client. Cataplexy is abrupt weakness or paralysis of voluntary muscles and is seen predominantly in the muscles of the arms, legs, and face. There are many gradations of the loss of voluntary skeletal contraction. The episode may be experienced as only a fleeting weakness or as the inability to move quickly. On the other hand, all the skeletal muscles may be paralyzed. The intraocular muscles are a frequent exception. The client may still be capable of perceiving his external environment. He may describe the attacks as "My knees buckled," "My jaws sagged," "I couldn't speak," "The muscles of my neck were twitching," or "I couldn't walk."

The cataplectic attack may last from a half second to 10 minutes, and the client may experience them only once or twice a year or as often as 100 times a day. The attacks appear to be triggered by strong emotion, loud noise, a startle reaction, or sudden fright. Hearty laughter has frequently been implicated as a stimulus to the episodes.

Hypnagogic hallucinations. These attacks may be described as dream episodes. They are generally disturbing or frightening dreams that occur as the client is falling asleep. The client describes the dream as very real—"As if I were right there"—and the feeling as one of being awake. This can occur in the normal individual.

Sleep paralysis. The phenomenon of sleep paralysis is a skeletal muscle paralysis of varying degrees that occurs when the client awakes. The client describes the arousal as one of waking and being aware of external conditions but unable to move or speak. If undisturbed, the client recovers gradually. However, if he is stimulated, as by touching, paralysis ameliorates quickly. It must be borne in mind that sleep paralysis may occur in as many as 2% to 3% of the normal population.

Relation to REM sleep. Although narcolepsy has been linked to epilepsy in the past because of similar EEG patterning, it is not the same; nor can narcolepsy be logically attributed to depression or schizophrenia. More acceptable in the light of research findings is that narcolepsy is related to REM sleep. REM activity can be recorded during sleep attacks. The victim has a REM period at the beginning of his long sleep period. Some individuals with cataplexy experience REM sleep prior to recovery. Both hypnagogic hallucinations and sleep paralysis in normal individuals has been associated with REM activity.

■ Secondary sleep disorders

Secondary sleep disorders are those sleep disturbances that occur in individuals who have clinical disorders. Those clinical entities most often accompanied by sleep disorders are hypothyroidism, chronic renal insufficiency, depression, schizophrenia, alcoholism, and anorexia nervosa.

Hypothyroidism. The client who has hypothyroidism has a decrease in stages 3 and 4 sleep.

Chronic renal insufficiency. The client who undergoes dialysis treatments for chronic renal insufficiency has been observed to have sleep disturbances that occur with greatest frequency just before dialysis and are improved after the dialysis. Investigation has shown that sleep disturbances correlate with the uremic condition.

Depression. Depression is both a mental illness and a symptom. Depression is seen in the grieving process over significant loss or when things otherwise go badly. The depressed client has prolonged latency in achieving sleep, more rapid transition from stage to stage, more frequent awakening, less slow-wave sleep, less total sleep time, and more REM activity.

Depression as a mental illness is that which is incurred without significant loss. A subgroup of depressives is made up of those individuals who alternate between periods of depression and mania. The classical clinical description of the sleep pattern in depression is that or early morning awakening. Stage 4 sleep decreases in both manic and depressive clients. During the manic phase the client is observed to have decreased total sleep time and decreased REM activity. Depressed periods are associated with normal sleep time.

Schizophrenia. Some investigators have reported anorexia and a reduction in REM sleep in the early phases of schizophrenia. Stages 3 and 4 sleep are also significantly reduced in the schizophrenic. Greater eye movement has been reported in hallucinating schizophrenics than in nonhallucinating individuals.

Alcoholism. Studies have shown that the subject who has drunk 6 oz of 95% alcohol prior to sleep shows REM deprivation during his sleep period, whereas the person who drinks small amounts of alcohol may not show changes in his sleep pattern. The client who drinks three to four drinks a day may feel tremulous in the morning and "need" a drink to calm down. Because alcohol is a CNS depressant, it may help the client get to sleep; but because it is a short-acting drug, it does not affect sleep maintenance. Furthermore, it may diminish REM sleep in the early hours of the sleep period and therefore contribute to a rebound increase of REM activity in the latter hours of sleep. Withdrawal studies of chronic alcoholics showed that sleep periods were made up almost entirely of REM sleep. These alcoholics frequently awakened from REM to experience hallucinations.

Both slow-wave and REM sleep appear to be decreased in acute alcoholic psychosis. Initially, slow-wave activity appears to increase whereas REM sleep is suppressed. As the condition progresses both may disappear. As mentioned above, REM rebound has been employed as an explanation for the hallucinations that occur on withdrawal of alcohol. The rebound of slow-wave sleep has been cited as the harbinger of recovery from the psychosis.

Anorexia nervosa. The individual experiencing anorexia nervosa has a protein calorie deficiency that is accompanied by a patterned sleep disturbance. There is a reduction of the deeper sleep stages, 3 and 4, as well as of REM sleep. Although stage 1 sleep is increased, there is a reduction in total sleep time.

■ Parasomnias

Parsomnia is the term used for those patterns of waking behavior that appear during sleep. Some of those most common behaviors are somnambulism (sleepwalking), sleeptalking, bruxism (teeth grinding), nocturnal erection, and enuresis (bedwetting).

Somnambulism. Sleepwalking and night terrors occur more often in children than in adults. Furthermore, boys are affected more frequently than girls. Both of these conditions occur during stages 3 and 4 sleep. The sleepwalker may not awaken during the episode if he is active less than 3 to 4 minutes but will show an awakening pattern if he stays up longer. The somnambulist is amnesic for the episode whether he wakens spontaneously or is aroused by someone else. During ambulation the sleeper functions at a low level of awareness and critical skill.

Sleep talking. The articulation of words during sleep appears to be a frequent occurrence. Talking during sleep generally occurs during NREM sleep and during body movement.

Nocturnal erections. Nocturnal erections occur during REM sleep and are said to occur at a frequency of approximately 80% in young men. While there is considerable variation in the frequency of penile erection in men in their 70s, with some individuals showing a marked decrement in REM sleep erection, many of these older men maintain the young adult frequency to age 80. The penile circumference during REM sleep erection is markedly decreased as frequency wans. Frequently the client who is impotent in the awake state can achieve an erection during sleep. However, the erection abates soon after awakening.

Although clients may report that the sleep they obtain following sexual intercourse is more relaxed and restful, no significant changes in EEG patterning have been noted.

Bruxism. The grinding of the teeth during the sleep period, called bruxism, may occur in as many as 15% of the population. Evidence of the practice may be seen in damaged teeth or supporting structures. EEG studies demonstrate that bruxism generally is seen during stage 2 sleep.

Enuresis. Enuresis refers to bedwetting during sleep by an individual who has physiological control of micturition. This is primarily a disorder of childhood that is identified in 5 to 15 percent of all preadolescent children, and may have a familial pattern. Enuresis has been observed to exist in some sample adult groups at a rate of 1% or 2%.

Enuresis occurs more frequently in boys than in girls. Research has demonstrated more frequent bladder contractions and greater heart rate during the entire sleep period of those individuals affected. The episode of bedwetting occurs during slow-wave sleep. Whereas primary enuresis may be the result of a pathophysiological defect, secondary enuresis may be reflected to psychological factors.

In assessing the enuretic child, one should explore the affective state surrounding this condition with both the child and his parents. Although data from sleep laboratories demonstrate that 90% of enuretic children are asleep when bedwetting occurs, in most cases studied the parents believed that the child had control over the occurrence. The parents punished the child, producing shame, embarrassment, guilt, or anxiety. To investigate how the episodes have been dealt with, the following questions might be used.

To the parents: "How have you felt about your child's wetting the bed?" If this question is nonproductive, more specific information might be gained by asking, "Do you feel he (she) could prevent the bedwetting?" or "Do you punish him (her) when he (she) wets the bed?"

To the child: "How do you feel when you wake up after wetting the bed?"

■ Sleep-provoked disorders: sleep patterns in chronic illness

The sleep-provoked disorders include symptoms and signs of chronic clinical diseases that are elicited during sleep.

Pain. Clients who experience chronic pain may complain of "tossing and turning all night." These clients awaken frequently and stay awake for long periods of time. What has been shown through observation of individuals with angina pectoris is that they tend to underestimate their actual number of movements. Clients with angina experience pain during REM sleep. On awakening they may or may not report an upsetting dream. A direct cause-and-effect relationship has not been established.

Duodenal ulcer. Clients with duodenal ulcer often awaken in the night and complain of epigastric pain, which is relieved by food or antacid. It has been shown that these incidents are correlated with an increased secretion of gastric hydrochloric acid, particularly related to REM sleep; normal subjects studied did not demonstrate this increase in secretion.

Cardiovascular symptoms. The pain of myocardial ischemia frequently accompanies REM sleep. Observations of patients with myocardial infarctions have shown that premature ventricular contractions (PVCs) are increased during or immediately following REM sleep. The horizontal position generally assumed during sleep results in an increased plasma volume as gravity

Table 6-3. Clinical observations associated with stages of sleep

Stage of sleep	Associated clinical condition
NREM sleep	
All stages	Enuresis—most episodes occur
	Bronchial asthma—except stage 4
Stage 2	Bruxism
Stage 4	Night terrors
	Sleep walking
	Hypothyroidism—metabolic rate most depressed
REM sleep	Sleep talking
	Nocturnal erection and emission
	Duodenal ulcer
	Migraine headaches
	Gastric acid secretion increased
	Coronary atherosclerosis, ECG changes, and anginal attacks increased
	Bronchial asthma attacks in children

effects on the fluid compartments are obviated. The increased cardiac onput may lead to left ventricular failure, resulting in pulmonary edema and dyspnea. Because many of the manifestations of heart disease do occur during the sleep period, many clients express a fear of going to sleep. This is particularly true of the client with angina pectoris or cardiac arrhythmia.

Respiratory alterations. Clients with emphysema have increased carbon dioxide tension and decreased oxygen saturation during sleep.

Children with asthma have been shown to have a decreased amount of stage 4 sleep as compared to normal children. In children asthmatic attacks originate in the late part of the sleep period, when the child is not in stage 4 sleep. In adults they may occur in any sleep stage.

Asthmatics frequently have bronchial spasm during REM sleep periods.

Metabolic disorders. Individuals with diabetes mellitus have been shown to have variable levels of blood glucose during the sleep period.

Rheumatoid arthritis. Early morning stiffness is a frequent symptom of the victim of rheumatoid arthritis.

Migraine headaches. Individuals with migraine headaches and with cluster headaches who suffered severe headache on awakening were monitored by EEG, which showed that the headache began during REM sleep.

ASSESSMENT OF SLEEP HABITS

In most cases it is more productive to allow the client to describe his sleep habits in his own words. An open-ended question may provide the stimulus to the client to give all the information pertinent to assessment. Examples of such questions are:

"How have you been sleeping?"
"Can you tell me about your sleeping habits?"
"Are you getting enough rest?"
"Tell me about your sleep problem."

There are times when the practitioner will have to ask more specific questions to understand the client's sleep habits. The suggested questions (see upper right column and p. 87) may serve as a guide for this assessment. Only those questions need be used that will elicit the information not given by the more general query.

A technique that might more clearly define the sleep-activity cycle of the client is to provide him with a graph form on which to record his hours of sleep. He should be encouraged to keep

Aspects of sleep pattern	Questions to elicit sleep pattern
Time retired	"What time do you usually go to bed?"
Initial insomnia	"Do you fall asleep right away?" "How long does it take you to fall asleep?" "How often do you have trouble falling asleep? Does it occur every night? Every other night? Just the weekend? Every Monday?" "How do you feel before you fall asleep?"
Maintenance insomnia	"Do you wake up in the night? How often does this occur?" "What wakes you up once you have fallen asleep? Is there something that helps you get back to sleep?"
Arousal terminal insomnia	"What time do you wake up? How often do you get up this early? What wakes you up at this early hour?" "What do you do once you wake up?"
Quality of sleep (affective response)	"How do you feel when you get up?" "Do you feel rested after a night's sleep?"
Dreams, night terrors	"Do you dream at night?" "Are your dreams ever frightening?" "Do your dreams ever wake you?" "How do you feel when you wake up from a bad dream?"
Bruxism	"Has anyone ever told you that you grind your teeth in your sleep?"
Somnambulism	"Has anyone ever told you that you walk in your sleep?" "Have you ever awakened in some place different than the one in which you went to sleep?" "Have you ever awakened to find furniture or other objects moved around in your home?"

Continued.

a record over a long enough period that the pattern is well demonstrated on the graph.

He might be taught to color code his various activities in order to give the examiner as well as himself a clearer picture of his circadian rhythm. Even a simple written daily record of the sleep-activity cycle may prove helpful. At any rate, a diary of several day's sleep-activity cycles will allow the examiner a broader data base from which to advise the client.

The medication the client has been taking must be assessed. Cases of insomnia due to drug interaction have been recorded, and many drugs currently prescribed for induction of sleep may change the EEG activity pattern. Some of these changes are summarized in Table 6-4. The drugs listed in this table should be given particular attention in assessing the client's sleep pattern.

Aspects of sleep pattern	Questions to elicit sleep pattern—cont'd
Daytime activity-work pattern	"What kind of work do you do?"
Recreation, exercise	"What kind of activity is involved?" "What do you do for fun?" "Are you engaged in any exercise?"
Home responsibilities	"Do you work at home? What kind of work do you do at home?"
Sleeping environment	
Bedding (mattress, pillows, blankets)	"Do you need any special bedding to help you sleep?" "How many pillows do you use?"
Light	"Do you sleep with the lights off?" "Does having a light on at night bother you?"
Noise	"Do you have to have it very quiet to sleep?" "Do noises keep you awake at night? Wake you up?"
Ventilation	"Do you open the window at night?"
Temperature	"Do you need the bedroom to be cold [warm] in order to sleep well?"
Special activities associated with sleep	
Bath, massage	"What do you do just before going to bed?"

Aspects of sleep pattern	Questions to elicit sleep pattern—cont'd
Food	"Do you eat before you go to bed?" "Do you like to have a snack before bed?"
Drink (warm milk, water)	"Do you like a drink before going to bed?" "What do you prefer as your bedtime beverage?"
Medication	"Do you take any medicine to help you sleep?" "Are you taking any medicine at all?"
Personal beliefs about sleep	"How much sleep do you think you should have to stay healthy?" "What will happen if you don't get enough sleep?"
Internal stimuli	"How does the way you sleep affect your family?"
Psychiatric disorders (anxiety, depression, schizophrenia)	"How have your spirits been?" "Have you had a lot of worries lately?"
Alteration due to physical condition (stimulus, electrolyte imbalance)	"How have you been sleeping?"

Table 6-4. Effects of pharmaceutical agents on the sleep cycle

Decrease time		Increase time		Allow normal time	
Drug	**Dosage**	**Drug**	**Dosage**	**Drug**	**Dosage**
REM sleep					
Placidyl	500 mg	Reserpine	1-2 mg	Chloral hydrate	0.5 gm
Doriden	500 mg	LSD	30 μg		1.0 gm
Seconal	100 mg				1.5 gm
Phenobarbital	200 mg				
Nembutal	100 mg			Dalmane	15-30 mg
Quaalude	300 mg			Quaalude	150 mg
Benadryl	50 mg			Librium	50-100 mg
Scopolamine	0.006 mg/kg			Valium	5-10 mg
Morphine				Caffeine	
Heroin					
Alcohol	1 gm/kg				
Tofranil	50 mg				
Elavil	50-75 mg				
Miltown	1,200 mg				
Amphetamine	15 mg				
Stage 4 sleep					
Doriden	500 mg	Antidepressants in the presence of depression			
Nembutal	100 mg				
Valium	10 mg				
Reserpine	0.14 mg/kg				
Chloral hydrate	1.5 gm				

BIBLIOGRAPHY

Aschoff, J.: Circadian systems in man and their implications, Hosp. Pract. 11:51, 1976.

Aschoff, J., Hoffmann, K., Pohl, H., and others: Reentrainment of circadian rhythms after phase-shifts of the zeitgeber, Chronobiologica 2:22, 1975.

Baker, R. M., Kales, A., Kallman, H., and others: Lots of things you should know (and probably were never taught) about sleep, Patient Care 4:24, 1970.

Brown, C. C., Hartmann, E. L., Usdin, G. L., and others: Sleep disorders; help for the patient who can't sleep, Patient Care 4:24, 1970.

Brown, F. A.: The "clocks" timing biological rhythms, Am. Sci. 60:756, 1972.

Bünning, E.: The physiological clock, London, 1973, The English Universities Press Ltd.

Conroy, R. T., and Mills, J. N.: Human circadian rhythms, London, 1970, J. and A. Churchill.

Folk, G. E.: Biological rhythms. In Folk, G. E., editor: Textbook of environmental physiology, Philadelphia, 1974, Lea & Febiger.

Freemon, F. R.: Sleep research: a critical review, Springfield, Ill., 1972, Charles C Thomas, Publisher.

Hartmann, E. L.: The functions of sleep, New Haven, 1973, Yale University Press.

Kales, A., editor: Sleep physiology and pathology, Philadelphia, 1969, J. B. Lippincott Co.

Kales, A., Beall, G. N., Berger, R. J., and others: Sleep and dreams; recent research on clinical aspects, Ann. Int. Med. 68:1078, 1968.

Kales, A., and Kales, J.: Sleep disorders, New Engl. J. Med. 290:487, 1974.

Kales, J. D.: Aging and sleep. In Goldmann, R., and Rockstein, M., editors: Physiology and pathology of human aging, New York, 1975, Academic Press, Inc.

Kiester, E., Jr.: I keep falling asleep; what's wrong with me? Today's Health 54:40, 1976.

Luce, G. C.: Biological rhythms in psychiatry and medicine, U.S. Department of Health, Education, and Welfare, National Institute of Mental Health, Public Health Service Publ. No. 2088, 1970, U.S. Government Printing Office.

Rechtschaffen, A., and Kales, A.: A manual of standardized terminology, techniques and scoring for sleep stages in human subjects (National Institute of Health Publ. No. 204), Washington, D.C., 1968, U.S. Government Printing Office.

Sollberger, A., Biological rhythm research, New York, 1965, Elsevier Publishing Co.

Usdin, G., editor: Sleep research and clinical practice, New York, 1973, Brunner/Mazel, Inc.

Webb, W.: Sleep; an experimental approach, New York, 1968, Macmillan Inc.

Wever, R.: Internal phase-angle differences in human circadian rhythms; causes for changes and problems of determinations, Int. J. Chronobiol. 1:371, 1973.

Williams, R. L., Karacan, I., and Hursch, C. J.: Electroencephalography (EEG) of human sleep; clinical applications, New York, 1974, John Wiley & Sons, Inc.

7 General assessment

THE SURVEY OR GENERAL INSPECTION

The survey or general inspection begins with those observations made of the client as he enters the room, during introductions, and as he follows instructions for seating before the interview begins. It is the overall impression of the client's general state of health and outstanding characteristics.

In some cases this initial looking over sets the focus of the interview and of the physical examination. For instance, some feature of the client's appearance may point immediately to his problem; sparse, fine hair, for example, may indicate the need to look further for the edema, the slow speech, the hoarse voice, and the sluggish movement of the hypothyroid individual.

There are certain characteristics that typically are noted in this section of the physical examination record: apparent age; sex; race; body type (constitution), stature, and symmetry; weight and nutritional status; posture and motor activity; mental status; speech; general skin condition; apparent state of health and signs of distress or disorder. These are factors that are not limited to a single system of the body but are instead parameters for the total or whole person—the general appearance.

The examiner observes thoroughly and discerningly. Many professionals experience some difficulty in gazing at the client without doing some task simultaneously. However, total absorption in the process of looking and perceiving must be achieved.

The practitioner perceives only that which he has prepared himself to attend to. Therefore, a plan should be kept in mind for the stimuli that should be perceived, associated, and responded to by the practitioner. Although the term inspection implies restriction to the visual stimuli, the examination may include smell, hearing, and touch, as well. In general, the survey proceeds in a cephalocaudal direction. The general observations continue throughout the interview.

An example of the record of the general survey might read:

Mr. A. is an alert, loquacious, asthenic 25-year-old white male who appears younger than his stated age and exhibits no indication of distress. He does not appear acutely or chronically ill.

Accurate observations can only be made in good light. This is particularly important in assessing skin color.

Although this initial survey may be considered a scanning procedure, the highlights gathered by the astute practitioner may be used as the basis for establishing the client's problem list.

■ The client as a whole

The general impression of wellness should be assessed. Historically, health and illness have been defined as opposites. For instance, the World Health Organization has defined health as "a state of complete physical, mental, and social well-being and not merely the absence of disease." By implication, any other condition is defined as illness. More recently, health and illness have been described in terms of a continuum. This conceptualization expresses the philosophy that the human being is never in a state of absolute wellness, or non-illness; that the person, in fact, varies from conditions of high-level wellness to markedly poor health, close to death. Illness is considered to exist when there is a disturbance or failure in either the biophysical or psychosocial function or development, so that observable (signs) or felt (symptoms) changes in the body are present. Mental or emotional illness is said to exist when the individual demonstrates inappropriate or inadequate behavior in a given social context.

Some terse but typical kinds of descriptions that have appeared as survey summaries are:

He appears acutely ill.
He appears chronically ill.
He appears frail.

The supporting documentation for these general terms makes the description more meaningful. For instance, the description of *chronically ill* might include terms such as *cachectic* or *dehydrated,* or other, more descriptive terms.

The practitioner should be aware of signs of distress in the patient. Detection of distress may predicate dealing with the underlying problem immediately and curtailing the full interview and physical examination for the present. Some of the signs that might require intervention are (1) anxiety that may be indicated by anxious or tense facies, fidgety movements, and cold, moist palms; (2) pain that may be indicated by drawn features, moaning, writhing, or guarding of the painful part; or (3) cardiopulmonary distress that may be signaled by labored breathing, wheezing, or coughing. Since the color of the skin is determined by the amount of oxygen-carrying hemoglobin and by the constriction or dilatation of the capillary beds, cyanosis and pallor are excellent indications of cardiopulmonary distress.

■ Body type and stature

A concise description of the client's bodily proportions should be included in the written record of the general survey.

Normal body types

Although the constitution is to some degree genetically determined in the sense that the endocrine control is inherited, the environment may play a significant role in altering the physiognomy. Several normal body types (constitutions) have been described by Draper, Dupertuis, and Caughey.

Sthenic type. The sthenic constitution is one of average height, well-developed musculature, wide shoulders with a subcostal angle that is approximately a right angle, and a flat abdomen. The most frequently observed type of face is ovoid in shape, and the dental arch is round and wide.

Hypersthenic type. The hypersthenic body build is short and stocky and the most likely of the body types to be obese. The chest is shorter and broader than is the sthenic build. The costal margin is a wider angle (obtuse). The heart is likely to lie in a transverse position. The abdominal wall is thicker than in the sthenic constitution. Roentgenographic examination reveals the stomach to be higher in the abdomen and more or less in a transverse configuration. The face is more rectangular in shape, as is the dental arch.

Hyposthenic type. The hyposthenic body build is often characterized as tall and willowy. The musculature is poorly developed. The subcostal angle is more acute than in the sthenic type. The chest is long and flat, with the heart in a more midline and vertical position. Since abdominal muscles are not as well developed, the abdominal wall may sag outward. The stomach is observed to be lower in the abdomen and more vertical in position. The neck is long. The face is triangular in shape (narrower and more pointed), as is the dental arch.

Asthenic type. The asthenic body build is an exaggeration of the hyposthenic constitution.

Gross abnormalities in body build

Marfan's syndrome. Elongated arms and limbs as compared to the trunk may indicate hypogonadism, or Marfan's syndrome.

Two rules of thumb that have been suggested in comparing body parts for appropriate development are (1) the distance from fingertip to fingertip of outstretched arms should equal the height; and (2) the distance from the crown to the pubic symphysis should roughly equal the distance from the pubic symphysis to the sole. Normally the ratio of the upper segment measurement to that of the lower segment is about 0.92 in whites and 0.85 in blacks.

In Marfan's syndrome, an inherited generalized disorder of connective tissue, the tubular bones are elongated and the ratio is lower. In addition, the arm span exceeds the height.

Hyposomatotropism. Dwarfism is the general term that has been used to mean an abnormally small person who has normal body proportions. Achondroplastic dwarfism refers to that individual who has abnormally small limbs but a normal-size trunk and head. This is the result of a disorder of cartilagenous growth.

Pituitary hyposomatic dwarfism. Pituitary dwarfism is the consequence of hyposecretion of growth hormone (GH). That deficiency in GH has little effect over fetal growth is evidenced by the relatively normal size at birth of babies who have no pituitary gland. However, the length at birth of the infant with hyposecretion of GH is less than that of the normal infant. The rate of growth declines in the first months of life and may be noticeable by the sixth month but more frequently is diagnosed between the age of around 3 years, at which time physical growth is half that of normal. However, because the epiphyseal closure is retarded, growth continues into the 40s and 50s, ending at the height of 4 or 5 feet. General health is maintained, and normal immune mechanisms are present. Mental development is usually normal for the chronological age. Males are affected twice as often as females. Many of the children appear obese, with adipose depositions over the iliac crest and lower abdomen. The eruption of secondary teeth is late. In adult life these dwarfs often develop wrinkles about the eyes and mouth and appear prematurely old.

Laron dwarfism. Laron dwarfism is a genetically transmitted (mendelian recessive) form of dwarfism that occurs in Orientals, Jews, and other Middle Eastern peoples. The condition is characterized by high levels of GH and low levels of somatomedin (SF), though metabolic response to GH hormones is subnormal.

Failure to thrive. Growth failure occurs in some children who suffer parental neglect or deprivation of love and affection. These children are characterized by distortions of appetite-feeding patterns and by the eating of food not usually considered nourishing or edible (pica). Bloating may be present, and clinical symptoms like those of malabsorption may be present.

Growth failure can follow any serious illness or nutritional deficiency in childhood. Prolonged corticosteroid therapy has been associated with early epiphyseal closure and growth lag. Some of the diseases associated with growth failure are Laurence-Moon Biedl syndrome, mongolism, achondroplasia, neurofibromatosis, severe congenital heart disease, congenital hemolytic anemia, and progeria.

African pigmy. The condition known as *African pigmy* is polygenically transmitted and is characterized by resistance to both GH and SF.

Hypothyroidism. Hypothyroidism, beginning in infancy, is called cretinism and is characterized by retarded bone maturation and multiple abnormal areas of epiphyseal ossification. Juvenile myxedema is also a cause of retarded growth.

Gonadal dysfunction. Gonadal dysplasia should be suspected in short girls with primary amenorrhea and congenital anomalies such as webbing of the neck, short metacarpal or metatarsal bones, or increased carrying angle of

the elbows (a cytological examination should be done for X chromosome defect).

Hypersomatotropism. Hypersomatotropism is characterized by abnormally enhanced secretion of GH.

Gigantism. The hypersecretion of GH occurring before puberty and prior to the ossification of the epiphyseal plates causes overgrowth of the long bones and gigantism results. The length of time of long-bone growth is also lengthened, since the gonadal secretion is depressed.

Acromegaly. Acromegaly is a disease caused by hypersecretion of GH; it is evidenced clinically in the fourth or fifth decade. In most instances growth of the acral (small) parts proceeds so slowly that their appreciation may not occur until the changes are well advanced. Bony and soft tissue growth is apparent clinically. Bony changes in the skull are most apparent. The mandible is increased in length and width. Prognathism or overbite of the lower incisors beyond the upper incisors by as much as a half inch is a characteristic of acromegaly. There is little increase in height since the epiphyseal plates have closed. The teeth become separated as the jaw elongates. The features are exaggerated due to the expansion of the facial, molar, and frontal bones. The skull itself, as well as the sinuses, may be markedly enlarged. However, in some individuals only a single feature appears grossly enlarged, such as the jaw of the supraorbital ridge. Arthralgia and arthritis are commonly present in acromegaly.

With the increased total mass of connective tissue that occurs concomitantly with retention of interstitial fluid, the skin appears coarse and leathery and the pores and markings of the skin appear enlarged. In addition, the hands are large with broad fingers and wide palms, thereby earning the description "spade hand." The tongue is frequently enlarged and furrowed. The body hair is coarse and increased in amount. On physical examination both cardiomegaly and hepatomegaly may be found.

Symmetry

The arrangement of most structures of the human body is symmetrical, that is, there is a correspondence in size and shape of parts. Inspection for obvious areas of lack of symmetry that can be investigated later should be performed in the survey.

Weight

The patient should be weighed and his height measured in order to compare these parameters to actuarial tables prepared by insurance companies of average weights and heights (refer to Tables 5-7 and 5-8).

Patterns of adiposity are described here in order that the typical fat deposits of obesity may be differentiated from those of disease states.

A sex difference is apparent in adipose deposition. Women are observed to have fat deposits over the shoulders, breasts, buttocks or lateral aspect of the thighs, and pubic symphysis. The fat deposits in men are more evenly dispersed throughout the body.

The fat deposition that is characteristic of Cushing's syndrome (hyperadrenalism) or administration of the glucocorticoid hormone is found in the facial, nuchal, truncal, and girdle areas. This kind of obesity has been termed centripetal or "buffalo" obesity.

In addition to fat deposition patterns, the following differences between simple obesity and Cushing's syndrome may be helpful in establishing the diagnosis:

Obesity	Cushing's syndrome
Thick skin	Thin skin
Pale striae	Purplish striae
Absence of plethora	Plethora
Preservation of muscle strength	Protein wasting resulting in muscle weakness
No evidence of osteoporosis	Evidence of osteoporosis

Growth is arrested in Cushing's syndrome; therefore, the obese child who is growing rapidly probably does not have this disease.

It is well to remember that the increased serum levels of the glucocorticoids may be due to delayed metabolism of these hormones by the liver or to increased production of estrogen.

■ Apparent age

There is great disparity in the apparent age of individuals at the same chronological age. These differences arise as a result of such influences as heredity, sex, past medical history, and life experiences.

Physical changes that have been associated with the aging process are elevations in blood pressure, decreased cardiac output and stroke volume, as well as lessened pulmonary reserve. However, those changes, like the "aches and pains" of old age, may be preventable or at least treatable with judicious exercise and hormone replacement. The kyphosis in women that once indicated the presence of osteoporosis may be

prevented with postmenopausal hormones and calcium balancing through diet and medication.

There are some indications that may help the practitioner in estimating the apparent age. Elastic fibers in the corium of the skin decline in number with advancing age. As the individual advances in age, the skin loses turgor, that is, its ability to return to its normal contour when released after being picked up between the examiner's fingers. The skin appears dull, moves less readily, sags, and wrinkles. These changes are noticeable in middle age and are first observable in the anterior neck and chin.

Hair begins to decline in amount in the middle years as the sex hormones decrease in amount.

Progeria is the term for premature senility occurring in childhood. The stature is small; the face looks old and wizened; the skin is dry and thin, and the hair is scanty; sexual organs are infantile.

Precocious puberty is the term for premature maturation of the gonads accompanied by secondary sexual characteristics.

■ Posture

The practitioner should develop a protocol for accurately observing the main postures of the body in all its common acts. Beginning observations are made by watching the client come into the room and seat himself and by observing the client while he is lying on the examining table. It is important to note whether the client sits tensely or slumps in the chair. Rigid positioning of the neck may be due to a fixated spine. Respiratory distress may result when the patient tries to lie flat. Hyperextension of the neck and muscular rigidity may indicate meningitis. Leaning to one side may be due to a fractured rib. Carcinoma of the tail of the pancreas may result in complaints of pain over the lower thoracic spine when the client is asked to lie flat.

■ Gait

The characteristics of the client's walk often provide clues to the pathophysiology involved in the client's problems. The client with a disorder in gait should be observed for his natural stance and for the attitude and dominant positions of the trunk, legs, and arms. The patient may be asked to walk a straight line. The rapidity or slowness of step may be noteworthy, as well as the style of movement. Table 7-1 presents various types of gait that are readily recognized.

Table 7-1. Diagnostic patterns of gait

Form	Description	Associated disorders
Spastic	Leg held stiffly—does not flex freely; jerking movements, poorly coordinated	Multiple sclerosis; syringomyelia; cerebral spastic diplegia
Scissors	Spasticity of adductor muscles of legs with legs held close together	Spastic paraplegia; paresis; cerebral palsy (choreoathetosis)
Sensory atactic	Uncertainty, irregularity, and stamping of feet	Interruption of afferent fibers for proprioception
Atactic	Staggering, reeling, steps uncertain; some shorter or longer than intended; may lurch to one side	Acute disease of cerebellum, cerebellar tracts of brain; severe alcohol and barbiturate intoxication
Slapping	Walks on broad base with feet wide apart; raises foot abnormally high—slapping noises as foot strikes floor; eyes on floor to observe where to place foot	Peripheral nerve disease; paralysis of pretibial and peroneal muscles; posterior column disease, tertiary syphilis
Foot dragging	Affected foot dragged in semicircle with toes outward; arms on affected side held rigidly against chest wall	Hemiplegia and paraplegia
Festinating	Body rigid, trunk bent forward—flexion; short, mincing steps barely clear ground—shuffling; arms carried ahead of body—do not swing; may make sudden hastening forward movement (propulsion) or backward movement (retropulsion)	Parkinsonism
Waddling or rolling	Steps regular, but uncertain; often lumbar lordosis, exaggerated elevation of one hip, depression of the other	Muscular dystrophy

■ Body movements

Bodily movements are observed for tremor occurring at rest or stimulated by voluntary movement. The amplitude of tremor or involuntary movement may be fine or coarse and may be confined to a single muscle or be generalized to the entire body. Examples of generalized involvement of skeletal muscles in involuntary contraction include the convulsive movements of epilepsy and the choreiform movements of Huntington's chorea. Asymmetry of body movement frequently occurs with damage to the central nervous system or with peripheral nerve damage.

■ Hair and hair growth patterns

Inspection for hair growth is made on the following body regions: scalp, beard, mustache, ears, hypogastric area, thoracic area, lower limbs, genital area, lumbosacral area, upper back, midphalangeal area, pubis, and axillae.

The hair is assessed for growth characteristics, distribution, density of growth, appearance, and hygiene.

In the present evolutionary state of *Homo sapiens*, hair growth patterns have a great deal of social value. Whereas in lower animals the

skin covering of hair may afford warmth and protection of exposed body parts from friction during motion, in man hair serves a decorative function.

Hair growth is influenced by hereditary and racial factors. Excessive hairiness is thought to be a dominant hereditary trait in the presence of androgens, whereas thinning or absence of hair is a recessive trait.

Although hair growth is continuous in some animals, in most animals, including man, hair growth is cyclic. Hair growth occurs in what is known as an anagen phase; it then enters a telogen, or resting, phase before it is pushed out and new hair grows in the follicle.

The anagen phase may continue for years in areas such as the scalp. This long phase of growth contributes to longer hairs. Pubic hair, on the other hand, grows for only a few months.

Hair growth can be described in terms of cycle, rate of growth, size, and density.

Hair grows at various rates. The most rapid rate of growth is that of the beard, followed by that of the scalp, axillae, thighs, and eyebrows. Long hairs regenerate most rapidly. In the male, more rapid regrowth is noted in scalp hair than for the female, but regrowth is slower in the axillae and on the thighs.

The rate of hair growth is affected by environmental temperature as well as by the general state of health. Extremely cold temperatures such as that experienced in the Antarctic impede hair growth, whereas hot climates appear to promote increased length.

General protein production is inhibited in starvation, and this is reflected in reduced hair growth and dullness in appearance. Chemotherapeutic drugs inhibit cell division and thereby inhibit hair growth. X-ray radiation causes hair to switch to the telogen phase as well as atrophy of perifollicular structures, resulting in hair loss.

White persons have more abundant and coarser bodily hair growth than do Asians. Facial hirsutism has been described for more than 40% of white women. Japanese women, on the other hand, do not develop excessive facial hair growth; and Japanese men have sparser beards than do white men. Blacks have kinky hair, whereas whites have straight or wavy to curly hair, and Mongolians and American Indians have straight hair.

A heavier distribution of hair is correlated with darker skin pigmentation (coloring); that is, the brunette individual is more likely to have more hair than the blonde person.

Some male hair growth characteristics may be normal for women of certain ethnic or familial groups, for instance, hair growth on the upper lip; sideburns; and hair growth on the intermammary periareolar area, abdomen, and lower limbs.

Because of the variations in hair growth patterns among individuals, it is more important to note marked changes in hair growth characteristics. Hair growth increases in normal sites have been associated with adrenal tumors.

Hair has been classified into three categories: primary, secondary, and terminal hair. Primary hair is the very fine, thinly pigmented short hair of the fetus. Secondary hair resembles primary hair structurally but appears postnatally. This secondary hair is generally distributed over the body and is the hair type involved in hypertrichosis. This hair is often termed lanuginous or vellus and is not hormonally influenced. Terminal hair is a coarser and more heavily pigmented growth that appears at the time of puberty. Axillary and pubic terminal hair is called ambosexual hair. Adrenal hormones initiate the growth of this coarse hair, which is also influenced by ovarian and testicular hormones. True sexual hair is that

Table 7-2. Morphological hair types in humans

Growth site	Description	Length
Head	Relatively small root; tapered tip; many variations	1,000 mm
Eyebrow and eyelash	Curved; smooth; coarse; punctate tip	10 mm
Beard and mustache	Relatively longer root than scalp hair; blunt tip	300 mm
Body	Fine; long tip	Up to 60 mm
Pubic	Coarse; irregular; asymmetrical; usually curved but may be spiral tufted	Up to 60 mm
Axillary	Coarse; straighter than pubic hair; may be spiral tufted in blacks	Up to 50 mm

which grows on the face, chest, abdomen, back, and extremities.

The hair may also be classified by the types of hormonal influences the growth receives:

1. Hair dependent on GH is that which grows on the head, eyelashes, eyebrows, midphalangeal area, distal portions of limbs, and to some extent, on the lumbosacral area.

2. Hair dependent on female hormones is that which grows on the pubic area, axillary limbs, and hypogastric area. The male hypogastric or pubic hair configuration is that of a diamond with its superior angle at the umbilicus, whereas the female pubic hair pattern is triangular with the base over the mons.

3. Hair dependent on male hormones is that of the beard, mustache, nasal tip, and ear, and body hair (particularly on the back).

Morphological characteristics of the hair found in various anatomical sites are described in Table 7-2.

Hirsutism. Hirsutism, the appearance of excessive hair in normal and abnormal sites, can be most disturbing to the affected female client. The degree of overgrowth need not be marked to pose a threat to the client's feelings of femininity.

On noting hirsutism in the female client, the examiner is alerted to note the presence of other virilizing signs, which include a deepening of the voice, clitoral enlargement, and changes in fat distribution.

Table 7-3. Classification of hirsutism

Stage	Site	Quantity, quality*
1	Languous hair Not in virilizing sites	D_1Q_1
2	Coarser hair in men Distribution sites: Upper lips Sideburns Intermammary area Periareolar area Midabdomen	D_1Q_2
3	Same sites as stage 2, as well as: Upper back Shoulders Inner thighs Ears, nose Supragluteal and gluteal areas Temporal recession	D_2Q_2 to D_3Q_3
4	Same sites as stage 3; in addition shows other signs of virilization	D_3Q_3

*D, quantity: D_1, mild; D_2, moderate; D_3, profuse. Q, quality: Q_1, fine; Q_2, coarse; Q_3, very coarse.

Hirsutism has been observed in the following pathophysiological conditions: bilateral polycystic ovary, Cushing's syndrome, and ovarian tumor.

Because of the identity confusion that may exist in the presence of hirsutism, the examiner approaches the investigation of the problem with sensitively phrased queries.

Description of the hirsute condition may be facilitated by Table 7-3.

Balding. Balding (alopecia) is more frequently noted in those individuals with abundant growth of coarse, or terminal, hair on the body and is thought to be related to testosterone production.

Generally, the man with a hairline that is low in the forehead does not bald. As a rule, women do not bald unless androgens are present in relatively increased amounts or the baldness occurs secondary to another disease.

■ **Odors**

The odor of the body and breath should be noted. The smell of alcohol on the client's breath alerts one to look for other effects of this CNS depressant. The fruity odor of acetone indicates that diabetes and starvation must be ruled out, whereas a fetid breath points to the possibility of an oral or pulmonary infection or may simply be the result of poor oral hygiene. The odor of ammonia may be detectable in the patient with uremia. Body odor may be related to the activities of the sweat and sebaceous glands and to the general cleanliness of the body.

■ **Nails**

The nails may be an indication of the level of concern and care the person has for his appearance. The nails are inspected with reference to the length, cleanliness, neatness of filing, and if a woman, the presence and condition of polish. The examiner further notes the texture recording thickness and ridging when present.

■ **Personal hygiene**

General cleanliness of the body is an important indication of the individual's self esteem and of the availability of necessary supplies to maintain good body care. Again, this is a socioculturally flavored value. It is important to note that deodorants are not used in all cultures. Although shaving of the legs is a norm in the United States, it is not done in India.

■ **Manner of dress**

The fit of the clothing should be noted, as well as the attendance to current style. In addition, the general cleanliness and press of clothing may provide further clues to the cultural or socioeconomic status, as well as to the ego strength of the individual. The unshaven or unwashed signs of neglect by relatives or others for the dependent client or of self-neglect should be carefully noted.

■ **Speech**

The manner of speech is the cornerstone to diagnosis of both emotional and physical illness. The characteristics that should be noted include:

1. *Pace:* A fast or rapid-fire manner of delivery may indicate hyperthyroidism, whereas slow speech and a thick, hoarse voice are typical of hypothyroidism.
2. *Clarity:* The ability to enunciate clearly may be lost in motor nerve disease of the tongue, jaws, or lips. Slurred speech can result from CNS damage.
3. *Vocabulary:* The choice of words may indicate the level of education of the client, and the accent he uses may indicate his socioeconomic class or the region of the country he stems from.
4. *Sentence structure:* The client's sentences

may give some indication of his cortical associative abilities.

5. *Tone of voice:* The voice should be observed for hoarseness, whining, or squeaky characteristics.

6. *Strength of voice:* Voice strength is evaluated in terms of loudness or softness in delivery of speech.

Some typical observations might be:

1. *Aphasia:* Inability to express oneself through speech (motor or expressive) or loss of verbal comprehension (receptive or sensory).

2. *Anarthria, dysarthria:* Loss of motor power to speak distinctly (stammering or stuttering).

3. *Aphonia, dysphonia:* Inability to produce sounds from the larynx. This is not due to a brain lesion. A possible cause might be laryngitis or malignancy.

In addition to observing the client's speech, one may find it useful to assess a sample of the client's writing for intactness of structures coordinating this complex act and for the client's ability to express his thoughts in this medium.

■ Mental status

The focus in this survey is to determine the client's problems in living and the psychodynamics underlying them. It is important that the client's own words be used in describing the problems.

The kind of information that is relevant will include the client's state of awareness from alertness to dullness to unconsciousness or coma. His ability to comprehend what he is told is described, as well as his level of education. The speed of responses to questions and reaction time in following instructions for motor activity may provide valuable clues. The length of attention span should be recorded. The facial expression should be observed at rest and during the early verbal interaction with the client for indications of anxiety, depression, apathy, and pain.

The client who slumps slowly into the chair should be watched for further indications of depression, such as carelessness in grooming and in dress.

The levels of cooperativeness can be described on a continuum from passive acceptance to rigid resistance. The level of aggressiveness may be described by descriptive terms relative to the client's relationship to things around him.

Mood has been described by such terms as hostility, resentment, depression, fearfulness, distrustfulness, elation, and euphoria. The difficulty in using these terms is that they may mean different things to the people who use them and to those who read the history. For instance, the client who sits looking at his hands while being interviewed might be described as "depressed," "withdrawn," "serious," or "thoughtful" by different observers. To obviate this confusion, it is best to describe the behavior that is observed.

The client's use of vocabulary and the complexity of sentence structure should be recorded, as well as his use of medical or other professional terminology.

Awareness is recorded in descriptive terms, relating the client's apparent perception of external stimuli and response to physiological stimuli.

The client's orientation for person, place, and time is assessed. It should be borne in mind that orientation usually is initially lost in the sphere of time, followed by place, and finally by person. Deviation from this order should be reported.

ASSESSMENT OF VITAL SIGNS

The clinical assessment of temperature, pulse, respiratory rate, and blood pressure are the most frequent clinical measurements made by the health practitioner. These measures of neural and circulatory function provide valuable data in the diagnosis of disease states. Irregularity of these parameters warrants further investigation. Because of the importance of these indicators in predicting the effectiveness of bodily function, they have been termed the *vital* or *cardinal* signs. Vital signs are assessed as the initial maneuver in any examination.

The history should be carefully attended for symptoms that would indicate alterations in the vital signs. These might include "pounding" of the heart, faintness, or dizziness.

The techniques utilized in the assessment of vital signs include inspection, palpation, and auscultation.

Inspection may reveal changes in color such as the flush of fever, the pallor in response to cold, or the dusky blueness of cyanosis. The bluish color observed as cyanosis results from an increased amount of reduced hemoglobin in superficial blood vessels. It is most readily identified in the vessels beneath the tongue or in the buccal mucosa. The examiner observes the chest for morphological changes that may indicate a pathological condition. For instance, in those individuals with chronic obstructive pulmonary disease, the anteroposterior diameter is often as great as the transverse diameter, and the ribs are observed to flare in the horizontal plane rather than downward. This structural change is thought to be due to the long period of overinflation of the lungs.

The chest is also observed for defects of the thoracic cage that might change the nature of respiration. Some of these are pigeon or chicken breast (the sternum is markedly protuberant, as in a bird), funnel chest or *pectus excavatum* (sternal retraction), and scoliosis.

Symmetry of thoracic expansion is noted. Bulging or retraction of the interspaces is recorded.

In addition to the assessment of pulsations, *palpation* may be used to determine temperature. Since the dorsal aspect of the hand is more sensitive to temperature variation, it is recommended that the backs of the fingers be used in this rough measure of temperature. Palpation may also reveal moisture and texture variations as well as the vibration of shivering.

Auscultation of the precordial area is employed to further evaluate the irregular pulse. Listening over the heart while simultaneously palpating a peripheral pulse is helpful in detecting a pulse deficit. Auscultation is the technique used to evaluate the sounds produced as a result of sphygmomanometer (Gr. *sphygmos*, pulse) manipulation.

The examiner must bear in mind that the assessment of vital signs is done in the interest of establishing a data base so that on future occasions the client may be compared to his own values—may be his own control.

Measurements of clinical significance are those that reveal variation from the client's basal value or from his last measurement. This is important in view of the considerable variability noted among individuals. The ranges of normal for temperature, for example, are 97° to 99.6° F (36.7° to 37.6° C).

The examiner must bear in mind the fact that his manner of approach to the client may alter the vital signs should the client react emotionally to the examiner's actions. For instance, a brusque, impatient, rude interaction or awkward handling of the instruments may prove upsetting to the client, increasing pulse rate, respiration, blood pressure, and even temperature if the interaction is prolonged.

■ Temperature

The optimal temperature for metabolic function of all cells of the human body is considered to be 98.6° F (37° C) for most individuals, and the core temperature of the human body is maintained at this level within very narrow limits. Although some individuals have a normal core temperature of 97° F and the range of normal extends to 99.6° F, the temperature of the individual shows little variation.

Temperature regulation is an excellent example of both homeostasis and biological rhythms. The accomplishment of the reasonably steady core temperature is a function of the hypothalamus, which serves as the thermostat. Two hypothalamic centers trigger heat-dissipating or heat-conserving mechanisms. The delivery of overwarmed blood to thermoreceptors in an anterior hypothalamic site results in sweating and redistribution of blood, so that surface capillaries are dilated (flushing). The loss of temperature from the skin is related to the delivery of blood flow to the skin and to the evaporation of sweat. This loss of heat is related to the difference in temperature between the skin and the external environment.

Conduction, convection, radiation, and evaporation are the physical phenomena involved. Heat is lost from the object of higher temperature to the object of lower temperature by *conduction*. *Convection* is the loss of heat to the molecules of air. Warm air rises, carrying the heat away. Conduction and convection cannot occur when external objects and ambient temperature are greater than that of the body.

Radiation is the loss of heat by electromagnetic infrared waves. The radiation does not heat the air through which it passes.

Evaporation is the conversion of liquid to gaseous form. The liquid involved is sweat. Perspiration in man is the insensible, thermal sweat from the eccrine glands and the autonomic, or emotional, sweat arising from the palms and soles. Insensible perspiration is moisture of diffusion principally noted from the corneum, from the sweat glands of the skin, and from the lungs. Insensible perspiration and thermal sweat are the most important in terms of heat loss. Evaporation of thermal sweat from the body requires 0.58 calories per 1 ml of sweat. Vaporization of perspiration is dependent on ambient humidity and does not occur when air is highly saturated with water.

When overcooled blood is delivered to thermoreceptors in a posterior hypothalamic site, heat-conserving mechanisms are instituted. These functions include reduction of blood flow to the distal extremities as a result of shunting via venae comitantes from large arteries to similar

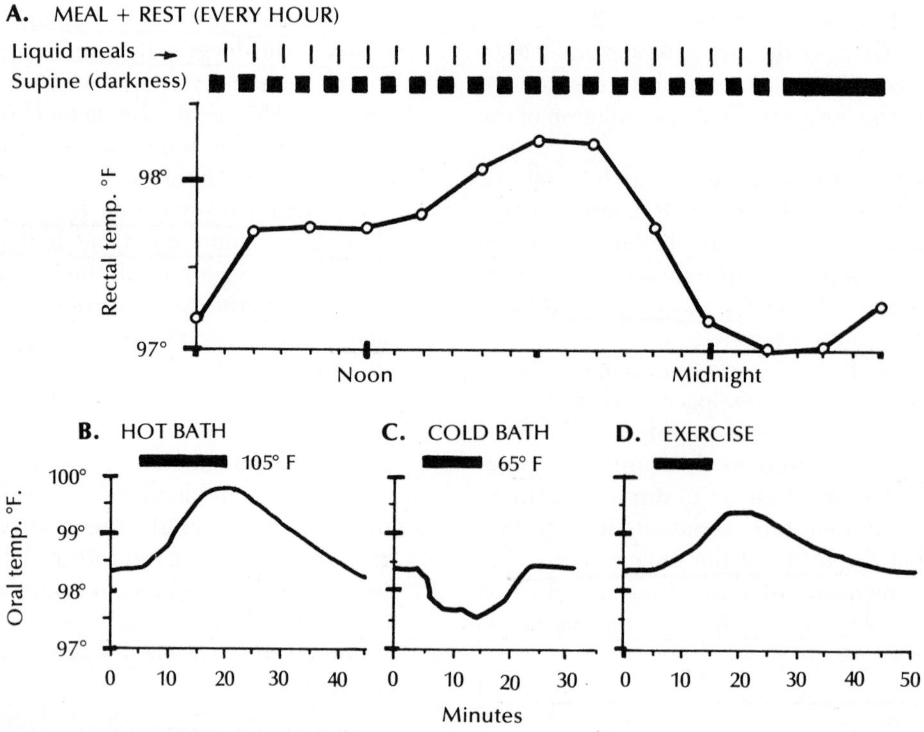

A. MEAL + REST (EVERY HOUR)

Liquid meals →
Supine (darkness)

Fig. 7-1. Factors influencing the body temperature of man. The body temperature is nicely regulated, but exact maintenance is altered by many factors, such as hot baths, cold water, and exercise. Also, there is a daily resetting of temperature regulation that persists in a resting individual if the influence of exercise or meals is removed. If standardized exercise is carried out at noon and at midnight, the day-night regulation is still apparent in the exercise body temperature. (From Folk, G. E.: Textbook of environmental physiology, ed. 2, Philadelphia, 1974, Lea & Febiger; in part from Green, J. H.: An introduction to human physiology, ed. 4, Oxford, 1976, Oxford University Press.)

veins and constriction of peripheral capillary beds (blanching). Compensatory heat production is enhanced both at the metabolic level (nonshivering thermogenesis) and through voluntary muscle contraction and shivering. Shivering occurs when vasoconstriction is ineffective in preventing heat loss.

Thermoreceptors in the skin sense ambient temperature and transmit neural signals to the spinal cord at all levels for relay through the spinothalamic tracts to the thalamus. These neural messages are thought to act as stimuli to the hypothalamic centers.

Factors influencing temperature

Biological rhythms are reflected in temperature assessment (Fig. 7-1). Diurnal variations of 1.0° to 1.5° F are observed; the trough occurs in the hours before waking and the peak in the late afternoon or early evening.

Secretion of hormones affects the body tem-

perature. Increased secretion of thyroid hormones is associated with increased heat production. Progesterone secretion at the time of ovulation is correlated with temperature increases of 0.5° to 1.0° F, which continues to the time of the menses. Both estrogen and testosterone may increase the rate of cellular metabolism.

There are some *environmental effects* on temperature. Although body temperature may be little altered by seasonal changes in environmental temperature, hot and cold baths are known to produce temporary changes in temperature, as shown in Fig. 7-1.

The physiological changes incurred in *exercise* are also known to increase body temperature (Fig. 7-2). The temperature rise associated with the *eating of food* is said to be due to the specific dynamic activity (SDA) of the food.

Drugs that alter circulation or metabolism will also affect body temperature.

Age is a factor in temperature assessment.

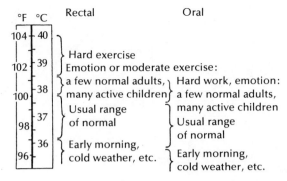

Fig. 7-2. Estimate of ranges in rectal and oral temperatures found in normal persons. This suggests that it would be wise to replace the little red arrow clinical thermometer by a red band covering the space between 96.5° and 99.3° F (33.7° to 37.8° C). (From DuBois, E. F.: Fever and the regulation of body temperature, American Lecture Series, Publ. No. 13, 1948. Courtesy of Charles C Thomas, Publisher, Springfield, Ill.)

Table 7-4. Metric-Fahrenheit equivalents for possible range of human temperature

Fahrenheit (degrees)	Centigrade (degrees)
93.2	34.0
95.0	35.0
96.8	36.0
98.6	37.0
100.4	38.0
102.2	39.0
104.0	40.0
105.8	41.0
107.6	42.0
109.4	43.0

Since heat control mechanisms are not as well established in the child as in the adult, considerable variation in temperature may occur.

Temperature recording

Body temperature is recorded in degrees of centigrade (°C) or in degrees of Fahrenheit (°F) according to the protocol of the agency. Since this country is committed to the future adoption of the metric system, the practitioner would do well to think of temperature in degrees of centigrade. Scales may be readily converted through the use of the following formulas:

$$°C = \frac{5}{9} \, (°F - 32)$$
$$°F = \frac{9}{5} \, °C + 32$$

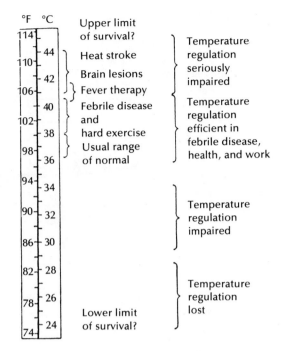

Fig. 7-3. Extremes of human body temperatures with an attempt to define the zones of temperature regulation. (From DuBois, E. F.: Fever and the regulation of body temperature, American Lecture Series, Publ. No. 13, 1948. Courtesy of Charles C Thomas, Publisher, Springfield, Ill.)

Table 7-4 equates Fahrenheit and centigrade temperatures in the range compatible with survival in the human being.

Temperature regulation

Temperature control may be altered in such a way that the mechanisms of control may be effective at a higher or lower level. An example of this might be seen in the individual exposed to marked exercise. During the first few days the core temperature may reach values of 102° F (38.9° C), but with adaptation the individual may undergo a decrease to 100° F (37.8° C), which will be maintained as long as the exercise is carried on.

Fever, or elevation of temperature due to the effect of pyrogens on the hypothalamus, also affects this type of core temperature resetting.

Temperature regulation becomes impaired or lost when extreme variations of temperature occur (Fig. 7-3).

Temperature regulation results from the balance of heat loss and heat conservation functions, these are summarized in Fig. 7-4.

99

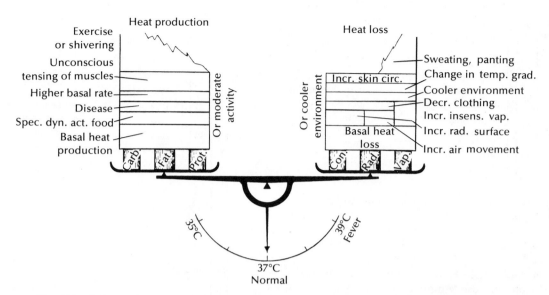

Fig. 7-4. Balance between factors increasing heat production and heat loss. (From DuBois, E. F.: Heat loss from the human body, Harvey Lecture, Bull. N.Y. Acad. Med. **15**:143, 1939.)

Temperature acclimatization

Clients who have spent a good deal of time in very cold climates show an increased ability to tolerate cold. Changes that have been measured in these individuals are (1) increased metabolic rate with increased rates of secretion of thyroid hormones, (2) reduction in shivering, and (3) growth of hair.

Adaptation to heat involves changes in the secretion of sweat. The amount of sweat produced declines from the profuse, dripping early response to a quantity that will evaporate on reaching the air.

Thermometry

Glass thermometry. The clinical glass thermometer has been in use since the fifteenth century. The thermometer reflects heat changes through the expansion of mercury. The accuracy of the instrument is determined by the amount and quality of the mercury and by the calibrations identified on the glass tube.

Recent studies have shown the glass thermometer to be subject to inaccuracy. Furthermore, in most subjects the oral thermometer must be left in place for 8 to 9 minutes in order to obtain full registration of the instrument. Thus, the readings obtained must be considered to be approximations of the actual temperature of the client.

Other disadvantages in the use of the glass thermometer are frequent breakage and danger to the client through the use of the rigid glass rod. Several instances of perforation of the rectal wall have occurred through inappropriate placement of a glass thermometer.

The examiner may also build in error through improper reading of the thermometer. The eyes must be at a 90° angle to the meniscus of the mercury to avoid parallax error.

Electronic thermometry. The electronic thermometer has been in use over the past decade. The advantages to be realized with the fully charged, correctly calibrated instrument are speed and accuracy of measurement. The probes used in these thermometers are unbreakable, thus obviating damage from broken glass and mercury ingestion, which are hazards with the traditional clinical thermometer.

Oral, rectal, and axillary temperature assessment

Differences in temperatures recorded from the mouth, rectum, or axilla have been shown to reflect the length of time the thermometer is allowed to register rather than actual variation in temperature from one site to another.

Oral temperature. The oral temperature registration is the most convenient method for the client. This site for temperature determination is the one used unless the client is an infant, unconscious, confused, or has shown erratic behavior.

A 5- to 15-minute wait is recommended before

temperature assessment if the client has ingested hot or iced liquids, to allow the temperature to stabilize. Small increases will occur if the client has smoked in the 2 minutes preceding the temperature assessment.

Rectal temperature. The rectal site for temperature registration is preferable for the confused or comatose client, the individual who is unable to close his mouth, or the client who is receiving oxygen.

The rectal temperature is routinely ordered as the general mode of temperature registration in some agencies.

The thermometer placed in the rectum will register adequately within a 2-minute time span in adults and within 3 minutes in premature infants.

Axillary temperature. Eleven minutes has been shown to be the maximum length of time necessary for the full registration of axillary temperature. This method has been shown to be safe and accurate for infants and small children.

Correlation of pulse and temperature

It should be noted that marked increases in temperature are accompanied by increments in pulse and respiratory rates, since oxygen requirements are known to increase 7% for every 1° F (10% per for every 1° C) rise in temperature. Since reducing cellular temperatures results in a decreased rate of cell metabolism, oxygen consumption is lessened in hypothermia; therefore, pulse and respiratory rates also decline.

Fever

Fever, or pyrexia, is the elevation of body temperature above normal limits as compared to a given individual's basal data. Fever may be a valid diagnosis when the temperature is found to be 98.6° F for a given client if his normal temperature ranges about 97° F.

Not all causes of fever are related to disease. Exercise may cause a temporary elevation of temperature, which subsides when the activity is stopped.

It has been suggested that a temperature above 97° F in a client who has been lying in bed (whose metabolism is basal) indicates the presence of disease. The association of an elevated temperature with disease is called fever.

Fever is caused by those conditions that contribute to heat production, that prevent heat loss, or that affect the heat-regulating centers of the CNS.

Fevers are described according to the chronological pattern of occurrence and amplitude. Frequently, the recognition of the pattern may help to establish the diagnosis. The following paragraphs present descriptions of fever.

A *continuous* or *sustained* fever is one in which there is a persistent elevation of temperature without a return to normal values for that individual. This pattern is typical of typhoid or typhus fever.

An *intermittent fever* is one in which there are major diurnal variations, so that there is a daily elevation of temperature with a drop to subnormal or normal values in the same 24-hour period. When there is a marked difference between the peaks and the troughs of the temperature, the fever is called *hectic* or *septic*. This type of fever is seen in pyrogenic infection.

Remittent fever is characterized by a temperature elevation that does not return to normal level but shows marked spikes of even further increased temperature on the febrile baseline. This appears in sustained or continuous fever, in which there are only slight variations from the elevated set point.

Relapsing fever is one in which febrile periods alternate with periods of normal temperature. This pattern of fever is seen in malaria, relapsing fever, and the Murchison-Pel-Ebstein fever of Hodgkin's disease.

Fever may also be described by the rate pattern of dissolution. *Lysis* is the gradual disappearance of fever, whereas *crisis* is the rapid (less than 36 hours) decrease of temperature to normal.

Stages or chronology of fever. The development of the febrile condition and its abatement have been described in three stages, called cold, hot, and defervescence.

The period of a developing increase in core temperature is characterized by heat conservation reactions. The affected individual has diminished cutaneous circulation, and the skin looks blanched and feels cold. Heat production is attested to by shivering and piloerection ("goose pimples"). Chills and rigor are the extremes of shivering that produce rapid increases in temperature.

The hot stage is the period after the fever has peaked (regulated at the new set point). During this stage blood flow to the periphery is increased. The affected individual's body radiates excess heat, feels hot, and is flushed.

The stage of defervescense is the period of fever abatement and is characterized by heat loss mechanisms; particularly prominent is vasodilation and sweating. Diaphoresis is diffuse perspiration, which may accompany fever abatement.

■ Respiratory pattern

The assessment of the respiratory pattern is discussed in Chapter 13 on Assessment of the respiratory system.

■ Pulsation

The assessment of central pulses discussed in Chapter 14 (Cardiovascular assessment: the heart and the neck vessels) should be read before this section.

Assessment of the peripheral arterial pulse has been a part of the health professional's armamentarium throughout recorded medical history. Although examination of the peripheral (radial) arterial pulsation gives less information concerning left ventricular ejection or aortic valvular function than does the assessment of the more central (carotid) arteries, the information obtained is a necessary part of the data base.

The peripheral pulses reveal important information regarding both cardiac function and peripheral perfusion. These peripheral pulsations are evaluated in terms of rate, amplitude (indicating volume), symmetry, and regularity of rhythm. The peripheral pulses are also auscultated for the presence of bruits.

Arterial pulses are examined while the client is reclining with the trunk of the body elevated about 15° to 30°.

The normal arterial pulse expands normal peripheral arteries only slightly.

Parameters of arterial pulsation

Visible pulsations result from diameter changes incurred through vessel filling as well as through straightening of the vessel. These pulsations are referred to as arterial pulse waves.

Pressure is applied to the wall of the artery through the overlying skin and subcutaneous tissue. The arterial pressure pulse wave is sensed through the pressure receptors in the pads of the examiner's fingers superimposed on the pressure exerted against the wall.

Rate. As defined by the American Heart Association, the heart rate is normal when it is between 50 and 100 beats per minute.

The pulse rate is counted for 1 full minute in order to evaluate rate, rhythm, and volume accurately. Some authorities recommend counting for 15 to 30 seconds for those pulses that are normal on palpation and to extend the period of evaluation only when irregularities are detected.

A diurnal rhythm is noted for pulse rate. The lowest rate is seen in the early morning hours,

Table 7-5. Chronological variations in pulse rate

Age	Pulse rate (beats per minute)
Birth	70-170
Neonate	120-140
1 year	80-140
2 years	80-130
3 years	80-120
4 years	70-115
Adult	60-100
Conditioned athlete	≅50

and the most rapid rates are observed in the late afternoon and evening.

Chronologically the pulse rate decreases from infancy through the middle years; there is a tendency for it to increase in the older client (Table 7-5).

A sex difference is noted in that women have demonstrated a rate 5 to 10 beats per minute faster than men.

Volume. Pulse volume is estimated from the feel of the vessel as blood flows through the vessel with each heartbeat. *Bounding* is the descriptive term used to describe the full pulse that is difficult to depress with the fingertips. *Weak,* *feeble,* and *thready* are descriptive words for a vessel that has low volume. The artery in this case is readily compressed.

Amplitude. The strength of the left ventricular contraction is reflected in the amplitude of the pulsation. This may be recorded as follows:

3+ Bounding, hyperkinetic
2+ Normal
1+ Weak, thready, hypokinetic
0 Absent

Elasticity of the arterial wall

Elasticity of the arterial wall is reflected by the expansibility or deformability of the artery as it is palpated by the examiner's fingers. The normal artery is soft and pliable, whereas the sclerotic vessel may be more resistant to occlusion, even hard and cordlike. The artery may feel beaded and tortuous to touch in the individual with arteriosclerosis.

Palpation of arterial pulses

Superficial temporal pulse. The superficial temporal artery is accessible to palpation and is frequently used in the clinical evaluation of pulsation.

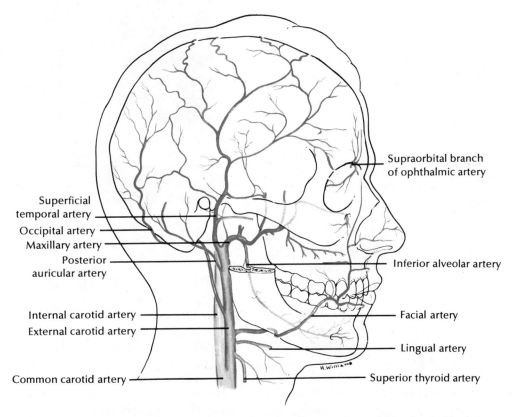

Superficial
temporal artery

Occipital artery

Maxillary artery

Posterior
auricular artery

Internal carotid artery

External carotid artery

Common carotid artery

Supraorbital branch
of ophthalmic artery

Inferior alveolar artery

Facial artery

Lingual artery

Superior thyroid artery

H.Williams

Fig. 7-5. Arteries of the head and neck. (From Frances, C. C., and Martin, A. H.: Introduction to human anatomy, ed. 7, St. Louis, 1975, The C. V. Mosby Co.)

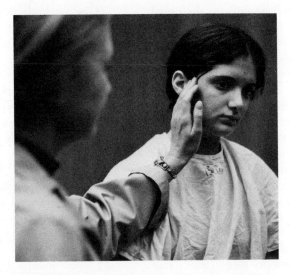

Fig. 7-6. Palpation of the superficial temporal artery.

Carotid pulse. Examination of the carotid and jugular pulse is described in Chapter 14. Fig. 7-7 shows one method of palpation of the carotid artery.

The carotid pulse is easily accessible and is frequently the pulse evaluated in emergency situations. The pulse is easily located by allowing the fingers to roll laterally off the trachea into the groove between the trachea and the sternocleidomastoid muscle. The carotid artery follows the lateral wall of the anterior triangle of the neck.

Radial pulse. The radial pulse is the one most frequently used as an initial indication of the rate and rhythm of pulsation, the pattern of pulsation, and the shape (consistency) of the arterial wall. This pulse is easily accessible to the examiner, and its evaluation causes little inconvenience to the client. Other pulses easily evaluated in the upper extremity are the ulnar and brachial pulses (Fig. 7-8).

The radial pulse is readily assessed by placing the pads of the examiner's second and third (or first, second, and third) fingers on the palmar surface of the relaxed and slightly flexed wrist medial to the radial styloid process (Fig. 7-9). Occasionally the arteries run a deeper and more lateral course. Both radial pulses should be felt simultaneously for an assessment of symmetry. The fingers should exert sufficient pressure to occlude the artery during diastole, yet allow the vessel to return to normal contour during systole.

Ulnar pulse. The ulnar artery may be compressed against the ulna on the palmar surface of the wrist. It is not used as frequently as the radial artery in evaluation (Fig. 7-9).

Brachial pulse. The brachial artery is palpated medial to the biceps tendon. The brachial artery may be used to determine the arterial waveform, as can the carotid artery. The waveform of more peripheral arteries may be distorted and therefore provide less valuable data.

Femoral pulse. The pads of the examiner's fingers explore the area just inferior to the midpoint of the inguinal ligament. This is also approximately midway between the anterior superior iliac spine and the symphysis pubis.

Popliteal pulse. Since the popliteal artery is situated relatively deeply in the soft tissues behind the knee, the knee should be flexed for examination of the pulsation in this artery. The pulse may be readily examined with the client in either the dorsal recumbent (Fig. 7-11) or prone position (Fig. 7-12). The fingertips are pressed deeply into the popliteal fossa.

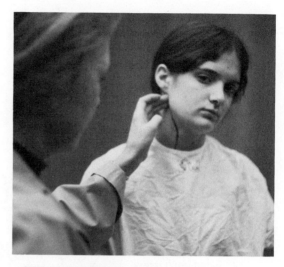

Fig. 7-7. Palpation of the carotid artery.

Dorsal pedal pulse. The pads of the examining fingers examine the dorsum of the foot. The foot should be dorsiflexed to obviate traction on the artery, preferably to 90° (Fig. 7-13).

When the dorsal pedal pulse is congenitally absent, pulsation may sometimes be discerned in the lateral tarsal artery, located in the proximal dorsum of the foot, or in the peroneal artery, anterior to the lateral malleolus.

Although only one pedal pulse can occasionally be palpated, this need not necessarily indicate arterial insufficiency; it may be due to clinically insignificant congenital variation in the arteries to the foot.

One or both dorsal pedal pulses have been noted to be absent in 12% of children and in 17% of adults. Whereas whites seldom show an absence of the posterior tibial pulse, a 9% incidence of absence has been found in black adults.

Posterior tibial pulse. The pads of the examining fingers palpate posterior or inferior to the tibial lateral malleolus while the client's foot is dorsiflexed, preferably to 90° (Fig. 7-14).

Irregularities in pulsation

Tachycardia. Rates persistently over 100 beats per minute (tachycardia) suggest some abnormality. However, hyperkinetic heart action can be the result of exercise, anger, anxiety, or fear in the normal client. Heart rates are increased during fever, anemia, hypoxia, and low volume states (shock).

Bradycardia. A slow heart rate less than 50 beats per minute is known as bradycardia. These

Text continued on p. 109.

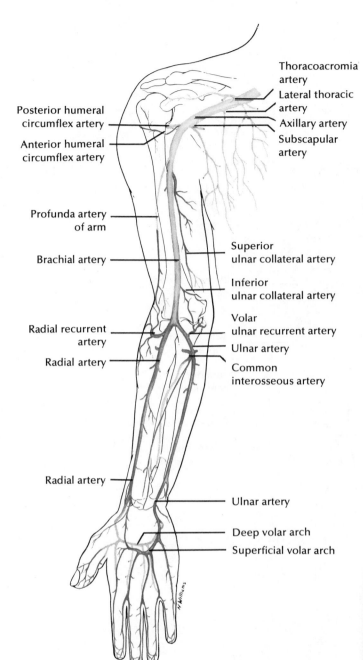

Posterior humeral circumflex artery

Anterior humeral circumflex artery

Profunda artery of arm

Brachial artery

Radial recurrent artery

Radial artery

Radial artery

Thoracoacromia artery

Lateral thoracic artery

Axillary artery

Subscapular artery

Superior ulnar collateral artery

Inferior ulnar collateral artery

Volar ulnar recurrent artery

Ulnar artery

Common interosseous artery

Ulnar artery

Deep volar arch

Superficial volar arch

Fig. 7-8. Arteries of the upper extremity. (From Frances, C. G., and Martin, A. H.: Introduction to human anatomy, ed. 7, St. Louis, 1975, The C. V. Mosby Co.)

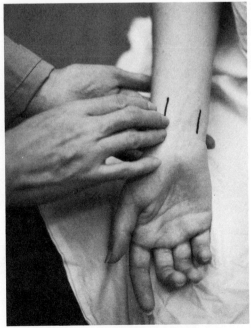

Fig. 7-9. Palpation of the radial pulse. The site for palpation of the ulnar artery is also marked.

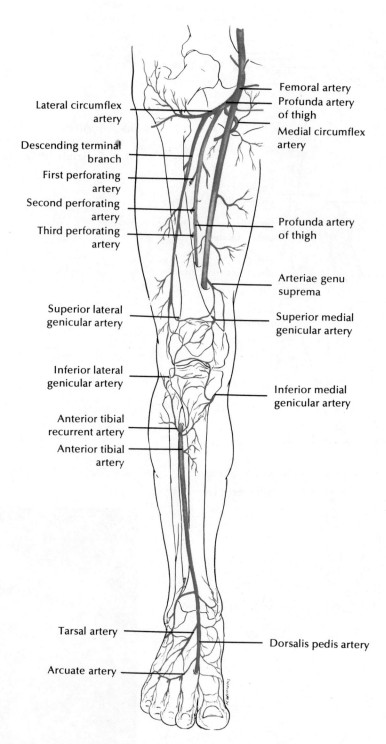

Lateral circumflex
artery

Descending terminal
branch

First perforating
artery

Second perforating
artery

Third perforating
artery

Superior lateral
genicular artery

Inferior lateral
genicular artery

Anterior tibial
recurrent artery

Anterior tibial
artery

Tarsal artery

Arcuate artery

Femoral artery

Profunda artery
of thigh

Medial circumflex
artery

Profunda artery
of thigh

Arteriae genu
suprema

Superior medial
genicular artery

Inferior medial
genicular artery

Dorsalis pedis artery

Fig. 7-10. Arteries of the lower extremity. (From Frances, C. C., and Martin, A. H.: Introduction to human anatomy, ed. 7, St. Louis, 1975, The C. V. Mosby Co.)

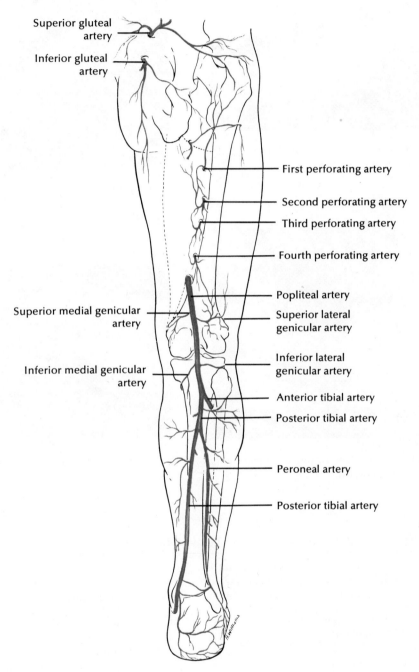

Superior gluteal artery

Inferior gluteal artery

First perforating artery

Second perforating artery

Third perforating artery

Fourth perforating artery

Popliteal artery

Superior medial genicular artery

Superior lateral genicular artery

Inferior medial genicular artery

Inferior lateral genicular artery

Anterior tibial artery

Posterior tibial artery

Peroneal artery

Posterior tibial artery

Fig. 7-10, cont'd. For legend see opposite page.

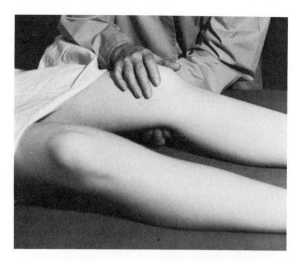

Fig. 7-11. Palpation of the popliteal pulse with client in the dorsal recumbent position.

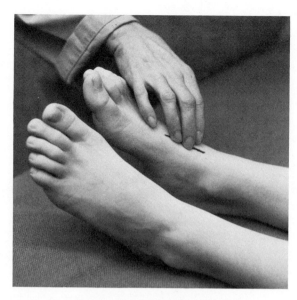

Fig. 7-13. Palpation of the dorsal pedal pulse.

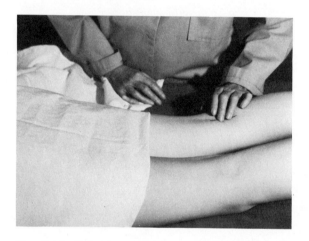

Fig. 7-12. Palpation of the popliteal pulse with client in the prone position.

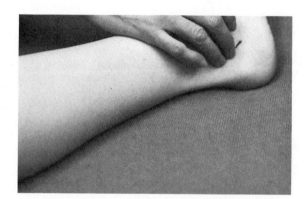

Fig. 7-14. Palpation of the posterior tibial pulse in the left leg.

Table 7-6. Characteristics of common forms of tachycardia

Type	Rhythm, amplitude	Most common ventricular rate (beats/min)	Onset	Termination	Effect of carotid sinus massage
Sinus tachy-cardia	Regular; constant amplitude	Usually 170	Gradual	Gradual	Gradual slowing and return to previous state
Paroxysmal atrial tachy-cardia (PAT)	Regular; constant amplitude	170	Abrupt	Abrupt	Sudden slowing of heart rate or no change
Paroxysmal atrial flutter	Flutter, regular; uniform ampli-tude	170	Abrupt		Sudden diminution of rate or temporarily irregular rythm
Ventricular tachy-cardia	Irregular; variable amplitude	140	Sudden		No effect

Table 7-7. Characteristics of common forms of bradycardia

Type	Rhythm, amplitude	Most common ventricular rate (beats/min)	Effect of exercise
Sinus bradycardia	Regular; constant amplitude	40	Rate increases appropriately through varying degrees of exercise
Incomplete heart block	Constant amplitude	40	May double or become irregular in response to exercise
Complete heart block		40	Increases only slightly in response to exercise

slow rates may indicate stimulation of the parasympathetic system or failure in the electrical conduction system of the heart. Bradycardia may be iatrogenically produced through overdoses of digitalis.

The well-trained athlete may have cardiac rates less than 50 beats per minute.

Atrial fibrillation. In atrial fibrillation, the number of pulsations reaching peripheral sites of pulsation may be less than the number of muscular contractions of the heart. This pulse deficit results in errors in calculations of rate as well as in an irregularity in rhythm.

Bigeminal pulse. A pulse that alternates in amplitude from beat to beat may be produced by a small, premature ventricular beat after a large beat, resulting from normal electrical cardiac conduction. The large pulse occurs after a long diastolic filling phase following the premature beat. This condition is called bigeminal pulse and can be identified by simultaneously palpating the radial pulse and listening at the precordium.

Pulsus paradoxus. The normal variation of the systolic blood pressure with respiration may sometimes be detected by palpation. However, the difference is more readily detected by sphygmomanometry. This slight change (10 mm Hg ± 5) is exaggerated in hypernea.

The change in cardiac filling occurs as the relatively increased negative pressure augments venous intrathoracic return to the heart but pools in the pulmonary circulation as the lung expands, thus ending in a decrease in left ventricular filling. Greater changes are referred to as pulsus paradoxus; causes of this variation in the pulse include superior vena cava obstruction, marked fluctuations of intrathoracic pressure, as in asthma, emphysema, and airway obstruction; congestive heart failure; and cardiac tamponade.

Palpitations. In the resting state the normal individual is unaware of the beating of his heart. Palpitation is the term used to record a descrip-

Table 7-8. Guide to causes of palpitations

Possible cause	Signs and symptoms
Menopausal symptom	Associated with heat "flashes" or perspiration
Drugs known to produce a hyperkinetic heart	History of ingestion of monamine oxidase inhibitors, thyroid replacement or stimulatory drugs, adrenergic drugs, alcohol, tea, coffee
Hemorrhage, hypoglycemia, pheochromocytoma	Sudden occurrence of palpitation not related to exercise or emotional arousal
Psychopathology	Clinical examination reveals no evidence of hyperkinetic heart or irregularity of rate
Postural hypotension	Palpitations occur when individual stands
Anemia, fever, atrial fibrillation, thyrotoxicosis, exposure to environmental heat	Clinical examination reveals hyperkinetic heart
Extra systoles	Irregular "skips"

tion given by the client of his perception of the feeling of his heartbeat. Such expressions as "pounding," "thudding," "fluttering," "flopping," and "skipping" are common descriptive terms used by clients to describe this phenomenon. The incidence of palpitation is more common just before falling asleep or during sleep.

Physiological palpitations may be experienced by the normal individual following strenuous exercise or when he is aroused emotionally or sexually. In this case the cardiac contraction is of greater rate and amplitude. Several pathophysiological states are also associated with a hyperkinetic heart (anemia, fever, hypoglycemia, and thyrotoxicosis). Irregularities in cardiac rhythm have also been associated with palpitations, particularly extra systoles and ectopic tachycardia. The chief complaint of palpitations is frequently correlated with psychopathology.

A common feature of the anxiety state, palpitations may be related to the increased adrenergic activity that is present in this arousal state. This relationship creates some problem for the examiner; since the presence of palpitations frequently creates anxiety, careful questions will be necessary to minimize this effect.

Arterial insufficiency

Assessment of the arterial pulsation is particularly important in those individuals suspected or diagnosed as having diseases known to compromise the arterial circulation. Some of these pathophysiological conditions are diabetes, atherosclerosis, Buerger's disease, Raynaud's disease, and arterial aneurysm.

Signs and symptoms of arterial insufficiency include intermittent claudication, increased pallor on elevation of the extremity, a prolonged venous filling time following elevation of the extremity, flush incurred by gravitational effect if the extremity is below the level of the heart, and tissue death (gangrene). Symptoms may also include easy fatigability. Ischemic pain may be incurred by simple resistance exercises. Intermittent claudication is the transient ischemic pain encountered by the client in his arms when he is working with them or in his legs when he is walking or standing.

Intermittent claudication in the arms may be confused with the pain of angina pectoris. The examiner must carefully define the fact that the pain occurred with work and disappeared with rest. Subclavian arterial insufficiency may result in dizziness and faintness.

Physical examination of the client thought to have arterial insufficiency includes auscultation of the arteries, palpation of the pulses and observations of cutaneous color; examination should be done before and after exercise.

Absence of pulsation in the femoral artery and at least one peripheral vessel is a criterion for the diagnosis of arterial insufficiency.

Arterial insufficiency in the arm, although generally thought to be less frequent than that of the leg, may frequently be demonstrated through changes in murmurs, pulses, and skin color after exercise.

Importance of exercise testing in determining arterial insufficiency of the extremities. Exercise testing of the poorly perfused limb is based on the inability of the occluded vessel to increase blood

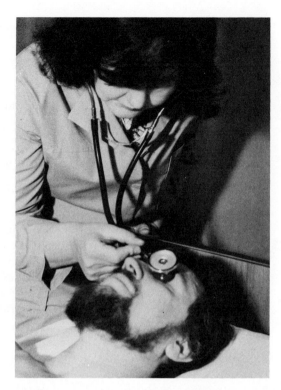

Fig. 7-15. Auscultation for bruits over the supraorbital branch of the ophthalmic artery.

flow to meet the increased demands for oxygen. Bruits that were present only in systole continue into diastole since there is a relatively decreased diastolic pressure distal to the obstruction, which promotes forward flow.

In clients with intermittent claudication the pulses diminish in amplitude following exercise. Cutaneous ischemia may be apparent.

The amount of exercise needed to produce these vascular changes is usually no more than that which is part of daily living. Flexion—extension exercises of the arms and legs (deep knee bends)—or walking may produce these changes.

Auscultation for arterial murmurs

All accessible arteries should be auscultated in the client suspected of arteriovascular disease. Murmurs are not present over major arteries in the normal adult, and only faint ones are heard in the normal child.

Arterial murmurs may result from hyperdynamic cardiac states or from irregularity of arterial walls.

The bell of the stethoscope is utilized to detect bruits over major vessels. The instrument is lightly held to avoid occluding the underlying

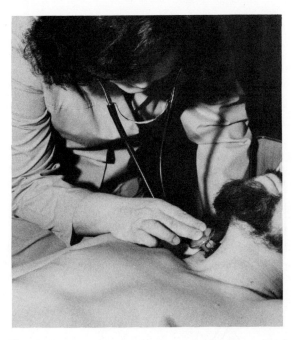

Fig. 7-16. Auscultation for bruits over the carotid artery.

vessel. Should the examiner detect a murmur, the limb is exercised if no contraindication exists, and the auscultation is repeated. The auscultation of a systolic murmur that extends into diastole in the postexercise state connotes some degree of arterial obstruction.

Sphygmomanometer detection of arterial flow

Failure to palpate pedal pulsation may indicate the use of the sphygmomanometer for detection of arterial flow. The pneumatic cuff is inflated to a pressure between the systolic and diastolic blood pressure. Oscillation of the needle (aneroid) or mercury column (mercury) on synchrony with the ventricular contraction is indicative of blood flow to the extremity. A disadvantage of this method is that it does not indicate the adequacy of the flow volume.

■ Blood pressure

The screening examination is especially important to the recognition of the client who has a disorder in blood pressure, particularly hypertension. Because hypertension may be present without symptoms, it is known as the silent disease. The client who does not feel ill does not usually present himself for health care. Thus, this examination may be instrumental in getting the hypertensive client into the therapeutic milieu in time to prevent some of the sequelae of hypertension.

A measure of the functions of the cardiovascular system may be accomplished through the assessment of peripheral arterial blood pressure. The peripheral blood pressure is the force exerted against the walls of the vessels and the force responsible for the flow of blood through the arteries, capillaries, and veins. The pressure is the result of the interaction of cardiac output and peripheral resistance and is dependent on the velocity of the arterial blood, the intravascular volume, and the elasticity of the arterial walls.

Stephen Hale made the first recorded direct measurement of blood pressure in 1733 when he cannulated the artery of a horse, allowing the blood to rise in a glass tube. He was also able to demonstrate the changes in blood pressure that occur in systole and diastole as he watched the blood rise and fall in the tube with each heartbeat. Almost a century later (1828), Poiseuille attached a mercury-filled tube to a cannulated artery. Since mercury is 13.6 times heavier than blood or water, the column in the tube was much shorter. Several instruments for the indirect method of blood pressure measurement were devised in the late 1800s.

The systemic arterial blood pressure may be assessed either by direct or indirect methods. The direct method requires cannulation of the artery but is the trusted method of measurement. Routine, direct arterial blood pressures are not measured, because of the potential sequelae, though the risks are small. Indirect blood pressure measurement can be made without opening the artery. The valid methods of indirect measurement are those that are closest in values to those made from direct techniques. Direct blood pressure standards are used to calibrate indirect pressure instruments.

Indirect measurement

Indirect methods of blood pressure measurement involve the following three physiological facts: (1) the arterial wall may be occluded by direct pressure, resulting in the obliteration of the pulse distal to the compression; (2) oscillations that vary directly with the amount of pressure being applied may be measured from the compressed artery; and (3) the normal extremity blanches (pales) when its arterial blood supply is occluded by pressure, and there is flushing or return of color when the pressure is removed.

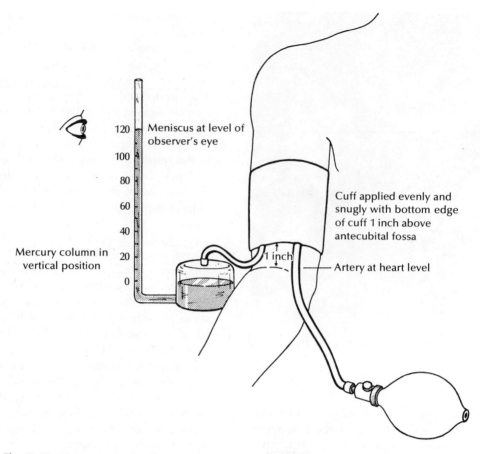

120 — Meniscus at level of observer's eye
100
80
60
40
Mercury column in vertical position — 20
0

Cuff applied evenly and snugly with bottom edge of cuff 1 inch above antecubital fossa

1 inch

Artery at heart level

Fig. 7-17. Mercury gravity manometer. (From Burch, G. E., and DePasquale, N. P.: Primer of clinical measurement of blood pressure, St. Louis, 1962, The C. V. Mosby Co.)

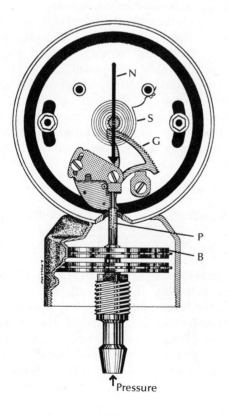

N
S
G
P
B
↑Pressure

Fig. 7-18. Anaeroid sphygmomanometer. Variations within the bellows (B) activate a pin (P), which sets a gear (G) into motion. The gear, in turn, operates the spring (S), which causes the needle (N) to move across the face of a calibrated dial. (From Burch, G. E., and DePasquale, N. P.: Primer of clinical measurement of blood pressure, St. Louis, 1962, The C. V. Mosby Co.)

The most commonly used method of indirect assessment of blood pressure is the auscultatory technique. The procedure utilizes a sphygmomanometer and a stethoscope.

The two types of sphygmomanometers used in the assessment of arterial blood pressure are the mercury gravity and the aneroid instruments. Each instrument includes a pressure manometer, an inflatable rubber bladder encased in a cloth cuff, and a rubber hand bulb with a pressure control valve.

The air distensible bladder encased in the cloth cuff is used to occlude an artery. The cuff is long enough to encircle the extremity and be fastened securely in place. The covering cuff must be made of an in elastic material so that pressure will be applied evenly to the limb.

The mercury gravity manometer (Fig. 7-17) is made up of a straight glass tube connected to a reservoir of mercury. The reservoir in turn is connected to the pressure bulb, so that pressure created on the bulb causes the mercury to rise in the tube. Because the weight of mercury is dependent on gravity, a given amount of pressure will always support a column of mercury of the same height, given the tube is straight and of uniform diameter. The mercury manometer does not need further calibration after the initial setting.

The aneroid sphygmomanometer (Fig. 7-18) is made up of a metal bellows connected to the compression cuff. Changes in pressure within the apparatus cause the bellows to expand and collapse. The movement of the bellows rotates a gear that moves a pointer across the calibrated dial. The aneroid sphygmomanometer is calibrated against a mercury manometer, since the more complex mechanisms have been shown to need frequent adjustment. This is simply done by using a connecting Y tube between the manometers.

Measurement of blood pressure by palpation. The brachial artery is palpated below the cuff, and the cuff is inflated to 30 mm Hg beyond the point at which the pulse is obliterated. The air pressure in the bladder is released at a rate of 2 to 3 mm Hg per heartbeat, and systemic blood pressure is recorded at the point at which pulsations first become palpable. The diastolic pressure is said to coincide with the cessation of vibrations in the artery. The diastolic value is difficult to obtain. In a test situation, more than 79% of the values obtained were within ±4 mm Hg of those obtained by auscultatory procedures.

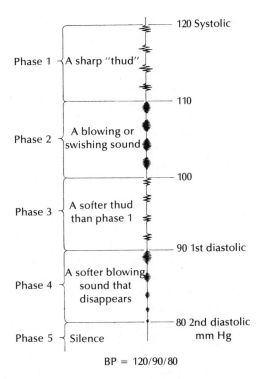

Fig. 7-19. Phases of the Korotkoff sounds. (From Burch, G. E., and DePasquale, N. P.: Primer of clinical measurement of blood pressure, St. Louis, 1962, The C. V. Mosby Co.)

Ausculatory method of arterial blood pressure assessment. When the cuff is properly placed on the limb, the arterial blood can flow past the cuff only when arterial pressure exceeds that in the cuff. Partial obstruction of arterial blood flow disturbs the laminar flow pattern, creating turbulence. This turbulence produces sounds called Korotkoff sounds and can be heard over arteries distal to the cuff through a stethoscope (Fig. 7-19).

The bell of the stethoscope is more effective than the diaphragm in transmitting the low-frequency Korotkoff sounds. The bell is applied snugly over the artery; care is taken not to press hard enough to close the artery.

The deflated cuff is applied, without wrinkles, snugly around the upper arm so that the edge of the cuff is 2 to 3 cm above the site at which the bell of the stethoscope is to be placed. The artery is palpated, and the cuff is inflated at a rate of 12 to 20 mm Hg per second to a peak of 30 mm Hg higher than the point at which the pulse was obliterated. The cuff is then deflated at a rate of 2 to 3 mm Hg per heartbeat. The level of the meniscus of the mercury column at which the Korotkoff sounds are changed is noted.

The _systolic blood pressure_ is recorded for that point at which the Korotkoff sounds are initially heard. This is also the beginning of _phase 1_, which starts with faint, clear, and rhythmic tapping or thumping noises that gradually increase in intensity. At this point the intraluminal pressure is the same as the cuff pressure but not great enough to produce a radial pulse.

Phase 2 is characterized by a murmur or swishing sound heard as the vessel distends with blood, creating eddies and producing vibration of the vessel wall. _Phase 3_ is the period during which the sounds are crisper and more intense. In this phase the vessel remains open in systole but obliterated in diastole.

The _muffling_ of the Korotkoff sounds is the guidepost for the beginning of _phase 4_ and the pressure at this point is felt by many authorities to be the closest to the _diastolic arterial pressure_ measured by a direct method. At this point the cuff pressure falls below the intraluminal pressure. It is frequently called the first diastolic pressure. The second diastolic pressure and _phase 5_ are said to be present when the Korotkoff sounds are no longer heard. Phase 5 marks the period wherein the vessel remains open during the entire cycle.

If muffling of the Korotkoff sounds is established as indicative of diastolic level, the value will be about 8 mm Hg greater than that obtained by the direct method.

Disappearance of the Korotkoff sounds is a risky criterion for diastolic pressure, since the sounds do not abate in some individuals until a pressure well below the diastolic value is reached.

Thus, three values are recorded: the systolic pressure, the point of muffling of the Korotkoff sounds, and the disappearance of the sounds. An example of the record might be 120/78/54. This method has the approval of the World Health Organization and the American Heart Association.

If the cuff is too narrow, the blood pressure reading will be erroneously high. A wide cuff increases the risk of an erroneously low reading.

The sphygmomanometer cuff should be 20% to 25% wider than the diameter of the extremity in which the blood pressure is being taken. Another recommendation is that the bladder width be equal to two fifths of the circumference of the limb. A more liberal approximation suggests that the cuff should cover two thirds of the upper arm. Ideally, the bladder should completely encircle the extremity and should be snugly applied. Cuffs may be obtained in the following sizes:

2.5×22.5 cm (neonate)
5×22.5 cm (toddler)
7×22.5 cm (1 year to 4 years)
9×22.5 cm (4 years to 8 years)
13×22.5 cm (standard adult)
14×40 cm (obese arm)
17.5×35 cm (thigh cuff and markedly obese arm)

Caution: The cuff size is determined by the diameter of the limb, not the age of the client.

The examiner's eye must be at a direct line with the level of the meniscus of the mercury column to avoid parallax error, and the mercury column must be kept in a vertical position.

The cuff should be deflated completely (0 mm Hg) between successive readings. At least a 15-second interval is allowed between readings, with the cuff completely deflated, to avoid spurious readings due to venous congestion.

The bladder and the pressure bulbs should be monitored for leaks. Erratic inflation or deflation usually indicates a leak.

Measurement of blood pressure in the leg. The blood pressure in the leg may be measured with the client in either the supine or prone position. The Korotkoff sounds are evaluated over the popliteal artery.

In the popliteal artery the systolic arterial blood pressure is higher (10 ± 5 mm Hg) than in the brachial artery, whereas the diastolic pressure is generally lower. This difference is magnified in aortic insufficiency and in some hyperdynamic states such as after exercise.

Increasing audibility of the Korotkoff sounds in infants and the flush test. Occasionally the Korotkoff sounds are not heard over the brachial artery in infants. A suggestion for making the sounds audible is to hold the infant's arm upright for 1 to 2 minutes with the cuff in place. The pressure is measured immediately on lowering the arm.

In the event that the Korotkoff sounds cannot be obtained, a flush pressure that approximates the mean blood pressure may be measured in the upper or lower extremity. The procedure for this test is as follows: The properly sized cuff is placed around the infant's wrist or ankle. An elasticized bandage is placed around the extremity distal to the cuff to promote vascular emptying. The bladder pressure of the sphygmomanometer is raised to approximately 150 mm Hg. The bandage is removed, and the cuff pressure is decreased at a rate of 2 to 3 mm Hg per heartbeat until a vascular flush (rubor) is observed. The appearance of the flush is correlated with the sphygmomanometer reading.

Auscultatory gap. Occasionally, as the pneumatic cuff is being deflated, the Korotkoff sounds disappear and then are heard 10 to 15 mm Hg later. This is called auscultatory gap. The examiner records systolic blood pressure at the onset of the first sound. Thus, the auscultatory gap will not be cause for error if the cuff was inflated to 20 mm Hg above the point at which the artery was occluded as determined by palpation.

Normal systolic and diastolic pressures. The systolic blood pressure shows a normal range of 95 to 140 mm Hg; 120 mm Hg is cited as average (when measured in the brachial artery).

Normal diastolic pressure ranges from 60 to 90 mm Hg; 80 mm Hg is average.

The systolic blood pressure in the noenatal period has a normal range of 20 to 60 mm Hg but then gradually increases until adolescence, when an accelerated rise is incurred. Thus, at about 17 or 18 years, blood pressure reaches adult levels.

The proper application of the auscultatory method yields values that are within ±4 to 5 mm Hg of the direct method of measurement.

Normal variations in blood pressure recordings. The blood pressure in a normal individual varies continually with respiration, autonomic state, emotional levels, and biological rhythms. Furthermore, successive readings of indirect measures of blood pressure by the same or different observers may differ by as much as 10 mm Hg.

In the normal individual, the *change from a supine to an erect position* causes a slight decrease in systolic blood pressure (less than 15 mm Hg) as well as in diastolic (less than 5 mm Hg) pressure. Marked drops in pressure (greater than 30 mm Hg) incurred when the individual stands may be indicative of a vasopressor defect or of hypovolemia.

The blood pressure also shows a *24-hour, or circadian, pattern.* Consistent with the other vital signs, the blood pressure has higher values in the afternoon and evening hours and lower values in the late hours of sleep.

Because blood pressure is readily altered by *stressful events,* an effort should be made to relax the client as much as possible before taking the blood pressure.

Food and exercise also affect the blood pressure. It is recommended that the individual should not eat or exercise in the 30 minutes before the determination is made. The extremity

should be at heart level for a period of approximately 5 minutes.

Differences in blood pressure indicating disease. The initial examination of blood pressure should include a measurement in both arms and one from the leg.

Differences in blood pressure between the two arms may be caused by aortic stenosis or by obstruction of the arteries of the upper arm.

Constriction or obstruction of the aorta may be suspected when the pressure assessed in the client's arms exceeds that in the legs, particularly when the differences are great.

Coarctation of the aorta must be suspected when the brachial pressure markedly exceeds that of the popliteal artery. This reversal of gradient may also accompany other obstructive lesions of the aorta or obstructive lesions in proximal arteries of the leg.

Assessment of pulsus paradoxus. Arterial blood pressure in normal man is known to vary as much as 10 mm Hg during relaxed respiration. The decrease with respiration may be 10 ± 5 mm Hg, whereas on inspiration a proportionate increase is noted. A difference greater than 15 mm Hg is indicative of pulsus paradoxus. These fluctuations may be more accurately assessed by allowing the cuff to deflate very slowly.

Assessment of pulsus alternans. Although the presence of pulsus alternans may be determined from palpation of the pulse, it may be more accurately assessed through the use of the sphygmomanometer. The cuff is inflated to 20 mm Hg above the systolic pressure as determined via palpation. On deflation to phase 1, only alternate beats are heard. Later all beats are audible and palpable. After still further deflation all beats are of equal intensity. The difference between this point and the peak systolic level is often used in determining the degree of pulsus alternans.

Pulse pressure. The pulse pressure is the difference between systolic and diastolic pressure. The normal value is generally 30 to 40 mm Hg. The heart rate may influence the pulse pressure. With a slowly beating heart the period of flow or "runoff" from the aorta to the periphery is lengthened, lowering the diastolic pressure. The net result is an increase in pulse pressure.

A wide pulse pressure accompanied by bradycardia frequently indicates increased intracranial pressure. The pulse pressure is also increased in hyperkinetic states such as hyperthyroidism or after vigorous exercise. Although the stroke volume may be greater, rapid runoff may result in low diastolic recordings.

With increased peripheral resistance, runoff to the peripheral circulation is less; thus, more blood accumulates in the aorta, and both systolic and diastolic blood pressure increase.

A small stroke volume will tend to decrease the pulse pressure.

Hypertension and hypotension

Hypertension. The World Health Organization defines hypertension as a persistent elevation of blood pressure greater than 140/90. The American Heart Association recommends that 160/95 be the defining point for hypertension in the client over 40 years of age. Elevation of either systolic or diastolic blood pressure is an indication for further diagnostic tests.

If the definition of hypertension in the adult is accepted as a diastolic pressure in excess of 90 mm Hg, then about 15% of whites and 30% of blacks in this country have hypertension. One study estimated that one half of these persons have not been identified.

The structures most frequently observed to suffer damage as peripheral resistance is increased are the heart, the kidneys, and the brain. Vessel changes are best observed in the retina. Sclerosis, hemorrhage, and exudates typify the alterations seen in hypertension.

The incidence of cardiovascular accident (CVA) is increased by high pressure in the vessels in the brain.

Increased cardiac work is required to pump the blood against the increased peripheral resistance. Thus, congestive heart failure, left ventricular hypertrophy, or angina pectoris may result from hypertension.

The examiner must bear in mind other signs and symptoms that accompany hypertension. These might include severe headache, blurred vision, and signs of renal disease.

Clinical assessment of hypertension in children. Although it is accepted that the routine measurement of blood pressure in all children from newborn through adolescence is imperative to the diagnosis of hypertension, this practice is frequently neglected. The screening examination may yield an incidence of hypertension of approximately 2.3% in children 4 to 15 years of age. Early detection of these hypertensive children may mean that diagnosis and treatment may be initiated in time to prevent the sequelae of the underlying disease process. It has been shown that 90% of adults are subject to essential or idiopathic hypertension, whereas this is true only for 20% of children. The blood pressure is re-

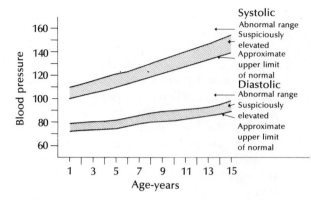

Fig. 7-20. Range of blood pressures measured in children. (From Gruskin, A.: Clinical evaluation of hypertension in children, Primary Care **1:**233, 1974.)

corded each time the child is seen and is considered with other developmental data.

Hypertension is said to exist in children when either the systolic or diastolic blood pressure is greater than the ninety-fifth percentile for age, that is, two standard deviations above the mean. Fig. 7-20 shows the range of blood pressures obtained in children. Note the progressive increase in blood pressure that is incurred from birth to age 15.

The findings of an elevated blood pressure in the pediatric client alert the examiner to look for indications of hypertensive encephalopathy (hyperactivity, excitability, and fundal changes).

Hypotension. Hypotension has been defined as a persistent blood pressure less than 95/60.

Hypotension in the absence of other signs or symptoms is generally innocent.

In hypovolemic or in endotoxic shock, the Korotkoff sounds will be less audible or absent. Since the peripheral blood pressure is an important parameter for determining the method of treatment, ultrasonic direct or invasive techniques of blood pressure assessment may be used.

Some other signs of shock might include increased pulse and respiratory rates, dizziness, confusion, blurred vision, diaphoresis, and cold and clammy skin.

Respiratory rate, volume, and rhythm assessment are described in Chapter 13 on Assessment of the respiratory system.

BIBLIOGRAPHY

Atkins, E., and Bodel, P.: Fever, N. Engl. J. Med. **286:**27, 1972.

Barnhorst, D. A., and Barner, H. B.: Prevalence of

congenitally absent pedal pulses, N. Engl. J. Med. **278:**264, 1969.

Draper, G., Dupertuis, C., and Caughey, J., Jr.: Human constitution in clinical medicine, New York, 1944, P. B. Hoeber, Inc.

DuBois, E. F.: Heat loss from the human body, Harvey Lecture, Bull. N.Y. Acad. Med. **15:**143, 1939.

DuBois, E. F.: Fever and the regulation of body temperature, Publ. No. 13, American Lecture Series, Springfield, Ill., 1948, Charles C Thomas, Publisher.

DuBois, E. F.: The many different temperatures of the human body and its parts, West. J. Surg. **59:**476, 1951.

Folk, C. E.: Temperature regulation. In Folk, G. E., editor: Textbook of environmental physiology, Philadelphia, 1974, Lea & Febiger.

Fowler, N. O.: Inspection and palpation of venous and arterial pulses, New York, 1970, American Heart Association.

Garn, S. M.: Types and distribution of hair on man, Ann. N.Y. Acad. Sci. **53:**498, 1951.

Garrison, G. E.: Floyd, W. L., and Orgain, E. S.: Exercise and the physical examination of peripheral arterial disease, Ann. Int. Med. **66:**587, 1967.

Geddes, L. A.: The direct and indirect measurement of blood pressure, Chicago, 1970, Year Book Medical Publishers, Inc.

Gold, J. J.: Hirsutism and virilism. In Gold, J. J., editor: Gynecologic endocrinology, New York, 1975, Harper & Row, Publishers.

Gruskin, A.: Clinical evaluation of hypertension in children, Primary Care **1:**233, 1974.

Hochberg, H. M., and Salomon, H.: Accuracy of an ultrasound blood monitor, Curr. Ther. Res. **13:**129, 1971.

Hurst, J. W., editor: The heart, ed. 4, New York, 1974, McGraw-Hill Book Co.

Karvenen, N. J., Telivuo, L. J., and Jarvinen, E. J.: Sphygmomanometer cuff size and accuracy of indirect measurement of blood pressure, Am. J. Cardiol. **13:**688, 1964.

King, G. E.: Errors in clinical measurement of blood pressure in obesity, Clin. Sci. **32:**233, 1967.

King, G. E.: Taking the blood pressure, J.A.M.A. **209:**1902, 1969.

Leon, M., Neves, E., Castro, M., and others: Biosynthesis of testosterone by a Stein-Leventhal ovary, Acta Endocrinol. **39:**411, 1962.

Londe, S.: Blood pressure in children as determined under office conditions, Clin. Pediatr. **5:**71, 1966.

Londe, S., Bourgoignie, J. J., Robson, A. M., and others: Hypertension in apparently normal children, J. Pediatr. **78:**569, 1971.

McCutcheon, E. P., and Rushmer, R. F.: Korotkoff sounds, Circ. Res. **20:**149, 1967.

Meninger, K.: A psychiatrist's world; the selected papers of Karl Meninger, M. D., New York, 1959, The Viking Press, Inc.

Nichols, G. A.: Taking adult temperatures; rectal measurement, Am. J. Nurs. **72:**1092, 1972.

Nichols, G. A., and Kucha, D. H.: Taking adult temperatures; oral measurements, Am. J. Nurs. **72:**1090, 1972.

O'Rourke, M. F.: The arterial pulse in health and disease, Am. Heart J. **82:**687, 1971.

Recommendations for human blood pressure determination by sphygmomanometer, New York, 1967, American Heart Association.

Simpson, J. A., Jamieson, G., Dickhaus, D. W., and others: Effect of size of cuff bladder on accuracy of measurement of direct blood pressure, Am. Heart J. **70:**208, 1965.

Sphygmomanometers; principles and precepts, Copiague, N.Y., 1965, W. A. Baum Co.

Ur, A., and Gordon, M.: Origin of Korotkoff sounds, Am. J. Physiol. **218:**524, 1970.

Williams, R.: Textbook of endocrinology, Philadelphia, 1974, W. B. Saunders Co.

Wu, R.: Behavior and illness, Englewood Cliffs, N.J., 1973, Prentice-Hall, Inc.

8 Assessment of the ears, nose, and throat

The examination of the ears, nose, and throat is an important part of every physical examination, since it provides the opportunity to inspect directly or indirectly most parts of the upper respiratory system and the first division of the digestive system. The clinical examination of these body orifices can provide information about the client's general health as well as information about significant local disease. The methods of examination are primarily inspection and palpation.

Discussion is focused on each of the three areas: the ears, the nose and paranasal sinuses, and the mouth and oropharynx. The portion of the chapter on each area includes a brief review of the anatomy and physiology, a description of the methods to be used in the examination, and some of the common findings of which the examiner should be aware when examining the particular area.

Ears

ANATOMY AND PHYSIOLOGY

The ear is a sensory organ that functions both in hearing and in equilibrium. It has three parts: the external ear, the middle ear, and the inner ear. Fig. 8-1 illustrates the structures of the ear.

The external ear has two divisions, the flap called the auricle or pinna and the canal called the external auditory canal or meatus. Stretching across the proximal portion of the canal is the tympanic membrane, which separates the external ear from the middle ear. The auricle is composed of cartilage, closely adherent perichondrium, and skin. The mastoid process is not part of the external ear but is a bony prominence found posterior to the lower part of the auricle.

The external auditory canal, which is about 1 inch in length with a slight curve, has a skeleton of cartilage in its outer third and a skeleton of bone in its inner two thirds. The skin of the inner part is exceedingly thin and sensitive.

The tympanic membrane, which covers the proximal end of the auditory canal, is made up of layers of skin, fibrous tissue, and mucous membrane (Fig. 8-2). The membrane is shiny, translucent, and of a pearl gray color. The position of the ear drum is oblique with respect to the ear canal. The anteroinferior quadrant is most distant from the examiner, which accounts for the cone of light or the light reflex. The membrane is slightly concave and is pulled inward at its center by one of the ossicles, the malleus, of the middle ear. The short process of the malleus protrudes into the eardrum superiorly, and the handle of the malleus extends downward from the short process to the umbo, the point of maximum concavity. Most of the membrane is taut and is known as the pars tensa. A small part superiorly is less taut and is known as the pars flaccida. The dense fibrose ring surrounding the tympanic membrane, with the exception of the anterior and posterior malleolar folds superiorly, is the annulus.

The middle ear is a small, air-filled cavity located in the temporal bone. It contains three small bones called the auditory ossicles: the malleus, the incus and the stapes. The middle ear cavity contains several openings. One is from the external auditory meatus and is covered by the tympanic membrane. There are two openings into the inner ear, the oval window into which the stapes fits and the round window covered by a membrane. Another opening connects the middle ear with the eustachian tube. The middle ear performs three functions: (1) it transmits sound vibrations across the ossicle chain to the inner

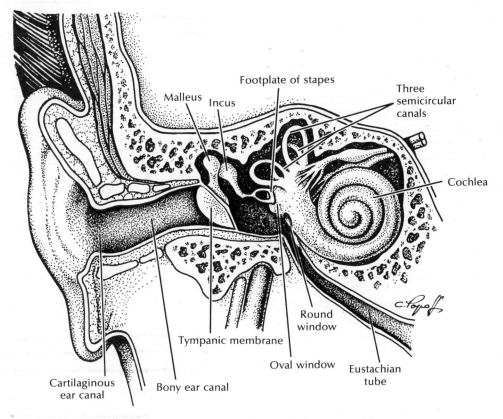

Fig. 8-1. External auditory canal, middle ear, and inner ear.

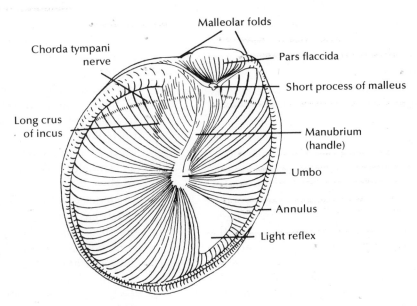

Fig. 8-2. Right tympanic membrane. (From Prior, J. A., and Silberstein, J. S.: Physical diagnosis; the history and examination of the patient, ed. 5, St. Louis, 1977, The C. V. Mosby Co.)

ear's oval window; (2) it protects the auditory apparatus from intense vibrations; and (3) it equalizes the air pressure on both sides of the dividing tympanic membrane to prevent the tympanic membrane from being ruptured.

The inner ear is made up of two parts, the bony labyrinth and, inside this structure, a membranous labyrinth. The bony labyrinth consists of three parts: the vestibule, the semicircular canals, and the cochlea. The vestibule and the semicircular canals comprise the organs of equilibrium. The cochlea comprises the organ of hearing. The cochlea is a coiled structure that contains the organ of Corti, which transmits stimuli to the cochlear branch of the auditory nerve (cranial nerve [CN] VIII).

Hearing occurs when sound waves enter the external auditory canal and strike the tympanic membrane, causing it to vibrate at the same rate as the sound waves striking it. The vibrations are transmitted through the auditory ossicles of the middle ear to the oval window. From the oval window the vibrations travel via the fluid of the cochlea, winding up at the round window, where they are dissipated. The vibrations of the membrane cause the delicate hair cells of the organ of Corti to impact against the membrane of Corti, acting as a stimuli setting up impulses in the sensory endings of the cochlear branch of the auditory nerve (CN VIII).

HEARING LOSS

There are several types of hearing loss. However, almost every form may be classified under one of three headings: conductive hearing loss, sensorineural or perceptive hearing loss, or mixed hearing loss.

Conductive hearing loss occurs when there are external or middle ear disorders such as impacted cerumen, perforation of the tympanic membrane, serum or pus in the middle ear, or a fusion of the ossicles. The vibrations are not adequately transmitted to the inner ear through the ear canal, tympanic membrane, middle ear, and ossicular chain; and a partial loss of hearing occurs.

Sensorineural, or perceptive, hearing loss occurs when there is a disorder in the inner ear, the auditory nerve, or the brain. Vibrations are transmitted to the inner ear, but an impairment of the cochlea or auditory nerve attenuates the nervous impulses from the cochlea to the brain.

Mixed hearing loss is a combination of conductive and sensorineural loss in the same ear.

EXAMINATION

The examination of the external ear begins with an inspection of both auricles to determine their position, size, and symmetry. Then the lateral and medial surfaces of each auricle and the surrounding tissues are inspected to determine the skin color and the presence of deformities, lesions, or nodules. The auricles and mastoid areas are palpated for evidence of swelling, tenderness, or nodules. Although fairly simple, this part of the examination is frequently neglected.

Examination of the external auditory canal and tympanic membrane requires additional lighting. It is suggested that the examiner become acquainted with the use and maintenance of the electric otoscope. For the otoscope to be effective, the batteries should be changed frequently to ensure optimal efficiency. The focus of light should be directed out of the end of the speculum. Some older models have a bulb carrier that can be bent, causing the light to be deflected to one side of the speculum.

Before inserting the speculum in the ear, one should inspect carefully the opening of the auditory canal for evidence of a foreign body. This is especially important when one is examining the ears of a child. Also, one should inspect for evidence of a discharge or inflammation. Any discharge should be described in terms of appearance and odor. A putrid odor is usually an indication of mastoid disease with bone destruction. Having completed this inspection, one should remember the following points when inserting the speculum:

1. Use the largest speculum that can be inserted in the ear without pain.
2. The client's head should be tipped toward the opposite shoulder for easy examination of the canal and tympanic membrane.
3. In adults the ear canal may be straightened by pulling the auricle upward and backward; in young children and infants it may be straightened by pulling the auricle downward.
4. The inner two thirds of the external meatus, which has a bony skeleton, is sensitive to pressure. Insert the speculum gently and not too far to avoid causing pain.
5. The angle at which the speculum is inserted into the meatus must be varied, or only a limited area of the tympanic membrane will be seen.

The auditory canal should be inspected for cerumen, redness, or swelling. The appearance

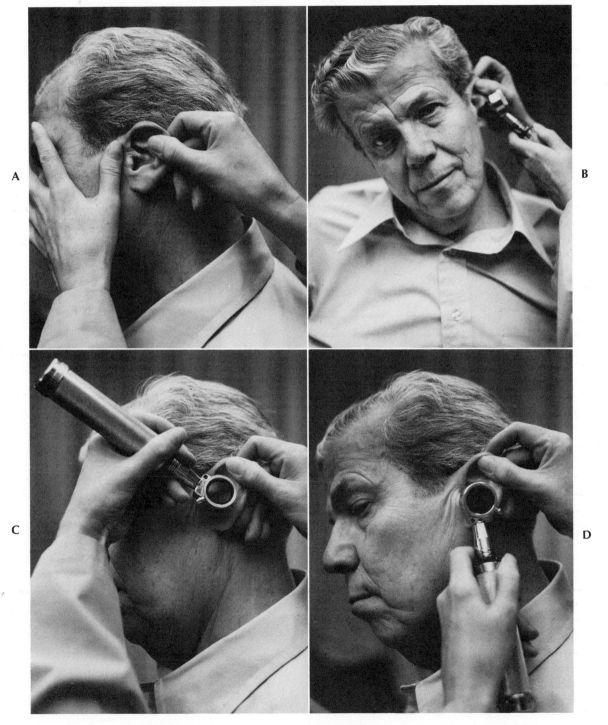

Fig. 8-3. Examination of the ear with the otoscope. **A,** Inspection of the meatus. **B,** Client's head is tipped toward the opposite shoulder. **C** and **D,** Two ways of holding the otoscope.

of the normal canal varies in regard to the diameter, the shape, and the growth of hairs. Hair growth is limited to the outer third of the canal, but the hairs may be numerous.

Another aspect of the examination of the auditory canal is the evaluation of cerumen, which is produced by the sebaceous glands and the apocrine sweat glands in the canal. There are apparently racial variations in color, and black or brown cerumen will be noted in the client with darker skin coloring. There is also some difference in the color of fresh cerumen as compared to older, drier cerumen; the former is a lighter, yellow or even pink color, and the latter is a darker, yellowish brown color. A small amount of cerumen will not interfere with the examination; the examiner can look past it and visualize the tympanic membrane. However, if the wax is excessive, it may be necessary to remove it. Two of the methods that can be used for the removal of wax are curettement or irrigation. *Curettement* is appropriate if the wax is soft or there is a question of perforation of the tympanic membrane. However, it should not be done except by a skilled clinician. The closeness of the blood vessels and nerves to the surface make it easy to cause bleeding and pain. *Irrigation* may be used when the wax is dry and hard but should not be carried out if there is a possibility that the membrane is perforated. Lukewarm water is used for the irrigation, which is done by repeatedly injecting the water from a syringe toward the posterosuperior canal wall. This procedure will cause the client to feel dizzy.

The examination of the tympanic membrane (Fig. 8-2) requires a careful assessment of the color of the membrane and the identification of landmarks. The membrane is usually a translucent pearl gray color; in disease the color may be yellow, white, or red. Some membranes have white flecks or dense white plaques that are the result of healed inflammatory disease. The landmarks are identified, beginning with the light reflex, which is a triangular cone of reflected light seen in the anteroinferior quadrant of the membrane. A diffuse or spotty light is not normal. At the top point of the light reflex toward the center of the membrane is the umbo, the inferior point of the handle of the malleus. Anterior and superior to the umbo is the long process of the malleus, which appears as a whitish line extending from the umbo to the juncture of the malleolar folds, where the small white projection of the short process of the malleus can be seen. The malleolar folds and the pars flaccida, the relaxed portion of the membrane, are superior and lateral to the short process. Finally, an attempt should be made to follow the annulus around the periphery of the pars tensa. It is in the areas close to the annulus that perforations are frequently noted.

Bulging of the tympanic membrane may occur when pus forms in the middle ear. The pressure increases, and the membrane may bulge outward in one part, or the entire membrane may bulge, resulting in obliteration of some or all of the landmarks. The light reflex is usually lost, and the membrane appears dull.

Retraction of the tympanic membrane occurs when pressure is reduced due to obstruction of the eustachian tube, usually associated with an upper respiratory system infection. The retraction of the membrane causes the landmarks to be accentuated. The light reflex may appear less prominent.

Normal tympanic membranes vary to some extent in size, shape, and color. It is only by examining many normal, healthy membranes that the ability to recognize the abnormal membrane is acquired.

■ Testing of auditory function

Clinical testing of auditory function is a process that starts early in the physical examination of the client. Understanding the spoken word is the principal use of hearing, and it may become apparent during the interview that there is an impairment or loss of auditory function. The actual testing of auditory function should be delayed until the end of the examination, after obvious problems related to hearing may have been identified.

Simple assessment of auditory acuity requires that only one ear be tested at a time. Therefore, it is necessary to mask the hearing in the ear not being tested. The examiner may occlude one of the client's ears by placing a finger against the opening of the auditory canal and moving the finger rapidly but gently.

Voice tests are frequently used in estimating the client's hearing. The testing is begun with a very low whisper; the lips of the examiner should be 1 or 2 feet away from the unoccluded ear. The examiner exhales and softly whispers numbers that the client is to repeat. If necessary, the intensity of the voice is increased to a medium whisper, and then to a loud whisper; then to a soft, then medium, then loud voice. To prevent lip reading, the examiner may find it necessary to shield his mouth from the client or ask the client to close his eyes.

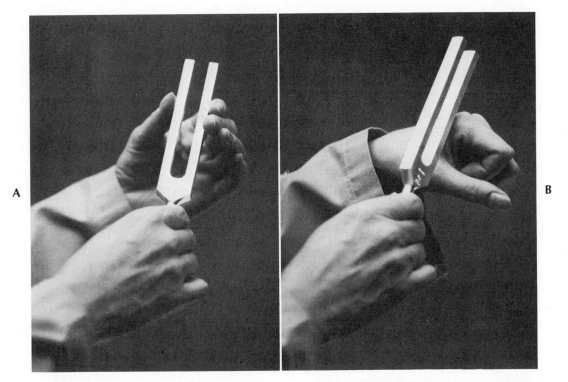

Fig. 8-4. Activating the tuning fork. **A,** Stroking the fork. **B,** Tapping the fork on the knuckle.

The watch tick is useful in testing but should not be used exclusively, because it provides only a high-frequency sound. The ticking watch is moved away from the ear until the client can no longer hear the sound.

Tuning fork tests are useful in determining whether the client has a conductive or a perceptive hearing loss. A fork with frequencies of 500 to 1,000 cycles per second (cps) is used because it can provide an estimate of hearing loss in the speech frequencies of roughly 500 to 2,000 cps. The tuning fork is held by the base and activated by gently stroking or tapping on the knuckle of the opposite hand (Fig. 8-4). It should be made to ring softly, not harshly.

The terms bone conduction and air conduction need to be clearly understood in the discussion of tuning fork tests. *Air conduction* implies the transmission of sound through the ear canal, tympanic membrane, and ossicular chain to the cochlea and auditory nerve. *Bone conduction* implies that sound is transmitted through the bones of the skull to the cochlea and auditory nerve. The client with normal auditory function will hear sound twice as long by air conduction, when the tuning fork is held opposite the external meatus, as he will by bone conduction, when the base of the tuning fork is placed on the mastoid bone.

The *Rinne test* makes use of air conduction and bone conduction (Fig. 8-5). The tuning fork is activated and held close to the auditory meatus until the client can no longer hear it. The base of the tuning fork is then immediately applied to the mastoid bone. If the client cannot hear it when it is placed on the mastoid bone, his Rinne test is considered normal or positive; sound is heard better by air conduction than by bone conduction. If the opposite is true and the client can hear the fork better by bone conduction, his Rinne test is negative and the deafness is due to a conductive hearing loss.

The *Weber test*, which makes use of bone conduction, is carried out by placing the base of the vibrating tuning fork on the vertex of the skull, on the forehead, or on the front teeth and asking the client if he hears the sound better in one ear or in the other (Fig. 8-6). In conductive deafness, the sound is referred to the deafer ear. This happens because the cochlea on that side will be undisturbed by extraneous sounds in the environment; these sounds are not transmitted, because of a problem or defect in the ear canal or middle ear. In perceptive deafness, the sound is referred to the better ear because the cochlea or auditory nerve is functioning more effectively.

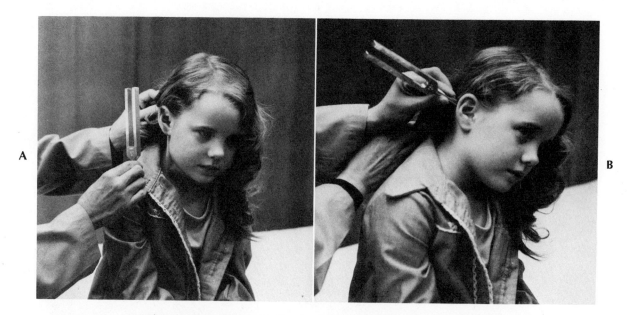

Fig. 8-5. Rinne test. **A,** Air conduction. **B,** Bone conduction.

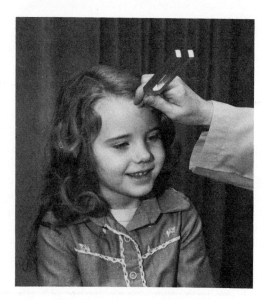

Fig. 8-6. Weber test.

Nose and paranasal sinuses

ANATOMY AND PHYSIOLOGY

The nose is the sensory organ for smell. It also warms, moistens, and filters the air inspired into the respiratory system.

The functions of the paranasal sinuses are not definitely known, but they may perform the same functions as the nose—that of warming, moisten-ing, and filtering air. They also aid in voice resonance.

The nose is divided into the external nose and the internal nose or nasal cavity (Fig. 8-7). The upper third of the nose is bone; the remainder of the nose is cartilaginous. The nasal cavity is divided by the septum into two narrow cavities. The cavities have two openings: the anterior cavity is the vestibule where the naris is located and is thickly lined with small hairs; the posterior opening, or choana, leads to the throat. The nasal septum forms the medial walls. The lateral walls are divided into the inferior, middle, and superior turbinate bones, which protude into the nasal cavity. The turbinates are covered by a highly vascular, mucous membrane. Below each turbinate is a meatus named according to the turbinate above it. The nasolacrimal duct drains into the inferior meatus, and most of the paranasal sinuses drain into the middle meatus. There is a plexus of blood vessels in the mucosa of the anterior nasal septum, which is a common site for epistaxis.

The receptors for smell are located in the olfactory area in the roof of the nasal cavity and upper third of the septum. The receptor cells, grouped as filaments, pass through openings of the cribiform plate, become the olfactory nerve (CN I), and transmit neural impulses for smell to the temporal lobe of the brain.

The paranasal sinuses are air-filled, paired, extensions of the nasal cavities within the bones of

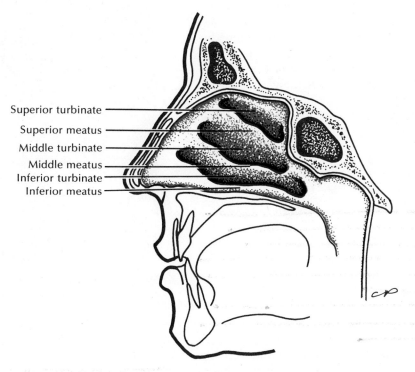

Superior turbinate
Superior meatus
Middle turbinate
Middle meatus
Inferior turbinate
Inferior meatus

Fig. 8-7. Lateral view of the left nasal cavity.

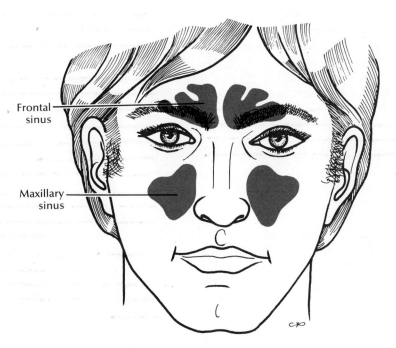

Frontal sinus

Maxillary sinus

Fig. 8-8. Anterior view of the frontal and maxillary sinuses.

the skull. They are the frontal, the maxillary, the ethmoidal, and the sphenoidal sinuses (Fig. 8-8). Their openings into the nasal cavity are narrow and easily obstructed. The frontal sinuses are located in the anterior part of the frontal bone. The maxillary sinuses, the largest of the paranasal sinuses, are located in the body of the maxilla. The ethmoidal sinuses are small and occupy the ethmoidal labyrinth between the orbit of the eye and the upper part of the cavity of the nose. The sphenoidal sinuses are found in the body of the sphenoid.

EXAMINATION

The external portion of the nose is inspected for any deviations in shape, size, or color; the nares are inspected for flaring or discharge. The ridge and soft tissues of the nose are palpated for displacement of the bone and cartilage and for tenderness or masses.

Examination of the nasal function includes determination of the ability to smell and the patency of the nasal cavities. To determine if the nasal cavities are patent, the client is asked to close his mouth, exert pressure on one naris with a finger and breathe through the opposite naris. The procedure is repeated to determine the patency of the opposite naris. To determine the adequacy of function of the olfactory nerve (CN I), the client is asked to close his eyes and occlude one naris again. The examiner places an aromatic substance, such as coffee or alcohol, close to the client's nose and asks the client to identify the odor. Each side is tested separately.

The examination of the nasal cavities may be carried out by using the electric otoscope with the short, broad nasal speculum or by using a nasal speculum and a penlight. Little of the interior of the nose can be seen unless the anterior naris is dilated. This is especially true in adults. The otoscope or speculum is held in the left hand, and the index finger is placed on the side of the nose to stabilize the position of the speculum and prevent displacement (Fig. 8-9). The right hand is used to position the head and hold the light. Care must be taken not to apply pressure on the nasal septum because of its great sensitivity; but, if a nasal speculum is being used, the blades must be opened as far as possible. In infants and young children the naris is wider and the vestibule more shallow; visualization of the interior of the nose can be accomplished without using a speculum by pressing the tip of the nose upward.

Examination of the nasal cavity through the an-

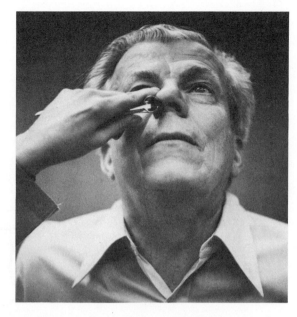

Fig. 8-9. Proper position for insertion of the nasal speculum with the index finger on the side of the nose.

terior naris is limited to the vestibule, the anterior portion of the septum, and the inferior and middle turbinates. It is necessary to change the position of the head several times during the examination to inspect the various areas. With the client's head tipped back, the inferior and middle turbinates can be seen (Fig. 8-10). The septum is inspected for deviation, exudate, and perforation. The septum is rarely straight. The lateral walls of the nasal cavities and the inferior and middle turbinates are examined for polyps, swelling, exudate, and change in color. The nasal mucosa is normally redder than the oral mucosa. Increased redness indicates infection; pale, boggy turbinates are typical of allergy. Any drainage from the middle meatus, which drains several of the paranasal sinuses, is important and should be described. The floor of the vestibule should be carefully inspected for evidence of a foreign body.

Examination of the paranasal sinuses is done indirectly. Information about their condition is gained by inspection and palpation of the overlying tissues or by transillumination. Only the frontal and maxillary sinuses are accessible for examination. Palpation for examination of the maxillary sinuses is performed on the maxillary areas of the cheeks, where tenderness may be elicited. By palpating both cheeks simultaneously, one can determine differences in tenderness. Swelling of the cheek rarely occurs in maxillary sinusitis. The

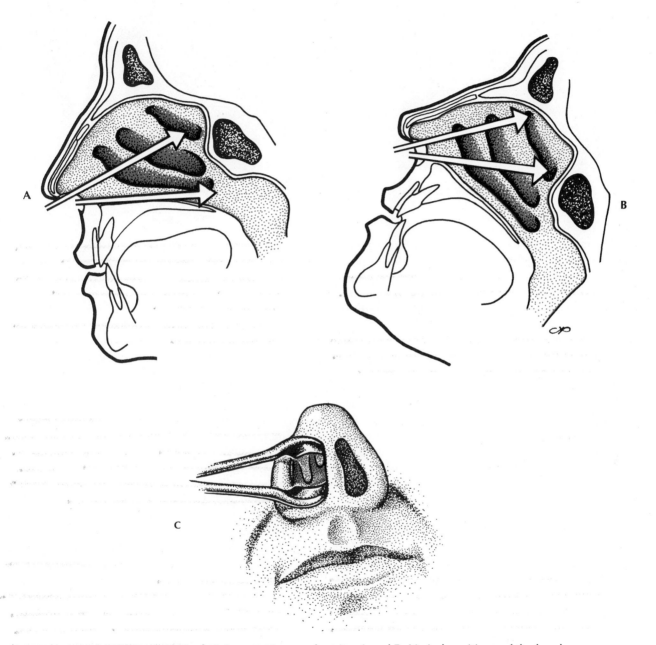

Fig. 8-10. Examination of the anterior nasal cavity. **A** and **B,** Varied positions of the head provide visualization of different areas of the cavity. **C,** View of the inferior and middle turbinates.

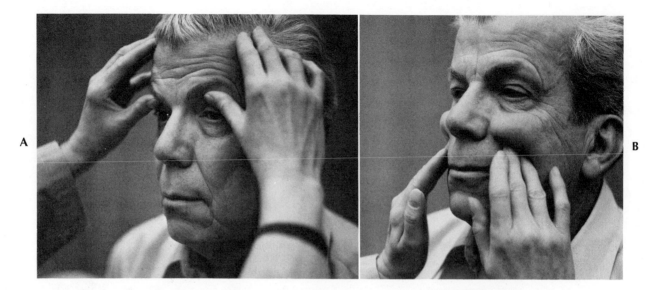

Fig. 8-11. Palpation of the frontal **(A)** and maxillary **(B)** sinuses.

frontal sinuses can be palpated by finger pressure below the eyebrows. Palpation of the sinuses is demonstrated in Fig. 8-11. Both the maxillary and frontal sinuses may also be percussed by lightly tapping with the index finger to determine if the client feels pain.

Transillumination of the maxillary sinuses is accomplished in a completely darkened room by shining a bright light in the client's mouth. The frontal sinus is transilluminated by shining a light through the medial aspect of the supraorbital rim.

Transillumination has limitations as a diagnostic tool and is not highly successful, since even normal sinuses will show differences in the amount of transillumination.

Mouth and oropharynx

ANATOMY AND PHYSIOLOGY

The mouth is the first division of the digestive tube and an entry site to the respiratory system. The oropharynx conducts air to and from the larynx and food to the esophagus from the mouth. The structures of the mouth and oropharynx are illustrated in Fig. 8-12.

The boundaries of the mouth are the lips anteriorly and the soft palate and uvula posteriorly. The floor is formed by the mandibular bone, which is covered by loose, mobile tissue. The roof of the oral cavity is formed by the hard and soft palates. They are distinctly different in color; the soft palate is pink, and the hard palate is white.

The uvula is a muscular organ that hangs down from the posterior margin of the soft palate. The muscles of mastication are innervated by two main nerves: the trigeminal nerve (CN V) and the facial nerve (CN VII).

The mouth contains the tongue, gums, teeth, and salivary glands. The tongue is composed of a mass of striated muscles interspersed with fat and many glands. The dorsal surface is rough in appearance due to the presence of papillae. The ventral surface toward the floor of the mouth is smooth and shows large veins. The fold of mucous membrane that joins the tongue to the floor of the mouth is the frenulum. The tongue is innervated by the hypoglossal nerve (CN XII). The sensory receptors for taste are the glossopharyngeal nerve (CN IX) and the facial nerve (CN VII).

The gums are composed of fibrous tissue covered with a smooth mucous membrane and are attached to the alveolar margins of the jaws and to the necks of the teeth. In the adult there are 32 teeth, 16 in each arch.

Three pairs of salivary glands secrete into the oral cavity. They are the parotid, submandibular, and sublingual salivary glands. The largest is the parotid gland, which lies in front of and below the external ear. The parotid (Stensen's) duct opens into the buccal membrane opposite the second molar. The submandibular gland lies below and in front of the parotid gland. The submandibular (Wharton's) duct opens at the side of the frenulum on the floor of the mouth. The sublingual gland is the smallest salivary gland and lies in the floor of the mouth. It raises the mucous mem-

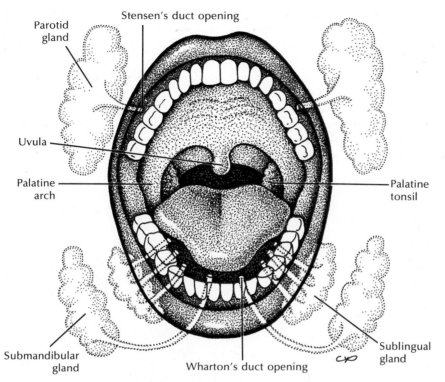

Fig. 8-12. Structures of the mouth.

brane, covering its superior surface to form the sublingual fold. It has numerous small openings, which open on the sublingual fold.

The oropharynx is the section of the pharynx that is posterior to the oral cavity and most accessible to examination. The nasopharynx lies behind the nasal cavities and is superior to the oropharynx. The laryngopharynx is inferior to the oropharynx. Along both lateral walls of the oropharynx are two palatine arches, and between them are the tonsils. The tonsils are usually the same color as the surrounding tissue and do not normally extend beyond the pillars. Tonsillar tissue in children enlarges until puberty and then shrinks back into the folds of the arches. Consequently, a child's tonsils may normally be larger than an adult's. The posterior pharyngeal wall that is visible during the clinical examination may show many small blood vessels and small areas of pink or red lymphoid tissue.

EXAMINATION

The examination is conducted from the anterior to the posterior areas of the mouth and begins with the external components of the mouth and jaw.

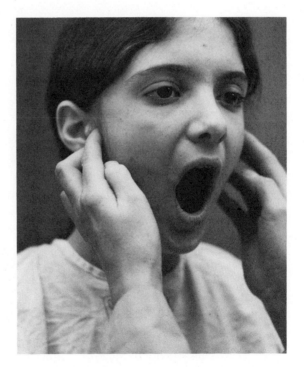

Fig. 8-13. Palpation of the temporomandibular joint.

The lips are inspected for symmetry, color, edema, or surface abnormalities. The client is asked to open and close his mouth to demonstrate the mobility of the mandible and the occlusion of the teeth. The temporomandibular joint is palpated while the mouth is opened wide and then closed, for any tenderness, crepitus, or deviation (Fig. 8-13). Pressure applied to the joint during closing of the mouth may result in referred pain to the ear; a common cause of the referred pain is malocclusion. The lips are palpated for induration.

The client is asked to remove dentures, if worn, for the rest of the mouth and throat examination. A good source of additional light is essential in examination of the mouth and throat.

The oral mucosal surfaces are normally light pink and are kept moist by saliva. The surfaces are examined systematically to ensure that all areas are inspected (Fig. 8-14). The examiner

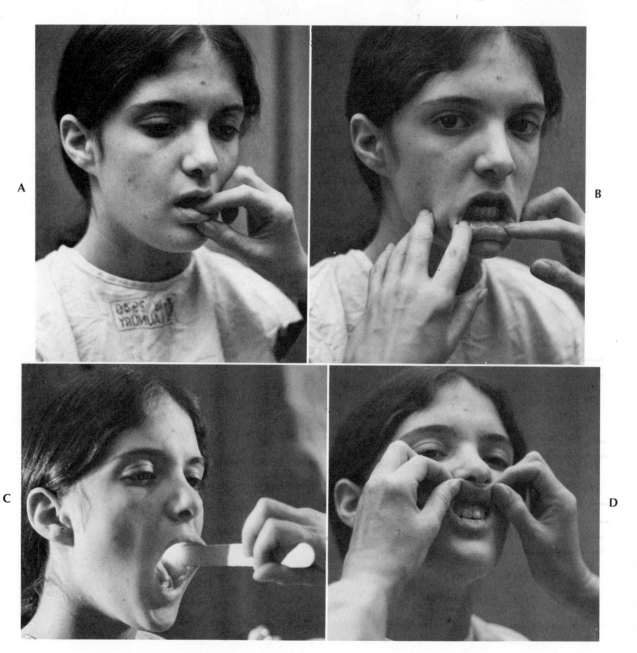

Fig. 8-14. Examination of the lips and oral mucosa. **A,** Palpation of the lips. **B,** Inspection of the mucosa of the lower anterior area. **C,** Inspection of mucosa of each cheek with identification of Stensen's duct opening. **D,** Inspection of mucosa of the upper anterior area.

may use two tongue depressors or the fingers as retractors. With the client's mouth partially open, the mucosa in the anteroinferior area between the lower lip and gum is examined. With the mouth wide open, the buccal mucosa and Stensen's duct (the opening to the parotid gland, opposite the upper second molar) of the right cheek are examined. The maxillary mucobuccal fold between the upper lip and gum is examined next; then the mucosa and Stensen's duct of the left cheek are examined.

The examination of the tongue begins with inspection of the dorsum for any swelling, variation in size or color, coating, or ulceration. The client is asked to extend the tongue in order to demonstrate any deviation, tremor, or limitation of movement; any of these would be indicative of impairment of the hypoglossal nerve (CN XII). To inspect the posterior and lateral areas of the tongue, a 4 × 4 piece of gauze is wrapped around the tip of the extended tongue and the examiner's hand is used to hold and position the tongue (Fig. 8-15). The tongue is swung to the left, and the right lateral border is inspected. The position is reversed, and the left lateral border is examined. The tongue is released, and the client is asked to touch the tip of the tongue to the palate. The ventral surface is observed for swelling or varicosities. The floor of the mouth is inspected for abnormalities or swelling; Wharton's ducts (the openings of the submandibular glands), the frenulum, and the sublingual ridge are identified. The entire tongue and the floor of the mouth are carefully palpated, because some diseases or tumors cause little change in the surface and can only be detected by palpation.

The teeth are inspected for caries and malocclusion. The gums are inspected for inflammation and bleeding. Pyorrhea starts as a simple inflammation; if it is treated early, advanced pyorrhea can be prevented. The gums gradually recede with age and expose a larger amount of the teeth.

With the client's head back, the palate and uvula are inspected. It may be necessary to depress the base of the tongue with a tongue depressor. The difference in color of the hard and soft palate are noted, as is any abnormality of architecture. An exostosis is frequently found in the midline of the palate. Such bony growths are benign. The uvula may be bifid and part of a submucosal cleft palate. The client is asked to say, "Ah," and the rise of the soft palate and uvula is noted. Any deviation or lack of movement indicates impairment of the vagus nerve (CN X).

The oropharynx is inspected while the client's head is back, and the base of the tongue is gently depressed with a tongue depressor. The anterior palatine arches and the posterior arches are inspected for inflammation or swelling. The size of the tonsils is estimated, and any exudate is noted. The posterior wall of the oropharynx is examined for any change in color. The glossopharyngeal nerve (CN IX) and the vagus nerve (CN X) are tested by touching the posterior wall of the pharynx on each side. The normal response is a gag reflex. A unilaterally impaired gag reflex usually indicates impairment of glossopharyngeal as well as vagal function.

Throughout the examination of the mouth and throat, attention should be given to mouth odors, which may result from systemic as well as oral disease.

BIBLIOGRAPHY

Ballantyne, J., and Groves, J.: Scott-Brown's diseases of the ear, nose and throat, vols. 1-4, Philadelphia, 1971, J. B. Lippincott Co.

DeWeese, D. D., and Saunders, W. H.: Textbook of Otolaryngology, ed. 4, St. Louis, 1973, The C. V. Mosby Co.

Foxen, E. H. M.: Lecture notes on diseases of the ear, nose and throat, ed. 3, Oxford, 1972, Blackwell Scientific Publications Ltd.

Romanes, G. J.: Cunningham's manual of practical anatomy, vol. 2, Head, neck and brain, ed. 13, New York, 1973, Oxford University Press, Inc.

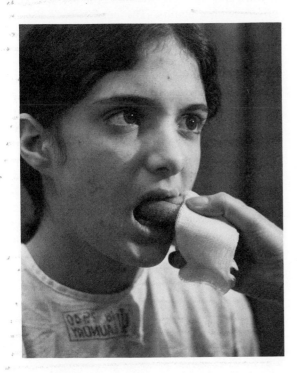

Fig. 8-15. Examination of the tongue.

9 Assessment of the head, face, and neck

A great variety of structures are located in the head and neck area, including several organs of special sensation. Although the examination of the entire head involves the examination of the special sense organs, those topics are covered in other chapters: Chapter 8 on Assessment of the ears, nose, and throat and Chapter 10 on Assessment of the eyes. This chapter deals with the remaining structures. Similarly, in the case of the neck examination, multiple structures are involved, some of which are covered in other chapters: Chapter 11 on Assessment of the lymphatic system, Chapter 13 on Assessment of the respiratory system, and Chapter 14 on Cardiovascular assessment: the heart and the neck vessels. This organization is presented so that the learner may better understand the examinations of complete body systems. Having learned this, the beginning practitioner must then proceed to organize and integrate the components of the physical examination by anatomical area.

The assessment techniques of inspection, palpation, and auscultation are utilized in the examination of the head and neck. Equipment requirements include a good light source, a glass of water, and a stethoscope.

Head

Those portions of the head examination covered here include assessment of the size and shape of the skull and assessment of the condition of the scalp and hair.

The shape of the skull is generally round with several prominences; the frontal areas are prominent anteriorly. The areas of the head take their names from the underlying bones, including the frontal, parietal, occipital, and mastoid bones; the maxilla; and the mandible (Fig. 9-1). There is a large range of normal-shaped skulls.

The skin overlying the superior, lateral, and posterior portions of the skull is called the scalp and is normally covered with hair.

The size and shape of the skull are assessed by inspection; the examiner also inspects the condition of the scalp by parting the hair in several areas. Obviously, wigs or other hairpieces must be removed to accomplish this assessment. The client should be carefully questioned regarding any previous head trauma, because the hair covering makes it difficult to assess the head and scalp completely. The examiner also notes the texture and amount of hair and the use of coloring or lubricating agents. The condition of the hair may be a useful indication of the client's emotional status, social group identification, and personal hygiene.

Several conditions may result in abnormalities of the skull. For example, an abnormally large head in children may result from the accumulation of fluid in the ventricles of the brain (hydrocephalus). In adults a large head may result from osteitis deformans, wherein the bony thickness increases, or from excessive growth hormone secretion (acromegaly), wherein the skull becomes enlarged and thickened, the length of the mandible increases, the nose and forehead are more prominent, and the facial features appear coarsened. Local deformities of the skull may result from trauma or from the surgical removal of portions of the skull.

Sebaceous cysts may develop on the scalp. These result from the occlusion of sebaceous gland ducts and are palpable as smooth, rounded nodules attached to the scalp. The scalp should also be assessed for dandruff and for the presence of parasites.

132

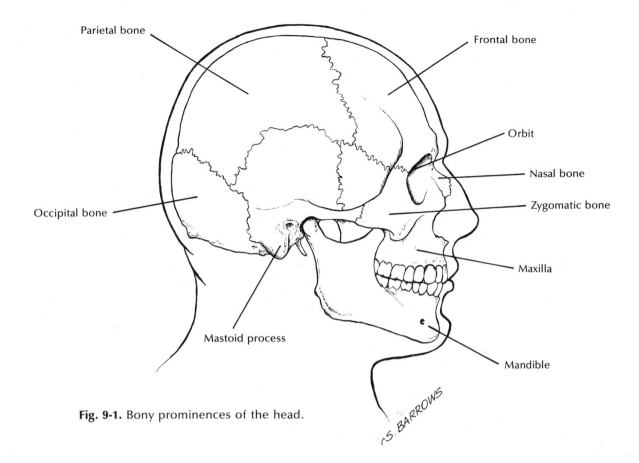

Parietal bone

Frontal bone

Orbit

Nasal bone

Zygomatic bone

Occipital bone

Maxilla

Mandible

Mastoid process

r.S. BARROWS

Fig. 9-1. Bony prominences of the head.

The hair is subject to the influence of altered metabolic conditions. The classic examples are the changes caused by thyroid disorders. In hypothyroidism, the hair is coarse, dry, and brittle; in hyperthyroidism, the hair becomes fine, silky, and soft. The thinning or loss of hair (alopecia) may be hereditary, especially in males, or a side effect of drugs used to treat malignant tumors. This condition may also accompany prolonged illness or emotional stress.

Face

The variations in facial appearance are as numerous as the earth's population. Furthermore, a client's facial expression at any moment is subject to change and often reveals much about his general feeling tone. In general, the examiner should observe the bilateral structures for symmetry in size, position, and movement.

In examining the face, the examiner observes the facial expression, the color and condition of the facial skin, and the shape and symmetry of the facial structures, including the eyebrows, eyes, nose, mouth, and ears. Normally the palpebral fissures, the distance between the eyelids, are

equal in size. The nasolabial folds, the creases extending from the angle of the nose to the corner of the mouth, are symmetrical (Fig. 9-2). Within the range of normal, there are many individuals with slightly asymmetrical characteristic expressions.

Sensation of the face is mediated by the trigeminal nerve (cranial nerve [CN] V), which has three sensory divisions. Its function is tested as part of the neurological examination for pain and touch. The muscles of facial expression are supplied by the facial nerve (CN VII). The examiner can test for facial muscle function by asking the client to elevate his eyebrows, frown or lower his eyebrows, close his eyes tightly, puff his cheeks, show his teeth, and smile.

The major accessible artery on the face is the temporal artery, which passes just anterior to the ear over the temporal muscle and into the forehead (Fig. 9-3). It is palpable in the temporal area just anterior to the tragus of the ear. Any thickening, hardness, or tenderness of the vessel should be noted.

Changes in color, shape, symmetry, hair distribution pattern, or movement of the face may occur. In situations where there is an increased amount of unsaturated hemoglobin in the body

133

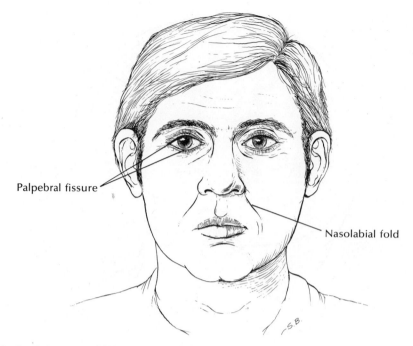

Fig. 9-2. Anterior view of the face showing the palpebral fissures and nasolabial folds.

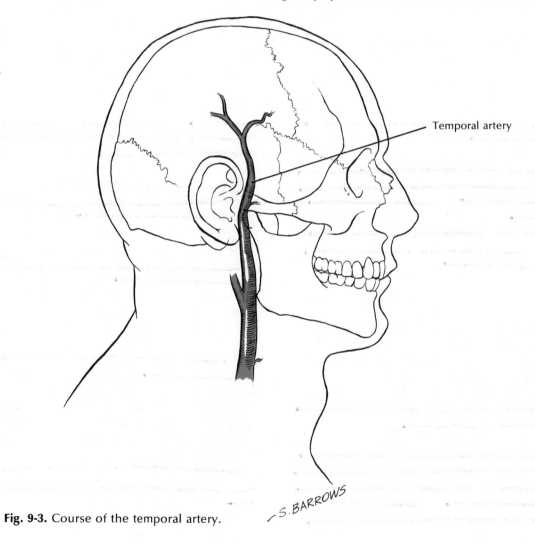

Fig. 9-3. Course of the temporal artery.

tissues, as may occur with cardiac or pulmonary disease, or where there is a local stasis of circulation, various facial and head structures, including the lips, nose, cheeks, ears, and oral mucosa, may become bluish, or cyanotic, in color. Facial pallor results from a decrease in circulating red blood cells, as in anemia, or from a decrease in local vascular supply, as in shock. The yellow color of jaundice results from an abnormal increase in bilirubin. Before jaundice is generally evident in the skin, it may be observed in the sclera and in the mucous membranes of the mouth under the tongue and on the palate. Localized color changes result from acne, moles, and scar tissue. More rare conditions associated with color alterations include lupus erythematosis, wherein an erythematous discoloration bridges the cheeks and nose, and conditions that alter the deposition of melanin, resulting in light or dark patchy areas.

Numerous situations may cause a change in facial shape. Edema, often initially evident in the eyelids, may result from cardiovascular or kidney disease. Thyroid disorders also affect the face: excessive function, hyperthyroidism, may be associated with an apparent protrusion of the eyeballs (exophthalmos) and with elevation of the upper lids, resulting in a staring or startled expression; diminished function, hypothyroidism, may lead to "myxedema facies," wherein the face is dull and puffy with dry skin and coarse features. As a result of increased adrenal hormone production (Cushing's syndrome) or secondary to the intake of synthetic adrenal hormones, "moon facies" may be observed, wherein the face is round and the cheeks quite red. Prolonged illness, dehydration, or starvation may produce a cachectic face, wherein the eyes, cheeks, and temples appear sunken, the nose appears sharp, and the skin is dry and rough.

Asymmetry or abnormal movements, or both, may result from facial nerve lesions. In Bell's palsy, a paralysis of the seventh nerve, the eye on the affected side cannot close completely, the lower eyelid droops, the nasolabial fold is lost, and the corner of the mouth droops. Slight weakness may be present but is not evident when the face is at rest, so the examiner should carefully check facial muscle function.

In the women of some ethnic groups, increased facial hair is a normal finding. Elevated production of adrenal hormones may lead to excessive hair growth in the moustache and sideburn areas and on the chin. Myxedema causes thinning of the scalp hair and eyebrows.

Neck

A complete examination of the neck includes assessment of the neck muscles and cervical vertebrae, the trachea, the thyroid gland, the carotid arteries and jugular veins, and the cervical lymph nodes. As mentioned earlier, this chapter covers only the muscles and the thyroid gland, since the other structures are discussed elsewhere in the text.

NECK MUSCLES

The major neck muscles are the sternocleidomastoid muscles and the trapezius muscles. Each sternocleidomastoid muscle extends from the upper sternum and proximal portion of the clavicle to the mastoid process behind the ear (Fig. 9-4). These muscles are involved in turning the head and in lateral flexion of the head. The two trapezius muscles are large, flat, and triangular in shape, and together they form a trapezoid shape. Each trapezius muscle extends from the occipital bone of the skull, the seventh cervical vertebra, and all the thoracic vertebrae to the clavicle and to the spine of the scapula (Fig. 9-5). The trapezius muscles are involved in the movements of shrugging the shoulders, pulling the scapulae downward and toward the vertebral column, drawing the head to the side, drawing the head backward, and elevating the chin. Both the sternocleidomastoid and the trapezius muscles are supplied by the spinal accessory nerve (CN XI).

The sternocleidomastoid muscles are used to describe areas of the neck. These muscles divide each side of the neck into two triangles, the anterior and posterior triangles (Fig. 9-4). The parameters of the anterior triangle are the mandible superiorly, the sternocleidomastoid muscle laterally, and the midline of the trachea medially. Within the anterior triangle lie the trachea, the thyroid gland, and the anterior cervical nodes; the carotid artery runs just anterior and parallel to the sternocleidomastoid muscle. The parameters of the posterior triangle are the sternocleidomastoid muscle laterally, the trapezius muscle medially, and the clavicle inferiorly. The posterior cervical lymph nodes are located here.

The neck muscles are inspected for symmetry of the musculature and for any abnormal masses or swellings. Their function is assessed by observing for the normal centered position of the head, by observing the active range of motion of the head, and by testing muscle strength against re-

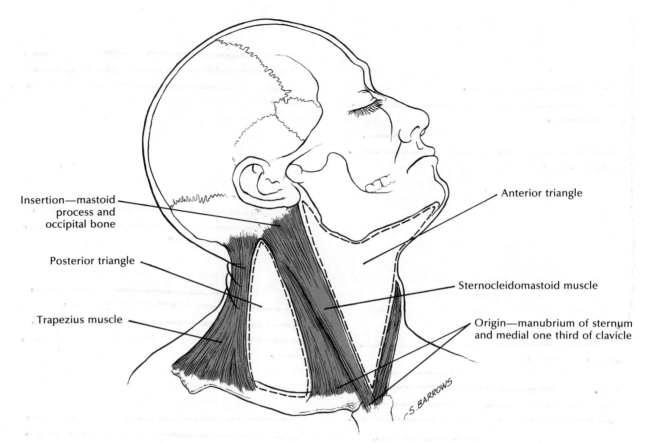

Insertion—mastoid process and occipital bone

Posterior triangle

Trapezius muscle

Anterior triangle

Sternocleidomastoid muscle

Origin—manubrium of sternum and medial one third of clavicle

—S. BARROWS

Fig. 9-4. Sternocleidomastoid muscle and the anterior and posterior triangles.

sistance. Normally, the head should flex until the chin rests on the chest with the mouth closed; the head should turn about 90° laterally and flex in that position until chin and shoulder touch; the head normally extends about 70° to 80° backward. Strength of the sternocleidomastoid muscles is tested by having the client turn his head to one side and then to the other against the resistance of the examiner's hand. Strength of the trapezius muscles is assessed by asking the client to shrug his shoulders against the resistance of the examiner's hands.

Common abnormalities of the neck muscles include stiffness and pain. In tense individuals, some degree of muscle spasm may occur and tenderness on palpation may be elicited over the affected muscles. Stiffness of the neck may also result from vertebral disease or meningitis. Cervical arthritis produces limitation of motion, and central nervous system disease involving irritation of the meninges is associated with pain on neck motion. *Note:* If there is any suspicion of traumatic neck injury, passive range of motion should never be done.

An abnormal position or tilting of the head may be due to shortening of the sternocleidomastoid muscle or may be secondary to visual difficulties. An abnormal up-and-down nodding movement of the head is seen with Parkinson's disease.

THYROID GLAND

The thyroid gland is the largest endocrine gland in the body and the only one accessible to direct physical examination.

An awareness of the midline neck structures is important in performing the examination of the thyroid gland (Fig. 9-6). Structures lying in the midline include:

1. The hyoid bone, which lies just below the mandible at the angle of the floor of the mouth.
2. The thyroid cartilage, which is shaped like a shield and which is the largest of the cartilagenous structures in the neck. The upper edge is notched, and its level corresponds to the level of bifurcation of the common carotid artery into the internal and external carotid arteries.

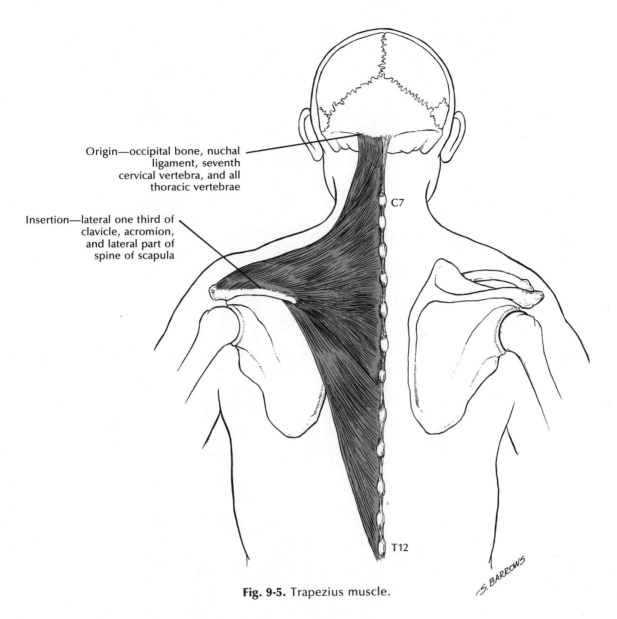

Origin—occipital bone, nuchal ligament, seventh cervical vertebra, and all thoracic vertebrae

Insertion—lateral one third of clavicle, acromion, and lateral part of spine of scapula

C7

T12

S. BARROWS

Fig. 9-5. Trapezius muscle.

3. The cricoid cartilage, which is the uppermost ring of the trachea. It is palpable just below the thyroid cartilage.

4. The tracheal rings.

5. The isthmus of the thyroid gland, which lies across the trachea below the cricoid cartilage.

The thyroid gland is butterfly shaped; it has two lateral lobes and a connecting isthmus that joins the lobes at their lower third area. The lobes are irregular and cone shaped, each about 5 cm long, 3 cm in diameter, and 2 cm thick. The average weight of the total gland is about 25 gm. The lobes curve posteriorly around the cartilages; the lateral portions are covered by the sternocleidomastoid muscles. Thyroid arteries supply the highly vascular thyroid tissue.

■ **Examination**

The techniques used to examine the thyroid gland include observation, palpation, and auscultation. It should be noted that observation of thyroid function or possible dysfunction includes more than observation of the area where the thyroid gland is located. The effects of thyroid activity are widespread; therefore, observations of behavior, appearance, skin, eyes, hair, and cardiovascular status are important.

To inspect the thyroid gland, the examiner stands before the client and observes particularly the lower half of the neck, first in normal position, next in slight extension, and then while the client swallows a sip of water (Fig. 9-7). The movements of the cartilages are easily observed. Any unusual bulging of thyroid tissue in the mid-

137

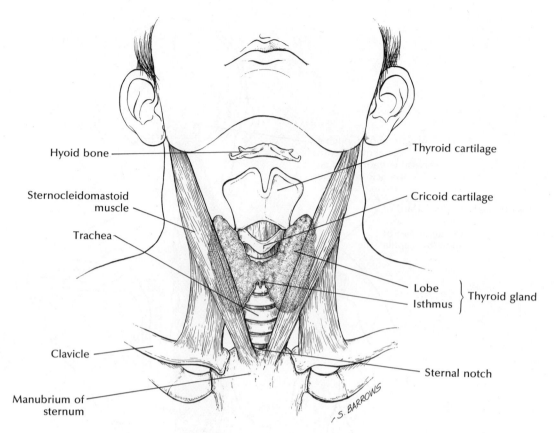

Hyoid bone

Thyroid cartilage

Sternocleidomastoid muscle

Cricoid cartilage

Trachea

Lobe
Isthmus } Thyroid gland

Clavicle

Sternal notch

Manubrium of sternum

Fig. 9-6. Midline neck structures.

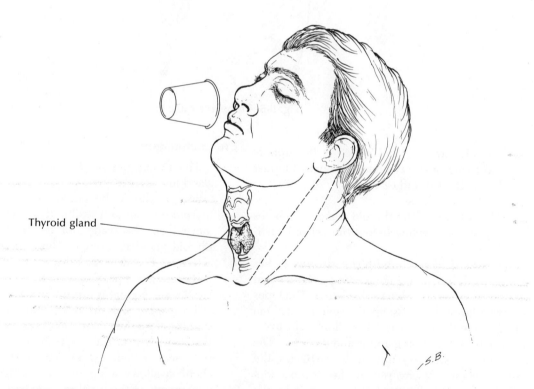

Thyroid gland

Fig. 9-7. Observation for the thyroid gland with the neck in slight extension. The structures of the thyroid gland are more distinct during swallowing.

line of the lobes or behind the sternocleidomastoid muscles should be noted; normally, none is seen. A good cross light is helpful for observing subtle neck movements or ascending masses.

Following observation, the neck is palpated for the presence of an enlarged thyroid, for consistency of the gland, and for any nodules. The normal thyroid gland is not palpable. However, in a thin neck, the isthmus is occasionally palpable; and in a short, stocky neck, even an enlarged gland may be difficult to palpate. Palpation may be done with the examiner standing either in front of or behind the client. Although there are several techniques utilized for palpation of the thyroid, the underlying principles for each technique include movement of the gland while the client swallows, adequate exposure of the gland by relaxation and manual displacement of surrounding structures, and comparison of one side of the gland with the other. The thyroid gland is fixed to the trachea and thus ascends during swallowing. This serves to distinguish thyroid structures from other neck masses.

Posterior approach. The client is seated on a chair or examining table while the examiner stands behind him. The client is requested to lower his chin in order to relax the neck muscles. The examining fingers are curved anteriorly, so that the tips rest on the lower half of the neck over the trachea (Fig. 9-8). The client is asked to swallow a sip of water while the examiner feels for any enlargement of the thyroid isthmus. To facilitate examination of each lobe, the client is asked to turn his head slightly toward the side to be examined with the chin still lowered. For example, to examine the right thyroid lobe, the examiner has the client lower his chin and turn his head slightly to the right. With the fingers of the left hand, the examiner displaces the thyroid cartilage slightly to the right while the fingers of the right hand palpate the area lateral to the cartilage where the thyroid lobe lies, for any enlargement (Fig. 9-9). The client is asked to swallow a sip of water as this procedure is being done. The examiner may also palpate for thyroid enlargement on the right side by placing the thumb deep to and behind the sternocleidomastoid muscle while the index and middle fingers are placed deep to and in front of the muscle (Fig. 9-10). This procedure is then repeated for the left lobe; the right hand displaces the cartilage, and the left hand palpates.

Anterior approach. The examiner stands in front of the client and with the palmar surfaces of the index and middle fingers palpates below the

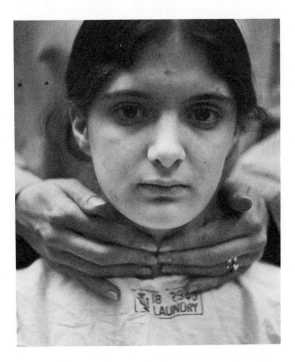

Fig. 9-8. Posterior approach to thyroid examination. Standing behind the client, the examiner palpates for the thyroid isthmus by placing the palmar aspects of the fingertips over the lower portion of the trachea.

cricoid cartilage for the thyroid isthmus as the client swallows a sip of water. In a procedure similar to the one used with the posterior approach, the client is asked to flex his head and turn it slightly to one side and then the other. The examiner palpates for the left lobe by displacing the thyroid cartilage slightly to the left with the left hand and examining for thyroid enlargement with the right hand (Fig. 9-11). Again, the examiner palpates the area and hooks thumb and fingers around the sternocleidomastoid muscle (Fig. 9-12). The procedure is repeated for the right side.

If enlargement of the thyroid gland is detected or suspected, the area over the gland is auscultated for a bruit. In a hyperplastic thyroid gland, the blood flow through the thyroid arteries is accelerated and produces vibrations that may be heard with the bell of the stethoscope as a soft, rushing sound, or bruit. (See Chapter 14 on Cardiovascular assessment: the heart and the neck vessels for further discussion of bruits.)

The thyroid gland may incur diffuse or local enlargement. Diffuse enlargement may occur to varying degrees. Symmetrical thyroid enlargement is not uncommon in areas where there is a

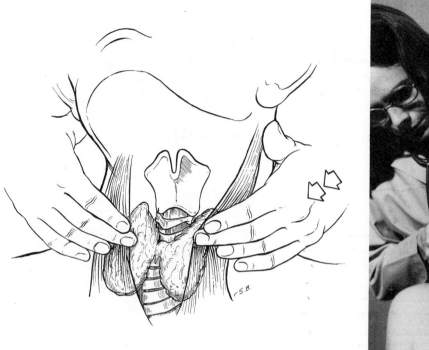

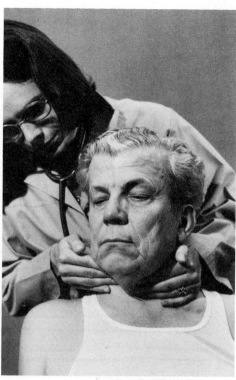

Fig. 9-9. Posterior approach to thyroid examination. In order to examine the right lobe of the thyroid gland, the examiner displaces the trachea slightly to the right with the fingers of the left hand and palpates for the right thyroid lobe with the fingers of the right hand.

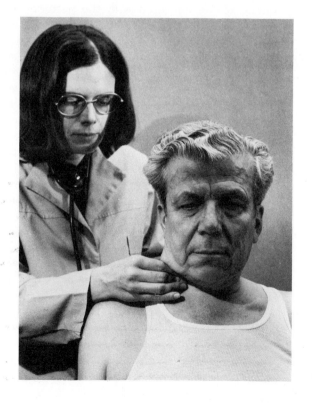

Fig. 9-10. Posterior approach to thyroid examination. Examining for an enlarged right thyroid lobe, the examiner grasps and palpates around and deep to the right sternocleidomastoid muscle.

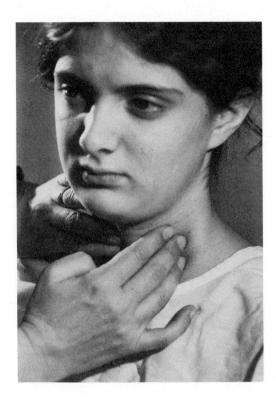

Fig. 9-11. Anterior approach to thyroid examination. Standing in front of the client, the examiner uses the fingers of the left hand to displace the trachea slightly to the left while the fingers of the right hand palpate for the left thyroid lobe.

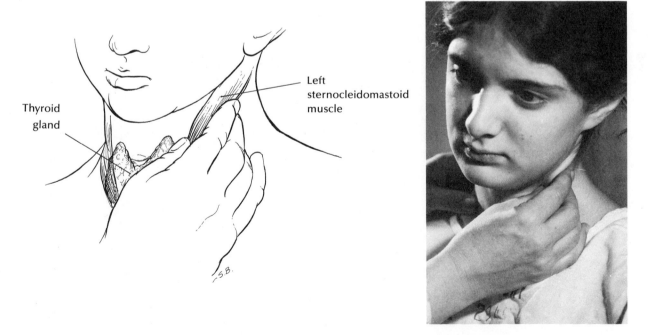

Thyroid gland

Left sternocleidomastoid muscle

Fig. 9-12. Anterior approach to thyroid examination. The examiner grasps around the left sternocleidomastoid muscle with the right hand to palpate for an enlarged left thyroid lobe.

deficiency of dietary iodine. Localized or nodular enlargement may consist of one or more nodules and may occur in either lobe or in the isthmus. Solitary nodules are suggestive of carcinoma, particularly in younger people.

Thyroid tissue located in the retrosternal area may also become enlarged. This is not discernible by physical examination but should be considered if other physical findings are suggestive of thyroid dysfunction.

BIBLIOGRAPHY

Werner, S. C.: Physical examination. In Werner, S. C., and Ingbar, S. H., editors: The thyroid; a fundamental and clinical text, ed. 3, New York, 1971, Harper & Row, Publishers.

10 Assessment of the eyes

Examination of the eyes is fascinating, beautiful and at least for a while, quite difficult. With much practice and great patience, the fundamentals of this complex examination can be mastered; the rewards for this effort are great. A thorough examination of the eyes can reveal something of the emotional status of the client, as well as information on both local and systemic health and disease processes.

The eye examination involves multiple components; students learning it should learn a reasonable arrangement of the various components in order to remember all portions. The ordering of these parts should focus both on completeness of the examination and on the comfortable positioning of the client.

This examination encompasses measurement of visual acuity, evaluation of visual fields, testing of ocular movements, inspection of the ocular structures, testing of nerve reflexes, and the ophthalmoscopic, or funduscopic, examination. To-

nometry should also be included, especially for persons over 40 years of age. The technique of inspection is the principal physical examination technique involved.

Because of the complexity of the eye examination, instead of presenting examination techniques with normal and abnormal findings together, the chapter is arranged as follows: first, a brief review of the anatomy of the eye and the normal appearance of the various structures is presented; then the examination technique and a method of organizing the examination are suggested; finally, some of the more common abnormal eye findings are discussed.

ANATOMY AND NORMAL FINDINGS
■ Ocular structures

The structures of the eyelid and the globe of the eye are shown in Figs. 10-1 and 10-2.

Eyelids and eyelashes. The eyelashes are

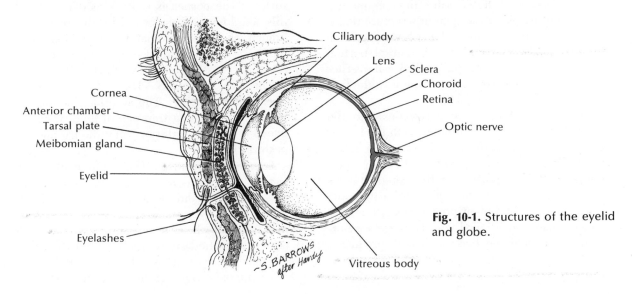

Fig. 10-1. Structures of the eyelid and globe.

Cornea
Anterior chamber
Tarsal plate
Meibomian gland
Eyelid
Eyelashes

Ciliary body
Lens
Sclera
Choroid
Retina
Optic nerve
Vitreous body

~S. BARROWS
after Hardy

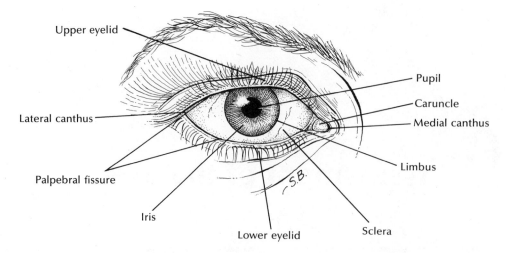

Fig. 10-2. Anterior view of the eye.

evenly distributed along the margin of the lids and curve outward. The eyelids serve a protective function, covering the anterior aspect of the eye and lubricating its surface. The lids should be able to close completely, so that the upper and lower lid margins approximate. When the eyes are open, the upper lid normally covers a small portion of the iris and the cornea overlying it, coming about midway between the limbus and the pupil. The margin of the lower lid lies at or just below the limbus. The limbus is the junction line where the cornea and sclera meet. The distance between the lid margins, called the palpebral fissure, should be equal in both eyes. The tarsal plates are thin strips of connective tissue that lie within the lid and give the lid some form and consistency.

Conjunctiva. Lining the lids and covering the anterior portion of the eyeball is the conjunctiva. This is a continuous, transparent structure that is divided into two portions: the palpebral portion and the bulbar portion. The palpebral portion lines the lids and is shiny pink or red as it overlies the fleshy vascular structures of the lids; the bulbar portion lies over the sclera.

The palpebral conjunctiva recesses into the folds of the lids and is continuous with the bulbar conjunctiva, which lies loosely over the sclera to the limbus, where it merges with the corneal epithelium. This portion of the conjunctiva is normally clear; the white color comes from the sclera below. The bulbar portion does, however contain many small blood vessels; these are normally visible and may become dilated, producing varying degrees of redness. A small fleshy elevation, the caruncle, is located in the nasal corner of the conjunctiva. Yellowish thickenings, called pinguecula, may occur in the bulbar conjunctiva near the limbus. The meibomian glands, which secrete an oily, lubricating substance, appear as vertical yellow striations on the palpebral conjunctiva.

Sclera. The sclera is the white portion of the eye visible anteriorly. Normally, several small, distinct conjunctival vessels are visible over the sclera, particularly around the periphery. In some dark-complected persons, small dark-pigmented dots may be visible on the sclera near the limbus.

Cornea. The cornea, like the bulbar conjunctiva, is a smooth, moist, transparent tissue. It covers the area over the pupil and iris and merges with the conjunctiva at the limbus. It is normally invisible except for the light reflections from its surface. The cornea is quite sensitive to touch; this sensation is transmitted by the ophthalmic branch of the trigeminal nerve (cranial nerve [CN] V). Stimulation of either cornea causes a blinking reflex in both eyes, which is transmitted by the facial nerve (CN VII).

Anterior chamber. The anterior chamber is a structure containing transparent fluid; it lies between the cornea anteriorly and the iris and lens posteriorly.

Lacrimal apparatus. The components of the lacrimal apparatus are illustrated in Fig. 10-3. The lacrimal gland, located above and slightly lateral to the eye, produces tears, which moisten and lubricate the conjunctiva and cornea. The tears are washed across the eye and then drain through the puncta, which are located on the nasal end of both upper and lower lids. The tears

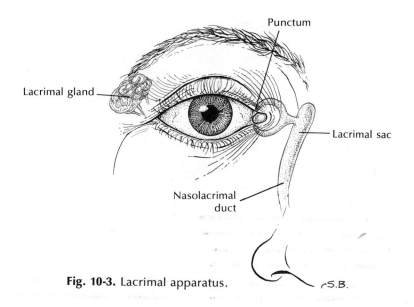

Fig. 10-3. Lacrimal apparatus.

then pass into the nasolacrimal sac, located in the medial portion of the orbit, and from there through the nasolacrimal duct to the nose. Of these several components of the lacrimal system, only the puncta are normally visible.

Iris. The iris is a circular, colored structure containing two involuntary muscles. The contraction and dilatation of the iris in response to light determines the size of the pupil. The color of the iris in each eye is the same or very similar.

Pupils. The pupils are normally round in shape and equal in size. A small percentage of individuals (about 5%) do have a slight but noticeable difference in the size of their pupils. Although this may be normal, the finding should be regarded with some suspicion. The size of the pupils is controlled by the autonomic nervous system. Stimulation of the parasympathetic fibers leads to constriction of the pupils; stimulation of the sympathetic fibers produces dilatation. The amount of ambient light influences the size; normally, increasing illumination causes pupillary constriction, whereas diminishing illumination causes dilatation. The pupils also constrict in response to accommodation, which is part of the adaptive mechanism of the eye for focusing on distant, then on close, objects.

The size of the pupils does vary in individuals exposed to the same degree of ambient light. Pupils tend to be smaller in infants and older persons; myopic (nearsighted) persons tend to have larger pupils, whereas hyperopic (farsighted) persons tend to have smaller pupils.

The constricting response of the pupils to a bright, direct light, a pupillary reflex, consists of both a direct and a consensual reaction. The direct reaction refers to the constriction of the pupil receiving the increased illumination. The constriction of the pupil that is not receiving increased illumination is the consensual reaction. The optic nerve (CN II) mediates the afferent arc of this reflex from each eye, and the oculomotor nerve (CN III) mediates the efferent arc to both eyes; thus, the presence of both direct and consensual responses indicates the functioning of these two cranial nerves.

The accommodation response of the pupils consists of convergence of the eyes and constriction of the pupils as the glance is shifted from a distant to a near object.

The rapidity of the responses to both light and accommodation varies in normal persons. What is important is the presence of the responses and the equality of the responses in both eyes.

Lens. Directly behind the iris and at the pupillary opening lies the lens, another normally transparent structure. The thickness of the lens is controlled by muscles of the ciliary body, and it is the changes in thickness of the lens that enable the eye to focus on objects both far and near. Thus, the coordinated functions of the muscles of the iris and the muscles of the ciliary body acting on the lens control the amount of light permitted to reach the neurosensory elements of the retina and the focusing of objects on the retina.

Retina. The eyeball is a spherical structure lined from the inside toward the outside by the retina, the choroid, and the sclera. Within this sphere lies yet another transparent fluid structure, the vitreous body.

The layers of the eyeball accessible to physical examination are the sclera anteriorly and the retina interiorly; the retina is visible by means of the ophthalmoscope.

The color of the retina is orangish red because of the deeper vascular supply and deeper-pigmented layers. The pigment present in the posterior layers of the retina also accounts for the slightly stippled appearance of the retina. Normally, the color of the retina is quite uniform throughout, with no patches of light or dark discoloration.

Observable on the retina are several important structures, including the optic disc, or nerve head of the optic nerve, with its physiological cup; the four sets of retinal vessels, which emerge from the optic disc and travel medially and laterally around the retina; the macular area, where central vision is concentrated; and the retinal background itself (Fig. 10-4).

Optic disc. The optic disc is located on the nasal half of the retina. Important characteristics of the disc include its size, shape, color, the nature of the margins, and the physiological cup. The optic disc is about 1.5 mm in diameter and its shape is round to vertically oval. Its color ranges from creamy yellow to pink; it is lighter in color than the surrounding retina. The color of both the disc and the retinal background vary from one individual to another; it is somewhat lighter in fair-complected, light-haired people and slightly darker in dark-complected, dark-haired people.

The margins of the disc are usually sharp and are clearly demarcated from the surrounding retina, though there are several normal variations that deserve comment. The nasal outline may normally be somewhat more blurred than the temporal outline. Dense pigment deposits may be situated about the disc margins, particularly in dark-complected people. A whitish to grayish crescent of scleral tissue may be present immediately adjacent to the disc, particularly on the temporal side.

Most discs have a small depression just temporal to the center of the disc; slightly lighter in color than the rest of the disc, this depression is yellowish white and is called the physiological cup or physiological depression. In normal individuals it does not extend completely to the disc margins but may occupy one fourth to one third of the area of the disc.

Retinal vessels. As shown in Fig. 10-4, four sets of retinal vessels emerge from the optic disc and wind outward, becoming smaller at the periphery. Each set includes an arteriole and a vein and is known by the quadrant of the retina that it supplies: superonasal, inferonasal, inferotemporal, or superotemporal. Important characteristics of the vessels include color, size, regularity of caliber, arteriolar light reflex, and the characteristics where one vessel crosses another.

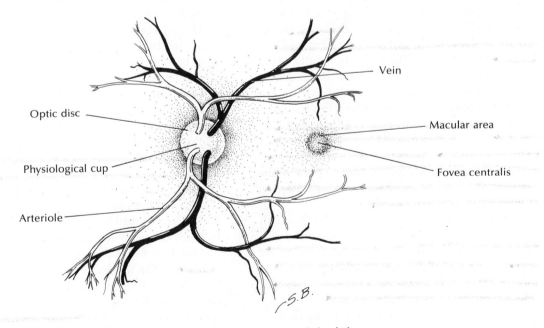

Fig. 10-4. Retinal structures of the left eye.

Optic disc

Physiological cup

Arteriole

Vein

Macular area

Fovea centralis

The vessel walls are normally quite transparent, and the "color" of the vessels describes the oxygenated or deoxygenated blood they carry. Thus, the arterioles are a brighter red than the veins, which are dark red. The arterioles are about 25% smaller than the veins; thus, an arteriole-to-vein (A:V) ratio of 2:3 or 4:5 is normal. When observed, arterioles have a narrow light reflex from the center of the vessel. Pulsations are sometimes visible in the veins near the optic disc and are caused by the forcing of blood out of the eye with each systole. Veins do not show a light reflex. Normally, both arterioles and veins show a gradually and regularly diminished diameter as they go from the disc to the periphery. They normally cross and intertwine each other; but where the vessels cross one another, there should be no change in the course or caliber of either vessel.

Retinal background and macular area. The neurosensory elements, rods and cones, are contained in the retina. At a point temporal to the disc at the posterior pole of the eye, there is a slight depression in the retina, known as the fovea centralis. The cones are most heavily concentrated here, making this the point of central vision and most-acute color vision. The retinal area immediately around this is called the macula. The macular area has no visible retinal vessels; it is nourished by choroidal vessels and appears slightly darker than the rest of the retinal background.

■ Visual pathway and visual fields

For a clear visual image to be perceived, light reflected from an object must pass through the cornea, the anterior chamber, the lens, and the vitreous fluid and then be focused on the retina. The images formed on the retina are reversed right to left and are upside down; thus, an object in the upper nasal field of vision will be formed on the lower temporal quadrant of the retina. The light stimulates neuron impulses that are conducted through the retina, the optic nerve, and the optic tract to the visual cortex of the occipital lobes.

The layout (spatial arrangement) of the nerve fibers in the retina are maintained in the optic nerve; that is, temporal (lateral) fibers run along the lateral side of the nerve, and nasal (medial) fibers run along the medial portion of the nerve. However, as the optic chiasm, the nasal or medial fibers cross over and join the temporal or lateral fibers of the opposite optic tract. Thus, the left optic tract contains fibers only from the left half of

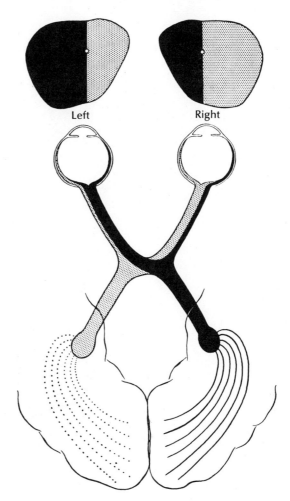

Fig. 10-5. Representation of the visual field in the optic pathways. (From Havener, W. H.: Synopsis of ophthalmology, ed. 4, St Louis, 1975, The C. V. Mosby Co.)

each retina (the right half of each field of vision), and the right optic tract contains fibers only from the right half of each retina (left half of each field of vision). By this sequence of pathways and events, conscious vision is produced. The relationship of visual pathways and fields of vision is illustrated in Fig. 10-5.

■ Neuromuscular aspects

Six muscles of each eye, working in a coordinated "yoked" fashion with the other eye, control eye movement, which normally occurs in conjugate, parallel fashion except during convergence, when a very close object is visualized. These six muscles include the superior, inferior, lateral and medial rectus muscles; the superior oblique muscle; and the inferior oblique muscle. This parallelism of the axis of the eye makes possible

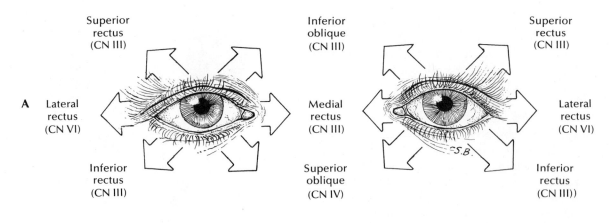

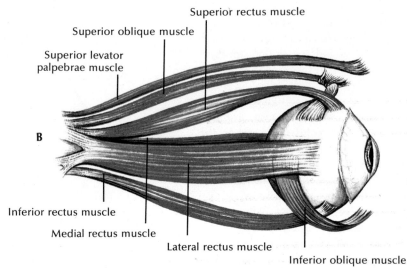

Fig. 10-6. A, Extraocular muscles. **B,** Muscles of the right orbit as viewed from the side. (**B,** From Anthony, C. P., and Kolthoff, N. J.: Textbook of anatomy and physiology, ed. 9, St. Louis, 1975, The C. V. Mosby Co.)

single-image, binocular vision. Thus, the yoked muscles are the muscles in each eye that work together to move the eyes in parallel motion to any given position of gaze. For example, the left lateral rectus and the right medial rectus are yoked muscles working concurrently to move the gaze to the left. The attachment of the muscles to the globe of the eye and the direction of their action are illustrated in Fig. 10-6.

These six eye muscles are innervated by three cranial nerves. The oculomotor nerve (CN III) innervates four muscles: the superior, inferior, and medial rectus muscles and the inferior oblique muscle. The trochlear nerve (CN IV) innervates the superior oblique muscle, and the abducens nerve (CN VI) innervates the lateral rectus muscle. A mnemonic device helpful for remembering this innervation is: LR_6SO_4.

Six of the 12 cranial nerves and portions of the

Table 10-1. Relationship of cranial nerves to eye structures

Cranial nerve	Activity
II Optic	Mediates vision
III Oculomotor	Innervates medial, superior, and inferior rectus muscles; inferior oblique muscle; musculature elevating the eyelid (levator palpebrae); and muscles of the iris and ciliary body
IV Trochlear	Innervates superior oblique muscle
V Trigeminal, ophthalmic division	Innervates sensory portion of corneal reflex
VI Abducens	Innervates lateral rectus muscle
VII Facial	Innervates lacrimal glands and musculature involved in lid closure (orbicularis oculi)

148

cerebral hemispheres are involved in the total neurological innervation of the eye and related structures. Table 10-1 summarizes the relationship of the six cranial nerves to the eye structures.

EXAMINATION

Examination of the functions and structures of the eyes involves multiple procedures and should be performed in a manner that provides efficient access to physical findings while maintaining the greatest degree of comfort for the client. There are, of course, numerous ways to organize this examination; the method suggested here is to examine initially the functions of visual acuity (central and peripheral) and ocular motility. This assessment of function is followed by the examination of ocular structures, starting with the outermost structures and working toward the retina. Finally, the estimation of intraocular tension should be performed as appropriate. This method allows the examiner to perform much of the ocular examination before touching any of the rather sensitive eye structures and reserves the somewhat uncomfortable procedures of ophthalmoscopic examination and tonometry until last.

Several pieces of equipment are required for the eye examination. These should be organized before the examination is begun:

Visual acuity chart

Newspaper clipping with several sizes of print for assessing near vision

Opaque card or eye cover for assessing visual acuity, visual fields, and muscle function

Penlight for assessing pupillary reflexes and external structures

Cotton-tipped applicator for eversion of the upper lid

Wisp of cotton for assessing corneal reflex

Ophthalmoscope for assessing ocular media and for the retinal examination

Tonometer for assessing ocular pressure

In addition to the equipment needed, there is an important environmental requirement, a room where the amount of lighting can be controlled by the examiner. A darkened room enables the examiner to assess the pupillary reflexes and to perform the funduscopic examination with greater ease.

In examination of the eye, the range of normal is broad and the variations from normal are numerous. Much time, patience, and practice is required to begin to assess the normal and common abnormal eye patterns.

■ Visual acuity

The assessment of visual acuity is a simple and rewarding test of ocular function. Findings in a normal range of visual acuity give the examiner an indication of the clarity of the transparent media (cornea, anterior body, lens, and vitreous body), the adequacy of macular or central vision, and the functioning of the nerve fibers from the macula to the occipital cortex.

Traditionally, Snellen's chart, with various sizes of letters or with the letter E facing various ways, is utilized. The chart has standardized numbers at the end of each line of letters; these numbers indicate the degree of visual acuity when measured from a distance of 20 feet. The numerator is 20, the distance in feet between the chart and the client, or the standard testing distance. The denominator is the distance from which the normal eye can read the lettering; therefore, the larger the denominator, the poorer the vision. It is important to note that although the terms numerator and denominator are commonly used, the measurement is not a fraction or a percentage of normal vision. Measurement of 20/20 vision in a client is an indication of a normal eye and optic pathway. Measurement of less than 20/20 vision is an indication of either a refractive error or some other optic disorder. Only one eye should be tested at a time; the other may be covered with an opaque card or eye cover, not with the client's fingers. A person who wears corrective lenses may be tested with and without them; this allows for an assessment of the adequacy of the correction. Reading glasses, however, do blur distant vision.

Persons who cannot see the largest letter on the chart (20/200) should be checked to see if they can perceive hand movements about 12 inches from their eyes or if they can perceive the light of the penlight directed into their eyes.

Assessment of near vision is performed if the client complains of reading difficulty and in persons over 40 years of age. The newspaper clipping with various sizes of print is used for this. With advancing age the lenses may become less flexible, resulting in difficulty with near vision. This condition is known as presbyopia.

■ Visual fields

The assessment of visual acuity is indicative of the functioning of the macular area, the area of central vision. However, it does not test the sensitivity of the other areas of the retina, which perceive the more peripheral stimuli. The visual

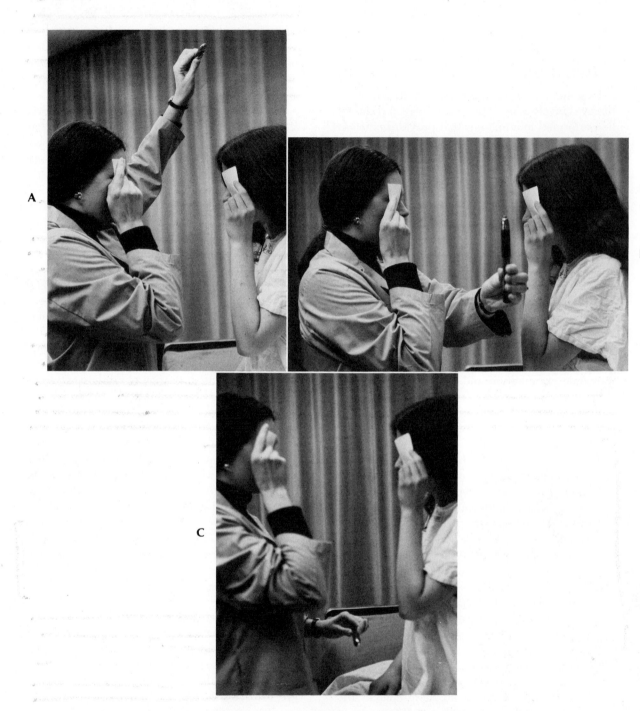

Fig. 10-7. In order to examine the visual fields, the examiner and client cover opposite eyes with an opaque card; the examiner brings in a penlight or other small object from the superior (**A**), nasal (**B**), inferior (**C**), and temporal fields of vision. (Temporal assessment not shown.)

field confrontation test provides a rather gross measurement of peripheral vision.

The performance of this test assumes that the examiner has normal visual fields, since the client's visual fields are compared with the examiner's. The examiner and the client sit opposite each other with their eyes at the same horizontal level at a distance of 1½ to 2 feet apart. The client covers one eye with an opaque card or eye cover, and the examiner covers his own eye opposite the client's covered eye; that is, if the client's right eye is covered, then the examiner's left eye is covered. This leaves the client's and the examiner's same field of vision open for inspection.

The client is asked to stare directly at the examiner's open eye while the examiner stares directly at the client's open eye. Neither looks out at the object approaching from the periphery. The examiner holds a small object, such as a pencil or penlight, in his hand and gradually moves it in from the periphery of both directions horizontally and from above and below. The object should be beyond the limits of the field of vision initially, held equidistant from both persons, and then advanced toward the center. The client and the examiner should be able to visualize the object at the same time. It is often difficult for the examiner to move the test object out far enough so that neither he nor the client can see it, especially in the temporal field. It may be necessary for the examiner to hold the object slightly farther from himself and closer to the client in the temporal field, moving it to a line equidistant between them as it is brought in (Fig. 10-7).

This test provides only a crude estimate of visual fields, and although it would pick up larger field defects, such as hemianopias, quadrantanopias, or large scotomas, it does not ascertain small lesions or changes. Thus, its clinical use is limited to gross screening. Any suspicions of decreasing peripheral vision, such as occurs with glaucoma and some brain lesions, should be referred for the more accurate quantitative measurements that can be performed with a perimeter or tangent screen. These tests are more useful for detecting, evaluating, and following visual pathway damage, whereas the confrontation method may fail to detect early evidence of damage, possibly delaying timely intervention.

■ Extraocular muscle function

There are several aspects to the assessment of extraocular muscle function: the corneal light reflex, the six cardinal positions of gaze, and the cover-uncover test. Basic to each of these is the observation of the parallelism of the eyes and ocular movements.

The parallelism, or alignment, of the anteroposterior axes of the two eyes can be assessed by observing the reflection of a light from the cornea. The client is requested to stare straight ahead while the examiner shines a penlight on the corneas. The bright dot of light reflected from the shiny surface of the corneas should be located at the same spot in each eye, for example, at the 1 o'clock position (Fig. 10-8). An asymmetrical reflex will indicate a deviating eye and a probable muscle imbalance. A weak or paralyzed extraocular muscle is a cause of ocular deviation.

The second mode of assessing muscle function is movement of the eyes through the six cardinal positions of gaze:

$$
\begin{array}{cccc}
SR \rightarrow IO & & IO \rightarrow SR \\
\nearrow 6 \quad 1 \searrow & \quad & \nearrow 6 \quad 1 \searrow \\
LR \; 5 \qquad 2 \; MR & 5 \qquad 2 \; LR \\
\nwarrow 4 \quad 3 \swarrow & \quad & \nwarrow 4 \quad 3 \swarrow \\
IR \leftarrow SO & & SO \leftarrow IR
\end{array}
$$

Right eye   **Left eye**

These six positions are used because the muscle indicated is weak or paralyzed if the eye will not turn to that particular position. As stated earlier, the normal eye muscles work in yoked fashion, so that when the left eye is moved to the upward and outward position, the right eye moves to the upward and inward position.

The client is asked to follow a small object held by the examiner, which is moved to each position

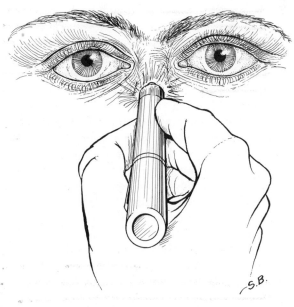

Fig. 10-8. Corneal light reflex.

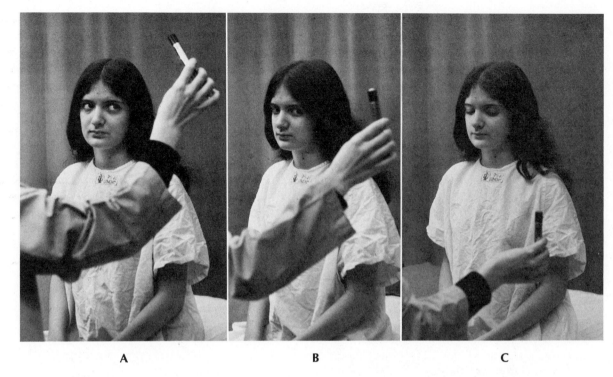

A   B   C

Fig. 10-9. To assess extraocular muscle function, the examiner directs the client's gaze into the six cardinal positions. Shown here: upward and left **(A)**; left lateral **(B)**; and downward and left **(C).** The client's gaze is then directed to the right in these three positions.

in a clockwise fashion. The client holds his head in a fixed position, and only his eyes follow the examiner's object. The examiner asks the client to fix his gaze momentarily in the extreme position of each of the six positions; and while the client is doing so, the examiner notes any jerking movements of the eye, or nystagmus. On extreme lateral gaze, some eyes will develop a rhythmic twitching motion, known as end-positional nystagmus. A few beats of nystagmus on extreme lateral gaze are normal, but any other nystagmus is abnormal. Three of the six positions of gaze are illustrated in Fig. 10-9.

After examining the extraocular muscles in the six cardinal positions, the examiner observes the relationship of the upper eyelid to the globe while directing the client's eyes from an upward to a downward gaze. The lid should overlap the iris slightly throughout this movement; no sclera should show between the iris and the lid.

A third, more delicate, method of assessing muscle function is the cover-uncover test. Maintenance of parallel eyes is a result of the fusion reflex, which makes binocular vision possible. If a muscle imbalance is present and the fusion reflex is blocked when one eye is covered, this weakness can be observed.

The examiner asks the client to look at a specific fixation point with both eyes. Then the examiner covers one eye with an opaque card or eye cover and while doing so observes the uncovered eye to see if it moves to fix on the object. If it does move, then it was not straight before the other eye was covered. The examiner then removes the opaque cover from the covered eye and observes for any movement of the eye just uncovered. When an eye is covered, the appearance of an object on that retina is suppressed. The eye relaxes, and if there is a weak tendency in one of the extrocular muscles, the eye drifts to another resting position. Then, when the client's eye is uncovered, the eye jerks back into the position where the visual image again appears on the retina.

The examiner then repeats this procedure on the other eye.

■ Ocular structures

The ocular structures to be examined include the eyelashes and eyelids, the conjunctiva, the cornea, the anterior chamber, the lacrimal apparatus, the sclera, the iris, the pupil, the lens, the vitreous body, and the retina.

Examination of outermost structures

Eyelids and eyelashes. The functions of the lids are to protect and lubricate the anterior portions of the globe. They are inspected for the ability to close completely, for position and color, and for any lesions, infection, or edema. When the lids do not close properly, drying of the cornea may result in serious damage.

The examiner observes for equality in the height of the palpebral fissures. The margins of the upper lids normally fall between the superior pupil margin and the superior limbus.

Raised yellow plaques, xanthelasma, may appear on the lids near the inner canthi; these grow slowly and may disappear spontaneously.

At this time the position of the globe, whether normal, prominent, or sunken, can be observed.

The distribution, condition, and position of the eyelashes are noted. The eyelashes should be evenly distributed and should curve outward.

Conjunctiva. The bulbar and palpebral portions of the conjunctiva are examined by separating the lids widely and having the client look up, down, and to each side. When separating the lids, the examiner should exert no pressure against the eyeball; rather, the examiner should hold the lids against the ridges of the bony orbit surrounding the eye (Fig. 10-10). The client is

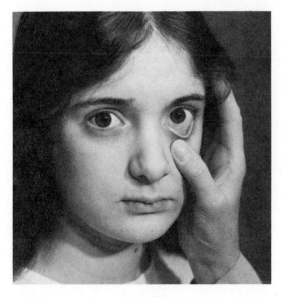

Fig. 10-10. The examiner inspects the conjunctiva by moving the lower lid downward over the bony orbit.

then instructed to direct his gaze upward and to each side. Many small blood vessels are normally visible through the clear conjunctiva. The white sclera is, of course, visible through the bulbar portion.

Although eversion of the upper lid is not a necessary part of the normal or screening examination, the beginning examiner should learn a careful technique for performing lid eversion when it is indicated. The entire procedure should be explained to the client before it is begun, and reassurance should be given during the process. In the absence of gentleness, carefulness, and reassurance, the client is very likely to become tense when the sensitive eye structures are manipulated, thereby making the examination much more difficult for both himself and the examiner.

Eversion of the upper eyelid is performed as follows (Fig. 10-11):

1. Ask the client to look down but to keep his eyes slightly open. This relaxes the levator muscle, whereas closing the eyes contracts the orbicularis muscle, preventing lid eversion.

2. Gently grasp the upper eyelashes and pull gently downward. Do not pull the lashes outward or upward; this, too, causes muscle contraction.

3. Place a cotton-tipped applicator about 1 cm above the lid margin on the upper tarsal border and push gently downward with the applicator while still holding the lashes. This everts the lid.

4. Hold the lashes of the everted lid against the upper ridge of the bony orbit, just beneath the eyebrow, never pushing against the eyeball.

5. Examine the lid for swelling, infection, a foreign object, and so on.

6. To return the lid to its normal position, move the lashes slightly forward and ask the client to look up and then to blink. The lid returns easily to a normal position.

Sclera. The sclera is easily observed during assessment of the conjunctiva. It is normally white, though some pigmented deposits are within the range of normal.

Cornea. The cornea is best observed by directing the light of a penlight at it obliquely from several positions. The cornea should be transparent, smooth, shiny, and bright. There should be no irregularities in the surface, and the features of the iris should be fully visible through the cornea. In older persons arcus senilis, a partial or com-

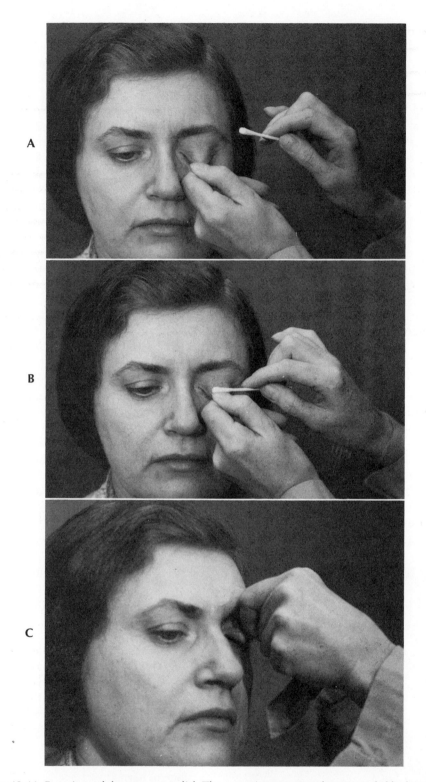

Fig. 10-11. Eversion of the upper eyelid. The examiner grasps the upper lid lashes, gently pulling downward and outward (**A**), then places the cotton-tipped applicator near the lower lid margin (**B**), and gently pulls the lashes upward over the applicator (**C**).

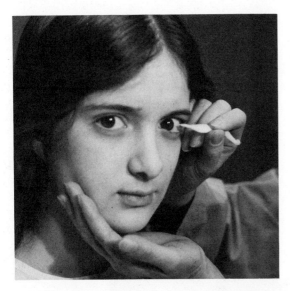

Fig. 10-12. Testing for corneal sensitivity, the examiner brings in a wisp of cotton from the side and lightly brushes it over the cornea.

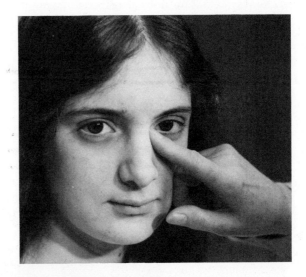

Fig. 10-13. To examine the lacrimal sac, the examiner presses with the index finger against the lower inner orbital rim, *not* against the nose.

plete white ring located around the periphery of the cornea, is normal.

Testing of the corneal reflex may be reserved for later in the eye examination, after the observation of all external structures is complete, but is discussed here as part of the complete assessment of the cornea. Corneal sensitivity is tested by bringing a wisp of cotton from the lateral side of the eye and brushing it lightly across the corneal surface (Fig. 10-12). The normal response is lid closure of both eyes when either eye is brushed.

Anterior chamber. The anterior chamber is easily observed in conjunction with the cornea. The technique of oblique illumination is also useful in assessing the anterior chamber. This, too, is a transparent structure. Any visible material in it is abnormal. The depth of the chamber should be noted by looking at the eye from the side instead of from directly in front. The depth is the distance between the cornea and the iris. From a side view, the iris should appear quite flat and should not be bulging forward.

Lacrimal apparatus. Of the various components of the lacrimal apparatus, including the lacrimal gland, the puncta, the lacrimal sac, and the nasolacrimal duct, only the puncta can normally be observed. These are located on the upper and lower nasal margins of the lids.

Blockage of the nasolacrimal duct can be checked by pressing against the lacrimal sac with the index finger inside the lower inner orbital rim, not against the side of the nose (Fig. 10-13). In the presence of blockage, this will cause regurgitation of material through the puncta.

Iris. The iris should be observed for shape and coloration.

Pupils. Examination of the pupils involves several observations, including assessment of their size, shape, reaction to light, and accommodation.

The pupils are normally round in shape and equal in size. The pupillary response to light consists of both a direct and a consensual reaction. The beam of a penlight is brought in from the side and directed on one eye at a time. The eye toward which the light is directed is observed for the direct response of constriction. Simultaneously, the other eye is observed for a consensual response of constriction. Each eye is observed for both the direct and consensual response. Normally, both responses are present; however, the rapidity with which the pupils respond does vary. A room that can be darkened to facilitate dilatation is helpful in assessing constriction in response to light; a sunny, well-lit room can make the assessment of constriction responses very difficult.

The test for pupillary accommodation is performed by asking the client to stare at an object across the room. Visualization of a distant object normally causes pupillary dilatation. The client is then asked to fix his gaze on the examiner's index finger, which is placed 5 to 6 inches from the client's nose. The normal response is pupillary constriction and convergence of the eyes. The rapidity of the response in individuals varies; the response is slower in older persons.

PERRLA stands for *pupils equal, round, react to light, and accommodation*.

Ophthalmoscopic examination

Examination of other ocular structures includes observation of the lens, the vitreous body, and the retinal structures and is performed with an ophthalmoscope. It is helpful to darken the room while performing the ophthalmoscopic examination, since this causes the pupils to dilate and thus facilitates the examination. If darkening the room does not adequately dilate the client's pupils, 10% phenylephine hydrochloride, 0.5% Mydriacyl, or 1% Cyclogel drops may be instilled in the client's eyes. Before utilizing dilating drops however, it is absolutely essential to rule out any suspicion of glaucoma. If the client wears corrective lenses, the examination may be done either with or without them. It is generally easier to perform the examination without the client's glasses on unless he has a high degree of astigmatism. Contact lenses may be left in place on the cornea.

Use of the ophthalmoscope. The head of the

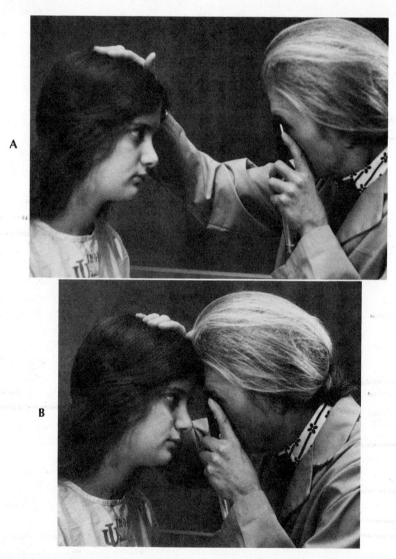

Fig. 10-14. A, The examiner uses the ophthalmoscope to inspect the lens and vitreous body from a distance of about 12 inches. The examiner uses the left eye and left hand to examine the client's left eye. **B,** Moving in closer to the client's eye, the examiner studies the retinal structures.

ophthalmoscope is equipped with a series of lenses that are changed by moving the round, white wheel. The 0 lens is clear glass; the red, or minus, numbers focus farther away; and the black, or positive, numbers focus closer to the ophthalmoscope. Several apertures and filters for the light are built into most ophthalmoscopes; however, the round aperture with white light is best for most examinations. The examiner should read the manual accompanying the ophthalmoscope for information on other apertures and filters. The light should be turned to maximum brightness unless the client cannot tolerate it.

The client's cooperation is essential to the performance of this examination. The client is asked to stare directly ahead at some object across the room, such as the light switch or the corner of a picture. This assists in two ways: staring at a distant point encourages dilatation of the pupils, and staring at one fixed point helps to prevent the eyes from rotating and moving about so much that it is impossible for the examiner to fix his view of any of the retinal structures.

The client is told that he may blink during the examination unless the blinking becomes so frequent that it is difficult to visualize the retinal structures. If this is the case, the examiner may elevate the upper lid and hold it against the upper orbital rim.

The examiner holds the ophthalmoscope in his right hand and to his right eye to examine the client's right eye, and in his left hand and to his left eye to examine the client's left eye. The examiner initially sets the ophthalmoscope lens at 0, holds the viewing aperture directly in front of his eye with the top of the ophthalmoscope against his forehead, and begins about 12 inches away from the client's eye (Fig. 10-14, A). The index finger of the hand holding the ophthalmoscope rests on the lens wheel to permit focusing during the exam. The bright circle of light is flashed on the eye through the pupil; a red glow, the red reflex, is visible through the pupil of the normal eye. While continuing to focus on the red reflex, the examiner moves close to the eye being examined (Fig. 10-14, B). If the examiner loses sight of the red reflex, it is usually because the light is no longer directed through the pupil and is resting instead on the iris or sclera. If this occurs, it is easiest to relocate the red reflex by backing away several inches and redirecting the beam of light. As the examiner moves close to the eye, the lenses are rotated to the positive numbers (+15 to +20), which focus on the near objects. At this setting the anterior chamber and lens are examined for transparency; there should be no clouding or opacities.

Gradually rotating the lens back toward 0, the examiner also observes the vitreous body for transparency. At this setting the examiner begins to look for some retinal structure, such as a vessel or the disc. Once some structure is located, the lens wheel is rotated until it is brought into focus. In a myopic or nearsighted person, whose eyeball is more elongated than normal, the more negative lenses will be needed to focus farther back. In a farsighted client the lens wheel is rotated toward the positive numbers. Focusing is quite individual and does depend on the refractive status of both the client and the examiner.

Often, a vessel is detected first and can be followed in toward the optic disc. If the examiner directs the beam of light through the pupil in a slightly nasalward direction, the beam will fall on or near the optic disc initially.

Retinal structures. Examination of the various retinal structures should be performed in a consistent and orderly fashion. The following order is recommended: (1) optic disc, (2) retinal vessels, (3) retinal background, and (4) macular area.

The disc is examined for its size, shape, color, the distinctness of its margins, and the physiological cup. The disc is also utilized as a standard measurement device. The distance from the disc and the size of other findings are estimated in terms of disc diameters (DD); for example, an alteration slightly larger than the disc situated in the upper portion of the fundus may be described as being 1 × 2 DD in size and 3 DD away from the disc at 1:30 in the left eye (Fig. 10-15).

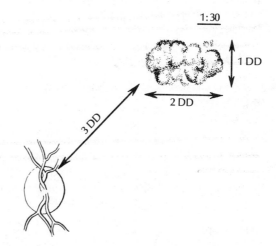

Fig. 10-15. Method of giving position and dimensions of a lesion in terms of disc diameters. (From Havener, W. H.: Synopsis of ophthalmology, ed. 4, St. Louis, 1975, The C. V. Mosby Co.)

The retinal vessels are examined for their color, the ratio in size of arterioles to veins is determined, arteriovenous crossings are examined for indentations, and the arterioles are examined for their light reflex. Each set of vessels should be followed out from the disc to the periphery. The retinal background is examined for its color and regularity of appearance and for any areas of light or dark color alterations. The more peripheral reaches of the vessels and retinal background can be examined by having the client direct his gaze upward, downward, and to each side. Observation of the macular area is reserved for last, because having a bright light directed at the center of most-acute vision is very uncomfortable for the client. The macula is about 1 DD in size and is located 2 DD temporal to the optic disc. It appears as an avascular area with the bright spot of light reflected from its center, the fovea. This area can be examined by having the client look directly at the examining light.

■ Intraocular pressure

Intraocular pressure is best measured by using the tonometer. This requires the installation of anesthetizing drops in the eye followed by the application of the tonometer foot to the anesthetized cornea. The tonometer should be checked regularly for accuracy.

Intraocular pressure may be grossly estimated by touch. The client is asked to look down but to keep his eyes open; the examiner than palpates over the sclera with a gentle to-and-fro motion using both index fingers. This maneuver gives only a rough estimate and is much less valuable than tonometry for measurement of intraocular pressure. All persons over 40 years of age should be checked regularly by tonometry; glaucoma is the single greatest cause of blindness in persons over 30 and is preventable.

PATHOLOGY
■ Visual acuity

Limited visual acuity may be an indication of a refractive error or of a more serious pathological condition. The determination of blindness cannot be made unless neither hand movements nor a bright beam of light can be perceived.

■ Visual fields

Visual field defects may be caused by lesions of the retina, by lesions at any point along the optic nerve or tract, or by lesions in the occipital lobes (Fig. 10-16). Damage to one optic nerve will af-

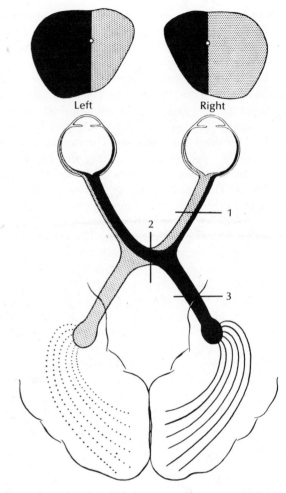

Fig. 10-16. Visual field defects. *1*, Blind right eye; *2*, bitemporal hemianopsia—no temporal vision; *3*, left homonymous hemianopsia—no vision in left field of either eye. (Adapted from Havener, W. H.: Synopsis of ophthalmology, ed. 4, St. Louis, 1975, The C. V. Mosby Co.)

fect the field of vision in that eye. Lesions occurring at the optic chiasm, optic tract, or in the brain usually affect the visual fields of both eyes because of the crossing of fibers at the chiasm. Lesions at the optic chiasm, as from a pituitary tumor, cause a loss of vision from the nasal portion of each retina, resulting in a loss of both temporal fields of vision. This condition is termed heteronomous or bitemporal hemianopsia.

Since nerves from both eyes mingle behind the chiasm in the optic tracts and in the brain, lesions along the optic tract or in the temporal parietal or occipital lobes will impair the same half of the field of vision in both eyes. For example, a lesion of the right optic tract or right side of the brain will result in visual field defects in the right nasal field and in the left temporal field. This condition is termed homonymous hemianopsia and may be caused by occlusion of the middle cerebral artery.

The location of disease on the retina determines the type of resultant visual field defects. Macular defects lead to a central blind area. Localized damage in other areas of the retina will cause a loss of vision corresponding to the involved area. A blind spot is known as a scotoma, that is, an area of blindness surrounded by an area of vision. Advanced diabetic retinopathy may cause macular damage, resulting in a loss of central vision. Glaucoma, or increased intraocular pressure, causes decreased peripheral vision due to the damage caused by the elevated pressure. As the disease advances, it may also cause a loss of central vision. A retinal detachment will cause of loss of vision from that portion of the retina.

Extraocular neuromuscular function

An asymmetrical corneal light reflex, an inability of the eyes to move in parallel fashion to the six cardinal positions of gaze, or an abnormal cover test indicates a weakness or paralysis of one or more of the extraocular muscles or a defect in the nerve supplying it. Table 10-2 indicates the muscle and cranial nerve involved when the eye will not turn to one of these six positions.

Examples of the effects of nerve lesions are:
1. *Oculomotor paralysis (CN III):* The eye turns down and out with drooping of the upper lid.
2. *Abducens paralysis (CN IV):* The eye turns in toward the nose because of unopposed action of the medial rectus.

Carrying the fixation point of the six cardinal positions out to the extremes will exaggerate a defect. A disparity of the anteroposterior axes of the eyes is call strabismus. Deviations in these axes may be detected during the cover test, which blocks the fusion reflex of the eyes. A mild weakness of the extraocular muscles is called phoria. If there is a weak tendency during the cover test, a definitely perceptible jerk of the eye is noted when the cover is removed. Tropia is a more pronounced imbalance producing a permanent disparity in the axes of the eyes. A mild outward deviation of the eye is called exophoria; an inward deviation is called esophoria. The rhythmic twitching motion of nystagmus may be normal at the end of the lateral position but is abnormal when the eyes are in any other position.

Ocular structures

Eyelids and eyelashes. Faulty positioning of the eyelids occurs in a variety of ways. The lid margins may fall above or below the middle part of the iris. A drooping lid margin (ptosis) that falls at the pupil or below may indicate an oculomotor nerve lesion or a congenital condition. If the lid margin falls above the limbus so that some sclera is visible, thyroid disease may be present. In the presence of thyroid disease the lid may lag behind the limbus as the gaze moves from an upward to a downward position (Fig. 10-17). Another type of faulty positioning of the lids is improper approximation of the lids to the eyeballs. The lids may be loose or lax and roll outward. This condition is called ectropion. Because the puncta cannot effectively drain the tears, epiphora (tearing) results. The lids may also roll inward because of lid spasm or the contraction of scar tissue. This condition is called entropion. Because the lashes are pulled inward, they may produce corneal irritation.

The tissues within the lids are loosely connected and collect excess fluid rather readily. Edema of the lids may be a manifestation of local or systemic disease. Examples of systemic problems that may cause lid edema include allergy, heart failure, nephrosis, and thyroid deficiency.

The glands of the lids may be sites of infection.

Table 10-2. Diagnostic clues to dysfunction of extraocular neuromuscular units

Position to which eye will not turn	Muscle	Cranial nerve
Straight nasal	Medial rectus	III
Up and nasal	Inferior oblique	III
Down and nasal	Superior oblique	IV
Straight temporal	Lateral rectus	VI
Up and temporal	Superior rectus	III
Down and temporal	Inferior rectus	III

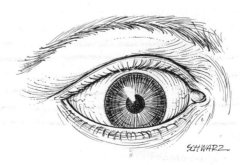

Fig. 10-17. Lid lag.

A localized infection of the small glands around the eyelashes in the hair follicle at the lid margin is a hordeolum, or sty (Fig. 10-18). The meibomian glands lying within the posterior portion of the lid may develop an infection or a retention cyst, known as a chalazion (Fig. 10-19); crusting or scaling at the lid margins may occur as a result of staphlococcal infection or seborrheic dermatitis. If a lid infection is present or suspected, the lids may be gently palpated by moving the examining finger across the lid surface. Pressure should never be exerted over the eye in an effort to separate the lids. As mentioned earlier, the bony orbital rims should be used as points over which to slide the lids.

Xanthelasma, the raised yellow plaques that may appear on the lids, may have no pathological significance, or they may be associated with hypercholesterolemia.

Conjunctiva. Infectious disease of the conjunctiva typically produces engorgement of the conjunctival vessels and a discharge. The infected vessels are usually more pronounced at the fornices. Small subconjunctival hemorrhages may result from more severe involvement, though in some persons these may also result from sneezing, coughing, or lifting.

Sclera. Changes in the color of the sclera may be indicative of systemic disease. For example, jaundice manifests its presence in the eyes as a yellow discoloration, scleral icterus. Excessive bilirubinemia may be evident as scleral icterus before jaundice of the skin becomes apparent. In the presence of osteogenesis imperfecta the sclera is bluish.

Cornea. The cornea is a very sensitive structure, and pain and photophobia are common manifestations of corneal disease. Any dullness, irregularities, or opacities of the cornea are abnormal. Two of the more frequent abnormalities affecting the cornea are abrasions and opacities. Although an abrasion may cause the surface to look irregular or may cast a shadow on the iris, it may be invisible and detectable only with fluorescein stain. Suspected corneal abrasion should be referred to an ophthalmologist.

Abnormal growth of tissue from the edge toward the center of the cornea, known as pterygium, may interfere with vision (Fig. 10-20).

Although the presence of arcus senilis is normal in elderly people, in younger individuals it may be associated with abnormal lipid metabolism.

Anterior chamber. Abnormalities observable in the anterior chamber are a decrease in depth

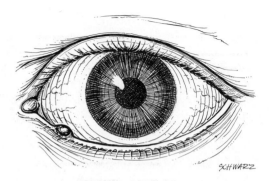

Fig. 10-18. Hordeolum or sty.

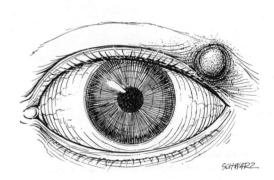

Fig. 10-19. Chalazion.

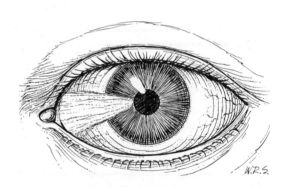

Fig. 10-20. Pterygium.

and any foreign material interrupting the normal transparency. A shallow anterior chamber may be a sign of glaucoma or may predispose the eye to glaucoma (Fig. 10-21). As the increased intraocular pressure causes the iris to become displaced anteriorly, there is less distance between the cornea and the iris. As a result of this anterior displacement, light directed obliquely from the temporal side will illuminate only the temporal side and the nasal side will appear darker or

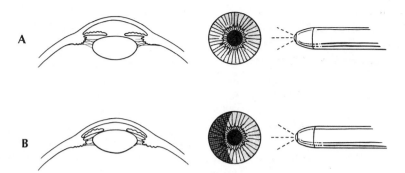

Fig. 10-21. A, Normal anterior chamber. **B,** Shallow anterior chamber. (From Havener, W. H.: Synopsis of ophthalmology, ed. 4, St. Louis, 1975, The C. V. Mosby Co.)

shadowed. The presence of a shallow anterior chamber is a contraindication to the use of dilating drops for the ophthalmoscopic examination.

Any cloudiness of the aqueous fluid or accumulation of blood (hyphemia) or purulent material (hypopyon) is abnormal.

Lacrimal apparatus. Both the lacrimal gland, which produces tears, and the system that drains the tears are subject to certain abnormalities. The lacrimal gland may be swollen as a result of infection or tumor. Infection with consequent blockage of the lacrimal sac or duct may occur with associated findings of swelling, redness, warmth, pain, and purulent discharge. The swelling tends to occur in the area below the inner canthus. The technique for examining for infection in the lacrimal sac is to press with the examining finger against the *inner* orbital rim (not against the nose), then to gently depress the lower lid over the lower orbital rim to observe for regurgitation of fluid through the puncta.

As mentioned earlier, ectropion may cause tearing because of inadequate drainage. Any unusual markings or growths should be noted.

Iris. Iritis, inflammation of the iris, results in throbbing pain and visual blurring and is associated with the findings of circumcorneal injection, a deep pinkish red flush about the cornea, and a constricted pupil. This is in contrast to conjunctivitis, wherein the infected vessels tend to extend from the periphery toward the center. If the lens has been removed, the normal support of the iris is absent and the iris will, with movements of the eye, have a tremulous fluttering motion.

Pupils. Abnormalities of the pupils include alterations in size and in reflexes. Although a slight but noticeable difference in pupil size does occur in about 5% of the population, this finding should be regarded with suspicion because it can be an indication of central nervous system (CNS) disease. Inequality in the size of the pupils is known as anisocoria.

Mydriasis, enlargement of the pupils, may result from emotional influences, recent or old local trauma, acute glaucoma, systemic reaction to parasympatholytic or sympathomimetic drugs, or the local use of dilating drops. A unilateral fixed enlarged pupil may be due to local trauma to the eye or to head injury. Fixed dilatation of both eyes occurs with deep anesthesia, CNS injury, and circulatory arrest.

Miosis, constriction of the pupils, is associated with iritis, use of morphine, and glaucoma treatment by pilocarpine and is seen physiologically with sleep.

Any irregularity in pupil contour is abnormal and may result from iritis, trauma, CNS syphilis, or congenital defects.

Failure of the pupils to react to light with preservation of the accommodation reaction is another characteristic of CNS syphilis. This is known as the Argyll Robertson pupil.

In the case of monocular blindness, the blind eye and optic tract will transmit no response to light and neither pupil will constrict. However, when the unaffected eye receives illumination, both pupils will constrict because the efferent pupil constriction stimuli are distributed evenly to both eyes.

Lens. Opacities in any of the clear portions of the eye (anterior chamber, lens or vitreous body) will appear as dark shadows on black spots within the red reflex on ophthalmoscopic examination because they prevent light from being reflected to the examiner's eye. Any clouding of the lens is an indication of cataract formation.

Retinal structures

Optic disc. Three of the major conditions causing alterations of the optic disc are papilledema, glaucoma, and optic atrophy. Papilledema, or swelling of the optic nerve head, causes the margins of the disc to become blurred and indistinct (Fig. 10-22). The nerve head appears out of focus with the surrounding retina. The degree of elevation can be assessed by focusing first on the disc and then on the surrounding retina and noting the difference in diopters on the ophthalmoscope.

Papilledema is a sign of increased intracranial pressure. This causes decreased venous drainage from the eye, hence venous stasis, or the accumulation and leakage of fluid, leading to edematous appearance of the disc. This condition may be associated with malignant hypertension, eclampsia, brain tumor, and hematoma.

The increased intraocular pressure of glaucoma gradually exerts pressure anteriorly against the iris, as mentioned earlier, and posteriorly against the optic disc, causing increased cupping (Fig. 10-23). This may be noted by observing the course of vessels as they emerge from the center and over the disc margins, since glaucoma may cause a vessel to seem to disappear from sight at the disc rim and then reappear at a slightly different site just past the rim. The pressure of glaucoma may also eventually cause pallor of the disc, a sign of optic atrophy. Advanced cupping and optic atrophy are late findings of the disease; the early findings are very subtle and are likely to be very difficult to recognize. Thus, the need for careful tonometry as a far more sensitive indicator is reemphasized.

Death of the optic nerve fibers leads to the disappearance of the tiny disc vessels that give the disc its normal pinkish color and results in optic pallor. The disc appears pale and white, either in a section or throughout. *Note:* The scleral crescent, a normal, crescent-shaped area around the rim of the disc only, should not be mistaken for disc pallor.

Retinal vessels. Changes in caliber and alterations at crossings can occur in the retinal vessels. Changes in these vascular structures are often indicative of systemic diseases, such as hypertension. Because any vessel caliber changes may or may not be evenly distributed along the course of the vessel, vessels should be observed from the disc to the periphery. Arterioles, normally about two thirds to three fourths the diameter of the corresponding veins, are subject to a decrease in diameter as a result of constriction of the vessels or reduced blood flow to the eye. In hyperten-

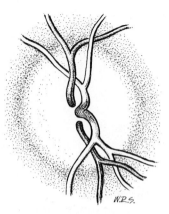

Fig. 10-22. Papilledema.

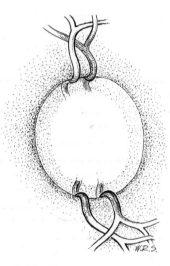

Fig. 10-23. Glaucomatous cupping.

sion, arterioles may become narrowed to a 3:5 or 2:4 or less ratio. More rarely, veins may increase in diameter as a result of conditions causing more blood to circulate to the eye or conditions impeding the exit of blood from the eye.

The condition of the arteriole vessel walls determines their color. Normally they are transparent and reflect the color of the column of blood within, but they may develop sclerotic or sheathing changes, causing them to become opaque and lighter in color. The width of the light reflex from the arteriolar wall also increases with arteriosclerosis to one third or more of the width of the vessel. In advanced stages, the vessels may appear as fine, silvery lines.

Changes at arteriolovenous crossings include an apparent narrowing or blocking of the vein where an arteriole crosses over it. This appearance is the result of some degree of concealment

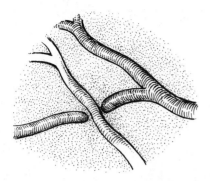

Fig. 10-24. Arteriovenous nicking.

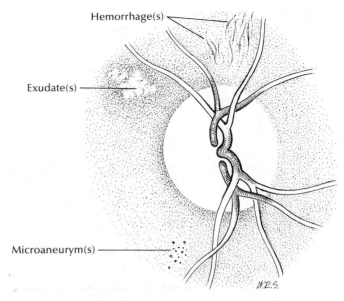

Fig. 10-25. Abnormalities of the retinal background: microaneurysms, exudates, and hemorrhages.

of the underlying vein by an abnormally opaque arteriole wall and occurs with long-standing hypertension; it is initially apparent as venous narrowing and later as a more complete interruption of the vessel. These changes are referred to as arteriovenous nicking (Fig. 10-24).

Emboli in a retinal vessel cause abrupt narrowing of arterioles and abrupt dilatation of a vein as it impedes return flow.

Retinal background. Among the more common abnormalities to appear on the retinal background are microaneurysms, exudates, and hemorrhages (Fig. 10-25). Microaneurysms, outpouchings in the walls of capillaries, appear as tiny bright red dots on the retina. These are frequently associated with diabetes mellitus.

Exudates are whitish yellow infiltrates that may occur alongside vessel walls. They are rather rounded in shape, appearing somewhat like a small cumulous cloud, and may have hazy or distinct edges. Exudates may be associated with systemic diseases, including diabetes mellitus and hypertension, and may occur with degenerative or inflammatory diseases of the retina. They may be resorbed over time.

Hemorrhages are bright-to-dark red, may be small and rounded in shape, as is commonly found with diabetes mellitus, or linear and flame-shaped, as in hypertension. Bleeding may occur from retinal or chloridal vessels into the preretinal, retinal, or choroidal areas.

In the case of any retinal abnormality, the color, shape, size, and proximity to the disc or vessels should be described.

Problems such as those just described may affect any part of the retinal background, including the macular area. Depending on the area affected, resultant difficulty with central or peripheral vision may occur.

BIBLIOGRAPHY

Albert, D. M.: Jaeger's atlas of diseases of the ocular fundus, Philadelphia, 1972, W. B. Saunders Co.

Becker, B., and Drews, R. C.: Current concepts in ophthalmology, vol. 1, St. Louis, 1967, The C. V. Mosby Co.

DeGowin, E. L., and DeGowin, R. L.: Bedside diagnostic examination, ed. 2, New York, 1970, Macmillan, Inc.

Jackson, C. R. S.: The eye in general practice, Baltimore, 1972, The Williams & Wilkins Co.

Newell, F. W., and Ernest, J. T.: Ophthalmology; principles and concepts, St. Louis, 1974, The C. V. Mosby Co.

Potts, A. M., editor: The assessment of visual function, St. Louis, 1972, The C. V. Mosby Co.

Vaughn, D., Cook, R., and Asbury, T.: General ophthalmology, Los Altos, Calif., 1968, Lange Medical Publications.

11 Assessment of the lymphatic system

The lymphatic capillary bed is very extensive. All tissues supplied with blood vessels also possess lymphatic vessels with the exception of the placenta. The lymphatic system is older in evolutionary history than the circulatory system. The function of the lymph is concerned with metabolic processes that have a slower pace than those of the blood circulatory system. The cardiovascular system was a phylogenetic development for a more active animal life wherein the transport of oxygen was necessary for the rapid processes of oxidation and reduction.

PHYSIOLOGY

The lymphatic system consists of a system of collecting ducts, the lymph fluid, and tissues; this tissue makes up the lymph nodes, the spleen, the thymus, the tonsils, and Peyer's patches in the intestines. Lymphoid aggregates are also found in bone marrow, in the lungs, and in gastric and appendiceal mucosa.

The lymphatic vessels originate as microscopic open-ended tubules termed capillaries. These capillaries merge to form larger collecting ducts, which drain to specific lymphatic tissue centers (nodes). Ducts from these lymph node centers eventually empty as trunks into the venous system at the subclavian veins (Fig. 11-1). The right subclavian vein receives the thin-walled lymphatic trunk, which drains from the right side of the head and neck, from the right arm, and from the right chest wall. The left subclavian vein is joined by the thoracic duct, which drains lymph from the remainder of the body. These vessels then return fluid and protein that has entered the lymphatic system from the interstitial space via the cardiovascular system.

Although the specific functions and properties of the lymphatic system are still imperfectly understood, the lymphocytic tissue has been ascribed responsibility for the immunological and various metabolic processes of the body and is implicated in the formation of corpuscular elements of the blood as well as in the extension of malignant disease.

Included in the functions of the lymphatic system are (1) the transport of lymph fluids, protein, and microorganisms for return to the cardiovascular system; (2) the production of lymphocytes in germinal centers of lymph nodes; (3) the production of antibodies (immune substances may be extracted from lymphocytes; lymphocytes contain at least one globulin identical with blood globulin); (4) phagocytosis by the reticuloendothelial cells lining the sinuses of the lymph nodes; (5) hematopoiesis in some pathological states; and (6) the absorption of fat and fat soluble materials from the intestine.

Lymphatic tissue in man is calculated to be 2% to 3% of the total body weight. Lymphatic capillaries and collecting ducts are the transport ducts of the system. The lymph channel section of the lymphatic system consists of lymphatic capillaries, lymph node precollecting ducts, lymph node postcollecting ducts, lymph nodes, and main lymphatic trunks. Lymphoid tissue is organized in its biological architecture to form nodes that are located at strategic points for filtering the lymph. Structurally the lymph node consists of the capsule, the cortex, and the medulla. The lymph and any substance that enters the lymph, including contrast media injected for lymphography, is filtered by the lymph nodes.

The lymph nodes are seldom found singly but are usually arranged in chains or clusters called lymph centers. The lymph nodes are found either in the subcutaneous connective tissue (superficial

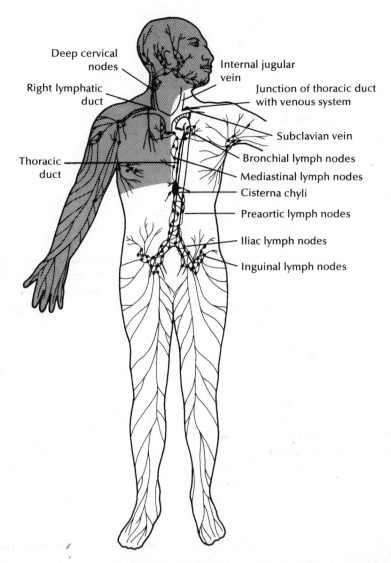

Deep cervical
nodes

Right lymphatic
duct

Thoracic
duct

Internal jugular
vein

Junction of thoracic duct
with venous system

Subclavian vein

Bronchial lymph nodes

Mediastinal lymph nodes

Cisterna chyli

Preaortic lymph nodes

Iliac lymph nodes

Inguinal lymph nodes

Fig. 11-1. Lymphatic drainage pathways. Shaded area of the body is drained via the right lymphatic duct, which is formed by the union of three vessels: the right jugular trunk, the right subclavian trunk, and the right bronchomediastinal trunk. Lymph from the remainder of the body enters the venous system by way of the thoracic duct. (From Francis, C. C., and Martin, A. H.: Introduction to human anatomy, ed. 7, St. Louis, 1975, The C. V. Mosby Co.)

lymph nodes) or beneath the muscular fascia and in the cavities of the body (deep lymph nodes). The nodes are disseminated along the course of the collecting ducts and are usually round or oval, though they are often observed as elongated and flattened to a cylindrical shape. Size is variable from small (almost invisible) to the size of a large pea or even an olive. Nodes found in children are comparatively larger than those found in adults.

Lymphocytes are mobile, spherical, mononuclear cells (6μ to 8μ in diameter) derived from reticular cells of the nodes. Lymphocytes may

evolve in one of three ways: (1) they may remain in lymphoid tissue and die there, (2) they may differentiate in lymphoid tissue, giving rise to other types of cells, or (3) they may leave lymphoid tissue, entering the lymph and then the blood and various organs.

Some of the processes carried on in this system have been clarified by inspecting the ducts with a radiopaque dye (lymphography). Three stages of lymphography have been described. During the first stage the afferent lymphatics, portions of the lymphoid sinuses, and the efferent lymphatics are filled with the contrast medium. The second stage is characterized by phagocytosis by the reticuloendothelial cell of the lipid soluble contrast media, and the third stage is the period during which the contrast media leaves the node. It can be assumed that all substances entering the lymphatic system undergo this fate.

Factors affecting the movement of lymph are (1) remitting compression of the lymphatic vessels by surrounding structures, especially contracting muscles; (2) respiratory movements that propel lymph from the cisterna chyli into the thoracic duct; (3) propulsive action of the smooth muscles contained in the walls of the lymphatic vessels, lymph nodes, and collecting ducts; (4) arterial pulsations (most of the lymphatic vessels course with the regional blood vessels; the deep lymphatic vessels accompany not only the veins but also the arteries, the pulsations of which can be transmitted to the lymphatic vessels); (5) negative pressure in the great vessels at the root of the neck, which determines the flow of lymph from the terminal parts of the jugular, subclavian, bronchial, mediastinal, and thoracic ducts into them; (6) peristaltic contractions of the intestines; (7) capillary blood pressure; and (8) force of gravity.

The formation and flow of lymph can be increased by the following processes: (1) an increase in capillary pressure due to increased venous pressure from venous stasis or obstruction; (2) an increase in permeability of the capillary walls due to an increase in temperature, a decrease in oxygen supply, or the administration of histamine; (3) increases in metabolic activity, the muscular pumping effect, or glandular activity (little lymph is formed when the client is exposed to anesthesia or absolute bed rest); (4) passive movements and massage, which facilitates the flow of lymph through the lymphatic vessels; and (5) hypertonic solutions, such as glucose and sodium chloride solutions.

PATHOPHYSIOLOGY

Pathological findings may be demonstrated for the lymphatic system as a result of (1) localized or systemic infection; (2) disorders in metabolism, particularly of lipids (storage-type adenopathy); (3) metastatic cancer; (4) infiltration of foreign substances; (5) primary hematopoietic disorders; and (6) hypersensitivity reactions.

The lymph nodes are the most significant parameters of the lymphatic system in physical diagnosis. The location and nature of involvement of diseased lymph nodes provide help in deter-

mining the site or origin of disease and the identity of the etiological agent.

The archaic term "swollen glands" is widely used by the lay populace. The early anatomists believed the lymph nodes were glands that functioned in a manner similar to true glands, such as the thyroid. Actual structure and function became apparent with the improved visualization afforded by light microscopy, but the continued use of the glandular reference will be apparent in both the chief complaint and the history.

Alterations in lymphatic flow patterns may also indicate disease.

■ Mechanical stasis of lymph

Any mechanical impediment to the flow of lymph results in deceleration or cessation of flow of lymph from that region. As a result of this impaired drainage, lymphatic vessels become dilated with the trapped lymphatic fluid. The valves become incompetent, causing a backflow of lymph within the interstitial space. Since the lymphatic system functions to return protein to the blood supply, colloid osmotic pressure increases as the interstitial protein concentration rises. Consequently, even more fluid is drawn into the extracellular spaces from the capillaries. In the absence of effective intervention, the extracellular protein precipitates and a fibrin reticulum forms. Proliferation of fibrocytes is stimulated. Subsequently, elastic and collagen fibers are formed and accumulate to give the connective tissue the characteristics of the so-called "brawny edema." This is followed by a fibrosclerotic end stage.

■ Lymphedema

Mechanical obstruction in the lymphatic system could result from extrinsic and intrinsic pressure, such as sclerosis, inflammation, neoplasm, surgical injuries, and functional lymphospasm. Compensating mechanisms are elicited that may result in complete or partial drainage of the lymph. The excess lymph of the dilated lymphatic vessels may be transuded back through the walls into the interstitial fluid and, as sufficient pressure builds up, back into the vascular system. Another compensating mechanism is the development of collateral anastomatic channels.

Lymphedema is the excessive accumulation of lymph in the interstitial spaces. Lymphedema results when the compensating mechanisms fail to provide drainage of all the lymph. Lymphedema is not accompanied by cyanosis, dilatation of veins, hyperpigmentation, or leathery indentation. It is usually firm and does not pit well. The more common pathological conditions leading to the formation of edema are inflammatory processes due to tuberculosis, syphilis or filariasis, thrombophlebitis, and trauma related to ionizing radiation or surgical operations.

Baseline measurement of edema should be as precise as possible. It is recommended that the circumference of the extremities be measured with a flexible measuring tape made of plastic or metal that will not stretch. It is important that the same reference point be used on subsequent measurements. This can be accomplished by measuring a certain number of inches or centimeters from a given point, such as the ankle or the knee. Some clinics have elected 10 cm as the distance always to be used in an effort to standardize these measurements.

■ Lymph nodes

As a general rule, the lymph nodes decrease in size from the periphery toward the center of the body. Thus, the axillary lymph nodes are larger than the supraclavicular lymph nodes, and the inguinal lymph nodes are larger than the iliac lymph nodes.

The number of lymph nodes varies from individual to individual; generally speaking, the smaller the nodes are, the more numerous they are. Some investigators have reported that the number of lymph nodes is diminished in older persons. Furthermore, the size of the lymph nodes decreases with aging because they lose some of their lymphoid elements. The nodes from older clients show fibrosis and fatty degeneration on sectioning.

Whereas in their normal state lymph nodes are round or oval, in pathological conditions their form may be greatly altered and they may assume an irregularly nodular (as in lymphadenitis) or horseshoe shape (as in senile involution).

Normally, lymph nodes cannot be felt or seen. Thus, the size of the lymph nodes is an important diagnostic feature, and any increase is considered pathological. Usually, the greatest increases are found in acute and chronic inflammatory conditions and in systemic neoplastic disease. The size of the lymph nodes is almost never increased in cases of metastasis unless inflammatory reaction changes are also present. On the other hand, children with otherwise negative physical findings frequently have enlarged neck nodes, which may not have clinical significance.

EXAMINATION

Examination of the lymphatic system is accomplished by incorporating the examination techniques into the regimen for each part of the body where lymph nodes are palpable. However, the information gained in these localized efforts must be integrated so that a general lymphadenopathy is not overlooked.

Inspection is the first step in regional lymph node examination. This is followed by palpation of the specific nodal regions for prominent nodes. Palpation of the lymph nodes is best accomplished through a gentle rotary motion of the palmar surface of the index and middle fingertips. One should exercise enough pressure that the skin moves in concert with the fingers, but not so much that underlying nodes are obscured in the deeper soft tissues.

Detected nodes are described according to *location, size, regularity, consistency, tenderness, fixation to surrounding tissues,* and *discreteness.*

Characteristics assessed in examination of lymph nodes or masses

Location	Be specific in describing the site. Use imaginary body lines or axes and bony prominences to relate findings. Draw pictures where appropriate.
Size	Define the volume in centimeters the three dimensions of length, width, and thickness. State the total volume. Describe the shape lucidly (round, cylindrical); if irregular, draw pictures.
Surface characteristics	Describe accurately as smooth, nodular, irregular.
Consistency	Describe as hard, firm, soft, resilient, spongy, cystic.
Symmetry	Used as a comparison with paired structures.
Fixation, mobility	Describe exact mobile parameters in centimeters. If mass is fixed in position, identify whether fixation is to underlying or overlying tissue.
Tenderness	Describe whether present without stimulation or elicited by palpation or movement. Indicate whether direct, referred, or rebound.
Erythema	Describe extent of color change if present.
Heat	Describe extent if present.
Pulsatile nature	Describe pulsations when they are usually not palpable at this locus. Ascultate all pulsating masses for bruits.
Increased vascularity	Describe prominence of overlying veins or cyanosis of the area.
Transillumination	If pathological structure is in an anatomical area that can be transilluminated, such as the scrotum, describe the results of the procedure.

as opposed to *matting*. There may be no significance in a few discrete, mobile lymph nodes that measure less than 1 cm in diameter in any of the nodal sites; however, these nodes ought to move easily beneath the fingers. The fixed, immobile node may signify malignancy, whereas nodes that have coalesced may indicate infection. On judging a node to be normal, one must examine the regions drained by this node for indications of infection or neoplasm. Furthermore, other lymph node regions should be investigated for the presence of enlarged nodes.

Whenever a primary cancer is found, the nodes draining the region must be examined as well as those of known patterns of metastasis. For this reason the description of superficial lymph nodes that are close enough to the surface to be palpated includes the origin of the collecting ducts entering the nodes and the destination of those ducts leaving the nodes. Matting of nodes may include a superimposed infection or invasion of the lymph node capsule.

REGIONAL LYMPHATIC SYSTEMS
Head and neck
Head

Lymphatic drainage from the integument of the head, ears, nose, cheeks, and lips is delivered by collecting ducts to the lymph centers of the head (Fig. 11-2).

The *suboccipital center* consists of three to six lymph nodes receiving the collecting ducts from the occipital region of the scalp and from the deep structures of the back of the neck. The efferent lymphatics from these lymph nodes reach the deep lymph nodes of the neck and spinal nerve chain.

The *postauricular, or mastoid, center* contains four or five lymph nodes over the outer surface of the mastoid process or under the sternomastoid muscle. The afferent lymphatic vessels drain the parietal region of the head as well as part of the ear. Those vessels leaving these nodes reach the parotid substernomastoid lymph nodes.

The *preauricular center* is made up of one or two lymph nodes situated in front of the tragus. The afferent ducts are from the forehead and upper face.

The nodes of the *parotid center* may be found on the surface of the gland, within the tissue of the gland, or under the parotid fascia. The nodes of both the preauricular and parotid centers receive collecting ducts from the side of the head and the parotid gland, as well as from the

forehead, cheek, eyelids, ear, nose, upper lip, and eustachian tube. These efferent ducts contribute to the lymph nodes of the internal jugular and subdigastric chains.

The *submandibular center* lies on the medial border of the mandible, where it receives collecting ducts from the chin, upper lip, cheek, nose, teeth, eyelids, part of the tongue, and floor of the mouth. The efferent vessels bring lymph to the internal jugular chain of the neck.

The nodes of the *retropharyngeal center* are found at the junction of the posterior and lateral walls of the pharynx near the location of the atlas. Lymph from the nasal cavity and lymph of the accessory sinuses of the nose, palate, epipharynx, and mesopharynx, and possibly of the middle ear, is delivered to these nodes; the lymph leaving this center reaches the internal jugular chain about at the level of the bifurcation of the carotid artery.

The *submental center* receives collecting ducts from the tongue.

Neck

The lymph nodes of the neck receive the lymph from the head as well as from the structures of the neck itself. The nodes are grouped serially and are referred to as chains.

The *superficial cervical chain* of four to six lymph nodes is located over the sternocleidomastoid muscle and near but deeper than the external jugular vein. The nodes are beneath the platysma muscle and superficial cervical fascia and receive lymph from the skin and neck.

The *deep cervical chain* is made up of four chains of lymph nodes: (1) the prelaryngeal chain, located anterior to the larynx; (2) the prethyroid chain, situated anterior to the thyroid gland; (3) the pretracheal and laterotracheal chain, located anterior and lateral to the trachea; and (4) recurrent chains, found along the course of the recurrent laryngeal nerve. These nodes receive lymph via the collecting ducts from the larynx, thyroid gland, trachea, and upper part of the esophagus. The efferent vessels go to the internal jugular chain, mediastinal lymph nodes, and the bracheocephalic trunk.

The finger must be bent or hooked around the sternocleidomastoid muscle to palpate the deep cervical nodes, which are frequently enlarged in rubella, infectious mononucleosis, and hepatitis.

The nodes of the *thyrolinguofacial chain* are found between the lower margins of the posterior head of the diagastric muscle and the thyrolinguofacial venous trunk. Lymph draining to this group

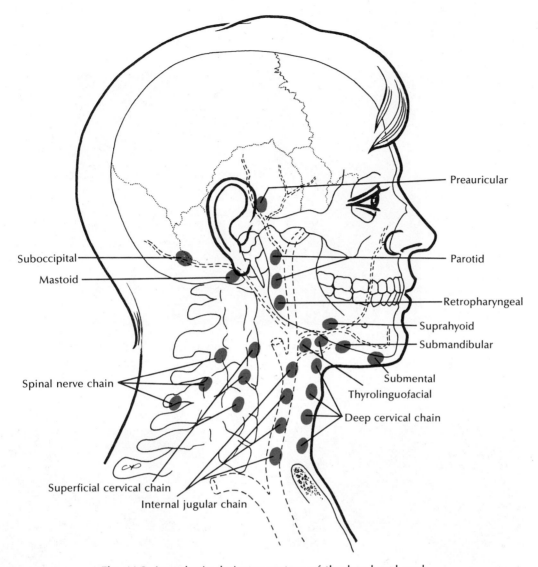

Preauricular

Suboccipital

Mastoid

Parotid

Retropharyngeal

Suprahyoid

Submandibular

Spinal nerve chain

Submental

Thyrolinguofacial

Deep cervical chain

Superficial cervical chain

Internal jugular chain

Fig. 11-2. Lymphatic drainage system of the head and neck.

is from the parotid, submaxillary retrolaryngeal, prelaryngeal, pretracheal, and recurrent areas as well as from the tongue, palate, tonsils, thyroid and submaxillary glands, nose, pharynx, and outer and middle ear.

The *internal jugular chain* is made up of many lymph nodes in contact with the jugular vein. The last of these nodes lie in contact with the thoracic duct.

The *chain of the spinal nerve* consists of 4 to 12 nodes lying in the upper part of the sterno-cleidomastoid muscle and following the external branch of the spinal nerve. Collecting ducts from the posterior and lateral regions of the neck reach these nodes as well as those of the occipital and mastoid regions of the head.

The *transverse cervical artery chain* of six to eight lymph nodes follows the transverse cervical artery and vein. This chain terminates in the great lymphatic trunk on the right side and in the thoracic duct on the left side. Lymph from the subclavian, laterocervical, anterothoracic, and internal mammary regions reaches these nodes.

The entire neck is lightly palpated for nodes (Fig. 11-3).

The anterior border of the sternocleidomastoid muscle is the dividing line for the anterior and posterior triangles of the neck. Description of locus may be facilitated through the use of these triangles.

Bending the client's head forward (Fig. 11-4) or to the side being examined (Fig. 11-5) will obviate tissue tension and permit more accurate palpation.

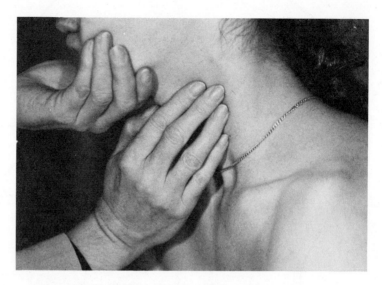

Fig. 11-3. The entire neck is lightly palpated for nodes.

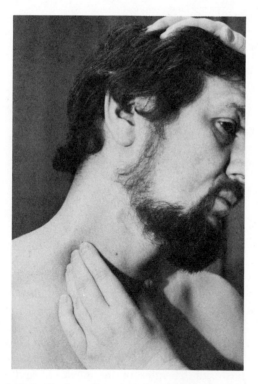

Fig. 11-4. Flexing the neck to obviate tissue tension, rendering any enlarged nodes more readily palpable.

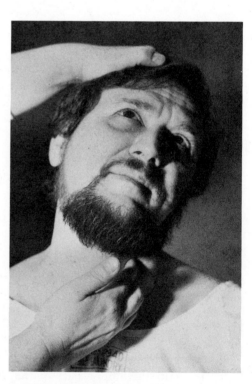

Fig. 11-5. Bending the head toward the side being examined to relax muscles and soft tissue, allowing more accurate palpation for lymph nodes.

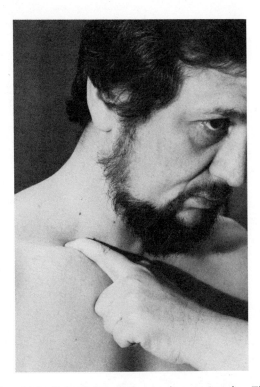

Fig. 11-6. Palpation of the scalene triangle. The client is encouraged to relax the musculature of the upper extremities, so that the clavicles are dropped. The examiner's free hand is used to flex the client's head forward in order to obtain relaxation of the soft tissues of the anterior neck. The left index finger is hooked over the clavicle lateral to the sternocleidomastoid muscle.

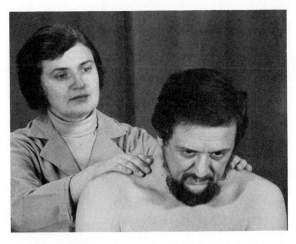

Fig. 11-7. Palpation of the posterior cervical nodes is accomplished while facing the client. The dorsal surfaces (pads) of the fingertips are placed along the anterior surface of the trapezius muscle and then moved slowly forward against the posterior surface of the sternocleidomastoid muscle.

Examination

The following maneuvers may be helpful in examining specific lymph node chains of the head and neck.

The *submental* and *submandibular nodes* can be examined by facing the client and placing the fingertips under the mandible on the side nearest the palpating hand. The skin and subcutaneous tissue is pulled laterally over the ramus of the mandible, and enlarged nodes can be felt as they roll over the mandibular surface beneath the examining fingers.

Another technique for the examination of the submandibular nodes is accomplished by placing one index finger in the floor of the mouth and the other fingers below the ramus of the mandible. The tissue between the fingers is gently rotated.

Palpation of the *scalene nodes* on the client's right side can be done by bending the left index finger over the clavicle and just lateral to the tendinous portion of the sternocleidomastoid muscle (Fig. 11-6). Moving the bent or hooked index finger in a rotary manner should allow nodes in the scalene triangle to be felt. The index finger should probe deeply into the triangle. To facilitate this entry, bending the client's head forward with the right hand will promote relaxation of the sternocleidomastoid muscle. The hand maneuver is reversed for the client's left scalene area.

The client is encouraged to generally relax the musculature of the upper extremities so that the clavicles will be pulled down, allowing the supraclavicular area to be explored thoroughly.

The posterior cervical nodes are examined from behind or while facing the client and by placing the dorsal surface of the fingertips along the anterior surface of the trapezius muscle and moving them slowly forward against the posterior surface of the sternocleidomastoid muscle (Fig. 11-7).

In some cases it is possible to determine the source of an infection from a characteristic pattern of lymph node involvement. For instance, infections of the tongue might produce enlargement of the submental, submandibular, suprahyoid, thyrolinguofacial, and internal jugular nodes (Fig. 11-8).

Another example would be infections of the ear that typically involve the preauricular, mastoid, parotid retropharyngeal, and deep cervical nodes (Fig. 11-9).

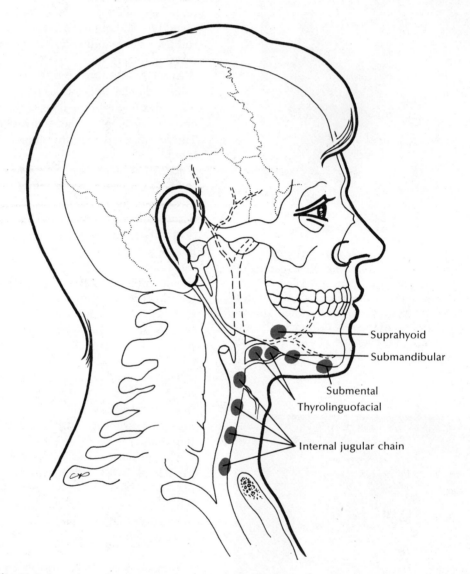

Suprahyoid

Submandibular

Submental

Thyrolinguofacial

Internal jugular chain

Fig. 11-8. Lymph nodes that may be potentially involved as a result of pathology of the tongue.

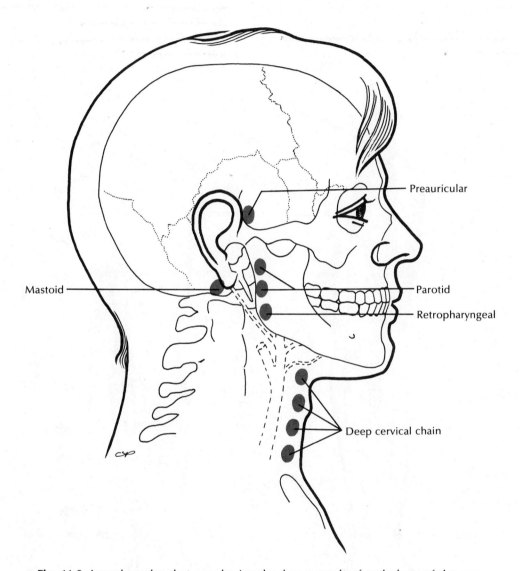

Fig. 11-9. Lymph nodes that may be involved as a result of pathology of the ear.

■ Upper extremity

A system of superficial and deep collecting ducts carry the lymph from the upper extremity to the subclavian lymphatic trunk (Fig. 11-10). The only peripheral lymph center is the epitrochlear center, which receives some of the collecting ducts from the pathway of the ulnar artery and nerve, and is located in a depression above and posterior to the medial condyle of the humerus (Fig. 11-11).

Enlargement of these nodes may be seen in secondary syphilis.

Lymphatics of the ulnar surface of the forearm, the little and ring fingers, and the medial surface of the middle finger drain into the epitrochlear nodes. Efferent ducts drain into the axillary or infraclavicular nodes, or both.

Axillary region

There are an average of 53 lymph nodes in the axillary fossa. Five groups of lymph nodes are distinguished in this area (Fig. 11-12).

The *center of the axillary or brachial veins*, or *lateral group*, consists of two to seven nodes lying

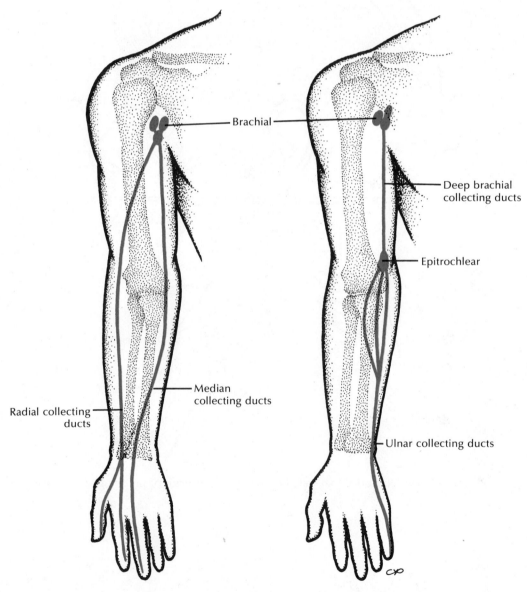

Brachial

Deep brachial collecting ducts

Epitrochlear

Median collecting ducts

Radial collecting ducts

Ulnar collecting ducts

Fig. 11-10. System of deep and superficial collecting ducts, carrying the lymph from the upper extremity to the subclavian lymphatic trunk. The only peripheral lymph center is the epitrochlear, which receives some of the collecting ducts from the pathway of the ulnar and radial nerves.

174

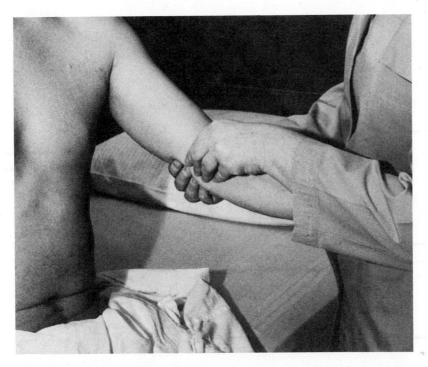

Fig. 11-11. Palpation for the epitrochlear lymph nodes is performed in the depression above and posterior to the medial condyle of the humerus.

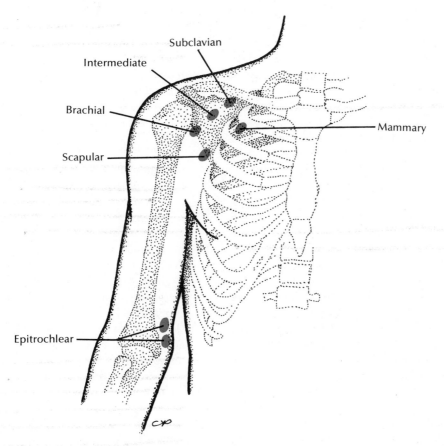

Fig. 11-12. Five groups of lymph nodes may be distinguished in the axillary fossa.

close to the axillary vein. These nodes receive collecting ducts from the upper extremity, deltoid region, and anterior wall of the chest, including the breast. Efferent ducts from this center terminate in the central lymph center, although some are known to connect with the subclavian lymph center.

The *scapular center, or posterior group,* consists of four or five nodes in contact with the inferior scapular vessels. The collecting ducts converging on these nodes are from the posterior wall of the chest and the posteroinferior neck. The efferent ducts drain to the central lymph center.

The *central or intermediate center* consists of eight to ten nodes and receives ducts from the brachial and scapular lymph centers as well as from the chest wall, breast, and arm. The ducts leaving these nodes go to the subclavian lymph center.

The *external mammary center, or anterior or pectoral group,* is a chain or nodes located along the course of the external mammary artery. A superior group of two or three nodes are found in the region of the third rib and the second and third intercostal spaces, and an inferior group is located over the fourth to sixth ribs. The ducts entering these nodes are from the breast and anterolateral chest wall and from the integument and muscles of the abdominal wall superior to the umbilicus. The efferent ducts from these nodes go to the subclavian center.

The *subclavian, or infraclavicular, center* may contain one to nine nodes situated in the tissues of the upper axilla. It receives lymph from all the other axillary centers, and ducts from this center empty into the venous junction of the jugular and subclavian veins.

Infections of the hand and arm may result in enlargement of these nodes.

Axillary examination is approached by regarding the area as a four-sided pyramid with its apex superior. The apex is located between the first rib and the clavicle. The apex in lay parlance is the armpit. The anterior border of the axilla is formed by the pectoral muscles; the posterior border is made up of back muscles, including the latissimus dorsi and subscapularis muscles; the medial border consists of the rib cage and serratus anterior muscle; and the lateral border, of the upper arm. Thus, the sides are anterior, posterior, medial, and lateral. Inspection and palpation must be done for each of the anatomical sides, first in a position of partial adduction of the subject's arms and then in abduction. The examination of the axillary area is accomplished by gently rolling the soft tissues against the chest wall and the muscles of the axilla (Fig. 11-13). Bimanual palpation is performed anteriorly to encompass the pectoralis muscle, as well as the posterior wall to include the back muscles.

Breast

The lymphatic system of the breast is particularly abundant. The lymphatic vessels drain to two major sites: the axillary and the internal mammary centers (Fig. 11-14). Lymph from the lower outer quadrant of the breast drains to the lateroinferior lymph nodes. Lymph from the areolar area, the upper outer quadrant, and the tail of the Spence drains to the mediosuperior axillary nodes. Lymph then courses through efferent ducts to the infraclavicular and supraclavicular nodes. The lymph from the inner aspect of the breast drains to the internal mammary nodes, which are three to four in number and inaccessible to palpation.

■ Lower extremity

As in the upper extremity, a system of superficial and deep collecting ducts drain the lymph from the leg (Fig. 11-15). Two or three nodes make up the *popliteal lymph center* in the back of the knee near the terminal portion of the saphenous vein. The afferent ducts to these nodes are, in fact, from the regions surrounding the external saphenous vein, that is, the heel and the outer aspect of the foot. However, the majority of the lymph is delivered to the inguinal nodes.

Superficial inguinal lymph center

A superior and inferior group of superficial inguinal nodes has been described.

The *inferior group* is a group of large lymph nodes that receive lymph from the superficial plexuses of the leg and foot (Fig. 11-16). They are the inguinal nodes below the junction of the saphenous and femoral veins. The superficial nodes lie along the course of the saphenous vein. The deep subinguinal nodes lie medial to the femoral vein and follow the vessel into the abdomen. Cloquet's gland, a node of this group, lies immediately above the saphenous opening. When this node is enlarged, incarcerated, or strangulated, femoral hernia may result.

The *superior group* is a center containing five or six nodes whose afferent ducts are from the abdominal wall inferior to the umbilicus, the buttocks, and the external genital organs as well as the efferent vessels from the inferior center (Fig.

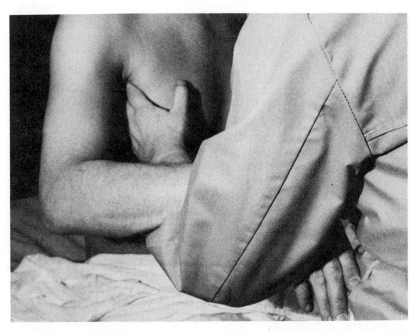

Fig. 11-13. The soft tissues of the axilla are gently rolled against the chest wall and the muscles surrounding the axilla.

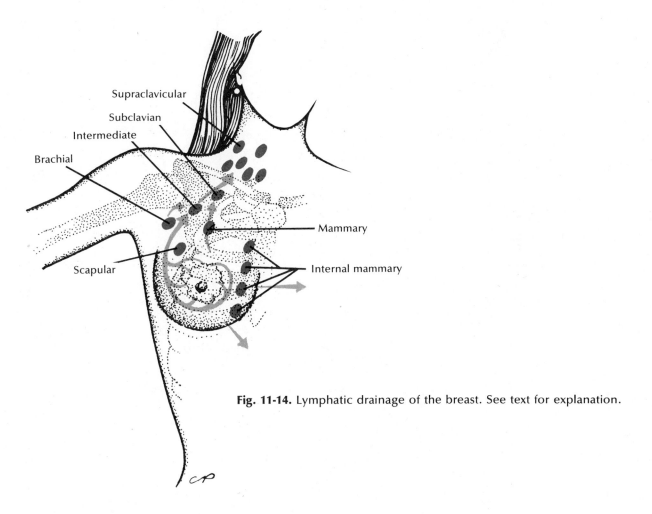

Fig. 11-14. Lymphatic drainage of the breast. See text for explanation.

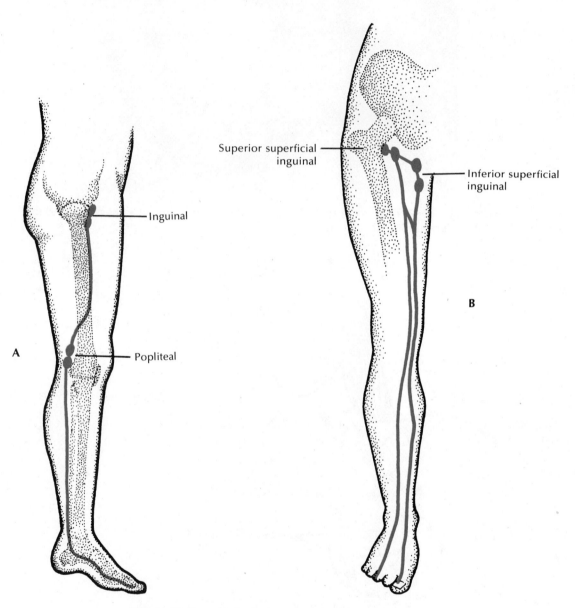

Fig. 11-15. Lymphatic drainage of the lower extremity.

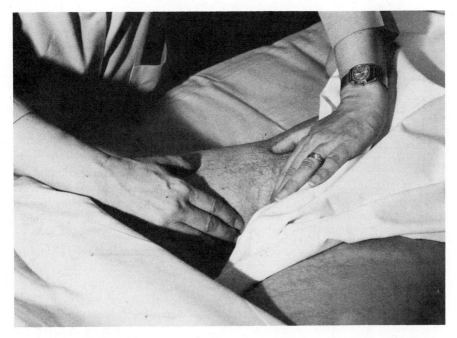

Fig. 11-16. Palpation of the inferior superficial inguinal lymph nodes.

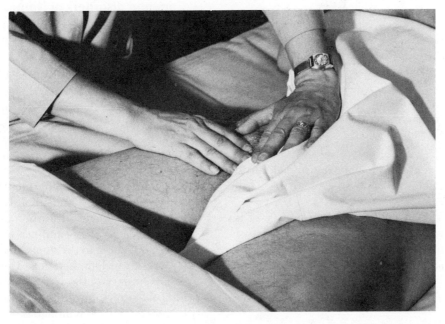

Fig. 11-17. Palpation of the superior superficial inguinal lymph nodes.

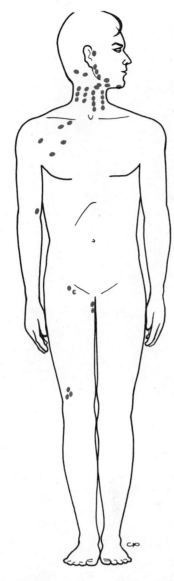

Fig. 11-18. Diagrammatic summary of the areas to be examined for lymph nodes during the course of the physical examination.

• • •

11-17). These nodes lie along and parallel to the inguinal ligament.

Fig. 11-18 is a diagrammatic summary of the areas where pathological lymph nodes may be identified by inspection and palpation. These are the sites to be assessed during the physical examination.

PATHOLOGY
■ Common diseases related to lymph node characteristics

The assessment parameters of pathological lymph nodes may combine to establish the diag-nosis of the disease process of the client. Some common findings related to specific diseases are described below.

Acute pyogenic infections. The nodes of acute infections are large, tender, and discrete. These alterations are accompanied by the classic signs of inflammation, which are *tumor* (swelling), *color* (redness and heat), and *dolor* (tenderness).

The nodes may become confluent if the infec-tion becomes chronic.

Tuberculosis. The lymph nodes of the tubercu-lar client may be soft and matted together. The nodes are generally nontender to the client. Oc-casionally sinus formation is present.

Metastatic cancer. Lymph nodes of metastatic cancer are described as discrete, nontender, of a firm to hard consistency, and unilateral in focus. They may be small or several centimeters in di-ameter.

Hodgkin's disease. Hodgkin's disease results in lymph node involvement in which the nodes are large, discrete, nontender, and of a firm, rubbery consistency.

Syphilis. A lymph node in the chain draining a syphilitic chancre is called a bubo. Characteristi-cally, the nodes are enlarged, hard, nonfluctuant, and painless. Such a node in the inguinal chain should prompt the practitioner to inspect thor-oughly for a genital chancre.

■ Common disorders of lymphatic vessels

Acute lymphangitis. The chief complaint of the client may include pain in the affected extremity. Elevation of temperature may be present, and the client may complain of malaise.

Inspection of the affected limb may reveal red-ness along the course of lymphatic collecting ducts, which appear as fine lines. The tubules may be palpable. The source of infection is sought. In the lower extremity interdigital spaces are carefully examined for cracks, which are often the site of entry for epidermophytosis.

Lymphedema. Congenital lymphedema may result in swelling or distortion of the extremities, caused by hypoplasia and maldevelopment of the system. Trauma to the ducts, leading to blockage, may result in lymphedema. This may be the re-sult of surgery of the regional lymph nodes, as in radical mastectomy or groin dissection. Extension of cancer to the lymphatics may also result in stasis of lymph flow. Infection may also block lymphatic ducts. (See also pp. 166-167.)

Elephantiasis. Elephantiasis is the term used for the massive accumulation of lymphedema. The condition may be the sequelae of congenital or acquired forms of lymphedema. The marked lymphedema predisposes the client to further infection and episodes of cellulitis. Recurrent infectious involvement leads to marked fibrosis of the edematous tissues.

REFERENCES

Battezatti, M., and Donini, I.: The lymphatic system, New York, 1973, John Wiley & Sons, Inc.

Brouse, N. L.: Response of lymphatics to sympathetic nerve stimulation, J. Physiol. **197:**25, 1968.

Haagensen, C. D., Fend, C. R., Herter, F. P., and others: The lymphatics in cancer, Philadelphia, 1972, W. B. Saunders Co.

Kinmonth, J. B.: The lymphatic diseases; lymphography and surgery, Baltimore, 1972, The Williams & Wilkins Co.

Mayerson, H. S.: Lymph and lymphatic system, Springfield, Ill., 1968, Charles C Thomas, Publisher.

Solnitzky, O. C., and Jeghers, H.: Lymphadenopathy and disorders of the lymphatic system. In McBride, C., and Blacklow, R., editors: Signs and symptoms; applied pathologic physiology and clinical interpretation, Philadelphia, 1970, J. B. Lippincott Co.

Yoffey, J. M., and Courtice, F. C.: Lymphatics; lymph and the lymphomyeloid complex, New York, 1970, Academic Press, Inc.

12 Assessment of the breasts

ANATOMY

The breast is a modified sebaceous gland that is paired and located on the anterior chest wall between the second and third ribs superiorly, the sixth and seventh costal cartilages inferiorly, the anterior axillary line laterally, and the sternal border medially.

The functional components of the breast consist of the acini or milk-producing glands, a ductal system, and a nipple (Fig. 12-1, *A*). The glandular tissue units are called lobes and are situated in circular, spokelike fashion around the nipple. There are 15 to 25 lobes per breast. Each lobe is composed of 20 to 40 lobules, each containing 10 to 100 acini.

Much of the bulk of the breast is composed of subcutaneous and retromammary fat. The breast is fairly mobile but is supported by a layer of subcutaneous connective tissue and by Cooper's ligaments (Fig. 12-1, *B*). The latter are multiple fibrous bands that begin at the breast's subcutaneous connective tissue layer and run through the breast, attaching to the muscle fascia.

Knowledge of the lymphatic drainage of the breast is critical because of the frequent dissemination of breast cancer through this system. There are three types of lymphatic drainage of the breast (Fig. 12-2).

Cutaneous lymphatic drainage is of lymph from the skin of the breast, excluding the areolar and nipple areas; this lymph flows into the ipsilateral axillary nodes (the mammary, scapular, brachial, and intermediate nodes). Lymph from the medial cutaneous breast area may flow to the opposite breast. Lymph from the inferior portion of the breast can reach the lymphatic plexus of the epigastric region and subsequently the liver and other abdominal regions and organs.

Areolar lymphatic drainage is of lymph formed in the areolar and nipple areas of the breast; this lymph flows into the anterior axillary group of nodes (the mammary nodes).

Deep lymphatic drainage is of lymph from the deep mammary tissues; this lymph flows into the anterior axillary nodes. Some of this lymph also flows into the apical, subclavian, infraclavicular, and supraclavicular nodes. Also, lymph from the retroareolar areas, medial glandular breast tissue areas, and lower glandular breast tissue areas communicates with lymphatic systems draining into the thorax and abdomen.

The largest portion of glandular breast tissue occurs in the upper lateral quadrant of each breast. From this quadrant there is an anatomical projection of breast tissue into the axilla. This projection is termed the axillary tail of Spence (Fig. 12-3). The majority of breast tumors are located in the upper lateral breast quadrant and in the tail of Spence.

Grossly, the normal breasts are reasonably symmetrical in size and shape, though not usually absolutely equal. This symmetry remains constant at rest and with movement. The skin of the breast is the same as that of the abdomen or back. There may be a small number of scattered hair follicles around the areola. In light-complected persons a horizontal or vertical vascular pattern may be observed. This pattern, when normally present, is symmetrical.

The areolae are pigmented areas surrounding the nipples. Their color varies from pink to brown, and their size varies greatly. Several or many sebaceous glands (termed Montgomery's tubercles or follicles) may be present on the areolar surface.

The nipples are round, hairless, pigmented, protuberant structures whose size and shape vary

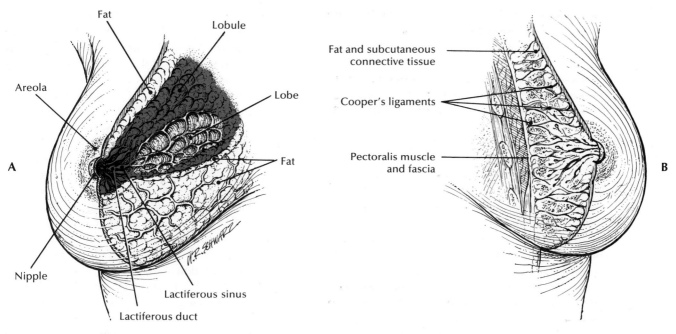

Fig. 12-1. Female breasts. **A,** Internal structures. **B,** Supportive tissue structures.

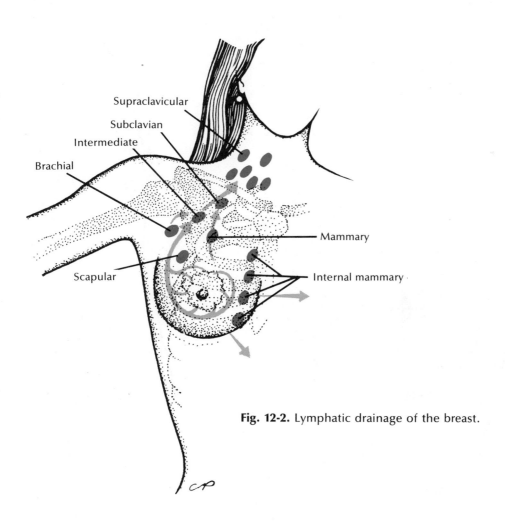

Fig. 12-2. Lymphatic drainage of the breast.

among women and in an individual woman depending on the state of contraction. Usually nipples are directed or "point" slightly upward and laterally.

Inversion of the nipple is an invagination or depression of its central portion. Inversion can occur congenitally or as a response to an invasive process.

During early embryonic development longitudinal ridges exist, extending from the axilla to the groin. Called "milk lines" (Fig. 12-4), these ridges usually atrophy, except at the level of the pectoral muscles, where a breast will eventually develop. In some women the ridges do not entirely disappear, and portions of the milk lines persist. This existence is manifested in the presence of a nipple, a nipple and a breast, or glandular breast tissue only. This congenital anomaly is termed a supernumerary breast or nipple.

The gross appearance and size of the normal female breast varies greatly. The following describes breast development through a woman's life span:

1. *Appearance before age 10:* There is little difference in the appearance of male and female breasts. The nipple is small, and there is no evidence of glandular tissue development.

2. *Development at approximately age 10:* A "mammary bud" develops on both breasts, and the breasts continue to progressively increase in size and shape through the early adolescent years. At this time the subareolar mammary tissues are prominent, and this area appears distinct from the rest of the breast. Breast development may begin or progress unilaterally; both breasts should be reasonably symmetrical in adulthood.

3. *Adult breast:* The breast is influenced by both estrogen and progesterone. The areolar "bud" recedes into the general contour of the breast, and the nipple protrudes. The size of the adult breast is influenced by heredity, individual sensitivity to hormones, and nutrition.

4. *Menstrual changes:* In response to hormonal changes during the menstrual cycle there is a pattern of breast size change, nodularity, and tenderness that is maximal just before the menses. The breast is small-

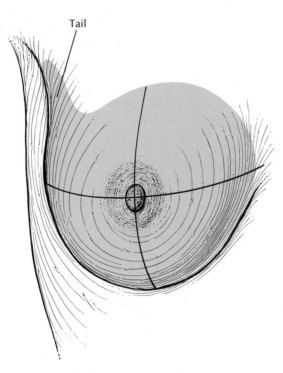

Fig. 12-3. Axillary tail of Spence.

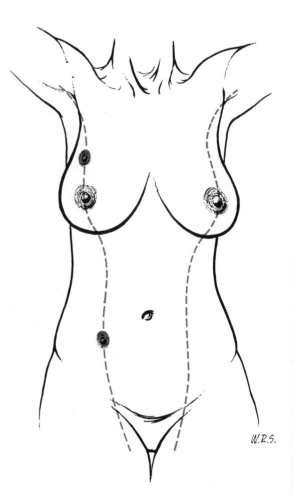

Fig. 12-4. Milk lines.

est in days 4 through 7 of the menstrual cycle. In days 3 to 4 before the onset of the menses, mammary tenseness, fullness, heaviness, tenderness, and pain are experienced by many women. The total breast volume is significantly increased.

5. *Changes in pregnancy:* The breast increases in size, sometimes to as large as two or three times the usual size. The areolae and nipples become more prominent and more deeply pigmented. The veins engorge, and striae are often observed.

6. *Menopausal changes.* After menopause, the breast's glandular tissue gradually involutes, and fat is deposited in the breasts. Breast form becomes flabby and flattened.

EXAMINATION
■ Inspection

Inspection and palpation are the techniques used in the examination of the breast. No special equipment is necessary. The client is uncovered to the waist and is seated on the side of an examining table. The breasts are observed for (1) symmetry of shape, color, size, and surface characteristics; (2) hyperpigmentation; (3) moles or nevi; (4) edema; (5) retraction or dimpling; (6) abnormal amount or distribution of hair; (7) presence of focal vascularity; and (8) lesions (Fig. 12-5).

Retraction, or dimpling, appears as a depression or pucker on the skin (Fig. 12-6, A). It usually is caused by the fibrotic shortening and immobilization of Cooper's ligament by an invasive process.

Whenever the skin of the breasts is stretched rapidly, damage to the elastic fibers or the dermis may occur and observable striae, or stretch marks, are produced. Newly created striae appear reddish; they become whitish with age.

Edema of the breasts produces exaggeration of the skin pores, creating an orange peel appearance of the breast, called peau d'orange (Fig. 12-6, B).

Vascular patterns should be diffuse and symmetrical. Focal or unilateral patterns are abnormal (Fig. 12-6, A).

The areolar area is inspected for size, shape, symmetry, color, surface characteristics, bulging, and lesions. As mentioned previously, size, shape, and color can normally vary greatly. Any asymmetry, mass, or lesion should be considered abnormal.

If the breasts are symmetrical, both nipples should be pointing laterally in the same way. The nipple is observed for size, shape, ability to erect, color, discharge, and lesions. The nipples should be round, equal in size, homogenous in color, and have convoluted surfaces, which give them a wrinkled appearance. Inversion of one or both nipples, if present from puberty, is normal; however, this condition may interfere with breastfeeding. Recent inversion of the nipple is probably retraction (Fig. 12-6, A) and should be investigated.

Paget's disease appears as a red glandular erosion on the nipple or as a nipple that is dry, scaly, or friable. The areola may also be affected. Paget's disease is a malignant condition requiring prompt therapy.

Breast secretions are normal in pregnancy or lactation. Other causes of discharge are mechan-

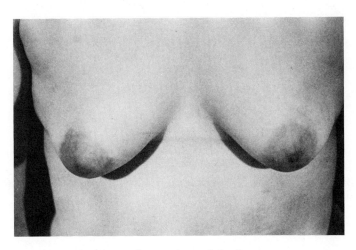

Fig. 12-5. Observation of the breasts.

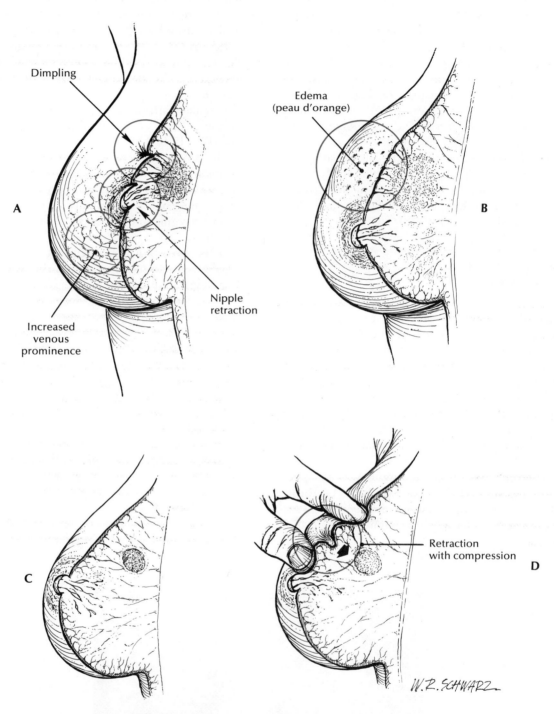

Fig. 12-6. Abnormalities of the breast. **A,** Breast with dimpling, nipple retraction, and increased venous prominence. **B,** Breast with edema (peau d'orange or pigskin appearance). **C,** Breast with tumor; no retraction is apparent. **D,** Breast with tumor; retraction is apparent with compression.

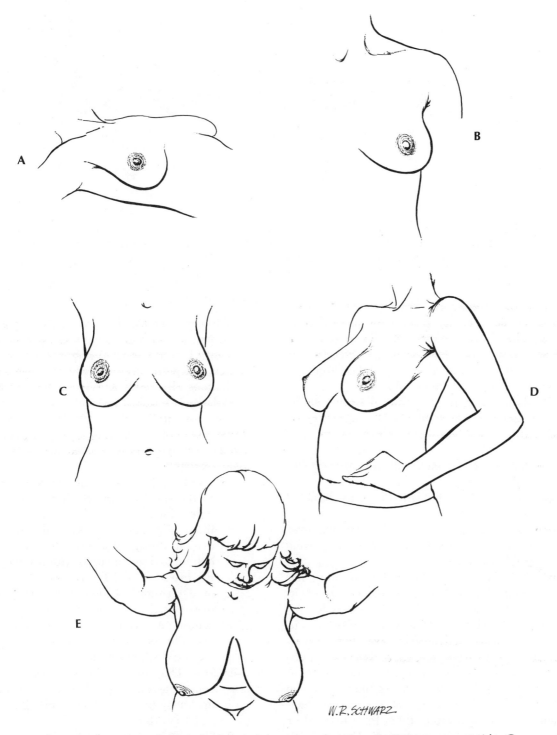

Fig. 12-7. Positions of client for breast inspection. **A,** Lying. **B,** Sitting, arms at side. **C,** Sitting, arms elevated. **D,** Sitting, pectoral contraction. **E,** Sitting, bending forward.

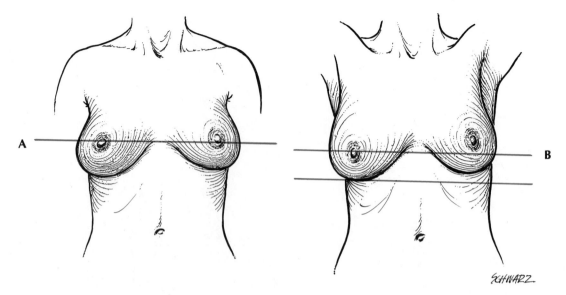

SCHWARZ

Fig. 12-8. A, Breasts appear symmetrical at rest. **B,** Breasts do not move symmetrically with arm elevation. The right breast is immobilized.

ical nipple stimulation, drug influence, hypothalamic and pituitary disorders, and malignant and benign breast lesions. The discharge can be milky, watery, purulent, serous, or bloody. The method for determining the site of discharge production is discussed under Palpation.

There are four major sitting positions of the client used for breast inspection. Every client should be examined in each position (Fig. 12-7):

1. The client is seated with her arms at her sides.
2. The client is seated with her arms abducted over her head.
3. The client is seated and is leaning over while the examiner assists in supporting and balancing her.
4. The client is seated and is pushing her hands into her hips, simultaneously eliciting contraction of the pectoral muscles.

While the client is performing these maneuvers, the breasts are carefully observed for symmetry, bulging, retraction, and fixation. An abnormality may not be apparent in the breasts at rest (Fig. 12-8, A), but a mass may cause the breasts, through invasion of suspensory ligaments, to fix, preventing them from upward or forward movement in positions 2 (Fig. 12-8, B) and 3. Position 4 specifically assists in eliciting dimpling if a mass has infiltrated and shortened suspensory ligaments.

The breasts are also observed with the client lying down, before the examiner palpates.

■ **Palpation**

The range of normal breast consistency is wide. The breasts feel homogenous in the young adolescent. The presence of progesterone in pregnancy and premenstrually causes the breasts to feel generally nodular. Hormonally induced nodularity is bilateral and diffuse.

The primary purpose for the palpation of breasts is to discover masses. If a mass is discovered, it is assessed according to the following characteristics:

1. *Location:* Masses are designated according to the quadrant in which they lie: upper outer, lower outer, upper inner, or lower inner (Fig. 12-9, A). When describing the mass in the client's record, one may find it helpful to draw the mass within a diagram of the breast (Fig. 12-9, B). Another method of describing location is to visualize the breast as the face of a clock; the nipple is center. A mass can be designated, for example, as being "5 cm from the nipple in the 8 o'clock position."
2. *Size:* The size should be approximated in centimeters in all its planes. For example, a mass may be ovoid, 3 cm wide, 2 cm long, and 1 cm thick.
3. *Shape:* The shape may be round, ovoid, irregular, or matted. Matting occurs in the presence of multiple lesions.
4. *Consistency:* A breast mass may be soft or hard, solid or cystic.
5. *Discreteness:* The borders of the mass are

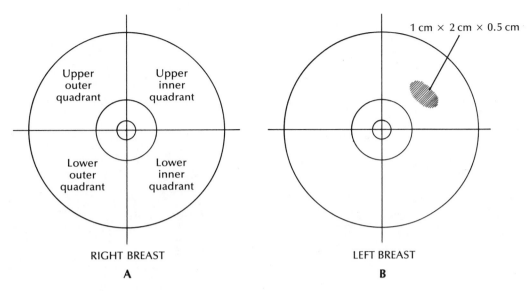

Fig. 12-9. A, The four quadrants of the breast. **B,** Diagram of a mass within a breast.

assessed to determine if they are sharp and well defined or irregular.

6. *Mobility:* The examiner attempts to move the mass over the chest wall. It is noted as being freely movable, movable, or fixed.

7. *Tenderness:* The client is questioned regarding any discomfort with palpation.

8. *Erythema:* The area of skin overlying the mass is inspected for erythema.

9. *Dimpling over the mass:* The tissue over the mass is compressed to determine if this maneuver produces dimpling (Fig. 12-6, *D*).

The palpation portion of the examination of the breast begins with palpation for axillary, subclavicular, and supraclavicular lymph nodes. This is most effectively performed with the client in a sitting position. The location and palpation of the axillary, subclavicular, and supraclavicular nodes are described in Chapter 11 on Assessment of the lymphatic system. To emphasize the importance of an adequate axillary area examination with each breast examination, this procedure is reviewed here.

In examining the axilla, the tissues can be best appreciated if the area muscles are relaxed. Contracted muscles may obscure slightly enlarged nodes. To achieve this relaxation while at the same time abducting the arm, the examiner supports the ipsilateral arm (Fig. 12-10).

The examiner should visualize the axilla as a four-sided pyramid and thoroughly palpate the following areas: (1) the edge of the pectoralis major muscle for the mammary group of nodes,

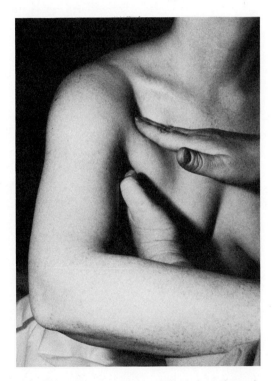

Fig. 12-10. Palpation of the axillary lymph nodes.

(2) the thoracic wall for the intermediate group of nodes, (3) the upper part of the humerus for the brachial axillary group of nodes, and (4) the anterior edge of the latissimus dorsi muscle for the subscapular group of nodes.

The breasts are most effectively palpated with the client in a supine position. Because of time constraints on most physical examinations, it is

189

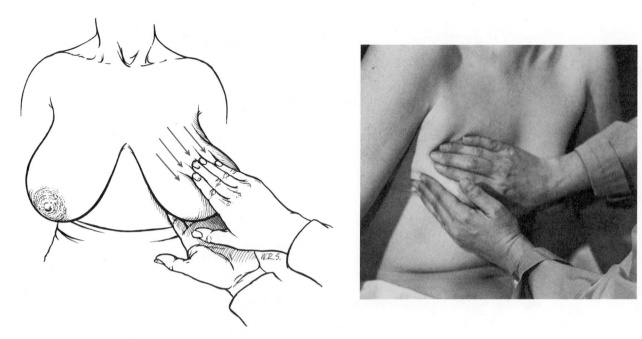

Fig. 12-11. Bimanual palpation of the breasts.

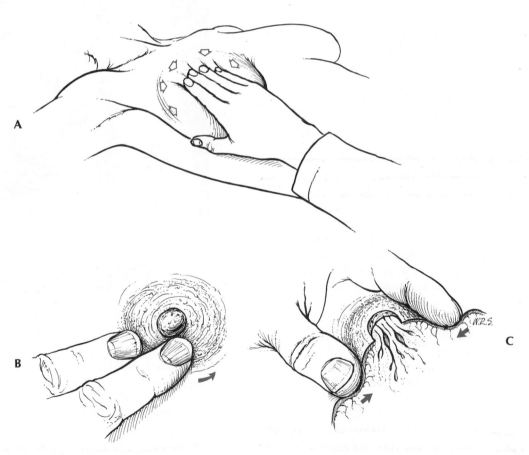

Fig. 12-12. Palpation of the breasts. **A,** Glandular area. **B,** Areolar area. **C,** Compression of the nipple.

not advised that all breasts be also palpated with the client in a sitting position. However, several groups of clients should also be examined in the sitting position: women with present or past complaints of breast masses, women at high risk of breast cancer, and women with pendulous breasts.

With the client in a sitting position, small breasts can be examined by using one hand to support the breast while the other hand palpates the tissue against the chest wall. Pendulous breasts are palpated using a bimanual technique (Fig. 12-11). The inferior portion of the breast is supported in one hand while the other palpates breast tissue against the supporting hand.

The client is then asked to lie down. The breasts are palpated while they are flattened against the rib cage. If the breasts are large, several mechanisms can be employed to enhance this flattening. A pillow can be placed under the ipsilateral shoulder, or the client can abduct the ipsilateral arm and place her hand under her neck. Both maneuvers shift the breast medially. The humerus should be at least slightly abducted to allow for thorough palpation of the tail of Spence.

The breasts are then thoroughly palpated (Fig. 12-12). The examiner should develop a system and habitually start and end at a fixed point on the breasts. The starting point is arbitrary. The breasts are palpated with the palmar surfaces of the fingers held together. The movements are smooth, and back and forth or circular. The breast is visualized as a bicycle wheel with six or eight spokes, and palpation occurs along each spoke until the breast has been thoroughly surveyed. Special attention is focused on the upper outer quadrant area and on the tail of Spence (Fig. 12-13).

An alternate method of breast palpation is to consider the breast as a group of concentric circles with the nipple as the center. Palpation occurs along the circumferences of the circle, starting at the outermost circle, until the total breast area is adequately surveyed.

The areolar areas are carefully palpated to determine the presence of underlying masses. Each nipple is gently compressed to assess for the presence of masses or discharge (Fig. 12-12, *C*). If discharge is noted, the breast is milked along its radii to identify the lobe from which the discharge is originating. Compression of the discharge-producing lobe will cause discharge to exude from the nipple.

If a client reports a breast nodule, the "normal" breast is examined first so that the baseline consistency of that breast will serve as a control when the reportedly abnormal one is palpated.

Mammary folds, crescent-shaped ridges of breast tissue found at the inferior portions of very large or pendulous breasts, may be confused with breast masses but are nonpathological.

■ Breast self-examination

The majority of breast masses are found by the clients themselves. Too often the malignant

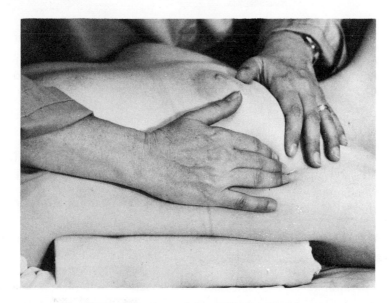

Fig. 12-13. Palpation of the axillary tail of Spence.

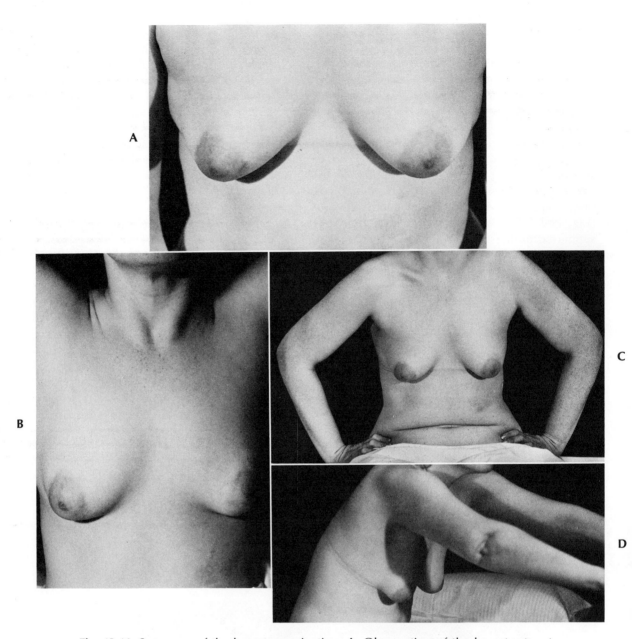

Fig. 12-14. Sequence of the breast examination. **A,** Observation of the breasts at rest. **B,** Observation with client's arms overhead. **C,** Observation with client contracting pectoral muscles. **D,** Observation with client leaning forward.

masses are found after extensive development and metastasis. While the practitioner is examining the client, he should review the rationale and process of the examination with the client and advise her to perform the examination at home during the period of the fourth to the seventh menstrual cycle day. During this time the breasts are smallest and the glandular tissue least congested.

The client can perform the breast self-examination in a manner similar to the one used by the examiner. For the axillary examination, it is recommended that she lie down with her arm abducted and supported by a bed.

■ **Special examination procedures**

Further evaluation of breast masses is accomplished through the use of several newly developed techniques.

Mammography is the technique of breast examination by the use of low-energy radiography.

Xerography is mammography using a xero-

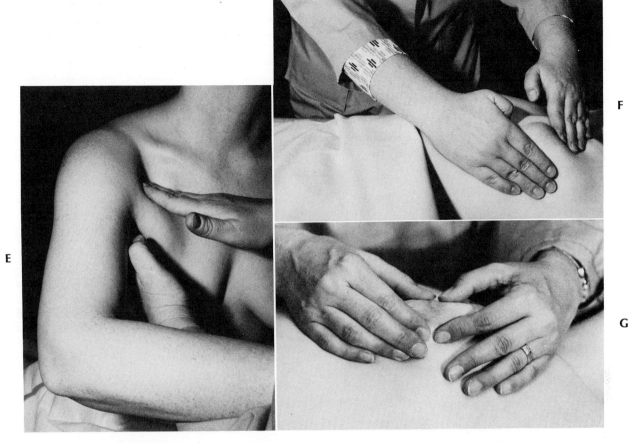

Fig. 12-14, cont'd. E, Palpation of axillary nodes. (Palpation of the supraclavicular and subclavicular areas is not illustrated). **F,** Palpation of the glandular area. **G,** Palpation of the nipple and areolar area.

graphic plate instead of film. The advantages of this technique are that radiation doses are smaller than with conventional mammography and the images produced are more distinct.

Thermography is a technique that measures the temperature distribution of the breast. Malignant lesions appear as "hot spots" in the breast.

PATHOLOGY
■ Breast cancer

Breast cancer is a leading cause of death in women in the United States and also a leading cause of cancer morbidity. Knowledge of factors indicating that a woman is at a higher than usual risk of cancer can assist in making decisions about screening programs and the frequency of general physical examinations. The following groups of women are at higher than usual risk of breast cancer:

1. Women who have never been pregnant
2. Women whose first full-term pregnancy was at age 30 or older
3. Women with a history of an early menarche or late menopause
4. Women with a history of chronic cystic mastitis
5. Women of North American or European descent
6. Women with a previous breast cancer
7. Women with a strong family history of breast cancer

These women should be taught to perform self-examination and should receive a professional physical examination at least once a year.

■ The male breast

Occurring most frequently in the areolar area, male breast cancer accounts for approximately 1% of all breast cancers. Every male client should be given a thorough breast examination with an adaptation of the technique used for female clients.

Gynecomastia, enlargement of the male breast, is a frequently occurring multicausal condition. Causes include pubertal changes, hormonal administration, cirrhosis, leukemia, thyrotoxicosis, and drugs.

SUMMARY

The following outline is a recommended sequence for the examination of the breast (Fig. 12-14):

1. Observation of the breasts at rest
2. Observation of the breasts in three additional positions
   A. Client with arms over her head
   B. Client leaning forward
   C. Client contracting pectoral muscles
3. Palpation of axillary node areas
4. Palpation of the supraclavicular and subclavicular areas
5. Palpation of the breasts with the client in a sitting position, if indicated
6. Observation of the breasts with the client lying down and the breasts shifted medially
7. Palpation of the breasts
   A. Glandular tissue areas
   B. Areolar areas
   C. Nipples
   D. Tail of Spence areas

Every female client should be taught to examine her breasts and should be advised to do this each month on the completion of the menses.

BIBLIOGRAPHY

Dunphy, J. E., and Botsford, T. W.: Physical examination of the surgical patient, ed. 4, Philadelphia, 1975, W. B. Saunders Co.

Evans, K. T., and Gravelle, I. H.: Mammography, thermography and ultrasonography in breast disease, Sevenoaks, Kent, 1973, Butterworth & Co. (Publishers) Ltd.

Kishner, R.: Breast cancer; a personal history and an investigative report, New York, 1975, Harcourt Brace Jovanovich, Inc.

Memorial Hospital for Cancer and Associated Diseases: Breast Cancer Monograph, New York, 1973, Memorial Hospital.

Papaioannou, A. N.: The etiology of human breast cancer, New York, 1974, Springer-Verlag New York Inc.

Rush, B.: Breast. In Schwartz, S. I., editor: Principles of surgery, ed. 2, New York, 1969, McGraw-Hill Book Co.

Vorherr, H.: The breast, New York, 1974, Academic Press, Inc.

Wolfe, J. N.: Zeroradiography of the breast, Springfield, Ill., 1972, Charles C Thomas, Publisher.

13 Assessment of the respiratory system

ANATOMY AND PHYSIOLOGY

The major purpose of the respiratory system is to supply the body with oxygen and eliminate carbon dioxide. This is accomplished through complex cooperation of many body systems which, in wellness, act in harmony. The actual transfer of oxygen and carbon dioxide between environmental gas and body liquid occurs in the alveoli, which are obviously not accessible to clinical examination. However, assessment of respiratory efficiency is accomplished by direct and indirect appraisal of structures supporting alveolar function.

The thoracic cage consists of a skeleton of 12 thoracic vertebrae, 12 pairs of ribs, the sternum, the diaphragm, and the intercostal muscles and is semirigid (Fig. 13-1). This cage is perpetually moving in the inspiratory and expiratory phases of respiration (Fig. 13-2). During inspiration the diaphragm descends and flattens. This maneuver produces differences in pressure among the areas of the mouth, the alveoli, and the pleural areas; and air moves into the lungs. The intrathoracic pressure is decreased, the lungs are expanded, and ribs flare, increasing the diameter of the thorax. The second to the sixth ribs move around two axes in a motion commonly termed the "pump handle" movement. The lower ribs move in a "bucket handle" motion. Because of the length and positioning of the lower ribs and because the lower interspaces are wider, the amplitude of movement is greater in the lower thorax.

Inspiration is opposed by the elastic properties of the respiratory system. At the end of respiration, the volume of inspired air equals the volume exchange of the thoracic cavity, the tidal volume. Expiration is a relatively passive phenomenon. At the completion of inspiration, the diaphragm relaxes and the elastic recoil properties of the lungs expel air and pull the diaphragm to its resting position.

The thoracic cavity is divided into right and left pleural cavities; lined by the pleural layers—the visceral (lung) layer and the parietal (wall) layer—the pleural cavity is the space between the pleura. It contains a lubricating fluid.

The lungs are paired, but not symmetrical, conical organs that conform to the thoracic cavity. The right lung contains three lobes, and the left lung contains two.

Air reaches the lungs via a system of flexible tubes. Air enters through the mouth or nose, traverses the respiratory portion of the larynx, and enters the trachea. The trachea begins at the lower border of the cricoid cartilage and divides into a left and right bronchus, usually at the level of thoracic vertebra 4 or 5 posteriorly and slightly below the manubriosternal joint anteriorly.

The right bronchus is shorter, wider, and more vertical than the left bronchus. The bronchial structures further subdivide into increasingly smaller bronchi and bronchioles. Each bronchiole opens into an alveolar duct from which multiple alveoli radiate (Fig. 13-3). Lungs in the adult contain approximately 300 million alveoli.

The bronchi have both transport and protective purposes. Their cavities contain mucus, which entraps foreign particles and is continuously swept by ciliary action into the throat, where it can be eliminated.

■ Topographical anatomy

Topographical (surface) landmarks of the thorax assist the examiner in identifying the location of the internal, underlying structures and in de-

Text continued on p. 200.

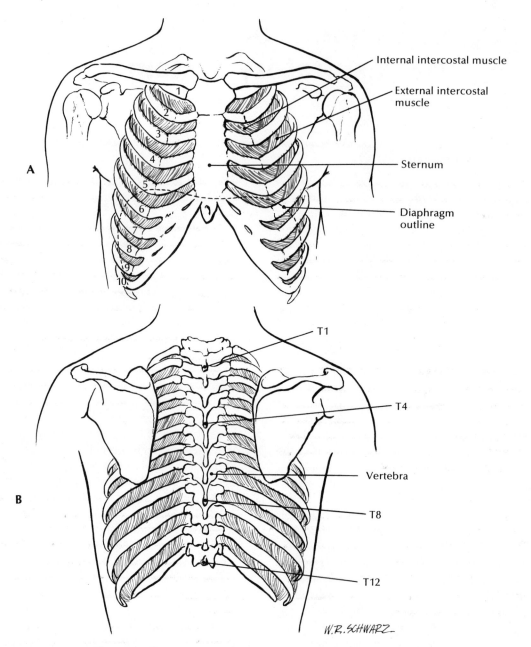

Fig. 13-1. Thoracic cage. **A,** Anterior thorax. **B,** Posterior thorax.

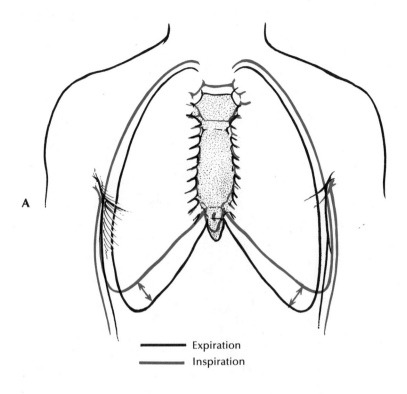

A

——— Expiration
——— Inspiration

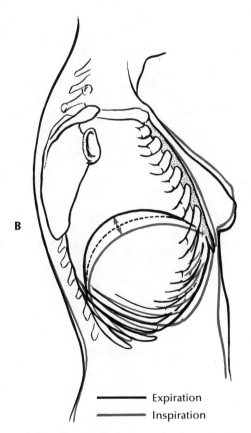

B

——— Expiration
——— Inspiration

Fig. 13-2. Movement of the thorax during respiration. **A,** Anterior thorax. **B,** Lateral thorax.

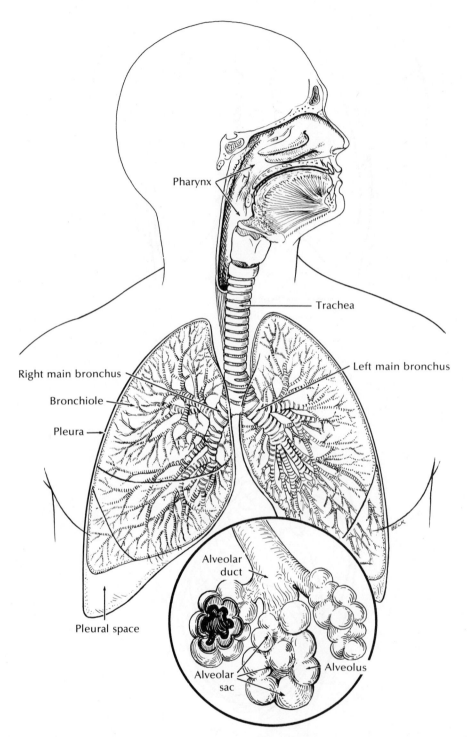

Fig. 13-3. Pharynx, trachea, and lungs. Alveolar sacs in inset. (From Anthony, C. P., and Kolthoff, N. J.: Anatomy and physiology, ed. 9, St. Louis, 1975, The C. V. Mosby Co.)

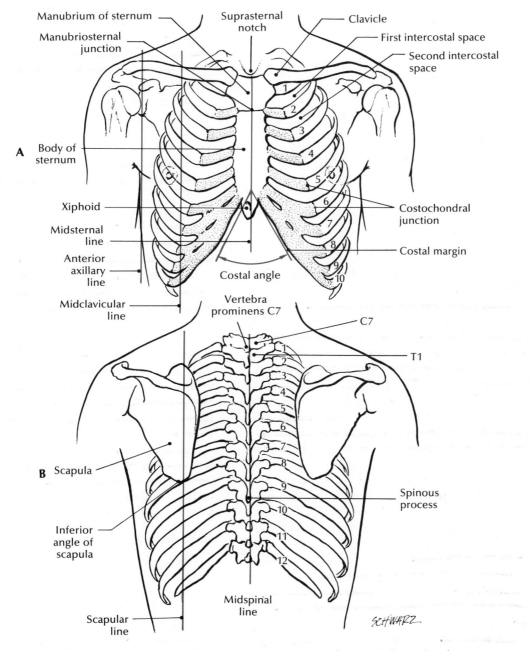

Fig. 13-4. Topographical landmarks. **A,** Anterior thorax. **B,** Posterior thorax.

Continued.

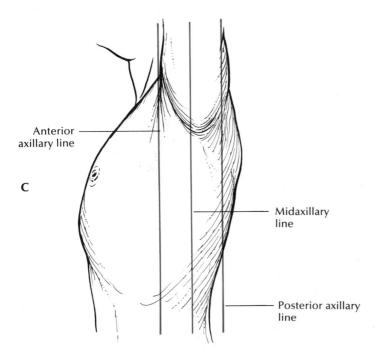

Anterior
axillary line

C

Midaxillary
line

Posterior axillary
line

Fig. 13-4, cont'd. C, Lateral thorax.

scribing the exact location of abnormalities (Fig. 13-4).

Manubriosternal junction (Louis's angle). The manubriosternal junction is an extremely useful aid in rib identification. It is a visible and palpable angulation of the sternum. The superior border of the second rib articulates with the sternum at the manubriosternal junction. The examiner can begin to palpate and count distal ribs and rib interspaces from this point. The intercostal spaces are numbered corresponding to the number of the rib immediately superior to the space. In palpation for rib identification, the examiner should palpate along the midclavicular line rather than at the sternal border because the rib cartilages are in very close proximity at the sternum, and the cartilages of only the first seven ribs attach directly to the sternum.

Suprasternal notch. The suprasternal notch is the depression above the manubrium.

Costal angle. The costal angle is the angle formed by the intersection of the costal margins.

Midsternal line. The midsternal line is an imaginary line drawn through the middle of the sternum.

Midclavicular lines. The midclavicular lines are left and right imaginary lines drawn through the midpoints of the clavicles and parallel to the midsternal line.

Anterior axillary lines. The anterior axillary lines are left and right imaginary lines drawn vertically from the anterior axillary folds, along the anterolateral chest, and parallel to the midsternal line.

Vertebra prominens (seventh cervical vertebra). When the client flexes his neck anteriorly and the posterior thorax is observed, a prominent spinous process can be observed and palpated. This is the spinous process of the seventh cervical vertebra. If two spinous processes are observed and palpated, the superior one is C7 and the inferior one is the spinous process of T1. The counting of ribs is more difficult on the posterior than on the anterior thorax. The spinous processes of the vertebrae can be counted relatively easily from C7 to T4. From T4 the spinous processes project obliquely, causing the spinous process of the vertebra not to lie over its correspondingly numbered rib, but over the rib below it. For example, the spinous process of T5 lies over the body of T6 and is adjacent to the sixth rib.

Midspinal line. The midspinal line is an imaginary line that runs vertically along the posterior spinous processes of the vertebrae.

Scapular lines. The scapular lines are left and right imaginary lines that lie vertically and are parallel to the midspinal line. They pass through the inferior angles of the scapulae when the client is erect and with arms at his sides.

Posterior axillary lines. The posterior axillary lines are the left and right imaginary lines drawn vertically from the posterior axillary folds along the posterolateral wall of the thorax when the lateral arm is abducted directly from the lateral chest wall.

Midaxillary lines. The midaxillary lines are the left and right imaginary lines drawn vertically from the apices of the axillae. They are approximately midway between the anterior and posterior axillary lines and parallel to them.

■ Underlying thoracic structures

When examining the respiratory system, the practitioner must maintain a mental image of the placement of organs and organ parts of the respiratory system and other systems sharing the thoracic area (Figs. 13-5 to 13-8).

Lung borders. In the anterior thorax, the apices of the lungs extend for approximately 1.5 inches above the clavicles. The inferior borders of the lungs cross the sixth ribs at the midclavicular line. In the posterior thorax, the apices extend to T1. The lower borders vary with respiration and usually extend from the spinous process of T10 on

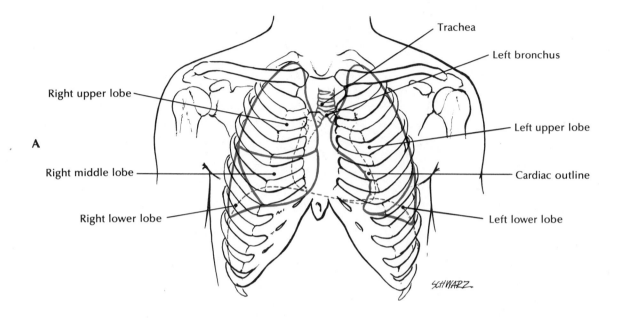

Trachea

Left bronchus

Right upper lobe

Left upper lobe

A

Right middle lobe

Cardiac outline

Right lower lobe

Left lower lobe

SCHWARZ

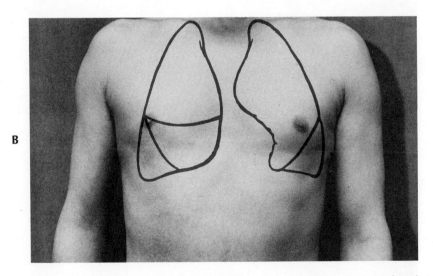

B

Fig. 13-5. Anterior thorax. **A,** Internal organs and structures. **B,** Lung borders.

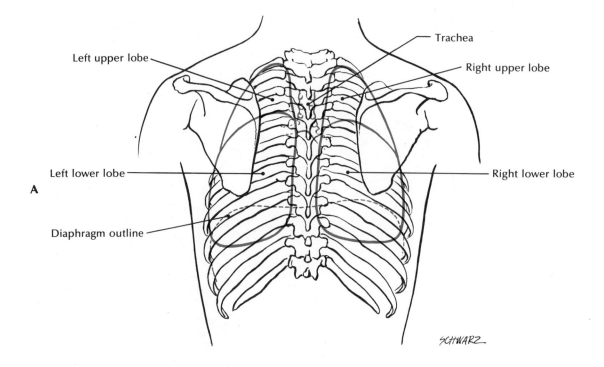

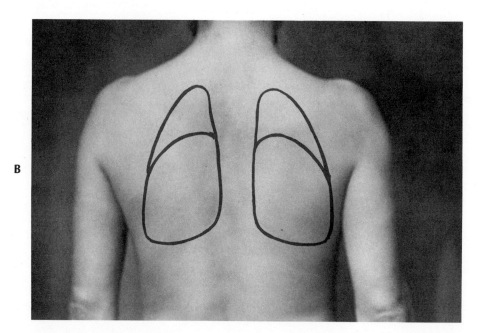

Fig. 13-6. Posterior thorax. **A,** Internal organs and structures. **B,** Lung borders.

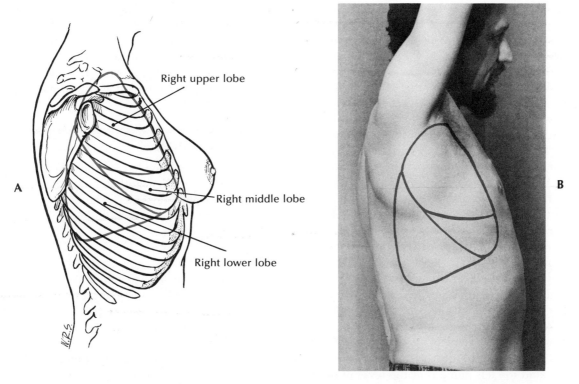

Fig. 13-7. Right lateral thorax. **A,** Internal organs and structures. **B,** Lung borders.

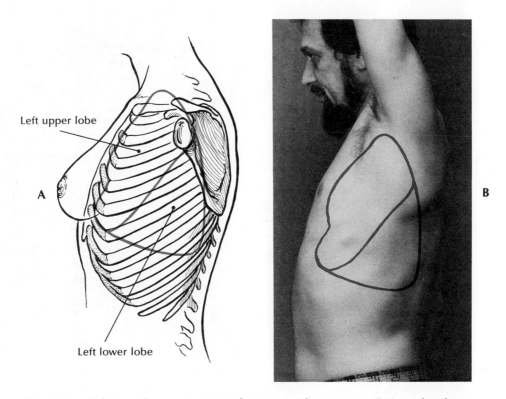

Fig. 13-8. Left lateral thorax. **A,** Internal organs and structures. **B,** Lung borders.

expiration to the spinous process of T12 on deep inspiration. In the lateral thorax, the lung extends from the apex of the axilla to the eighth rib of the midaxillary line.

Lung fissures. The right oblique (diagonal) fissure extends from the area of the spinous process of the third thoracic vertebra laterally and downward until it crosses the fifth rib at the right midaxillary line. It then continues anteriorly and medially to end at the sixth rib at the right and left midclavicular lines. The right horizontal fissure extends from the fifth rib slightly posterior to the right midaxillary line and runs horizontally to the area of the fourth rib at the right sternal border. The left oblique (diagonal) fissure extends from the spinous process of the third thoracic vertebra laterally and downward to the left midaxillary line at the fifth rib and continues anteriorly and medially until it terminates at the sixth rib in the left midclavicular line.

Border of the diaphragm. Anteriorly, on expiration, the right dome of the diaphragm is located at the level of the fifth rib at the midclavicular line and the left dome is at the level of the sixth rib. Posteriorly, on expiration, the diaphragm is at the level of the spinous process of T10; laterally, it is at the eighth rib at the midaxillary line.

Trachea. The bifurcation of the trachea occurs approximately just below the manubriosternal junction anteriorly and at the spinous process of T4 posteriorly.

EXAMINATION

Equipment needed for the respiratory system examination are a stethoscope, a marking pencil, and a centimeter ruler. The examination should be performed in a well-illuminated area that allows for privacy.

■ Inspection

For adequate inspection of the thorax, the client should be sitting upright, without support and uncovered to the waist. It is essential that the room lighting be adequate and that there be available a mechanism for supplementary lighting, used in the close inspection of small areas. It is critical that the client be warm and not ob-

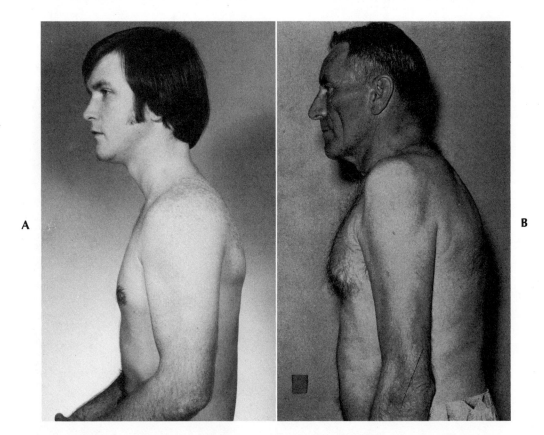

Fig. 13-9. A, Anteroposterior diameter of a normal subject. **B,** Subject with increased anteroposterior diameter. (From Prior, J. A., and Silberstein, J. S.: Physical diagnosis; the history and examination of the patient, ed. 5, St. Louis, 1977, The C. V. Mosby Co.)

served by persons extraneous to the examination. The examiner first observes the general shape of the thorax and its symmetry. Although no individual is absolutely symmetrical in both body hemispheres, most individuals are reasonably similar side to side. Using the client as his own control whenever paired parts are examined is an excellent habit and will often yield significant findings.

Thoracic configuration. The anteroposterior diameter of the thorax in the normal adult is less than the transverse diameter at approximately a ratio of 1:2 to 5:7 (Fig. 13-9). In the normal infant, in some adults with pulmonary disease, or in aged adults the thorax is approximately round. This condition is called barrel chest. Other observed abnormalities of thoracic shape might include:

1. Retraction of the thorax. The retraction is unilateral, or of one side.
2. Pigeon or chicken chest (pectus carinatum), sternal protrusion anteriorly. The anteroposterior diameter of the chest is increased,

and the resultant configuration resembles the thorax of a fowl.

3. Funnel chest (pectus excavatum), depression of part or all of the sternum. If the depression is deep, it may interfere with both respiratory and cardiac function.
4. Spinal deformities. While the client is uncovered and the examiner is behind him, the spine should be examined for deformities. (See Chapter 18 on Musculoskeletal assessment for the specific techniques of spinal examination.)

The approach to the physical examination is a regional and integrated one. The examination of systems is combined in body regions when appropriate. Since the client is uncovered to the waist during the examination, a large portion of the skin and tissue is accessible to inspection. The observation of the skin and underlying tissue provides the examiner with knowledge of the general nutrition of the patient. Common thoracic skin findings are the spider nevi associated with cirrhosis and seborrheic derma-

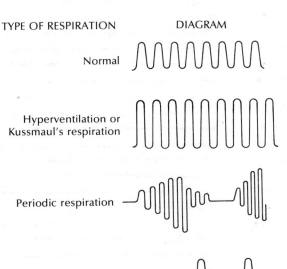

TYPE OF RESPIRATION	DIAGRAM	DISCUSSION
Normal		16-20/min; regular in rhythm; ratio of respiratory rate to pulse rate is 1:4
Hyperventilation or Kussmaul's respiration		Increase in both rate and depth; hyperpnea is an increase in depth only
Periodic respiration		Alternating hyperpnea, shallow respiration and apnea; sometimes called Cheyne-Stokes breathing; frequently occurs in the severely ill
Sighing respiration		Deep and audible; audible portion sounds like a sigh
Air trapping		Present in obstructive pulmonary diseases; air is trapped in the lungs; respiratory level rises, and breathing becomes shallow
Biot's breathing		Shallow breathing interrupted by apnea; seen in some CNS disorders and in healthy persons

Fig. 13-10. Characteristics of commonly observed respiratory patterns.

titis. (See Chapter 9 on Assessment of the skin.)

Ribs and interspaces. The reaction of interspaces on inspiration may be indicative of some obstruction of free air inflow. Bulging of interspaces on expiration occurs when there is obstruction to air outflow or may be the result of tumor, aneurysm, or cardiac enlargement. Normally the costal angle is less than 90°, and the ribs are inserted into the spine at about a 45° angle (Fig. 13-1). In clients with obstructive lung diseases these angles are widened.

Pattern of respiration. Normally men and children breathe diaphragmatically, and women breathe thoracically or costally. A change in this pattern might be significant. If the client appears to have labored respiration, the examiner observes for the use of the accessory muscles of respiration—the sternocleidomastoid and trapezius muscles—and for supraclavicular retraction. Impedance to air inflow is often accompanied by retraction of intercostal spaces during inspiration. An excessively long expiratory phase of respiration accompanies outflow impedance.

The normal respiratory rate is 16 to 21 breaths per minute and is regular. The ratio of respiratory rate to pulse rate normally is 1:4. Tachypnea is an adult respiratory rate of over 20 breaths per minute; bradypnea is an adult respiratory rate of less than 10 breaths per minute.

There are many abnormal patterns of respiration. Some of the commonly seen patterns are outlined in Fig. 13-10. Dyspnea is a subjective phenomenon of inadequate or distressful respiration.

Lips and nails. Inspection in the respiratory system examination includes observation of lips and nail beds for color and observation of the nails for clubbing. These phenomena are discussed in Chapter 7 on General assessment and in Chapter 14 on Cardiovascular assessment: the heart and the neck vessels.

■ Palpation

Palpation is performed in order to (1) further assess abnormalities suggested by the history or observation, such as tenderness, pulsations, masses, or skin lesions; (2) assess the skin and subcutaneous structures; (3) assess the thoracic expansion; (4) assess vocal (tactile) fremitus; and (5) assess the tracheal position.

General palpation. The examiner should specifically palpate any areas of abnormality. The temperature and turgor of the skin should be generally assessed. The examiner then palpates

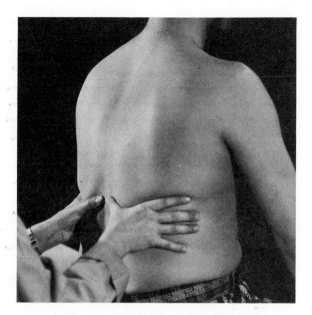

Fig. 13-11. Palpation for thoracic excursion.

the muscle mass and the thoracic skeleton. If the client has no complaints in relation to the respiratory system, a rapid, general survey of anterior, lateral, and posterior thoracic areas is sufficient. If the client does have complaints, all chest areas should be meticulously palpated for tenderness, bulges, or abnormal movements.

Assessment of thoracic expansion (Fig. 13-11). The degree of thoracic expansion can be assessed from the anterior or posterior chest. Anteriorly, the examiner's hands are placed over the anterolateral chest with the thumbs extended along the costal margin, pointing to the xiphoid process. Posteriorly, the thumbs are placed at the level of the tenth rib and the palms are placed on the posterolateral chest. The examiner feels the amount of the thoracic expansion during quiet and deep respiration and observes for divergence of the thumbs on expiration. There should be symmetry of respiration between the left and right hemithoraces.

Assessment of fremitus. Fremitus is vibration perceptible on palpation. Vocal or tactile fremitus is palpable vibration of the thoracic wall, produced by phonation.

The client is asked to repeat "one, two, three" or "ninety-nine" while the examiner systematically palpates the thorax (Fig. 13-12). The examiner can use the palmer bases of the fingers, the ulnar aspect of the hand, or the ulnar aspect of the closed fist. If one hand is used, it should be moved from one side of the chest to the corresponding area on the other side. If two hands are

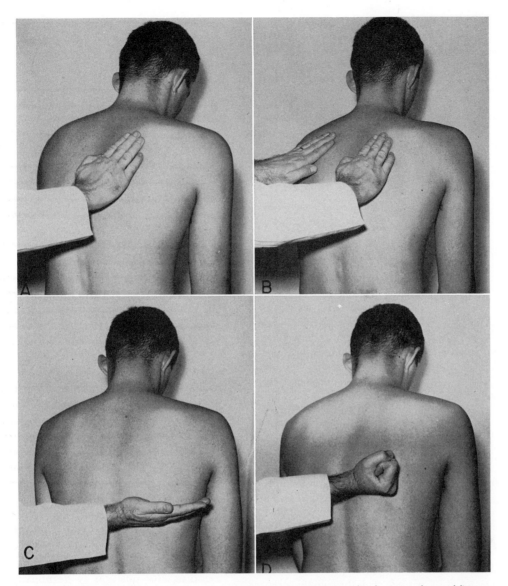

Fig. 13-12. Palpation for assessment of vocal fremitus. **A,** Use of palmar surface of fingertips. **B,** Simultaneous application of the fingertips of both hands. **C,** Use of ulnar aspect of the hand. **D,** Use of ulnar aspect of the closed fist. (From Prior, J. A., and Silberstein, J. S.: Physical diagnosis; the history and examination of the patient, ed. 4, St. Louis, 1973, The C. V. Mosby Co.)

used for examination, they should be simultaneously placed on the corresponding areas of each thoracic side. Types of fremitus are outlined in Table 13-1.

Whenever the practitioner examines the thorax, he must be mindful of the fact that there are four parts for examination: the posterior chest, the anterior chest, the right and left lateral thoracic areas, and the apices. The examiner should move from the area of one hemisphere to the matching corresponding area on the other (right to left, left to right) until all four major parts

are surveyed. During palpation for assessing fremitus and all subsequent procedures for the examination of the respiratory system, all areas must be meticulously and systematically examined. Usually the apices, posterior chest, and lateral areas can be examined with the practitioner standing behind the client.

Assessment of tracheal deviation. The trachea should be assessed by palpation for any deviation. The examiner places a finger on the trachea in the suprasternal notch. He then moves his finger laterally left and right in the spaces between the

Table 13-1. Characteristics of normal and abnormal tactile fremitus

Type of fremitus	Discussion of characteristics
Normal fremitus	Varies greatly from person to person and is dependent on the intensity and pitch of the voice, the position and distance of the bronchi in relation to the chest wall, and the thickness of the chest wall. Fremitus is most intense in the second intercostal spaces at the sternal border near the area of bronchial bifurcation.
Increased vocal fremitus	May occur in pneumonia, compressed lung, lung tumor, or pulmonary fibrosis. (A solid medium of uniform structure conducts vibrations with greater intensity than a porous medium.)
Decreased or absent vocal fremitus	Occurs when there is a diminished production of sounds, a diminished transmission of sounds, or the addition of a medium through which sounds must pass before reaching the thoracic wall as, for example, in pleural effusion, pleural thickening, pneumothorax, bronchial obstruction, or emphysema.
Pleural friction rub	Vibration produced by inflamed pleural surfaces rubbing together. It is felt as a grating, is synchronous with respiratory movements, and is more commonly felt on inspiration.
Rhonchal fremitus	Coarse vibrations produced by the passage of air through thick exudates in the large air passages. These can be cleared or altered by coughing.

clavicle, the inner aspect of the sternocleidomastoid muscle, and the trachea. These spaces should be equal on both sides. In diseases such as atelectasis and pulmonary fibrosis the trachea may be deviated toward the abnormal side. The trachea may be deviated toward the normal side in conditions such as neck tumors, thyroid enlargement, enlarged lymph nodes, pleural effusion, unilateral emphysema, and pneumothorax.

Crepitations. In subcutaneous emphysema, the subcutaneous tissue contains fine beads of air. As this tissue is palpated, audible crackling sounds are heard. These sounds are termed crepitations.

■ Percussion

Percussion is the tapping of an object in order to set underlying structures in motion and consequently to produce a sound called a percussion note and a palpable vibration. Percussion penetrates to a depth of approximately 5 to 7 cm. Percussion is utilized in the thoracic examination to determine the relative amounts of air, liquid, or solid material in the underlying lung and to determine the positions and boundaries of organs.

Two techniques of percussion are immediate, or direct, percussion and mediate, or indirect, percussion. In *immediate, or direct, percussion,* the examiner strikes the object to be percussed directly with the palmar aspect of two, three, or four fingers held together or with the palmar aspect of the tip of the middle finger. The strikes are rapid and downward; movement of the hand from the wrist is in rapid strokes. This type of percussion is not normally utilized in thoracic examination. It is useful in the examination of the thorax in the infant and the sinuses in the adult. *Mediate, or indirect, percussion* is the striking of an object held against the area to be examined (Fig. 13-13). The middle finger of the examiner's left hand (if the examiner is right handed) is the pleximeter. The distal phalanx and joint are placed firmly on the surface to be percussed. The other parts of the hand are held off of the skin. The plexor is the index finger of the examiner's right hand or the index and middle fingers held together. Its position is demonstrated in Fig. 13-13.

With the forearm and shoulder stationary and all movement at the wrist, the pleximeter is struck sharply with the plexor. The blow is aimed at the distal interphalangeal joint, and the plexor is immediately withdrawn. The plexor strikes with the tip of the finger at right angles to the pleximeter. One or two rapid blows are struck in each area. Bony areas are avoided; interspaces are used for percussion. The examiner compares one side of the thorax with the other.

With experience and study the practitioner will be able to differentiate among the five percussion tones commonly elicited on the human body. In the study of tones, the determination of four characteristics will assist in assessment and labeling:

1. *Intensity (amplitude):* The loudness or softness of the tone.
2. *Pitch (frequency):* Relates to the number of

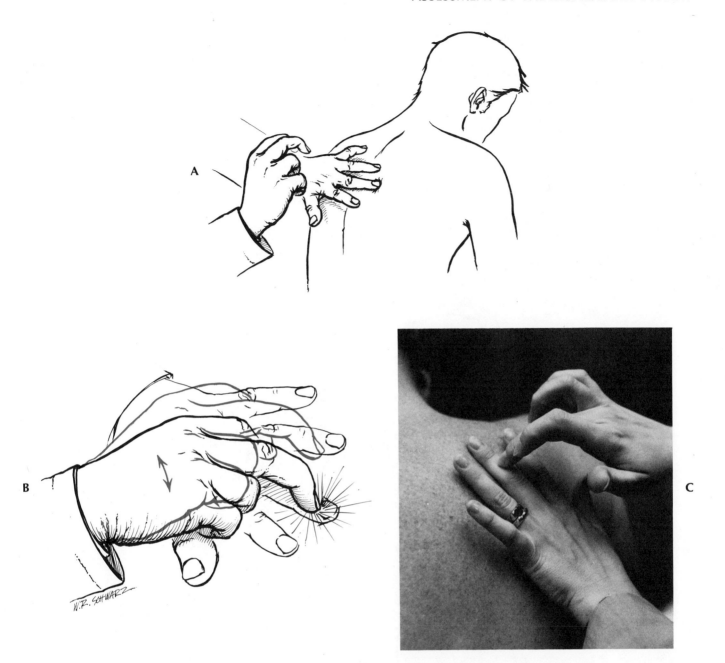

Fig. 13-13. Percussion. **A,** Positioning of the hands. **B,** Hand movement. **C,** Percussion of the posterior thorax.

vibrations per second. Rapid vibrations produce high-pitched tones; slow vibrations produce low-pitched tones. The greater the density of an object, the higher the frequency.

3. *Quality:* A subjective phenomena relating to the innate characteristics of the object being percussed.

4. *Duration:* The amount of time a note is sustained.

Table 13-2 describes the commonly used de-scriptive terms for percussion tones elicited by physical examination.

Fig. 13-14 is a percussion map for the normal chest.

The following is the procedure for thoracic percussion:

1. Percuss the apices to determine if the normal 5-cm area of resonance is present between the neck and shoulder muscles (Fig. 13-14).

2. Position the client with his head bent and

Table 13-2. Description of percussion notes

Note	Intensity	Pitch	Duration	Quality	Normal location
Resonance	Moderate to loud	Low	Long	Hollow	Peripheral lung
Hyperresonance	Very loud	Very low	Very long	Booming	Child's lung
Tympany	Loud	High	Moderate	Musical, drumlike	Air-filled stomach
Dullness	Soft	High	Moderate	Thud like	Liver
Flatness	Soft	High	Short	Extreme dullness	Thigh

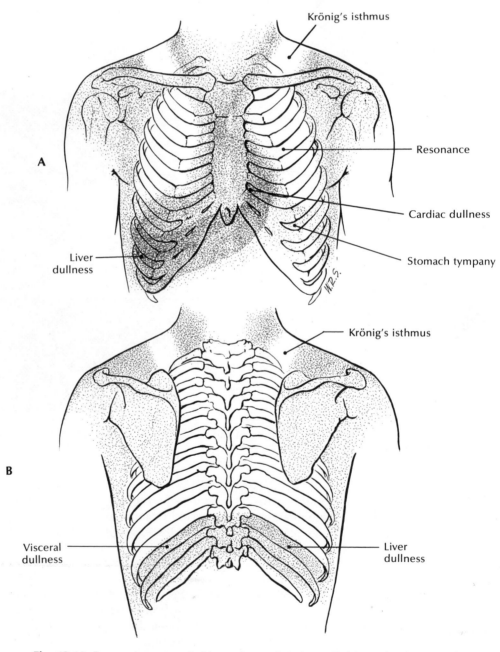

Fig. 13-14. Percussion area. **A,** Normal anterior chest. **B,** Normal posterior chest.

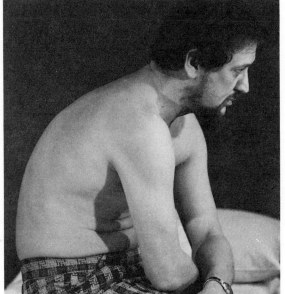

Fig. 13-15. Position of client for examination of the posterior thorax.

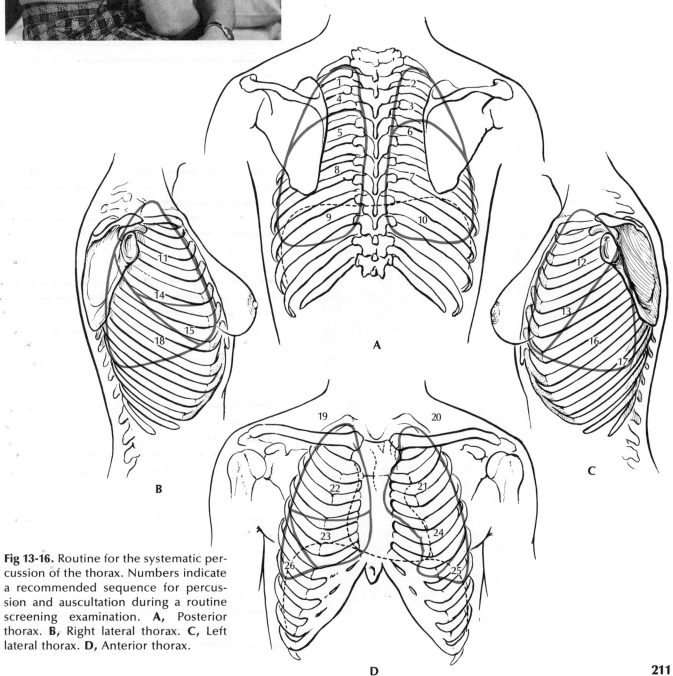

Fig 13-16. Routine for the systematic percussion of the thorax. Numbers indicate a recommended sequence for percussion and auscultation during a routine screening examination. **A,** Posterior thorax. **B,** Right lateral thorax. **C,** Left lateral thorax. **D,** Anterior thorax.

his arm folded over his chest (Fig. 13-15). With this maneuver, the scapulae move laterally and more lung area is accessible to examination.

3. On the posterior chest percuss systematically at about every 5-cm intervals from the upper to lower chest, moving left to right, right to left, and avoiding scapular and other bony areas; percuss the lateral chest with the client's arms positioned over his head (Fig. 13-16).

4. Measure the diaphragmatic excursion. Instruct the client to inhale deeply and hold his breath in. Percuss along the scapular line on each side until the lower edge of the lung is identified. Sound will change from resonance to dullness. Mark the point of change on each side at the scapular line. Then instruct the client to take a few normal respirations. Next, instruct the client to exhale completely and hold his expiration. Proceed to percuss up from the marked point at the midscapular line to determine the diaphragmatic excursion in deep expiration. Measure and record the distance between the upper and lower points in cen-

timeters. The diaphragm is usually slightly higher on the right side and excursion is normally 3 to 5 cm. Diaphragmatic excursion is usually measured only on the posterior chest (Fig. 13-17).

In the actual examination, the practitioner would complete the examination of the apices and the posterior and lateral chest and would then percuss the anterior chest.

■ Auscultation

Through auscultation, the practitioner obtains information about the functioning of the respiratory system and about the presence of any obstruction in the passages. Auscultation of the lungs is accomplished by the use of a stethoscope. The diaphragm of the stethoscope is usually used for the thoracic examination because it covers a larger surface than the bell. The stethoscope is placed firmly on the skin. Client or stethoscope movement are avoided because movements of muscle under the skin or movements of the stethoscope over hair will produce confusing extrinsic sounds.

Before beginning auscultation, the examiner should instruct the client to breathe through his mouth and more deeply and slowly than in usual respiration. The examiner systematically auscultates the apices and the posterior, lateral, and anterior chest (Fig. 13-16). At each application of the stethoscope, the examiner listens to at least one complete respiration. The examiner should observe the client for signs of hyperventilation and stop the procedure if the client becomes light-headed or faint. The process of auscultation includes (1) the analysis of breath sounds, (2) the detection of any abnormal sounds, and (3) the examination of the sounds produced by the spoken voice.

Breath sounds. Breath sounds are the sounds produced by the movement of air through the tracheobronchoalveolar system. These sounds are analyzed according to pitch, intensity, quality, and relative duration of inspiratory and expiratory phases. Table 13-3 outlines the types of sounds heard over the normal and abnormal lung.

Absent or decreased breath sounds can occur in (1) any condition that causes the deposition of foreign matter in the pleural space, (2) bronchial obstruction, (3) emphysema, or (4) shallow breathing.

Increased breath sounds can occur in any condition that causes a consolidation of lung tissue.

Abnormal or adventitious sounds. Adventitious sounds are not alterations in breath sounds

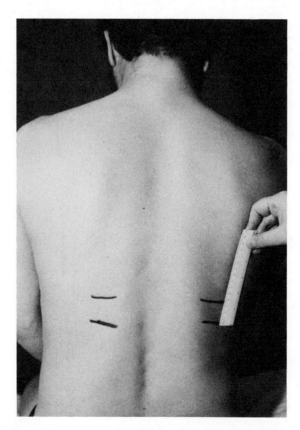

Fig. 13-17. Assessment of diaphragmatic excursion.

Table 13-3. Characteristics of breath sounds

Sound	Duration of inspiration and expiration	Diagram of sound	Pitch	Intensity	Normal location	Abnormal location
Vesicular	Inspiration > expiration 5:2		Low	Soft	Peripheral lung	Not applicable
Broncho-vesicular	Inspiration = expiration 1:1		Moderate	Moderate	First and second intercostal spaces at the sternal border over major bronchi	Peripheral lung
Bronchial (tubular)	Inspiration < expiration		High	Loud	Over trachea	Lung area

Table 13-4. Origin and characteristics of adventitious sounds

Sound	Origin	Characteristics
Rales—fine to medium	Air passing through moisture in small air passages and alveoli	Discrete, noncontinuous; inspiratory; have a dry or wet crackling quality; not cleared by coughing; sound is simulated by rolling a lock of hair near the ear
Rales—medium to course	Air passing through moisture in the broncioles, bronchi, and trachea	As above; louder than fine rales
Ronchi-sibilant (wheezes)	Air passing through air passages narrowed by secretions, swelling, tumors, and so on	Continuous sounds; originate in the small air passages; may be inspiratory and expiratory but usually predominate in expiration; high-pitched, wheezing sounds
Ronchi-sonorous	Same as wheezes	Continuous sounds; originate in large air passages; may be inspiratory and expiratory but usually predominate in expiration; low-pitched, moaning or snoring quality; coughing may alter sounds
Friction rubs	Rubbing together of inflamed and roughened pleural surfaces	Creaking or grating quality; superficial sounding; inspiratory and expiratory; heard most often in the lower anterolateral chest (area of greatest thoracic expansion); coughing has no effect

but sounds superimposed on breath sounds. Classification of these sounds varies among authorities; consequently, nomenclatures are arbitrary. Commonly utilized terms for adventitious sounds are described in Table 13-4.

If the client has rales, the examiner listens for several respirations in the areas in which the rales are heard to determine the effects of deep breathing. Also, the client is asked to cough, and the changes in adventitious sounds are noted after coughing.

If the client has complained of respiratory difficulty and no adventitious sounds are heard, he is asked to cough; often, adventitious sounds are noted in post-tussive breathing.

Voice sounds. Vocal resonance is produced by the same mechanism that produces vocal fremitus. It is transmitted voice sounds as heard by the stethoscope on the chest wall. Normal vocal resonance is heard as muffled, nondistinct sounds; it is loudest medially and is less intense at the periphery of the lung. Vocal resonance is assessed if there has been any respiratory abnormality detected on observation, palpation, percussion, or auscultation. The routine utilized is the same systematic one that has been previously utilized in the respiratory examination. The client says "one, two, three" or "ninety-nine" while the examiner surveys the thorax.

The increase in loudness and clarity of vocal

resonance is termed bronchophony. Special vocal resonance techniques are used when resonance is increased. These include tests for whispered pectoriloquy and egophony.

Whispered pectoriloquy is exaggerated bronchophony. The client is instructed to whisper a series of words. The words as heard through the stethoscope on the chest wall are distinct and understandable.

In *egophony*, the intensity of the spoken voice, as heard through the stethoscope applied to the chest wall, is increased and the voice has a nasal or bleating quality. If the client says "e- e- e," the transmitted sound will be "a- a- a."

Decreased vocal resonance occurs in the same clinical situations as the ones in which vocal fremitus is decreased and breath sounds are absent. Vocal resonance is increased and whispered pectoriloquy and egophony may be present in any condition that causes a consolidation of lung tissue.

■ **Respiratory distress syndrome**

Despite the heavy reliance on laboratory and x-ray findings in the diagnosis of respiratory prob-

lems, the examiner can derive reasonably sound diagnostic probabilities by compiling and analyzing the physical assessment data. Table 13-5 outlines the usual assessment findings in a variety of common problems.

SUMMARY

The following is an outline for the performance of a respiratory system screening examination:

I. Observation
   A. Thoracic configuration
      1. Anteroposterior diameter
      2. Skin and subcutaneous tissue
   B. Ribs and interspaces
   C. Respiratory pattern
      1. Accessory muscles of respiration
      2. Oxygenation
      3. Respiratory rate
II. Palpation
   A. General palpation
      1. Areas of observed abnormality
      2. Tissue and bony structures
   B. Assessment of thoracic expansion

Table 13-5. Assessment findings frequently associated with common lung conditions

Condition	General inspection and palpation	Vocal fremitus	Percussion	Voice sounds	Breath sounds	Other
Consolidation	Guarding, less motion on affected side; palpable limitation of expansion	Increased	Dull to flat	Increased intensity, bronchophony, whispered pectoriloquy	Increased intensity; bronchial or bronchovesicular sounds	Medium to coarse inspiratory rales; friction rub common
Pneumothorax	Tracheal shift; less respiratory motion	Decreased or absent	Hyperresonant	Diminished intensity	Diminished or absent	
Emphysema	Barrel chest; ribs horizontal, increased anteroposterior diameter	Normal or decreased	Resonant to hyperresonant; diaphragm low and motion decreased	Normal or diminished	Diminished intensity	Sibilant rhonchi; prolonged expiration
Pleural effusion	Less definition of intercostal spaces on affected side; decreased excursion unilaterally	Decreased or absent	Flat to dull	Diminished or absent	Diminished intensity	Usually no adventitious sounds
Atelectasis	Tracheal shift; less motion on affected side	Usually absent	Dull to flat over consolidated area; hyperresonance over remainder of hemithorax	Variable intensity	Absent or diminished intensity; bronchial breathing may be present	Transient fine rales
Congestive failure without effusion	Not remarkable	Normal	Normal	Normal	Normal	Fine to medium rales, usually at lung bases
Acute bronchitis	Normal	Normal	Normal	Normal	Normal	Localized rales, rhonchi, wheezes

C. Assessment of tactile fremitus
D. Assessment of tracheal deviation
III. Percussion
    A. Systematic survey
        1. Apices
        2. Lateral chest
        3. Posterior chest
        4. Anterior chest
    B. Diaphragmatic excursion
IV. Auscultation
    A. Systematic survey (same as for percussion)
    B. Analysis of breath sounds
    C. Identification of adventitious sounds
    D. Vocal resonance (assessed if tactile fremitus or breath sounds are increased)
        1. Test for whisper pectoriloquy
        2. Test for egophony

BIBLIOGRAPHY

Burrows, B., Knudson, R. J., and Kettel, L. J.: Respiratory insufficiency, Chicago, 1975, Yearbook Medical Publishers, Inc.

Druger, G.: The chest; its signs and sounds, Los Angeles, 1973, Humetrics Corp.

Geschickter, C. F.: The lung in health and disease, Philadelphia, 1973, J. B. Lippincott Co.

Holman, C. W., and Muschenheim, C.: Bronchopulmonary diseases and related disorders, vols. 1 and 2, Hagerstown, Md., 1972, Harper & Row, Publishers.

Kao, F.: An introduction to respiratory physiology, ed. 2, Amsterdam, Excerpta medica, 1972.

Slonim, N. B., and Hamilton, L. H.: Respiratory physiology, ed. 2, St. Louis, 1971, The C. V. Mosby Co.

14 Cardiovascular assessment: the heart and the neck vessels

This chapter covers those portions of the cardiovascular examination dealing with examination of the heart and the major neck vessels—the jugular veins and the carotid arteries. A brief review of the anatomy and physiology of the heart precedes the description of examination techniques and findings. Assessment of the peripheral pulses and blood pressure measurement, also integral components of the cardiovascular examination, are described in Chapter 7 on General assessment.

The heart

ANATOMY AND PHYSIOLOGY

In the examination of the heart and the subsequent description of findings, several anterior chest wall landmarks are important. These include the midsternal line; the midclavicular line; the anterior, middle, and posterior axillary lines; the suprasternal notch; and the ribs and intercostal spaces. The area of the chest overlying the heart and pericardium is known as the precordium. These landmarks are illustrated in Fig. 14-1.

The heart lies in the thoracic cavity within the mediastinum. The upper portion, consisting of both atria, lies at the top behind the upper portion of the body of the sternum; the lower portion, composed of both ventricles, is directed downward and toward the left. The upper portion is referred to as the base of the heart, and the lower left portion is referred to as the apex. The aorta, pulmonary arteries, and great veins are located around the upper portion, or base, of the heart.

■ Heart chambers

Most of the anterior cardiac surface consists of the right ventricle, which lies behind the sternum and extends to the left of it. The left ventricle lies posterior to the right ventricle and extends further to the left, thus forming the left border of the heart and making up a small portion of the anterior cardiac surface. The right atrium lies slightly above and to the right of the right ventricle, and the left atrium occupies a posterior portion of the heart (Fig. 14-2). It is the contraction and thrust of the left ventricle that produces the normal apical impulse, sometimes referred to as the point of maximum impulse, that is located at or just medial to the midclavicular line in the fifth left intercostal space.

■ Heart valves

The atrioventricular (AV) valves lie between the atria and ventricles; the right AV valve is the tricuspid valve, and the left is the mitral valve. The semilunar valves separate the ventricles from the great vessels, the aorta, and the pulmonary artery. On the right the pulmonic valve separates the right ventricle from the pulmonary artery, and on the left the aortic valve separates the left ventricle from the aorta. It is basically the closure of the heart valves that produces the normal heart sounds. (There is much discussion as to the actual mechanism of heart sound production; it is thought that tensing of the muscular structures and flow of blood may be involved, as well as valve closure.)

Although the four valves are actually located rather close to each other in a small area behind the sternum, the areas on the chest wall where their closure is best heard are not located directly over the valves (Fig. 14-3). The sound produced

216

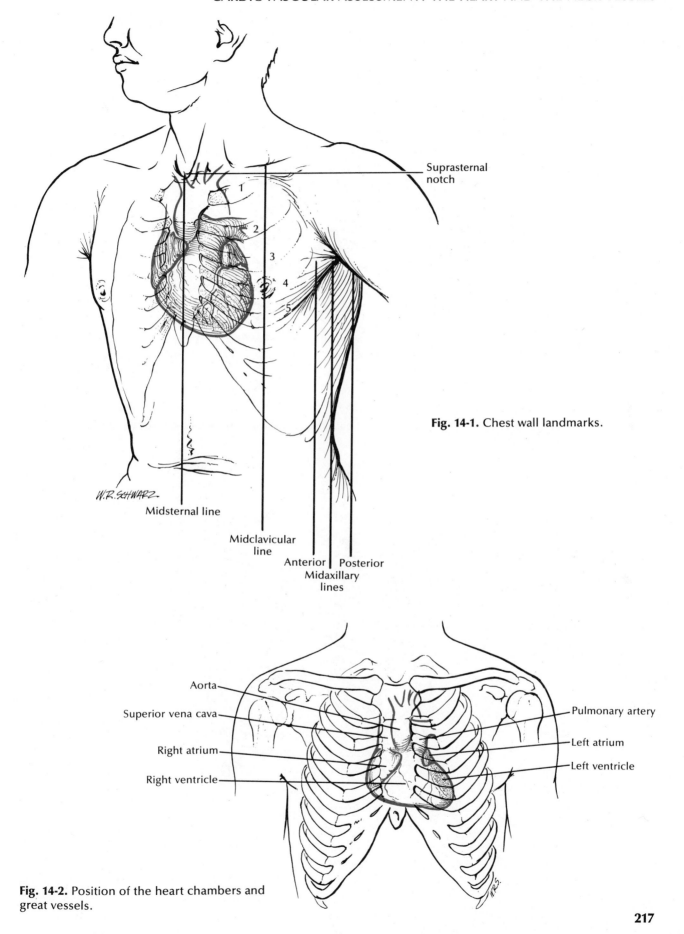

Fig. 14-1. Chest wall landmarks.

Suprasternal notch

Midsternal line

Midclavicular line

Anterior | Posterior
Midaxillary lines

Aorta

Superior vena cava

Right atrium

Right ventricle

Pulmonary artery

Left atrium

Left ventricle

Fig. 14-2. Position of the heart chambers and great vessels.

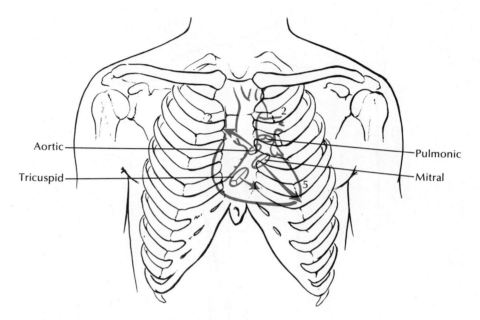

Fig. 14-3. Anatomical location of the heart valves and transmission of sounds produced by valve closure.

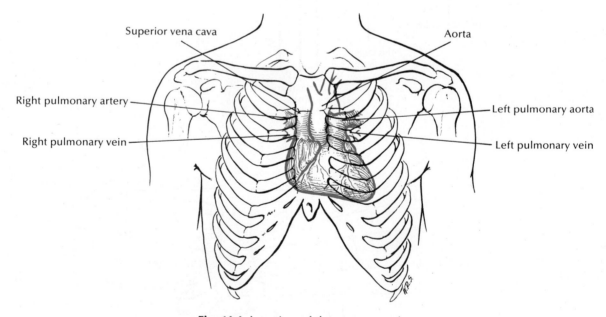

Fig. 14-4. Location of the great vessels.

by closure of the mitral valve is best heard at the apex, at the fifth left intercostal space in the midclavicular line; the sound produced by closure of the tricuspid valve is best heard along the lower left sternal border at the fourth left intercostal space; the sound produced by the aortic valve is heard best at the second right intercostal space at the sternal border; and the sound produced by the pulmonic valve is best heard at the second left intercostal space at the sternal border. The auscultatory valve areas can be summarized as follows:

Mitral valve: Fifth LICS at MCL.
Tricuspid valve: Fourth LICS at LSB.
Aortic valve: Second RICS at SB.
Pulmonic valve: Second LICS at SB.

■ The great vessels

As mentioned earlier, the great vessels lie at the top, or base, of the heart. The pulmonary artery extending from the right ventricle bifurcates quickly into its left and right branches. The aorta, extending from the left ventricle, curves upward over the heart, then backward and down. The superior and inferior vena cava empty into the right atrium, and the pulmonary veins return blood to the left atrium. The relationship of these vessels to the heart chambers is shown in Fig. 14-4.

■ Pericardium

The pericardium is a tough, double-walled, fibrous sac encasing and protecting the heart. Several cubic centimeters of fluid are present between the inner and outer layers of the pericardium, providing for easy, low-friction movement. The outer layer of the pericardium is firmly attached to the diaphragm, sternum, pleura, esophagus, and aorta.

■ Variable position of the heart

The position of the heart in the thorax has a large range of normal and varies considerably with different body builds, chest configurations, and diaphragm levels. In an average-size person, the heart lies obliquely; one third of it lies to the right of the midsternal line, and two thirds of it lies to the left of it. In short, stocky persons the heart may tend to lie more horizontally; in tall, slender persons it may hang more vertically.

■ Cycle of cardiac events

The flow of blood, movements of the chambers and valves, pressure relationships, and electrical stimulation are discussed here briefly.

The cardiac cycle may be said to begin with the return of blood from the systemic circulation via the superior and inferior vena cavae to the right atrium and with the return of oxygenated blood from the lungs via the pulmonary veins to the left atrium. Following ventricular systole, during which blood has been ejected from the ventricles, the AV valves open, allowing blood that has been collected in the atria to flow into the ventricle. Toward the end of this passive filling phase, or ventricular diastole, the atria contract, ejecting the remaining blood into the ventricles. Then ventricular contraction begins. As intraventricular pressure increases, the AV valves are forced closed, preventing regurgitation of blood to the atria and producing the first heart sound (S_1). During the early part of contraction, the volume of blood in the ventricle remains the same; this is called the period of isovolumic contraction. As the pressure continues to rise during ventricular contraction, a point is reached when the pressure in the left ventricle exceeds the pressure in the aorta; the semilunar valves are forced open, and blood is ejected into the aorta. (Events on the left side of the heart are used for describing the cycle. Right-sided events are similar but occur at much lower pressures.)

At the end of ejection, the ventricle relaxes, the pressure in the ventricle drops below the pressure in the aorta, and the semilunar valves snap shut, producing the second heart sound (S_2). Meanwhile, during ventricular systole the atria have been filling; as the ventricular pressure drops, the AV valves open, permitting the flow of blood into the ventricles once again. Because of the manner in which myocardial depolarization occurs, events on the left side of the heart normally occur slightly before events on the right side. Therefore, in the production of S_1, mitral valve closure briefly precedes tricuspid valve closure. Similarly, in the production of S_2, aortic valve closure precedes pulmonic valve closure. The pressure relationships and points of valve closure are illustrated in Fig. 14-5.

Normally, ventricular systole, the contraction phase, is slightly shorter than ventricular diastole, the relaxation or filling phase. At heart rates of about 120 per minute, the phases become nearly equal in length.

The electrical events stimulating and coordinating the mechanical events just described begin with an electrical discharge originating at the sinoatrial (SA) node, located in the right atrium. This electrical discharge then flows through the atria, producing atrial contraction. The impulse then travels to the AV node, located in the low

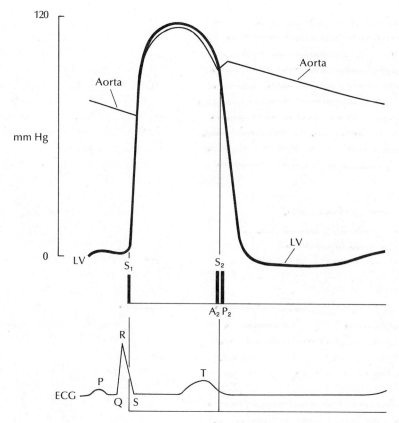

Fig. 14-5. Pressure curves of the left ventricle and aorta, S₁ and S₂, and the ECG.

atrial septum, and on through the bundle of His and its branches in the myocardium, stimulating ventricular contraction. The SA node is the cardiac pacemaker, normally discharging between 60 and 100 impulses per minute. The passage of the electrical impulses is shown in the electrocardiogram (ECG) tracing below the pressure diagram in Fig. 14-5. The P wave represents spread of the impulse through the atria; the QRS complex represents spread of the impulse through the ventricles; and the T wave represents repolarization of the ventricles. Electrical stimulation briefly precedes the mechanical response.

■ Characteristics of cardiovascular sounds

All sounds, including those of cardiovascular origin, can be characterized by their frequency (pitch), intensity (loudness), duration, and their timing in the cardiac cycle. All cardiovascular sounds are of relatively low frequency and require special concentration for perception by the human ear. Examples of heart sounds in the lower frequencies include the diastolic murmur of mitral stenosis and a third heart sound (S₃); the

normal S₂ is of a slightly higher frequency, and the diastolic murmur of aortic or pulmonic valve insufficiency is of yet a higher frequency.

The intensity of cardiovascular sounds is widely variable. The range extends from sounds that can be heard only with great concentration and by careful "tuning in" to those that can be heard with the edge of the stethoscope not touching the chest wall.

The duration of most cardiovascular sounds is very brief, usually much less than 1 second. In cardiac auscultation, both the duration of sounds and the periods of silence are important. Normally, S₁ and S₂ are very brief, lasting only fractions of a second; the intervals of silence, that is, systole and diastole, are longer. Diastole is longer than systole at a heart rate below 120 per minute; at faster rates the duration of diastole is diminished, and systole and diastole become about equal in duration.

The timing of any additional cardiac sounds is designated as occurring during either systole or diastole. Systole begins with S₁ and extends to S₂; diastole begins with S₂ and extends to the next S₁. A helpful method for determining S₁ and S₂ and

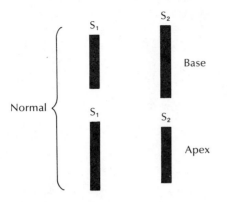

Fig. 14-6. Relative loudness of S_1 and S_2 as heard over the base and apex of the heart.

thus differentiating systole and diastole is to palpate the carotid pulse while auscultating the heart. The carotid pulsation and S_1 are very nearly synchronous; S_1 only briefly precedes the carotid impulse.

Heart sounds are illustrated by vertical bars on a horizontal line. The height of the bar indicates the relative loudness of the sound, and the width of the bar indicates the duration. For example, S_1 and S_2 as heard at the base and apex of the heart are illustrated as shown in Fig. 14-6.

The audibility of cardiac sounds is modified by the amount of interposed tissue between the sound at its point of origin and the outer chest wall. Large amounts of fat, muscle, or air, as in the obese, muscular, or emphysematous client, tend to dampen or diminish the heart sounds and cause them to sound more distant.

The heart sounds

First heart sound. The AV valves are forced closed as ventricular pressure rises, producing S_1. This sequence of events is similar on both sides of the heart, but pressures and pressure gradients are much greater on the left side, and the sounds produced by left-sided events are usually louder. Events on the left side usually slightly precede those on the right side because the left ventricular myocardium begins depolarization slightly earlier. S_1 can be heard over the entire precordium but is heard best at the apex and is usually louder than S_2 there (Fig. 14-6). At the base of the heart S_1 is usually louder on the left than on the right and on both sides is quieter than S_2. Usually both components of S_1, mitral and tricuspid valve closure, are heard as one sound. As a result of slight asynchrony in valve closure, however, a split S_1 may be audible and may be

heard in the area where tricuspid valve closure is best transmitted, that is, at the fourth left intercostal space at the sternal border. Tricuspid valve closure may become louder as a result of pulmonary hypertension because of the increased right-sided pressures. Splitting of S_1 is neither as commonly nor as easily heard as splitting of S_2.

The frequency of S_1 is slightly lower than that of S_2, and its duration is slightly longer. Its occurrence can be timed with the apical impulse or with the carotid pulsation; it should not be timed with the radial pulse, because the time lapse is too great and leads to confusion.

Alterations in the first heart sound. Factors altering or influencing the loudness of S_1 may be extracardiac or cardiac. Extracardiac factors usually affect both S_1 and S_2. An increase in the amount of tissue interposed between the heart and the stethoscope, as found in obesity, emphysema, or the accumulation of pericardial fluid will diminish the intensity of both S_1 and S_2. Cardiac factors influencing the intensity of S_1 consist of the position of the AV valves at the time of ventricular contraction, the structure of the valves, and the force and abruptness of ventricular contraction. If ventricular systole begins when the AV valves are still wide open, before they have time to "drift" or "float" close together, a loud S_1 results. This situation occurs when the P-R interval is short, as accompanies hyperkinetic states such as exercise, anemia, and hyperthyroidism. Conversely, a prolonged P-R interval, during which the AV valves may begin to close and ventricular contraction is delayed, may result in a faint S_1. Even with a normal P-R interval, S_1 may be diminished. With forceful atrial contraction into a noncompliant ventricle, a situation that may exist with hypertension, the pressure rise in the ventricle may cause the valve to close sooner; the valve may already be partially closed at the onset of ventricular contraction.

Changes in valve leaflet structure may alter the intensity of S_1. As a result of rheumatic fever, the mitral valve may become so fibrosed and calcified that only limited motion is possible and S_1 is diminished. However, if the valve leaflets retain some mobility, as they may with mitral stenosis, S_1 may be accentuated. Significant mitral stenosis may also increase S_1 because of the greater ventricular pressure needed to overcome the increase in atrial pressure. This produces an increased closing pressure and more abrupt closure. Abrupt ventricular contractions producing a more intense S_1 may also result from the hyperkinetic states mentioned earlier, including exercise, fever, thyrotoxicosis, and anemia.

In the presence of a complete heart block, where the length of the P-R interval is frequently changing, variation in the intensity of S_1 will occur.

Second heart sound. As ventricular systole is completed, pressure in the aorta and pulmonary artery exceeds ventricular pressure and the semilunar valves close. Vibrations produced by closure of the aortic and pulmonic valves are primarily responsible for S_2. Closure of the aortic valve is the loudest component of S_2 at both the right and left second intercostal spaces and is referred to as A_2; the sound produced by the pulmonic valve, referred to as P_2, is normally heard only in a small area centering around the second left interspace and can be identified as separate from the component of S_2 caused by aortic valve closure only when splitting of S_2 occurs. In children and adolescents P_2 may normally be accentuated, causing an increase in S_2 heard in the pulmonic area. It should be reemphasized that A_2 and P_2 refer to the two components of S_2; they do not refer to any anatomical location on the chest wall.

S_2 is audible over the entire precordium but is best heard at the base of the heart and is louder there than S_1; at the apex it is quieter than S_1 (Fig. 14-6). S_2 marks the beginning of diastole, normally the longer interval. It is slightly higher in frequency and shorter in duration than S_1.

Normal physiological splitting of the second heart sound. Right ventricular systolic ejection time is very slightly longer than left ventricular systolic ejection time. Therefore, pulmonic valve closure, which marks the end of right ventricular ejection, occurs slightly later than aortic valve closure. This normal asynchrony of valve closure is increased during inspiration because of the decrease in intrathoracic pressure, which facilitates increased venous return to the right side of the heart and a further delay in pulmonic valve closure. During expiration, the disparity between left and right ejection times is decreased and splitting becomes less pronounced or nonexistent as the valves close nearly synchronously, producing a single sound (Fig. 14-7). Inspiratory splitting is commonly most marked at the peak of the inspiratory phase of respiration and is best determined during ordinary respiration. If the breath is held in inspiration, rather than sustaining the splitting, the ejection times again equalize and the split sound becomes single. Splitting will be evident only where pulmonic as well as aortic

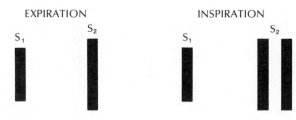

Fig. 14-7. Normal splitting of S_2.

closure can be heard, that is, at the second left interspace.

The degree of splitting varies from one individual to another. In some individuals two distinct sounds are quite clear though very close in sequence (the splitting seems more like two parts of a single sound), whereas in others no splitting can be recognized. In some individuals clear splitting may be audible during inspiration and a very slight degree of splitting is audible during expiration.

Variations in S_2 include changes in loudness as well as variations in splitting. In general, louder closure sounds result from higher closing pressure. In systemic hypertension, for example, louder aortic closure sounds occur; S_2 may become ringing or tambourlike in quality and may become louder than S_1 at the apex. Exercise and excitement may also increase the pressure in the aorta and thus increase the aortic S_2. Conditions associated with pulmonary hypertension, including mitral stenosis and congestive heart failure, may produce an increased pulmonic S_2. A fall in systemic blood pressure, as occurs with shock, will produce a diminished aortic S_2. As was the case with S_1, pathological changes in the valves will also affect the intensity of S_2. Semilunar valves that are injured but still flexible may increase S_2, whereas injured valves that have become markedly thickened and calcified may diminish it.

Variations in splitting of S_2 include wide splitting, fixed splitting, and paradoxical splitting (Fig. 14-8). Conditions causing delayed electrical activation, on contraction or emptying, or both, of the right ventricle, for example, right bundle branch block, also cause a delay in pulmonic valve closure. Wide splitting of S_2 exists with expiration; on inspiration, the splitting is even wider. Fixed splitting is associated with large atrial septal defects. Here, pulmonic closure is delayed because with each beat, the right ventricle is ejecting a larger volume than is the left ventricle. Presumably, right-sided filling

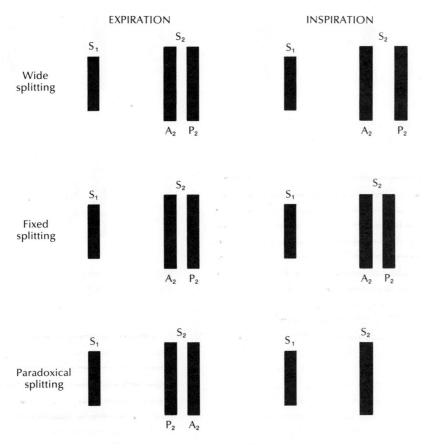

Fig. 14-8. Variations in splitting of S₂.

cannot be further increased by inspiration, so the split sound remains relatively fixed. In contrast to delayed closure of the pulmonic valve with its resultant wide splitting, delayed closure of the aortic valve in a left bundle branch block may result in narrowed splitting or splitting where the normal sequence of sounds is reversed, so that pulmonic closure precedes aortic closure. This produces a paradoxical situation wherein inspiration results in the two sounds coming closer together and even fusing to a single sound and expiration results in more widely separated sounds. On expiration, pulmonic closure occurs first, followed by aortic closure; then on inspiration, when pulmonary valve closure is normally delayed, the pulmonic sound merges with the aortic sound.

Third heart sound. During diastole there are two phases of rapid ventricular filling. The first is in early diastole and is a passive, rapid filling phase. When the AV valves open, after S_2, the blood stored in the atria flows rapidly into the ventricles. This rapid distention of the ventricles causes vibrations of the ventricular walls to occur.

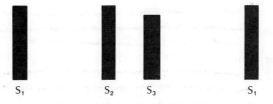

Fig. 14-9. S_3: an early diastolic sound.

Known as the third heart sound (S_3) (Fig. 14-9), these vibrations are low in frequency and intensity and are best heard at the apex with the bell of the stethoscope. The sound may be accentuated by having the client assume the left lateral decubitus position. This sound is commonly heard in normal children and young adults and in such instances is known as a physiological S_3. However, in other circumstances, an S_3 is abnormal. For example, in an older person with heart disease an S_3 often signifies myocardial failure. In such a case S_3 contributes to the production of a ventricular or protodiastolic gallop.

Fourth heart sound. The second phase of rapid

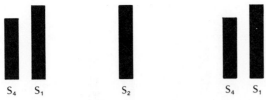

Fig. 14-10. S₄: a late diastolic sound.

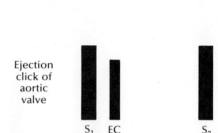

Fig. 14-11. Opening snap of the mitral valve following S₂ and ejection click of the aortic valve following S₁.

ventricular filling occurs after the first phase of passive filling. In late diastole, with atrial systolic ejection of blood into the ventricle, the second, active rapid filling phase occurs, just before S_1. The inflow of this phase, too, may cause vibrations of the valves, supporting structures, or ventricular walls, resulting in a late diastolic filling, or fourth, heart sound (S_4) (Fig. 14-10). It may be heard physiologically, especially in a young person with a thin chest wall, but is more rare in a normal client than a physiological S_3. An abnormal S_4 results from an increased resistance to filling secondary to either a change in compliance of the ventricle or to an increase in volume. Therefore, it may be associated with hypertensive cardiovascular disease, coronary artery disease, or aortic stenosis, wherein there may be decreased left ventricular compliance. It may be associated with severe anemia or hyperthyroidism, wherein there is an increased stroke volume.

S_4 is also a low-frequency, low-intensity sound, heard best with the bell at the apex shortly before S_4. It may also be well heard at the base. Care must be taken not to confuse an S_4 with a split S_1. The presence of an S_4 produces a sequence of sounds known as a presystolic gallop because of its timing in the cardiac cycle.

Summation gallop. When both phases of rapid ventricular filling become audible events as an S_3 and S_4, a quadruple rhythm results. As the heart rate increases and diastole become shorter, the two sounds come closer together and may be heard as one sound in diastole. Then there are three cardiac sounds: S_1 and S_2 and the summation sound of S_3 and S_4. This is known as a summation gallop.

Abnormal extra heart sounds. There are two extra heart sounds that always indicate an abnormality. Both of these sounds are produced by the opening of diseased valves. They are the opening snap of the mitral valve and the ejection click, or opening snap, of a semilunar valve. Pericardial friction rub also produces an extra cardiac sound.

Opening snap of the mitral valve. Opening of the mitral valves, normally a silent event, may become audible if it becomes thickened or otherwise altered, as by rheumatic heart disease. This sound occurs early in diastole, is high pitched, brief, and of a snapping or clicking quality (Fig. 14-11). It is usually best heard medial to the apex and toward the lower left sternal border and may radiate toward the base. It is always associated with a good, and often accentuated, S_1. It can be differentiated from an S_3 because it occurs earlier (temporally, mitral valve opening is before ventricular filling), is sharper and higher pitched, and radiates more widely. In the pulmonic area, the opening snap must be differentiated from a split S_2. A split S_2 is best heard in the second left intercostal space, and an opening snap is best heard between the apex and the lower left sternal border. Whereas respiration affects the splitting of S_2, an opening snap is not affected by respiration and will remain at a fixed interval after the aortic component of S_2.

The loudness of the opening snap is affected by the pressure in the left atrium and by the flexibility of the mitral valve. Higher left atrial pressures increase the loudness of the opening snap. Marked fibrosis and calcification of the valve decrease the mobility, and consequently, the sound produced.

Ejection click. Semilunar valve changes may also be associated with an opening sound. This sound occurs early in systole at the end of isovolumic contraction when the semilunar valves open (Fig. 14-11). The aortic ejection click, the more common of the two, is heard both at the

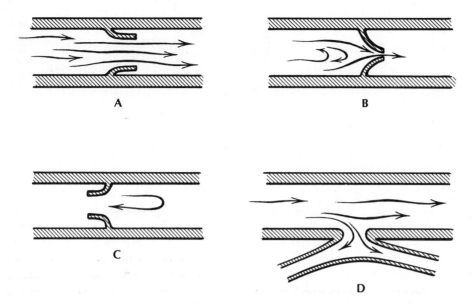

Fig. 14-12. Mechanisms of murmur production. **A,** Increased flow across a normal valve. **B,** Forward flow through a stenotic valve. **C,** Backflow through an incompetent valve. **D,** Flow through a septal defect or arteriovenous fistula.

base and at the apex and does not change with respiration. Pulmonary ejection clicks are heard best at the second left interspace, radiate poorly, and change in intensity with respiration, increasing with expiration and decreasing with inspiration.

Pericardial friction rub. Inflammation of the pericardial sac causes the parietal and visceral surfaces of the roughened pericardium to rub against each other. This produces an extra cardiac sound of to-and-fro character with both systolic and diastolic components. One, two, or three components of a pericardial friction rub may be audible. A three-component rub indicates the presence of pericarditis and serves to distinguish a pericardial rub from a pleural friction rub, which ordinarily has two components. It resembles the sound of squeaky leather and is often described as grating, scratching, or rasping. The sound seems very close to the ear and may seem louder than or may even mask the other heart sounds. Friction rubs are usually best heard between the apex and sternum but may be widespread.

Heart murmurs

A variety of conditions may result in the production of the more prolonged sound during systole or diastole known as a murmur. These are abnormal sounds produced by vibrations within the heart or in the walls of the large vessels. They tend to originate in the vicinity of the heart valve

and are often best heard around the area of the valve responsible for their production.

Mechanisms of production. Three main factors related to murmur production are (1) increased flow rate of blood across normal valves, (2) forward flow through an irregular or constricted valve or into a dilated vessel or chamber, and (3) backflow or regurgitant flow through an incompetent or insufficient valve, a septal defect, or a patent ductus arteriosus (Fig. 14-12). In addition, a combination of these factors may prevail.

Murmurs are illustrated in a manner similar to the way in which they appear in a phonocardiogram, that is, with a series of vertical lines in systole between S_1 and S_2 or in diastole between S_2 and S_1. The lines are drawn in such a way as to indicate the level of, and increase or decrease in, intensity of the sound. For example, a midsystolic ejection murmur that is crescendo-decrescendo in nature, is shown in Fig. 14-13, *A;* a holosystolic regurgitant murmur is shown in Fig. 14-13, *B.*

Valve alterations. The adequacy of opening and closure of the valves and of the orifice size determines many of the characteristics of murmurs. Heart valves that are functioning normally and competently permit the forward flow of blood and prevent backflow or regurgitation. It is essential to understand the stations of the valves and flow patterns during systole and diastole. During ventricular systole, the mitral and tricuspid valves are closed, preventing backflow, and the

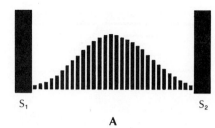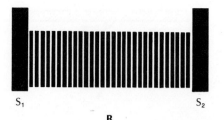

S₁ S₂   A   S₁ S₂   B

Fig. 14-13. Systolic murmurs. **A,** Crescendo-decrescendo systolic ejection murmur. **B,** Holosystolic regurgitant murmur.

aortic and pulmonic valves are open, permitting forward flow. During ventricular diastole, the mitral and tricuspid valves are open, permitting forward flow, and the aortic and pulmonic valves are closed, preventing backflow.

Stenotic valves prevent adequate forward flow; thus, a stenosed mitral valve interferes with normal flow during diastole, when the atrium empties blood into the ventricle. Mitral stenosis produces a diastolic murmur. A stenosed aortic valve prevents adequate forward flow of blood during ventricular systole, when the blood is being forced from the ventricle into the aorta; thus, aortic stenosis produces a systolic murmur. Blood flowing through such a narrowed orifice meets resistance and produces vibrations.

Incompetent or insufficient valves fail to close completely during that phase of the cardiac cycle when their leaflets should be firmly approximated; they leave an aperture through which blood flows inappropriately back from the ventricles to the atria or from the aorta or pulmonary artery back to the ventricles. This regurgitation, or backflow, of blood produces vibrations of the valve and of parts of the myocardium, producing a murmur. An incompetent mitral valve permits the inappropriate backflow of blood from the left ventricle to the left atrium during ventricular systole, producing a systolic murmur. An insufficient aortic valve permits the backflow of blood from the aorta to the left ventricle during ventricular diastole, producing a diastolic murmur.

Characteristics. Murmurs are classified and described according to several characteristics, including timing (systolic or diastolic), frequency, location, intensity, radiation, quality, and effects of respiration.

Timing. The timing of murmurs is according to their occurrence during either diastole or systole. At times, murmurs may occur during both phases of the cycle. The timing of the murmur may be further characterized as occurring during the entire phase of a cycle, or for instance, during early, mid, or late systole. Murmurs that endure throughout systole are known as holosystolic or pansystolic murmurs; the same is true for diastolic murmurs. Early diastolic murmurs are known as protodiastolic, and late diastolic murmurs are called presystolic.

In general, systolic murmurs are caused by stenosed aortic or pulmonic valves or by incompetent mitral or tricuspid valves, and diastolic murmurs are produced by stenosed mitral or tricuspid valves or by incompetent aortic or pulmonic valves. It is important to remember, however, that not all murmurs result from valve defects; they may also be produced by alteration in the velocity of flow, by changes in the vessels, and by defects in the myocardium.

Frequency. The frequency, or pitch, or murmurs varies from high to low. The main determining factor is the velocity of blood flow. Generally, when the rate of flow is rapid, a high pitch results; when the velocity is slow, the pitch is low. The pitch of a murmur is classified as high, medium, or low.

Location. A murmur is described by means of anatomical landmarks according to where it is best heard. Some are localized to small areas, whereas others are heard over large portions of the precordium. The location of a murmur is significant in terms of its size of production. The murmurs originating from valvular alterations are usually best heard in the area to which sounds from that valve are transmitted.

Intensity. The loudness of a murmur is described on a scale of one to six; one is the softest, and six is the loudest. The description of each level of loudness is as follows:

Grade I: Barely audible, very faint; can be heard only with special effort.

Grade II: Clearly audible but quiet.

Grade III: Moderately loud.

Grade IV: Loud.

Grade V: Very loud; may be heard with stethoscope partly off the chest.

Grade VI: Loudest possible; audible with the stethoscope just removed from contact with the chest wall.

It is important to note that though the grading of the loudness of a murmur is helpful, it is also a rather subjective description, dependent on the auditory acuity of the listener.

The terms crescendo and decrescendo are used to describe the pattern of intensity reflecting changes in the flow rate. A crescendo-decrescendo murmur, for example, increases from quiet to louder and then decreases again, forming a diamond-shaped pattern. In the case of aortic stenosis, for example, the flow rate increases, reaches a peak, and then decreases, producing a crescendo-decrescendo systolic murmur with a rather harsh quality. The diastolic murmur of aortic insufficiency is a decrescendo, high-pitched, blowing murmur. The flow rate of blood leaking back into the ventricle from the aorta is approximately proportional to the decreasing pressure gradient between the aorta and the ventricle. Although the patterns of the various murmurs may not be that easily determined with the stethoscope, the murmurs do appear that way on the phonocardiogram.

Radiation. Some murmurs radiate in the direction of the bloodstream by which they are produced. For example, the diastolic murmur of aortic insufficiency may be heard along the left sternal border. In this case, the blood leaks back from the aorta into the left ventricle. Other factors, such as the variation in sound transmission through various tissues, also influence radiation.

Quality. Several descriptive terms are often used to characterize a murmur; these include *musical*, *blowing*, *harsh*, and *rumbling*. For example, the murmur of aortic stenosis may be described as harsh; the murmur of mitral insufficiency may be described as a long, blowing sound; and the murmur of mitral stenosis tends to be of a low, rumbling quality.

Effect of respiration. As mentioned earlier in this chapter, certain events on the right side of the heart are affected by respiration due to intrathoracic pressure changes and right-sided filling changes. Murmurs that originate on the right side of the heart are also subject to influence by these factors. The murmur of tricuspid insufficiency, for example, may increase with inspiration.

EXAMINATION

The division of the cardiac examination into the techniques of inspection, palpation, and auscultation is useful. Because the findings of inspection and palpation are closely related and complimentary to one another, these techniques are discussed together. Auscultation provides much valuable information about cardiac dynamics, but the practitioner must be cautious not to apply the stethoscope to the chest wall before performing the visual and palpatory examinations.

Several environmental considerations are basic to the cardiac examination. A quiet room is essential, because cardiac sounds are for the most part subtle and low pitched and are thus easily missed if outside noises prevail. A good light source that can be directed tangentially across the chest wall is important for adequate observation.

Examination of the precordium is most effectively performed with the examiner standing on the client's right side. The complete assessment requires that the client be examined in the sitting, supine, and left lateral recumbent positions. Whereas inspection and palpation are performed primarily with the client in the supine position, thorough auscultation should be performed with the client in all three positions. Sitting forward and lying in the left lateral position both bring various parts of the heart closer to the chest wall, thus enhancing certain auditory findings.

■ Inspection and palpation

The purpose of both inspection and palpation is to determine the presence and extent of normal and abnormal pulsations over the precordium. These pulsations may be manifested as the apex beat (or apical impulse) or as heaves or lifts of the chest; they provide some reflection of myocardial and hemodynamic activity. Inspection and palpation together provide a useful method of assessing left, right, and combined ventricular hypertrophy. The visibility and palpability of those movements are affected by the thickness of the chest wall and by the type and amount of tissue through which the vibrations must travel.

Inspection

The chest wall and epigastrium are inspected while the client is in the supine position. A tangential light is helpful for observing subtle movements of the chest. The examiner stands on the client's right side and observes the chest for size and symmetry and then for any pulsations, lifts or heaves, or retractions. The location and timing of all impulses should be noted.

Apical impulse. The thrust of the contracting left ventricle may produce a visible pulsation in the area of the midclavicular line in the fifth left intercostal space. This is the normal apical impulse, and it is visibly evident in about half of the normal adult population. It occurs nearly synchronously with the carotid impulse, and simultaneous palpation of a carotid artery is helpful in identifying it.

When visible, the apical impulse helps to identify an area very near the cardiac apex, thus giving some indication of cardiac size. In the case of left ventricular hypertrophy or dilatation, or both, as may occur with systemic hypertension, the apical impulse may be located more laterally or inferiorly, or both; for example, it may be located at the left anterior axillary line in the sixth left intercostal space.

Retractions. A slight retraction of the chest wall just medial to the midclavicular line in the fifth interspace is a normal finding. Marked or actual retraction of the rib is abnormal and may be due to pericardial disease. Left ventricular

hypertrophy is often accompanied by a systolic thrust, producing a "rocking" movement.

Heaves or lifts. When the work and forcefulness of the right ventricle is greatly increased, a diffuse lifting impulse is often produced along the left sternal border with each beat. This is referred to as a lift or heave; these terms are generally used interchangeably.

Palpation

The technique of palpation builds on and expands the findings gleaned from inspection. The entire precordium is palpated methodically, beginning at the apex, moving to the left sternal border, and then to the base of the heart (Fig. 14-14). Other areas may also be included if indicated, including the left axillary area, the epigastrium, and the right sternal border. During palpation the examiner is searching for the apical impulse at or near the apex and for any abnormal heaves, thrills, or retractions elsewhere on the precordium, indicating cardiac hypertrophy, dilatation, or murmurs. The abnormal flow of blood resulting in an audible murmur may also result in the palpatory sensation known as a thrill. It is rather like a rushing sensation beneath the

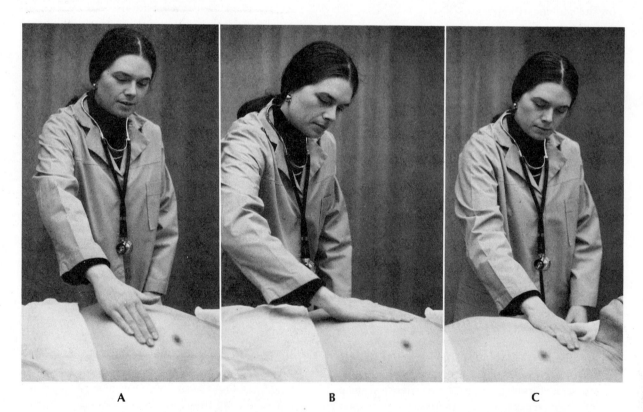

| A | B | C |

Fig. 14-14. Palpation of the precordium. The examiner palpates three areas of the precordium: **A,** over the apex; **B,** over the left sternal border; **C,** over the base of the heart.

fingers and has been likened to the feeling transmitted to the fingers placed over the larynx of a purring cat. As with inspection, the shape and thickness of the chest wall are important variables.

The client is in the supine position for this portion of the cardiac examination. The examiner should take adequate time to "tune in" or "warm up" to movements over the precordium, because many are faint and subtle and are perceived only after a "warming up" period. It is important to describe pulsations in relation to their timing in the cardiac cycle. This is facilitated by simultaneously palpating the carotid pulsation with the left hand while palpating the precordium with the right. All pulsations should be described in terms of their location in an interspace and their distance from the midsternal, midclavicular, or axillary lines.

Apical impulse. Although the thrust noted over the apex of the heart is sometimes referred to as the point of maximum impulse (PMI), this term is not recommended, because the actual point or area of maximum impulse may or may not be located over the apical area. The term apical impulse is preferred. The presence, location, size, and character of the apical impulse should be assessed. The apical impulse is palpable in about half the normal adult population.

Standing to the right of the client and using the finger tips and palmar aspect of his right hand, the examiner palpates first over the apex, particularly in the area of the fifth interspace in the midclavicular line. Normally, the apical impulse is palpable in or just medial to the midclavicular line and is felt as a faint, short-duration, localized tap less than 2 cm in diameter. On occasion the apical impulse may be normally located lateral to the midclavicular line, for example, in association with a high diaphragm, as occurs with pregnancy. The outward movement of the normal impulse is not excessively forceful and is palpable only during the first part of systole. The amplitude of the apical impulse may seem to be increased in normal individuals with thin chest walls. Turning the client to the left lateral position may cause a normal impulse to seem abnormal in both amplitude and duration, since the apex is brought closer to the chest wall, thus accentuating its activities. In obese persons or those with an increased anteroposterior chest diameter, the apical impulse is not likely to be palpable. Conditions such as anxiety, anemia, fever, and hyperthyroidism may produce an apical impulse increased in force and duration. Normally, systolic ejection may be as-

sociated with a slight retraction of the lower left parasternal area.

Apex area: left ventricular hypertrophy. Hypertrophy of the left ventricle typically produces an abnormally forceful and sustained outward movement during ventricular systole. In addition, the apex impulse may be displaced laterally and downward and may be increased in size. For example, the apical impulse may be found 4 cm lateral to the midclavicular line in the sixth intercostal space and may be 4 cm in diameter.

Generally, the degree of displacement of the impulse correlates with the extent of cardiac enlargement. In addition to an alteration in location and size, the impulse may become more diffuse and palpable in more than one interspace; also, the amplitude or forcefulness may be increased. Displacement tends to be maximal when there is both dilatation and hypertrophy. Conditions associated with a volume overload, such as mitral and aortic regurgitation and left-to-right shunts, tend to produce such dilatation and hypertrophy. Hypertrophy of the left ventricle without dilatation, as may occur with aortic stenosis and systemic hypertension, results in an apical impulse that is increased in force and duration but not necessarily displaced laterally; it may still be located in the midclavicular line. In some persons with left ventricular hypertrophy, the increased force and prolonged duration of the apical impulse produces a lifting sensation under the examiner's fingers.

Left sternal border: right ventricular hypertrophy. Right ventricular hypertrophy is less common than left ventricular hypertrophy. It may be detected on palpation as a diffuse, lifting systolic impulse along the lower left sternal border. This finding may be associated with a systolic retraction at the apex, resulting from displacement and rotation of the left ventricle posteriorly by the enlarged right ventricle. A diffuse lift, or heave, along the lower left sternum is associated, for example, with pulmonary valve disease, pulmonary hypertension, and chronic lung disease. A thrill may also be palpated in this area and is associated with ventricular septal defects. The palmar aspect of the examiner's right hand is placed over the left sternal border.

Base of the heart. The examiner's right hand then rests over the base of the heart at the second left and right intercostal spaces at the sternal borders and feels for pulsations, thrills, or the vibrations of semilunar valve closure. Normally, the base is fairly "quiet" to palpation.

Aortic stenosis may be associated with a thrill palpable in the first and third right interspaces as well as in the second right interspace. In persons with systemic hypertension, it may be possible to palpate the accentuated vibration of aortic valve closure at the time of S_2.

Pulmonic valve stenosis may be associated with a thrill in the second and third left interspaces near the sternum. In persons with pulmonary hypertension, pulsations may be palpated in the same area. The most common causes of abnormal pulsations in the pulmonary artery area are increases in pressure or flow in the pulmonary artery, such as in pulmonary hypertension or atrial septal defect. In some normal people with thin chest walls, it is possible to palpate a brief, slight pulsation in this area. Conditions such as anemia, fever, exertion, and pregnancy would accentuate this pulsation.

Percussion

The technique of percussion is of limited value in cardiac assessment. In the past, percussion was used to determine the borders of cardiac dullness, but the actual size of the heart is much more accurately determined by a chest roentgenogram, and ventricular hypertrophy is better determined by combined inspection and palpation. Variations in chest wall configuration and the type and amount of interposed tissue, such as air or fat tissue, alter and limit the accuracy of this procedure. The value of percussion is further limited in the assessment of right ventricular enlargement, since this condition causes substernal and anteroposterior enlargement, which is not accessible to the percussion note.

Auscultation

The stethoscope is a device that gathers and slightly amplifies sound before it is transmitted to the ears. A comfortable and properly fitting stethoscope is essential for adequate auscultation. Although the selection of proper earpieces for comfort and the best sound transmission is a matter of individual preference, there are several general guidelines that are useful in making that selection. The earpieces should be large enough to provide a snug fit in the external canal and to block out extraneous room noises. Enough tension should be present to hold the earpieces tightly in place. The rigid metal tubing leading to the earpieces should be bent so as to angle in the same direction as the ear canal, that is, forward. The flexible tubing may be made of rubber or plastic, and it should be thick enough to keep out

extraneous sounds; it should also be reasonably short, about 1 foot, because added length dampens the sound and decreases the efficiency of the stethoscope in transmitting higher frequencies.

The stethoscope chestpiece should be equipped with both a bell and a diaphragm, each of which selectively transmits different frequencies of sound. The valve facilitating a change between the two should be tight fitting, permitting a change without the admission of outside sound. The diaphragm accentuates the higher-frequency sounds. It should be made of a fairly rigid substance and pressed firmly against the skin during auscultation, further enhancing faint, high-frequency sounds. In contrast to the diaphragm, the bell brings out the low-frequency sounds and filters out the high-frequency ones. It should be placed very lightly on the chest wall with just enough pressure applied to seal the edge. If greater pressure is applied to the bell against the chest wall, the skin becomes a relatively tight diaphragm, filtering out the lower-pitched sounds. Alternating the application of light and heavy pressure to the bell may be a helpful maneuver when listening to low-pitched murmurs or filling sounds. Most low-pitched sounds are diastolic filling sounds or murmurs and are often best heard with the client lying down, since orthostatic pooling on standing may cause such sounds to diminish in intensity. Although heart sounds are referred to as being of "high" or "low" frequency, these terms are relative. All heart sounds are generally low pitched (low frequency) and are in a range ordinarily difficult for the human ear to hear. Thus, any technique that improves audibility should be carefully utilized.

Satisfactory auscultation requires a quiet room; mechanical and conversational noises must be minimized. The room should be comfortably warm for the client so that shivering and subsequent muscular noises are avoided. The anterior chest should be exposed to the waist. The examining table should be adequately large for the client to change positions from sitting to supine to left lateral recumbent with ease. Examination in only one position is not adequate.

A systematic method of auscultation is essential; all precordial areas and each sound and pause must be attended to. One recommended system is to begin at the apex and "inch" the stethoscope toward the left sternal border and up the sternal border to the second left and then to the second right intercostal space. Another method consists of beginning the examination at the base of the heart at the second right intercostal space, where

S_2 is always the loudest of the two heart sounds. This is particularly helpful if the heart sounds are heard as nearly equal in intensity at the apex. Auscultation should be performed using both the bell and the diaphragm and should cover the entire precordium and areas of radiation, such as the axillary area or carotid arteries, when indicated.

In each area examined, the examiner listens selectively to each component of the cardiac cycle; as with palpation, this usually requires a period of "warming up" or "tuning in" to the various cardiac events. First, the examiner notes the rate and rhythm of the heartbeat. Then, at each auscultatory area, he concentrates initially on S_1, noting its intensity and variations therein, possible duplication, and the effects of respiration. The examiner then selects out S_2 and focuses on the same characteristics. Next, he concentrates on systole, then on diastole, listening first for any extra sounds and then for murmurs. The examiner must listen selectively for each component; it is impossible to listen for everything at once.

If the initial part of the examination was done on the client lying in a supine position, the client is now asked to roll to his left side; the examiner applies the bell lightly at the apex and listens for the presence or absence of low-frequency diastolic sounds, such as a filling sound or a mitral valve murmur. The client is then asked to sit up and lean slightly forward. Pressing the diaphragm firmly against the chest, the examiner listens at both the second left and right intercostal spaces at the sternal border to detect the presence or absence of high-pitched diastolic murmurs of aortic or pulmonic valve insufficiency (Fig. 14-15). Listening is done during normal respiration and then with the client's breath held in deep expiration.

Neck vessels

The vascular structures of the neck accessible for and included in the cardiovascular examination are the jugular veins and the carotid arteries. Examination of these vessels provides information on local states and also reflects the activity of the heart. The jugular veins are observed for pulse waves and pressure level; the carotid arteries are examined by inspection, palpation, and auscultation to assess the characteristics of their pulsations.

JUGULAR VEINS

Venous pulse waves and venous pressure are assessed at the external and internal jugular veins. The external jugular veins lie superficially and are visible above the clavicle close to the insertion of the sternocleidomastoid muscles. The internal jugular veins are larger and lie deep to the sternocleidomastoid muscles near the carotid arteries; reflections of their activity may be visible on the skin overlying these vessels. Blood from the jugular veins flows directly into the superior vena cava. Fig. 14-16 illustrates the location of the external and internal jugular veins.

Venous return and the filling volume are important determinants of cardiac performance. These cannot be directly assessed on physical examination, but a general estimate can be made from observation of the jugular veins. The veins leading to the right side of the heart may be

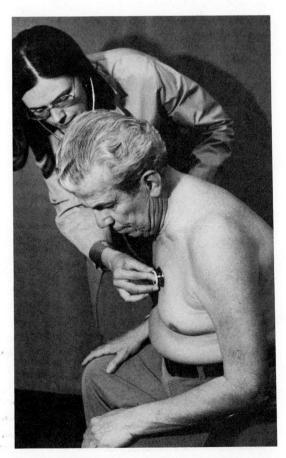

Fig. 14-15. Using the diaphragm of the stethoscope while the client leans forward and holds his breath in full expiration, the examiner listens for high-pitched murmurs at the base of the heart.

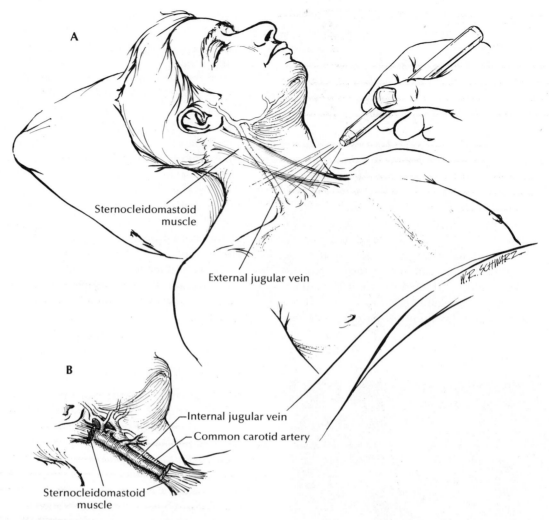

A

Sternocleidomastoid
muscle

External jugular vein

W.R. SCHWARZ

B

Internal jugular vein
Common carotid artery

Sternocleidomastoid
muscle

Fig. 14-16. A, Inspection of the external jugular vein. **B,** Location of the internal jugular vein and common carotid artery.

thought of as a system of distensible tubes with partially competent valves. Therefore, some judgment of the filling pressure of the heart may be made by observing the pressure level and the waveforms transmitted from the heart. Observation of the two components of pressure level and pulse waves in the veins gives an indication of the dynamics of the right side of the heart.

In the examination of the jugular veins the client is in the supine position. If this position is uncomfortable, the client's trunk may be elevated to a 45° angle. If the veins are very distended, it is best to examine them with the client in a sitting position. The veins or venous pulsations are more readily visible if the client's neck is slightly turned away from the side being examined, and the veins are observed with tangential lighting so that small shadows are cast. Clothing should be

removed from the neck and upper thorax so that there is no constriction. The head and neck may rest comfortably on a pillow, but the neck should not be sharply flexed.

■ **Jugular venous pulse**

When the normal person is in the sitting position, no jugular venous pulsations are visible; with the trunk elevated 45° from horizontal, the jugular venous pulse does not rise more than 1 to 2 cm above the level of the manubrium. When the normal person is in the reclining position, the venous pulse becomes evident because gravity no longer prevents backflow from the heart and the veins become filled.

The normal venous pulse consists of three positive components—the a, c, and v waves—and two negative slopes—the x and y descents (Fig.

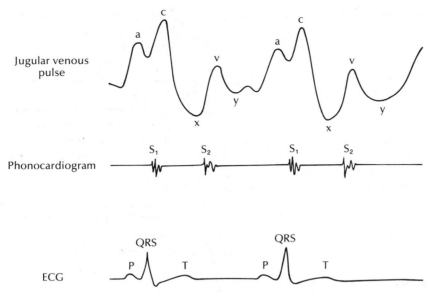

Fig. 14-17. Jugular venous pulse waves in relation to S_1 and S_2 and the ECG.

14-17). The a wave is frequently the highest part of the total pulse wave and is produced by atrial contraction. As the right atrium contracts, ejecting blood into the right ventricle, there is also a brief backflow of blood into the vena cava. This retrograde pulse wave is reflected in the jugular veins as the a wave. This wave occurs just before S_1; if an S_4 is present, it occurs at the peak of the a wave.

Two simultaneous events contribute to the production of the c wave: the impact of the adjacent carotid artery pulsation and the retrograde transmission of a pulse wave, caused by right ventricular systole and bulging of the closed tricuspid valve. The c wave occurs at the end of S_1.

The tricuspid valve remains closed during ventricular systole while blood from the systemic circulation continues to fill the vena cava and the right atrium. The increased volume in these structures leads to a pressure increase reflected in the jugular veins as the v, or passive filling, wave. This wave reaches a peak during late ventricular systole. Following this, the pressure in the right atrium begins to fall as the bulging of the tricuspid valve decreases, first during relaxation of the right ventricle and then as the tricuspid valve opens.

The x descent following the c wave is produced by downward displacement of the base of the ventricles (including the tricuspid valve) during ventricular systole and by atrial diastole. The y

descent following the v wave is produced by the opening of the tricuspid valve and the subsequent rapid flow of blood from the right atrium to the right ventricle.

It is usually possible to discern the three positive and two negative waves of the jugular venous pulse when the heart rate is below 90 beats per minute and the P-Q interval is normal. At more rapid heart rates, there is often a fusion or overlapping of some of the waves and analysis of the waveform is difficult.

Abnormalities of waves

The a wave. The a wave, which may be the highest or most pronounced of the three positive waves, is increased when it becomes more difficult for the contracting right atrium to empty into the right ventricle. For example, in tricuspid valve stenosis, the a wave is more prominent. When there is right ventricular enlargement due to severe pulmonary stenosis or pulmonary hypertension and the right atrium must contract more forcefully to fill it, an enlarged a wave also results.

Irregularly enlarged a waves result from a complete AV block. When the atrium contracts against a closed tricuspid valve, giant (cannon) a waves are produced. In ventricular tachycardia, the cannon waves may occur irregularly, since the cause of their production—simultaneous atrial and ventricular systole and a closed tricuspid valve—does not accompany each beat.

The x descent, and c and v waves. When the tricuspid valve is insufficient, backflow of blood from the right ventricle to the right atrium occurs during ventricular systole. This causes the x slope to become obliterated or replaced by the positive waves, the c and v waves, which then form the c-v wave. Thus, with the obliteration of a negative slope and the accentuation of the two positive waves, a large jugular venous pulse wave is produced. The c-v wave may become so enlarged as to resemble exaggerated arterial pulsations. Tricuspid insufficiency may be organic, resulting from rheumatic heart disease; or it may be produced in clients with generalized cardiac failure, wherein the right ventricle becomes so dilated that the tricuspid ring is stretched and regurgitation ensues.

The y descent. The tricuspid valve opens shortly after S_2, and the rapid filling phase of ventricular diastole begins. The characteristics of the y descent depend on several factors, including pressure and volume circumstances in the great vessels, the right atrium, and the right ventricle, and resistance to flow across the tricuspid valve. Tricuspid stenosis, therefore, would produce a slow y descent because it presents obstruction to right atrial emptying. In clients with severe heart failure in which the venous pressure is extremely high, a sharp, exaggerated y wave is produced.

Differentiation from carotid arterial pulsations

Because the internal jugular vein lies deep to the sternocleidomastoid muscle and close to the carotid artery, its pulsations may be confused with those produced by the common carotid artery. There are several means of differentiating these pulsations.

Quality and character of the pulse. In normal sinus rhythm, the jugular venous pulse has three positive waves and the carotid pulse has one positive wave. Usually, the venous pulse waves are more undulating than the brisk arterial waves. The examiner may be assisted in differentiating the two by palpating the carotid pulse on one side of the neck and observing the jugular venous pulse on the other.

Effect of respiration. With normal inspiration, intrathoracic pressure decreases, blood flow into the right atrium increases, and the level of the pulse wave in the neck veins descends. The opposite occurs during expiration. Respiration does not have this effect on the carotid pulsations.

Effect of changing position. Pulsations in the neck veins become more prominent when the client assumes the recumbent position and less prominent when the client is in the sitting position. Carotid pulsations are not affected by posture.

Effect of venous compression. The pulsations of the jugular veins are rather easily eliminated by applying gentle pressure over the vein at the base of the neck above the clavicle. This blocks the retrograde transmission of the venous pulse wave, leaving only the arterial pulsations.

Effect of abdominal pressure. Pressure applied by the examiner's hand over the client's abdomen may cause an increased prominence of the venous pulsations. The examiner presses, using the palm of his hand and applying moderately firm pressure over the upper right quadrant of the abdomen for 30 to 60 seconds. In normal persons there is slight, if any, increase in the venous pulsations. However, if there is right-sided heart failure, the jugular venous pulsations and distention may markedly increase as venous return to the heart is increased. Normally this maneuver produces no change in the carotid pulsations.

■ Jugular venous pressure

The level of the column of blood in the jugular veins reflects the volume and pressure circumstances on the right side of the heart. Both the external and internal jugular veins can be assessed. Although other mechanical techniques are available for the evaluation of venous pressure, inspection on physical examination remains a useful and reliable maneuver.

In a normal client examined in the supine position, full neck veins are normally visible. When the normal person is examined with the thorax elevated to a 45° angle from horizontal, the venous pulses should ascend no more than a few millimeters above the clavicle. With markedly elevated venous pressure, the neck veins may be distended as high as the angle of the jaw, even when the person is in the upright sitting position. The height of venous pressure may be estimated by measuring the distance that the veins are distended above the manubrium sterni.

The examiner should inspect the veins on both sides of the neck. When the venous pressure is generally increased, distention is noted on both sides; unilateral distention may occur as a result of kinking in the left innominate vein in some older clients. The level to which distention is observed and the position of the client should be noted.

Elevation of venous pressure may be an indication of congestive heart failure, constrictive pericarditis, or obstruction of the superior vena cava. The most common cause of elevated venous pressure is failure of the right ventricle secondary to left ventricular failure. As described earlier, the effect of applying increased abdominal pressure may increase the amount of venous distention in the presence of right-sided heart failure.

CAROTID ARTERIES

The techniques of inspection, palpation, and auscultation are utilized in examining the carotid arteries. The neck is observed for unusually large or bounding carotid pulses. The carotid arterial pulses are then palpated bilaterally, as are all the pulses, for rate, rhythm, equality, amplitude, and contour. The examiner palpates with his forefinger below and just medial to the angle of the jaw (Fig. 14-18). Only one side is examined at a time in order to avoid excessive carotid sinus massage, thus preventing unnecessary slowing of the pulse, and to avoid further embarrassment of borderline circulation in older clients. The head should be rotated slightly toward the side being examined in order to relax the sternocleidomastoid muscle. The heart sounds may be used as reference points, and simultaneous auscultation of the heart is then helpful. S_1 and the carotid impulse are very nearly simultaneous events. The carotid arteries are auscultated with the bell of the stethoscope for bruits indicating local obstruction or for the sound of transmitted cardiac murmurs.

■ Carotid arterial pulse

The carotid arteries are the best arteries in which to assess several characteristics of the arterial pulse, for example, whether the force is strong or weak, the rise and collapse rapid or slow, and the impulse double or single in nature.

The normal carotid pulse consists of a single positive wave followed by a dicrotic notch (Fig. 14-19). The upstroke is smooth and rapid, the

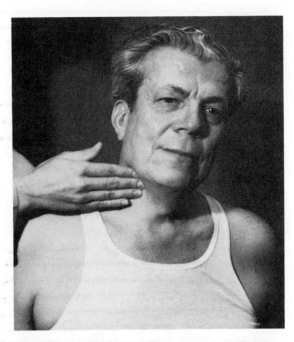

Fig. 14-18. The examiner palpates the carotid pulse below and just medial to the angle of the jaw.

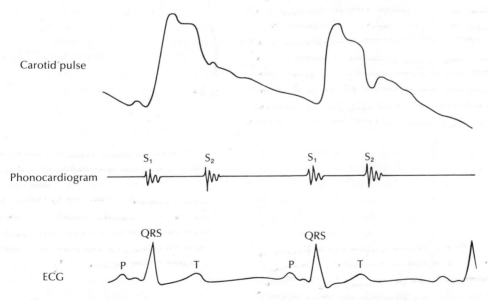

Carotid pulse

Phonocardiogram S_1 S_2 S_1 S_2

ECG QRS P T QRS P T

Fig. 14-19. The carotid pulse wave in relation to S_1 and S_2 and the ECG.

summit is dome shaped, and the downstroke is less steep than the upstroke. The dicrotic notch on the downstroke may not be palpable or may be only slightly palpable. It is often definitely felt in the otherwise normal client during exercise, excitement, or fever.

The size or amplitude of the arterial pulse is determined by a variety of factors, including left ventricular stroke volume and ejection rate, peripheral resistance or distensibility, and pulse pressure. Clinically, abnormalities of the pulse size may be divided into two groups: exaggerated, or hyperkinetic, pulses and weak, or hypokinetic, pulses. During palpation, the examiner may gain an impression of the height of the pulse and the rate of change on the upstroke and downstroke.

Situations associated with a widened arterial pulse pressure—an increased stroke volume and a deceased peripheral resistance—produce a hyperkinetic carotid pulse. The pulse may be large and strong with a normal contour (bounding pulse), or it may be characterized by a markedly high and rapid upstroke (water-hammer pulse) or by an extremely rapid downstroke (collapsing pulse). In the latter two cases, the peak of the pulse is short and rapid. The hyperkinetic pulse may be produced as the result of hyperdynamic or high-output states, such as occur with anxiety, exercise, fever, or pregnancy; as the result of hyperthyroidism or anemia; or as the result of abnormally rapid runoff of blood from the arterial system, such as occurs with abnormal shunting of blood (patent ductus arteriosus or septal defects) or with aortic insufficiency. Aortic insufficiency is a common organic cause of the hyperkinetic pulse in adults. With severe regurgitation, the pulse is described as water hammer and collapsing; a large volume of blood is rapidly ejected from and then returns to the left ventricle across the incompetent valve. Another cause of the hyperkinetic pulse in adults is a complete heart block with bradycardia and increased stroke volume.

The hypokinetic carotid pulse is associated with conditions wherein there is a diminished stroke volume of the left ventricle, increased peripheral vascular resistance, a narrowed pulse pressure, or resistance to flow across the cardiac valves. Examples of causes of a hypokinetic pulse include left ventricular failure due to myocardial infarction, constrictive pericarditis, and moderate or severe valvular aortic stenosis. In aortic stenosis, the pulse may demonstrate a slow upstroke, a delayed peak, and a small volume.

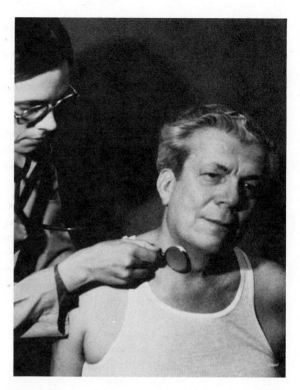

Fig. 14-20. The examiner listens with the bell of the stethoscope for bruits over the carotid artery.

Pulses with double, rather than single, pulsations may be produced by combined aortic stenosis and insufficiency (pulsus bisferiens) or by lowered peripheral resistance and lowered diastolic pressure (dicrotic pulse).

A pulse that occurs at regular intervals but varies in amplitude (pulsus alternans) is produced by alterations in left ventricular contractile force, as may occur with left ventricular failure. Premature ventricular contractions coupled with previous normal beats produce a bigeminal pulse; that is, every alternate beat is premature.

■ Auscultation

Several conditions may produce a palpable carotid thrill associated with an audible bruit. These conditions include local obstruction of a carotid artery, a jugular vein–carotid artery fistula, and a high-output state, such as occurs with severe anemia and thyrotoxicosis. Aortic valvular stenosis may cause a thrill to be referred to the carotid arteries. The bruits are heard by placing the bell of the stethoscope on the skin overlying the carotid artery and listening while the client holds his breath (Fig. 14-20).

BIBLIOGRAPHY

Burch, G. E.: A primer of cardiology, Philadelphia, 1971, Lea & Febiger.

Butterworth, J. S., and others: Cardiac auscultations, New York, 1960, Grune & Stratton, Inc.

Carson, P.: Cardiac diagnosis, New York, 1969, McGraw-Hill Book Co.

Examination of the heart (series of four), New York, 1967, American Heart Association.

Fowler, N. O.: Physical diagnosis of heart disease, New York, 1962, MacMillan, Inc.

Friedburg, C. K.: Diseases of the heart, ed. 3, Philadelphia, 1966, W. B. Saunders Co.

Hurst, J. W., editor: The heart, ed. 3, New York, 1974, McGraw-Hill Book Co.

Ravin, A.: Auscultation of the heart, Chicago, 1958, Yearbook Medical Publishers, Inc.

15 Assessment of the abdomen and rectosigmoid region

Abdomen

Although physical assessment of the abdomen includes all of the four methods of examination (inspection, auscultation, percussion, and palpation), palpation is the technique that is most useful in detecting abdominal pathological conditions. Inspection is done first, followed by auscultation, since the movement or stimulation by pressure on the bowel occasioned by palpation and percussion are known to alter the motility of the bowel and generally to heighten the sounds.

The only special equipment necessary for examination of the abdomen is a stethoscope; a metal, cloth, or plastic ruler or tape measure that will not stretch; and a skin-marking pencil.

INSPECTION

The optimal position of the patient for inspection of the abdomen is supine with the abdominal muscles as relaxed as possible. Tension in these muscles is best avoided by placing the client's arms comfortably at his sides as opposed to extending them upward, as in placing them behind the head. Contraction may be further avoided by placing a small pillow beneath the knee to maintain the legs in slight flexion. Again, a small pillow placed beneath the head may add to the comfort of the client.

The room should be sufficiently warm that the draped client does not shiver, thereby tensing the abdominal wall. A further advantage may be obtained by instructing the client to relax and to breathe quietly and slowly through the mouth. Words of explanation and support may help to ease tension.

The entire abdomen must be free of clothing. An examination gown may be folded up over the chest, or a small towel may be used to cover the breasts of women. A sheet may be folded downward to the level of the mons.

A single source of light is used in inspection of the abdomen (Fig. 15-1). The light may be directed at a right angle to the long axis of the client or may be focused lengthwise over him, shining from the foot to the head. The examiner assumes a sitting position generally at the right side of the client; the examiner's head is only slightly higher than the client's abdomen. The resultant shadow will be high, so that even small changes in contour will be highlighted, thereby increasing the likelihood of detection of a pathological condition. The examiner should carefully focus his attention on the abdomen for several minutes in order to accurately describe the presence or absence of symmetry, distention, masses, visible peristaltic waves, and respiratory movements.

The client is instructed to take a deep breath, forcing the diaphragm downward and decreasing the size of the abdominal cavity. In this manner, masses such as the enlarged liver or spleen are made more obvious.

The examiner should then inspect the abdomen from a standing position at the foot of the bed or examining table. Asymmetry of the abdominal contour may be more readily detected from this position.

■ Anatomical mapping

Definitive description of signs and symptoms of the abdomen is facilitated through two commonly used methods of subdivision. The most frequently used method divides the abdomen into four quadrants (Fig. 15-2). An imaginary perpendicular line is dropped from the sternum to the pubic bone through the umbilicus, and a second

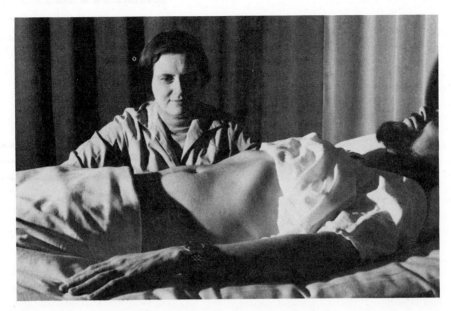

Fig. 15-1. Inspection of the abdomen with the examining light focused to provide the greatest amount of contrast for the abdominal terrain.

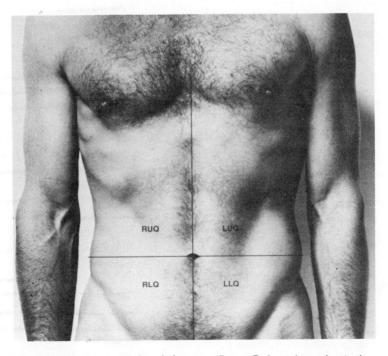

Fig. 15-2. The four quadrants of the abdomen. (From G. I. series; physical examination of the abdomen, part 1, Inspection, Richmond, Va., 1969, A. H. Robins Co.)

line is dropped at a right angle to the first through the umbilicus.

For the most part, abdominal structures will be located in these quadrants as shown below.

Loops of the small bowel are found in all four quadrants. The bladder and the uterus are located at the lower midline.

Right upper quadrant	Left upper quadrant
Liver and gallbladder	Left lobe of liver
Pylorus	Spleen
Duodenum	Stomach
Head of pancreas	Body of pancreas
Right adrenal gland	Left adrenal gland
Portion of right kidney	Portion of left kidney
Hepatic flexure of colon	Splenic flexure of colon
Portions of ascending and transverse colon	Portions of transverse and descending colon
Right lower quadrant	**Left lower quadrant**
Lower pole of right kidney	Lower pole of left kidney
Cecum and appendix	Sigmoid colon
Portion of ascending colon	Portion of descending colon
Bladder (if distended)	Bladder (if distended)
Ovary and salpinx	Ovary and salpinx
Uterus (if enlarged)	Uterus (if enlarged)
Right spermatic cord	Left spermatic cord
Right ureter	Left ureter

Right hypochondriac	Epigastric	Left hypochondriac
Right lobe of liver	Pyloric end of stomach	Stomach
Gallbladder	Duodenum	Spleen
Portion of duodenum	Pancreas	Tail of pancreas
Hepatic flexure of colon	Portion of liver	Splenic flexure of colon
Portion of right kidney		Upper pole of left kidney
Suprarenal gland		Suprarenal gland
Right lumbar	**Umbilical**	**Left lumbar**
Ascending colon	Omentum	Descending colon
Lower half of right kidney	Mesentery	Lower half of left kidney
Portion of duodenum and jejunum	Lower part of duodenum	Portions of jejunum and ileum
	Jejunum and ileum	
Right inguinal	**Hypogastric**	**Left inguinal**
Cecum	Ileum	Sigmoid colon
Appendix	Bladder	Left ureter
Lower end of ileum	Uterus (in pregnancy)	Left spermatic cord
Right ureter		Left ovary
Right spermatic cord		
Right ovary		

The second method of establishing zones of the abdomen results in nine sections (Fig. 15-3). This is accomplished by dropping two imaginary vertical lines from the midclavicles to the middle of Poupart's ligament, analogous to the lateral borders of the rectus abdominis muscles. At right angles to these lines, two imaginary parallel lines cross the border of the costal margin and the anterosuperior spine of the iliac bones. Essentially, the abdominal structures correlate with the zones shown in the lower left column.

Certain anatomical structures have been used as landmarks to facilitate the description of abdominal signs and symptoms (Fig. 15-4). The following landmarks have been useful for this purpose: the ensiform process of the sternum, the costal margin, the midline—drawn from the tip of the sternum through the umbilicus to the pubic bone, the umbilicus, the anterosuperior iliac spine, Poupart's ligament, and the superior margin of the os pubis.

■ Skin

Attention is directed to the skin. The abdomen is an especially valuable area for observation of the skin since it encompasses a relatively large expanse of skin. Inspection of the abdominal skin for pigmentation, lesions, striae, scars, dehydration, general nutritional status, and venous patterns may yield valuable information regarding the client's general state of health.

Pigmentation. Because the skin of the abdomen is frequently protected from the sun by clothing, it may serve as a baseline for comparison with the pigmentation of the more tanned areas. Jaundice is more readily observed in this less exposed skin. Irregular patches of faint pigmentation may be due to von Recklinghausen's disease.

Lesions. The observation of skin lesions is of particular significance since gastrointestinal alterations are frequently associated with skin changes.

Generally, the skin lesions are secondary to gastrointestinal disease. However, skin lesions and gastrointestinal disease may arise from the same cause; they may also occur without interrelationship.

Although the presence of small, hard, painless nodules over a wide area of the abdomen may be due to metastasis of malignancy, they are generally not due to carcinoma of the abdominal viscera.

Tense and glistening skin is often correlated with ascites or edema of the abdominal wall.

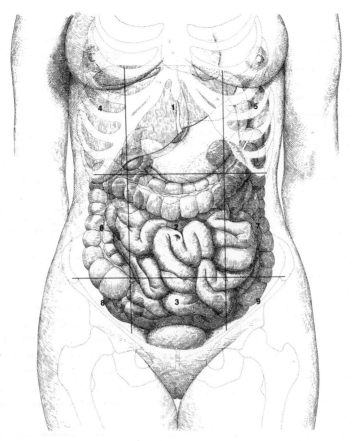

Fig. 15-3. The nine regions of the abdomen. *1,* Epigastric; *2,* umbilical; *3,* pubic; *4* and *5,* right and left hypochondriac; *6* and *7,* right and left lumbar; *8* and *9,* right and left inguinal. (From G. I. series; physical examination of the abdomen, part 1, Inspection, Richmond, Va., 1969, A. H. Robins Co.)

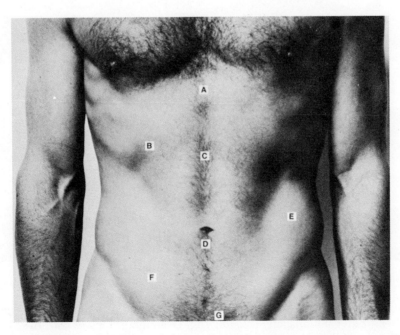

Fig. 15-4. Landmarks of the abdomen. *A,* Ensiform process of the sternum; *B,* costal margin; *C,* midline; *D,* umbilicus; *E,* anterosuperior iliac spine; *F,* Poupart's ligament; *G,* superior margin of the os pubis. (From G. I. series; physical examination of the abdomen, part 1, Inspection, Richmond, Va., 1969, A. H. Robins Co.)

Striae. Linea albicantes, or striae, are atrophic lines or streaks that may be seen in the skin of the abdomen following such rapid or prolonged stretching of the skin that the elastic fibers of the reticular layer of the cutis are disrupted. Striae of recent origin are pink or blue in hue but progress to a silvery white color. Striae occuring as a result of Cushing's disease, however, remain purple. The stretching of abdominal skin may occur as a result of an abdominal tumor, ascites, obesity, or pregnancy.

Scars. Inspection of the abdomen for scars may yield valuable data concerning previous surgery or trauma. The size and shape of scars are best described through the use of a drawing of the abdomen on which the landmarks or quadrants are shown and the dimensions noted in centimeters, as in the following:

If the cause of the scar was not elicited in the history, the information is sought during inspection. The fact that the client has experienced a previous surgery should alert the examiner to the possibility that adhesions may be present.

Deep, irregular scars may indicate burns. Some individuals produce a dense overgrowth of fibrous tissue in the healing process. This overgrowth is called a keloid and consists of large, essentially parallel bands of dense collagenous material, separated by bands of cellular fibrous tissue. Keloid formation most frequently occurs following a traumatic injury or burn. Increased prevalence of keloid formation has been noted in black individuals and those of Asian extraction.

■ **Contour**

Contralateral areas of the normal abdomen are symmetrical in contour and appearance. The contour of the normal abdomen is described as flat, rounded, or scaphoid. Contour is a description of the profile line from the rib margin to the pubic bone, viewed from a right angle to the umbilicus with the client in a recumbent position (Fig. 15-5).

A flat contour is one wherein the abdominal

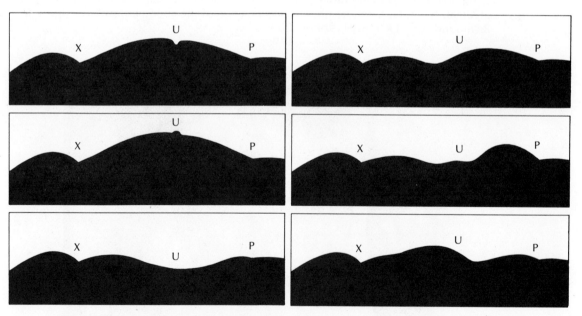

Fig. 15-5. Abdominal profiles. *Left. Top,* Generalized distention, with umbilicus inverted: obesity or recent distention from gas. *Middle,* Generalized distention with umbilicus everted, chronic ascites, tumor, or umbilical hernia. *Bottom,* Scaphoid abdomen from malnourishment. *Right. Top,* Distention of lower half: ovarian tumor, pregnancy, or bladder. *Middle,* Distention of lower third: ovarian tumor, uterine fibroids, pregnancy, or bladder. *Bottom,* Distention of upper half: carcinomatosis, pancreatic cyst, gastric dilatation. *X,* xiphoid; *U,* umbilicus; *P,* pubis. (From G. I. series; physical examination of the abdomen, part 1, Inspection, Richmond, Va., 1969, A. H. Robins Co.)

wall is viewed as an essentially horizontal plane from the rib margins to the pubic bone. The flat contour is seen in the muscularly competent and well-nourished individual.

A rounded contour is the description given the convex profile made by the abdominal wall to the horizontal plane. With the individual in the recumbent position, the maximum height of the convexity is at the umbilicus. However, when the individual stands, the convexity has its greatest height between the umbilicus and the symphysis pubis because of the pull of gravity. The rounded abdomen is normal in the young child, but in the adult it is generally due to poor muscle tone or excessive subcutaneous fat deposits, or both. The rounded abdomen is often called the "spare tire" or "bay window" of middle age.

A scaphoid contour depicts a concave profile to the horizontal plane and may be seen in thin clients of all ages. The scaphoid contour reflects a decrease in fat deposits in the abdominal wall, as well as a relaxed or flaccid abdominal musculature.

If an umbilical or incisional hernia or diastasis recti abdominis is suspected, the client is instructed to raise his head from the pillow, increasing the intra-abdominal pressure, which may cause the hernia to protrude. The rectus muscles will contract, and a separation will be revealed.

Distention. Distention is the term used for unusual stretching of the abdominal wall. The presence of distention generally implies disease and therefore warrants further investigation. *Asymmetrical distention* of the abdominal wall may be due to hernia, tumor, cysts, or bowel obstruction. A mnemonic device for classifying the six common causes of distention are fluid, flatulence, fat, feces, fetus, and fibroid tumor.

Generalized, or symmetrical, distention of the abdomen with the umbilicus in its normal inverted position is generally due to obesity or recent pressure of fluid or gas within the hollow viscera. If the umbilicus is observed to be everted (umbilical hernia), ascites or underlying tumor may be the cause. Ovarian tumor, distended bladder, or pregnancy may be suspected if the distention is confined to the area between the umbilicus and the symphysis pubis; distention of the lower third of the abdomen suggests ovarian tumor, uterine fibroid tumor, pregnancy, or bladder enlargement (Fig. 15-5). Possible causes of distention of the upper half of the abdominal wall include pancreatic cyst or tumor and gastric dilatation.

■ Movement

Respiratory movement. Observation of respiratory movement has more significance in the male client since the female client manages gaseous exchange mainly with costal movement. On the other hand, the male client evidences essentially abdominal respiratory movement at rest. Peritonitis or other abdominal infection and disease may limit this abdominal respiratory action in the male client.

Whereas abdominal breathing is the mode in the child who is less than 6 or 7 years of age, the presence of abdominal respiratory movements in an older child may indicate respiratory problems. The absence of abdominal respiratory movements in the child who is less than 6 is suggestive of peritoneal irritation. Retraction of the abdominal wall on inspiration is called Czerny's sign and is associated with some central nervous system (CNS) diseases, such as chorea.

Visible peristalsis. Motility of the stomach and intestines may be reflected in movement of the abdominal wall in lean individuals, even in the absence of disease. However, when strong contractions are visible through an abdominal wall of average thickness, the possibility of bowel obstruction should be investigated. The abdomen is observed for several minutes from just above the level of the abdominal profile while the examiner sits at the client's side, gazing across the abdomen. Weak peristalsis may be augmented by percussing the abdomen. Peristaltic waves of the stomach and small intestine may be seen as elevated oblique bands in the upper left quadrant that move downward to the right. Several of these peristaltic waves occurring in rapid succession may produce a series of parallel bands or a "ladder effect."

Reverse peristalsis, observed in the upper abdomen in an infant, is seen as an undulation moving from left to right. This observation indicates the presence of pyloric stenosis or, more rarely, duodenal stenosis or malrotation of the bowel.

Before touching the abdomen, the examiner asks the client whether any of the abdominal areas are painful or tender. If the answer is positive, the areas the client indicates are treated with gentleness.

AUSCULTATION

Auscultatory findings of diagnostic significance are those sounds originating from the viscera, the arterial system, the venous system, muscular activity, or parietal friction rubs. Light pressure on

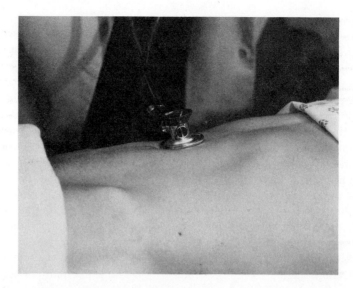

Fig. 15-6. Auscultation for bowel sounds. Intestinal sounds are relatively high pitched; the diaphragm of the stethoscope is used.

the stethoscope is sufficient to detect bowel sounds as well as bruits (Fig. 15-6). Because the abdominal intestinal sounds are relatively high pitched, the diaphragm of the stethoscope, which accentuates the higher-pitched sounds, should be used. However, the bell may be used in exploring certain arterial murmurs and venous hums.

■ Peristaltic sounds

The use of the stethoscope to hear the sounds of air and fluid as they move through the gastrointestinal tract can provide valuable diagnostic clues relevant to the motility of the bowel. Normal bowel sounds occur approximately every 5 to 15 seconds. Some authorities suggest that the number is as high as 15 to 20 per minute, or roughly, 1 bowel sound for each breath sound. However, peristaltic sounds may be quite irregular. Thus, it is recommended that the examiner listen for at least 5 minutes before concluding that no bowel sounds are present. The duration of a single sound may be less than a second or may extend over several seconds. The frequency of sounds is related to the presence of food in the gastrointestinal tract or to the state of digestion. Uninterrupted bowel sounds may be heard over the ileocecal valve 4 to 7 hours following a meal. A silent abdomen, that is, the absence of bowel sounds, indicates the arrest of intestinal motility. Stimulation of peristalsis may be achieved by flicking the abdominal wall with a finger or by dropping ether on the skin.

Stomach sounds may be heard in a well child

by rocking him back and forth. The presence of fluid within the stomach may produce a splash.

The two significant alterations in bowel sounds are (1) the absence of any sound or extremely soft and widely separated sounds; and (2) increased sounds with a characteristically high-pitched, loud, rushing sound.

Decreased bowel sounds. Inhibition of motility of the bowel is accompanied by diminished or absent bowel sounds. Decreased motility occurs with inflammation, gangrene, or reflex ileus. Peritonitis, electrolyte disturbances, the aftermath of surgical manipulation of the bowel, and late bowel obstruction are frequently accompanied by decreased peristalsis. In addition, diminished bowel sounds are often correlated with pneumonia.

Increased bowel sounds. Loud, gurgling borborygmi accompany increased motility of the bowel. Sounds of loud volume also are heard over areas of a stenotic bowel. Sounds resulting from an early bowel obstruction are high pitched. These may be splash sounds, like that of the emptying of a bottle into a hollow vessel. Fine metallic, tinkling sounds are emitted as tiny gas bubbles break through the surface of intestinal juices. Increased motility may be the result of a laxative or gastroenteritis. Common pathological conditions associated with increased bowel sounds are gastroenteritis and subsiding ileus.

■ Vascular sounds

Arterial sounds. A bruit that is heard while the client is in a variety of positions and with the bell

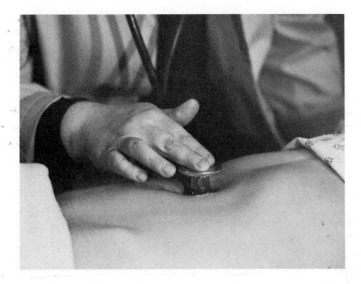

Fig. 15-7. Auscultation for bruits is performed with the bell of the stethoscope held lightly against the abdomen.

Fig. 15-8. Scratch test in assessment of liver size. The stethoscope is placed over the liver while the other hand scratches lightly over the abdominal surface with short, transverse strokes; when the scratch is done over the liver, the sound is magnified.

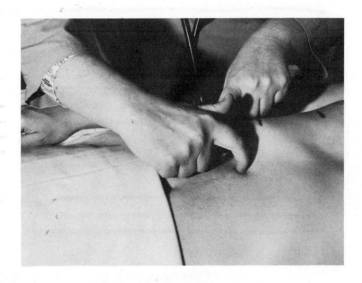

of the stethoscope held lightly against the abdomen may indicate a dilated, tortuous, or constricted vessel (Fig. 15-7). Loud bruits detected over the aorta may indicate the presence of an aneurysm. Soft, medium- to low-pitched murmurs due to renal arterial stenosis may be heard over the midline or toward the flank. For the hypertensive client, particular care is devoted to listening over the center and posterior flank for a bruit in the arterial tree.

Venous hums. A normal hum originating from the inferior vena cava and its large tributaries is continuously audible through the stethoscope. Its tone is medium pitched in quality and is similar to a muscular fibrillary hum. In the presence of obstructed portal circulation, as from a cirrhotic liver, an abnormal venous hum may be detected in the periumbilical region. Pressure on the bell

of the stethoscope must be avoided since this may obscure the hum. The hum may be accompanied by a palpable thrill.

Another pathological hum accompanies the dilated periumbilical circulation of Cruveilheir-Baumgarten disease. The hum may be detected near the midline between the umbilicus and the xiphoid process. Hepatic angiomas may produce hums that can be auscultated over the liver.

■ Scratch test

The scratch test utilizes the difference in sound over solid as opposed to hollow organs. It is occasionally used to assess the size of the liver. The stethoscope is placed over the liver while the opposite hand scratches lightly over the abdominal surface with short, transverse strokes (Fig. 15-8). When the scratch occurs over the liver, the sound is magnified. Although the test is of questionable accuracy, it is thought to be of some value in assessing the individual with abdominal distention or spastic abdominal muscles.

■ Peritoneal friction rub

Peritoneal friction rub provides a rough, grating sound described as like that of two pieces of leather being rubbed together. Because the liver and spleen have large surface areas in contact with the peritoneum, these two structures are most often the originating sites of the peritoneal friction rubs.

Common causes of friction rubs include splenic infection, abscess, or tumor; these are heard best over the lower rib cage in the anterior axillary line. Deep respiration may emphasize the sound. Liver tumor and abscess are the usual causes of peritoneal friction rubs located over the lower right rib cage.

■ Muscular activity sounds

A fibrillating muscle produces a hum that can be heard with a stethoscope. Both voluntary and involuntary contraction (as in muscle guarding of a painful area) produces this sound. The hum is often accentuated by palpation of the tender area.

PERCUSSION

Percussion of the abdomen is aimed at detecting fluid, gaseous distention, and masses and in assessing solid structures within the abdomen

(Fig. 15-9). The major contribution of this technique, in the absence of disease, is the delineation of the position and size of the liver and spleen.

The entire abdomen should be percussed lightly for a general picture of the areas of tympany and dullness. Tympany will predominate because of the presence of gas in the large and small bowel. Solid masses will percuss as dull, as will the distended bladder.

To lessen the chance of omitting any portion of the examination, the practitioner should establish a definite pattern or route that he habitually uses in percussing abdominal structures.

■ Assessment of the liver span

Percussion done to determine the size of the liver is begun in the right midclavicular line at a level below the umbilicus (Fig. 15-10). The percussion is done over a region of gas-filled bowel (tympanitic) and progressed upward toward the liver. The lower border of the liver is indicated by the first dull percussion note, and the site is marked on the abdomen. The upper border of liver dullness is ascertained by starting the percussion in the midclavicular line and examining caudally from an area of the lung resonance to the first dull percussion note (generally the fifth to seventh interspace). This spot is duly marked, and the distance between the two marks is measured in centimeters (Fig. 15-11). Other sites for measurement are the anterior axillary line and the midsternal line.

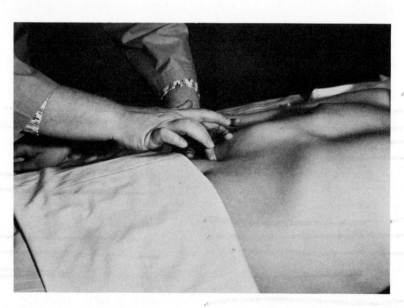

Fig. 15-9. Percussion of the abdomen for evaluation of fluid, gaseous distention, and masses within the abdominal cavity.

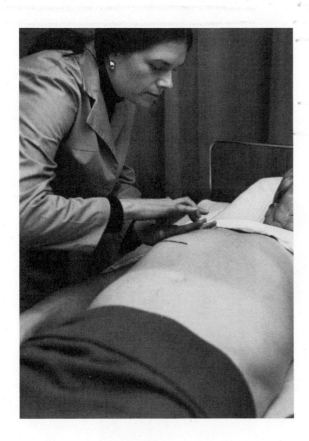

Fig. 15-10. Percussion method of estimating the size of the liver. Lower border percussion is begun over a region of air- or gas-filled bowel and carried upward to the dull percussion note of the liver. The spot is marked. Upper border percussion is performed over the midclavicular line from an area of lung resonance to the first dull percussion note (generally the fifth to seventh interspace). The spot is marked.

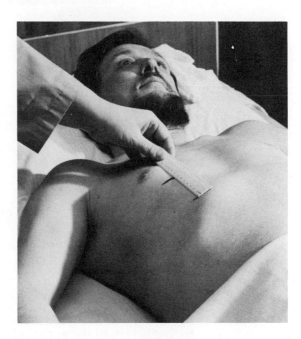

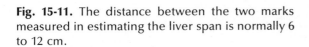

Fig. 15-11. The distance between the two marks measured in estimating the liver span is normally 6 to 12 cm.

Suggested values for normal are 6 to 12 cm in the midclavicular line and 4 to 8 cm in the midsternal line. A liver span greater than 11 cm in the midclavicular line is considered indicative of hepatomegaly. A less accurate sign of an enlarged liver is the percussion or palpation of the liver edge 2 or 3 cm below the costal margin in the midclavicular line. The liver span is seen to be greater in men than in women and in the tall as opposed to the short individual. Error in estimating the liver span can occur when pleural effusion or lung consolidation obscures the upper liver border or when gas in the colon obscures the lower border.

On inspiration the diaphragm moves downward; thus, the span of liver dullness will normally be shifted inferiorly 2 to 3 cm. Pulmonary edema may also displace the liver caudally, whereas ascites, massive tumors, or pregnancy may push the liver upward.

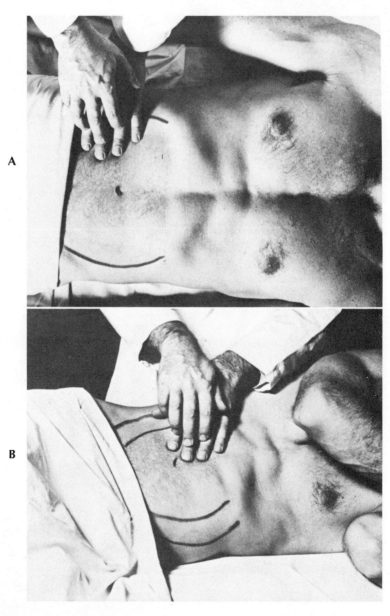

Fig. 15-12. Test for shifting dullness. **A,** With the client on his back, the line of dullness is marked in both flanks. **B,** The client is rotated on one side and then the other, and the new levels of dullness are marked each time. (From G. I. series; physical examination of the abdomen, part 3, Percussion, Richmond, Va., 1972, A. H. Robins Co.)

■ Percussion for tympany and dullness

Spleen. Splenic dullness may be percussed at the level of the sixth to the tenth rib just posterior to the midaxillary line.

Stomach. A lower-pitched tympany than that of the intestine is typical of the percussion note of the gastric air bubble. Percussion is performed in the area of the left lower anterior rib cage and in the left epigastric region to define the region occupied by the bubble.

Test for shifting dullness. A technique for differentiating ascites from cysts or edema fluid in the abdominal wall is the percussion test for shifting dullness (Fig. 15-12).

The client is placed in the supine position, and fluid dullness is percussed laterally in the flank while the abdomen medial to the dullness is tym-

panic due to the presence of gas within the bowel. The line of demarcation between the dull and tympanitic sounds is marked, and the client is instructed to lie on his side. The ascites fluid will flow via gravity to shift the line of dullness closer to the umbilicus. A new line is marked, and the change is measured in centimeters. Subsequently, the client is turned to the opposite side and the change recorded. The test enables the examiner to detect free fluid as well as make a rough estimate of the volume.

Knee-chest position. Percussion of the periumbilical region of a client in the knee-chest position enables the examiner to detect smaller amounts of fluid than is possible with the individual supine.

Puddle sign. After maintaining the client in the

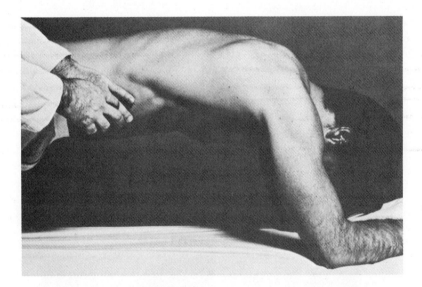

Fig. 15-13. Elicitation of the puddle sign. (From G. I. series; physical examination of the abdomen, part 3, Percussion, Richmond, Va., 1972, A. H. Robins Co.)

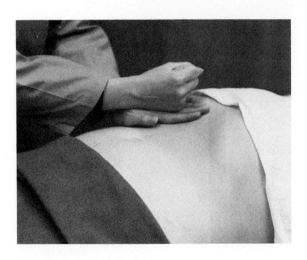

Fig. 15-14. Fist percussion of the liver. The palm of the hand is placed over the region of liver dullness and is struck a light blow with the fisted right hand. Tenderness elicited by this method is usually due to hepatitis or cholecystitis. Fist percussion may be used over the costovertebral junction to elicit renal tenderness.

knee-chest position for several minutes so that ascitic fluid puddles over the umbilicus by gravity, the examiner percusses the umbilical area for the dull notes of fluid (Fig. 15-13).

■ Fist percussion

Another use of percussion in the abdominal examination is the use of fist percussion to vibrate the tissue rather than produce sound (Fig. 15-14). The palm of the left hand is placed over the region of liver dullness and is struck a light blow by the fisted right hand. Tenderness elicited by this method is usually associated with hepatitis or cholecystitis. Fist percussion at the costovertebral junction is also useful in assessing renal tenderness.

PALPATION

Following careful visual scrutiny, auscultation, and percussion, palpation is used to substantiate findings and to further explore the abdomen. Palpation is used to evaluate the major organs of the abdomen; these organs are examined with respect to shape, position and mobility, size, consistency, and tension. Thorough and systematic screening is performed to detect areas of tenderness, muscular spasm, masses, or fluid.

The client's position is checked to make sure that maximum relaxation has been achieved. The examiner's hands should be warm, and the examiner should use techniques for enhancing bodily and psychological relaxation. Observation that the client does not relax the abdominal muscles in spite of these maneuvers may justify the use of the technique wherein the examiner exerts downward pressure on the lower sternum with his left hand while palpating with the other. The deeper inspiration that results inhibits abdominal muscle contraction. A suggestion for achieving relaxation in children is that of putting them into a tub of warm water. The examiner is at the right side of the client, and the fingers of the examining hand are approximated. Measurements are more accurately recorded in centimeters. The older method of describing distance in finger breadths invites error since the finger of examiners are of varying diameters.

■ Light palpation

Light palpation is gentle exploration performed with the hand parallel to the floor, the palm lying lightly on the abdomen, and the fingers approximated (Fig. 15-15). The fingers depress the abdominal wall approximately 1 cm without digging. This method of palpation is best for eliciting slight tenderness, large masses, and muscle guarding. Frequently an enlarged or distended structure may be appreciated with this light touch as a sense of resistance.

Areas of tenderness or guarding, or both, defined by light palpation will alert the examiner to proceed with caution in the application of more

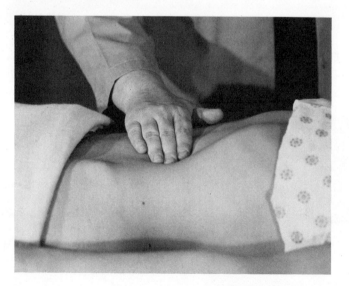

Fig. 15-15. Light palpation is performed with the hand parallel to the floor and the fingers approximated. The fingers depress the abdominal wall about 1 cm. This method of palpation is recommended for eliciting slight tenderness, large masses, and muscle guarding.

vigorous manipulation of these structures during the remainder of the examination.

■ Assessment of hypersensitivity

Zones of hypersensitivity of sensory nerve fibers of the skin have been described and are thought to reflect specific zones of peritoneal irritation. These are called Head's zones of cutaneous hypersensitivity (Fig. 15-16). Although the research has not provided proof for all of the zones, clinical reliance has been demonstrated for the zone shown for the appendix in cases of appendicitis and for the midepigastrium in the individual with peptic ulcer.

Evaluation of this hypersensitivity may be achieved in two ways. One method is to stimulate gently with the sharp end of an open safety pin, a wisp of cotton, or the finger nail (Fig. 15-17). The second method is to gently lift a fold of skin away from the underlying musculature (Fig. 15-18). The alert patient may be able to describe his reaction to this stimulation, or changes in facial expression (grimacing) may indicate the increased sensation the individual is experiencing.

■ Assessment of muscle spasticity

Involuntary muscle contraction or spasticity may indicate peritoneal irritation. Further palpation is done to determine whether the spasticity is unilateral or on both sides of the abdomen. Generalized and boardlike contraction is thought to be typical of peritonitis. Further definition is achieved by asking the client to raise his trunk from a horizontal position without arm support. The experience of unilateral pain in response to this maneuver may further pinpoint the areas of spasticity. This mechanism may also help to differentiate muscle contraction from abdominal mass; as the head is raised, the hand would be moved away from an abdominal mass. Rigidity and tenderness over McBurney's point and in some cases over the entire right side is strongly suggestive of appendicitis. Acute cholecystitis is frequently accompanied by rigidity of the right hypochondrium.

■ Moderate palpation

The side of the hand rather than the fingertips is used in moderate palpation (Fig. 15-19). This

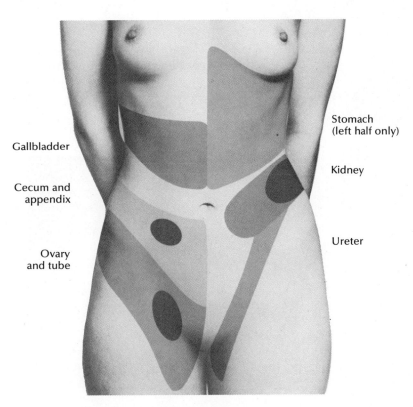

Fig. 15-16. Head's zones of cutaneous hypersensitivity. (From G. I. series; physical examination of the abdomen, part 2, Palpation, Richmond, Va., 1972, A. H. Robins Co.)

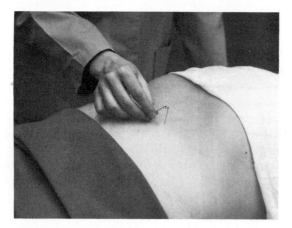

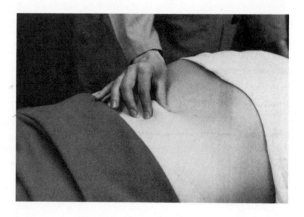

Fig. 15-17. Assessment of superficial pain sensation of the abdomen.

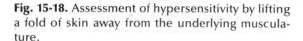

Fig. 15-18. Assessment of hypersensitivity by lifting a fold of skin away from the underlying musculature.

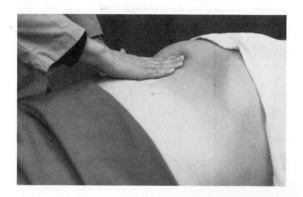

Fig. 15-19. Moderate palpation is performed with the side of the hand. This method of palpation is particularly useful in assessing organs that move with respiration, such as the liver and spleen.

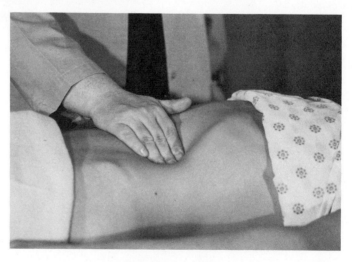

Fig. 15-20. Deep palpation is performed by pressing the distal half of the palmar surfaces of the fingers into the abdominal wall. Deep structures such as the retroperitoneal organs are assessed by deep palpation.

method obviates the tendency to dig into the abdomen with the fingertips as well as the resultant discomfort and involuntary guarding that may accompany such focal probing.

The sensation produced by palpating with the side of the hand is particularly useful in assessing organs that move with respiration, such as the liver and the spleen. The organ is felt during normal breathing cycles and then as the client takes a deep breath. On inspiration the organ will be pushed downward against the examining hand.

Tenderness not elicited by gentle palpation may be perceived by the client on deeper pressure.

Deep palpation

Deep palpation is indentation of the abdomen performed by pressing the distal half of the palmar surfaces of the fingers into the abdominal wall (Fig. 15-20). The abdominal wall may slide back and forth while the fingers are moving back and forth over the organ being examined. Deeper structures, such as retroperitoneal organs (the kidneys), or masses may be felt with this method. Tenderness of organs not elicited by light or moderate palpation may be uncovered with this method. In the absence of disease, the pressure produced by deep palpation may produce tenderness over the cecum, the sigmoid colon, and the aorta.

The technique of deep palpation may help to give more specific information concerning a lesion or mass detected by lighter palpation.

Bimanual palpation

Superimposition of one hand. Bimanual palpation with superimposition of one hand may be used when additional pressure is necessary to overcome resistance or to examine a deep abdominal structure. In this method one hand is superimposed over the other, so that pressure is exerted by the upper hand while the lower hand remains relaxed and sensitive to the tactile sensation produced by the structure being examined. Generally, for the right-handed examiner the left hand is the lower, or examining, hand while the right hand applies pressure exerted by the tips of the left fingers on the terminal interphalangeal points of the examining fingers (Fig. 15-21). The technique is recommended because the palpating hand is less sensitive if it has to be used to exert pressure at the same time.

Trapping technique. Both hands may be used to establish the size of a mass. The mass is trapped between the examining hands for measurement.

Detection of a pulsatile mass. Pulsation may be sensed in the fingertips of both hands as they are pushed apart as a pulsatile flow expands a structure such as the aorta; pulsation may also be felt in a mass held between the examining hands. This palpatory finding indicates that the structure being felt is pulsating rather than transmitting pulsation. The normal aorta is approximately 2.5 to 4 cm wide, whereas an aneurysm is a good deal broader. As noted previously, a bruit is generally heard over an aneurysm. The most common

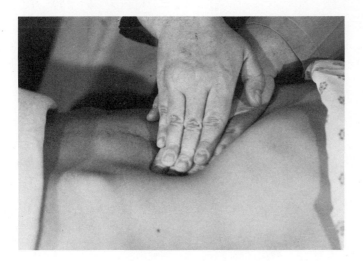

Fig. 15-21. Bimanual palpation with superimposition of one hand. Pressure is exerted by the upper hand while the lower hand remains relaxed and sensitive to tactile stimulation.

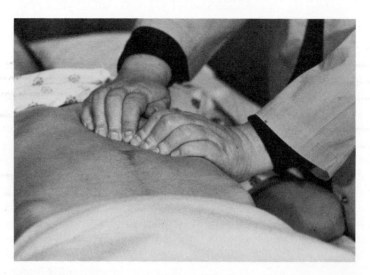

Fig. 15-22. Bimanual palpation with the hands side by side. Descent of the liver or spleen is often measured by hooking the fingers over the costal margin from above.

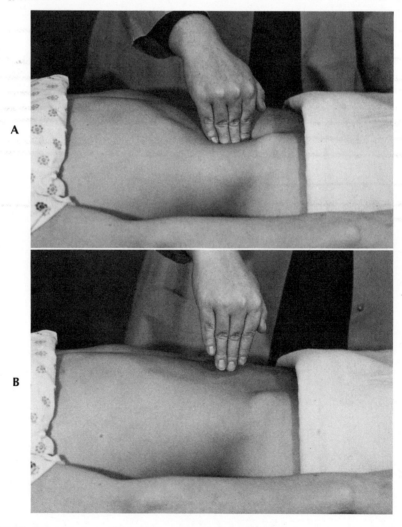

Fig. 15-23. Palpation to elicit rebound tenderness. **A,** Deep pressure is applied to the abdominal wall. **B,** On release of pressure, a sensation of pain would indicate peritoneal irritation.

physical finding in clients with an abdominal aneurysm is the presence of an expansile, pulsating mass, more than 95% of which are located inferior to the renal arteries but generally at or above the umbilicus. Femoral pulses are usually present but are markedly damped in amplitude. More than half of clients with abdominal aneurysms are asymptomatic; thus, the mass might be discovered during a screening physical. Although more than 80% of abdominal aneurysms can be palpated, small aneurysms in the markedly obese client may not be felt.

Hands approximated (side by side). Minimal descent of the liver or spleen below the costal margin is occasionally detected by hooking the fingers over the costal margin from above while standing beside the thorax, facing the client's feet (Fig. 15-22).

The outline of a tubular structure such as the sigmoid colon or cecum can frequently be more specifically outlined with the hands side by side, rolling the fingers over the structure.

■ Palpation to elicit rebound tenderness

To provoke rebound tenderness, the approximated fingers are pushed gently but deeply in a region remote from that suspected of tenderness and then rapidly removed (Fig. 15-23). The rebound of the structures indented by palpation causes a sharp stabbing sensation of pain on the side of the inflammation. This sensation of pain following the withdrawal of pressure is a sign of peritoneal irritation. The test may be repeated over to the side of the suspected disease. The test is best performed near the conclusion of the examination, since the production of severe pain or muscle spasm may interfere with subsequent examination. Voluntary coughing by the client may produce the same results.

■ Ballottement (Fig. 15-24)

Single-handed ballottement. Single-handed ballottement is performed with the fingers extended in a straight line with the forearm and at a right angle to the abdomen. The fingers are moved quickly toward the mass or organ to be examined and held there. As fluid or other structures are displaced, the mass will move upward and be felt at the fingertips. Some examiners prefer this technique for examination of the spleen.

Bimanual ballottement. Bimanual ballottement is accomplished by using one hand to push on the anterior abdominal wall to displace contents to the flank while the other receives the mass or structure pushed against it and feels the dimensions.

■ Demonstration of ascites

The presence of large amounts of fluid within the peritoneal cavity allows the elicitation of a

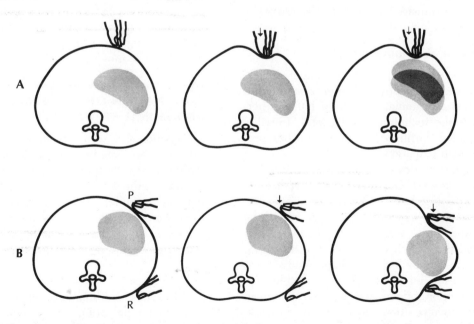

Fig. 15-24. Ballottement. **A,** Single-handed ballottement. **B,** Bimanual ballottement: *P,* pushing hand; *R,* receiving hand. (From G. I. series; physical examination of the abdomen, part 2, Palpation, Richmond, Va., 1972, A. H. Robins Co.)

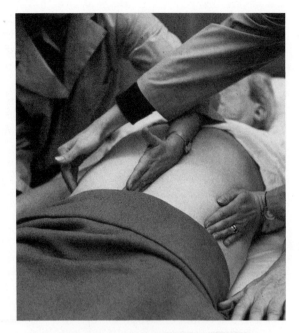

Fig. 15-25. Test for presence of a fluid wave.

Table 15-1. Characteristics of abdominal masses related to common pathological conditions

Description of mass	Possible pathological condition
Descends on inspiration	Liver, spleen, or kidney mass
Pulsatile mass	Abdominal aneurysm, tortuous aorta
Movable from side to side, not head to foot	Mesenteric or small bowel mass
Complete fixation	Tumor of pancreatic or retroperitoneal origin

cavity will be more difficult to feel or will be pushed out of reach altogether.

Normal abdominal structures occasionally mistaken for masses are:

Lateral borders of the rectus abdominis muscles
Uterus
Feces-filled ascending colon
Feces-filled descending colon and sigmoid colon
Aorta
Common iliac artery
Sacral promontory

Palpable bowel segments. The presence of feces within the bowel frequently contributes to the examiner's ability to palpate the cecum, the ascending colon, the descending colon, and the sigmoid colon. The feces-filled cecum and ascending colon produce a sensation suggestive of a soft, boggy, rounded mass. The client may complain of cramps resulting from stimulation of the bowel by the movements of palpation.

fluid wave (Fig. 15-25). To test for the presence of a fluid wave, the client is placed in a supine position. The examiner places the palmar surface of one hand firmly against the lateral abdominal wall and taps the contralateral wall with his other hand. An assistant places the edge of his hand and lower arm firmly in the vertical midline of the client's abdomen to damp vibrations that might otherwise be transmitted through the tissues of the anterior abdominal wall.

■ Palpation for abdominal masses

All of the quadrants of the abdomen are examined systematically by palpation. For the most part, bimanual examination with the hands superimposed is the technique most useful. Initially, light palpation is utilized; the examiner then proceeds to deep palpation.

The characteristics of an abdominal mass are carefully described. Of particular importance are consistency, regularity of contour movement with respiration, and mobility. A sketch of the anterior abdominal wall with all of its bony landmarks and the umbilicus may be the most efficient way to convey location, shape, and size.

Difficulties in determining that a palpable mass is in the anterior abdominal wall rather than in an intra-abdominal position may be resolved by asking the client to flex the abdominal muscles. Masses in the subcutaneous tissue will continue to be palpable, whereas those in the peritoneal

EXAMINATION OF THE SPECIFIC ABDOMINAL STRUCTURES

Palpation is a useful technique for identification and assessment of the specific abdominal structures. A systematic approach, always beginning at the same area, is suggested in order that the examiner not skip any part of the abdomen. Since most examiners approach the client from the right, the liver may prove to be the most convenient structure to palpate first.

■ Liver

Two types of bimanual palpation are recommended for palpation of the liver. The first of these is superimposition of the right hand over the left hand. The client is asked to breathe normally for two or three breaths. Then he is asked

Table 15-2. Characteristics of hepatomegaly related to common pathological conditions

Description of liver	Possible pathological condition
Smooth, nontender	Portal cirrhosis
	Lymphoma
	Passive congestion of the liver
	Portal obstruction
	Obstruction of the vena cava
	Lymphocytic leukemia
	Ricketts
	Amyloidosis
	Schistosomiasis
Smooth, tender	Acute hepatitis
	Amebic hepatitis or abscess
	Early congestive cardiac failure
Nodular	Late portal cirrhosis
	Tertiary syphilis
	Metastatic carcinoma
Hard	Carcinomatosis

to breathe deeply. The diaphragm is exerted downward in inspiration and will push the liver toward the examining hand. The liver usually cannot be palpated in the normal adult. However, in extremely thin but otherwise well individuals, it may be felt at the costal margin. When the normal liver margin is palpated, it feels regular in contour and somewhat sharp.

In the second technique, the left hand is placed beneath the client at the level of the eleventh and twelfth ribs and upward pressure applied in order to throw the liver forward toward the examining right hand. The palmar surface of the examiner's right hand is placed parallel to the right costal margin. As the client inspires, the liver may be felt to slip beneath the examining fingers.

Tenderness over the liver may be demonstrated by placing the palm of one hand over the lateral costal margin and delivering a blow to that hand with the ulnar surface of the other hand, which has been curled into a fist.

Gallbladder

Whereas the normal gallbladder cannot be felt, a distended gallbladder may be palpated below the liver margin at the lateral border of the rectus muscle. The cystic nature of the mass helps in the identification of the gallbladder. There is, however, a good deal of variation in the location of the left border; it may be found either more medially or more laterally.

An enlarged, tender gallbladder is indicative of cholecystitis, whereas a large but nontender gallbladder portends of obstruction of the common bile duct.

Murphy's sign: inspiratory arrest. Murphy's sign is helpful in determining the presence of cholecystitis through bimanual examination. While performing deep palpation, the examiner asks the client to take a deep breath. As the descending liver brings the gallbladder in contact with the examining hand, the client with cholecystitis will experience pain and stop the inspiratory movement. Pain may also occur in the client with hepatitis.

Spleen

The spleen is generally not palpable in the normal adult. Since the spleen is generally soft and is located retroperitoneally, it is frequently difficult to palpate. Turning the client on his right side brings the spleen closer to the abdominal wall and is frequently employed in the examination.

With the client in the supine position, three techniques of palpation are useful. In the first technique, the right hand is placed flat on the client's abdomen in the upper left quadrant with the fingers delving beneath the costal margin and toward the anterior axillary line (Fig. 15-26). The left hand is stretched over the client's abdomen and brought posterior to the client in the flank below the costal margin. This hand is used to exert an upward pressure that will displace the spleen anteriorly.

The Middleton technique for examination of the spleen is performed with the examiner standing on the client's left side, facing the client's feet. The fingers are hooked over the costal margin, pressing upward and inward at the anterior axillary line (Fig. 15-22). On inspiration the spleen may be felt at the fingertips. The client may assist by placing his left fist under the left eleventh rib.

Either of these techniques may be used with the client on the left side to throw the spleen forward and with the knees flexed to relax the abdomen.

The technique of one hand superimposed over the other may also be used to palpate the spleen. Again, the examiner stands at the client's left side, facing the client's feet. The fingers are hooked over the costal margin, and the uppermost hand is used to apply pressure while the lower hand is used as a sensing device. Again, the client is asked to breathe in and out while the ex-

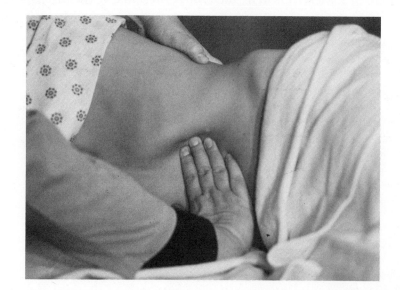

Fig. 15-26. Assessment of the spleen.

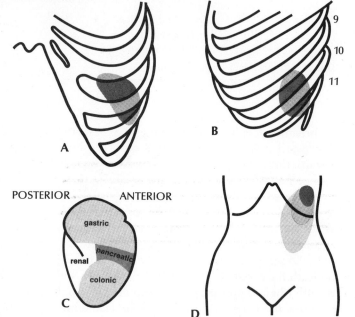

Fig. 15-27. Normal (**A, B, C**) and enlarged (**D**) spleen. **A,** Anterior view. **B,** Left lateral view. **C,** Regions of spleen (anterior view) that touch other viscera. **D,** Directions of splenic enlargement. (From G. I. series; physical examination of the abdomen, part 2, Palpation, Richmond, Va., 1972, A. H. Robins Co.)

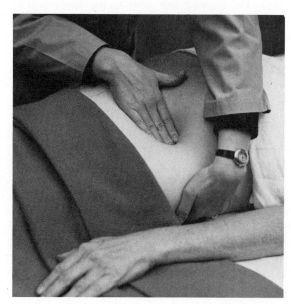

Fig. 15-28. Assessment of the left kidney.

aminer focuses on the inspiratory phase in an attempt to feel the contour of the spleen.

The spleen may also be percussed. When the spleen has normal dimensions, resonance may be percussed over the lowest left intercostal space between the anterior and midaxillary lines both during inspiration and expiration. However, a finding of resonance on expiration and dullness on inspiration probably denotes splenic hypertrophy. Normally, splenic dullness may be percussed from the ninth to the eleventh ribs in the midaxillary line.

Enlargement of the spleen may best be described by a drawing of the anterior abdomen indicating the relative site and shape of the spleen in relation to the costal border and the umbilicus (Fig. 15-27).

Pancreas

The pancreas cannot be palpated in the normal client because of its small size and retroperitoneal position. However, a mass of the pancreas may occasionally be felt as a vague sensation of fullness in the epigastrium.

Kidney

Palpation of the kidney is best accomplished with the client in the supine position and with the examiner standing on the client's right side. For the left kidney, the examiner reaches across the client with his left arm, placing his hand behind the client's left flank (Fig. 15-28). The left flank is elevated with the examiner's fingers, displacing the kidney anteriorly. With the kidney optimally positioned, the right palmar surface of the examiner's hand is used in deep palpation through the abdominal wall. The left kidney is generally not palpable.

The examiner remains on the client's right side to examine the right kidney. The right flank is similarly elevated with the left hand, and the right hand is used to palpate deeply for the right kidney. The lower pole of the right kidney may be felt as a smooth, rounded mass that descends on inspiration.

Differentiation between splenic and kidney enlargement may be accomplished by percussion. The percussion note over the spleen is dull since the bowel is displaced downward, whereas resonance is heard over the kidney because of the intervening bowel (Fig. 29). In addition, the free edge of the spleen is sharper in contour and tends to enlarge caudally and to the right.

Urinary bladder

The urinary bladder is not palpable in the normal client unless it is distended with urine. When the bladder is distended with urine, it may be felt as a smooth, round, and rather tense mass. Percussion may be used to define the outline of the distended bladder, which may extend up as far as the umbilicus.

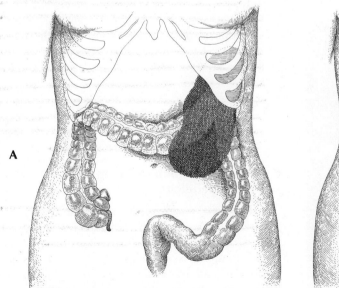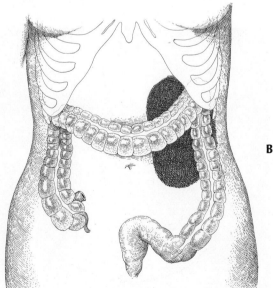

Fig. 15-29. Differentiation of enlarged spleen **(A)** from enlarged left kidney **(B)**. (From G. I. series; physical examination of the abdomen, part 3, Percussion, Richmond, Va., 1972, A. H. Robins Co.)

■ Umbilicus

Umbilical hernia. Whereas umbilical hernia noted in children is seen directly at the umbilical opening centrally located in the linea alba, the adult defect is often apparent above an incomplete umbilical ring and may be called paraumbilical.

The examination for hernia is done by pressing the index finger into the navel. The fascial opening may feel like a sharp ring, and there is a soft center. The umbilicus may be everted by marked intra-abdominal pressure from masses, pregnancy, or large amounts of ascitic fluid.

St. Mary Joseph's nodule. Carcinoma originating in the abdomen and particularly in the stomach may metastasize to the navel. The metastatic lesion is called St. Mary Joseph's nodule.

Patent urachus. On occasion the urinary tract of the fetus, which extends from the apex of the bladder to the umbilicus, does not fibrose. The result is a umbilicourinary fistula called a patent urachus. The client may report dampness or the smell of urine at the umbilicus.

Cullen's sign. Free blood in the peritoneal cavity may produce a blue hue at the umbilical opening, which is known as Cullen's sign.

■ Abdominal reflexes

A key, a longitudinally broken tongue blade, the base end of an applicator, or a fingernail is drawn gently across the skin, moving toward the umbilicus or the midline. The reflex is elicited by

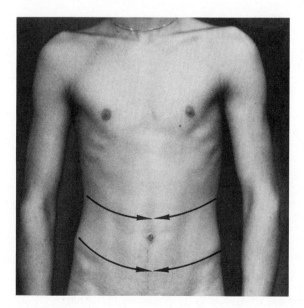

Fig. 15-30. Stimulus sites for abdominal reflexes. All four quadrants must be tested.

gently stroking the abdominal skin over the lateral borders of the rectus abdominis muscles toward the midline (Fig. 15-30). This maneuver is repeated in each quadrant. With each stroke, contraction of the rectus abdominis muscles is observed coupled with pulling of the umbilicus to the stimulated side.

The reflex may be weak or absent in the individual who has sustained a good deal of stretching of the abdominal musculature. Thus, the practitioner may be unable to obtain the abdominal reflex in the multiparous or obese client. The reflex may also be absent in the normal, aging client. Absence of the reflex may indicate a pyramidal tract lesion.

■ Changes in vascular patterns: venous engorgement

In health, the veins of the abdominal wall are not prominent, but in the malnourished individual the veins are more easily visible because of decreased adipose tissue. The venous return to the heart is cephalad in the veins above the umbilicus and caudal below the navel. Direction of flow may be demonstrated by placing the index fingers side by side over a vein, pressing laterally, and separating the fingers (Fig. 15-31). A section of the vein may be emptied. One finger is removed, and the time for filling is measured. The blood is milked from a short section of the vein, the other index finger is removed, and the time for filling from this side is measured.

Reversal of flow or an upward venous flow in the veins below the umbilicus accompanies obstruction of the inferior vena cava, whereas superior vena cava obstruction promotes downward flow in the veins above the navel. A pattern of engorged veins around the umbilicus is called caput medusae and is occasionally seen as an accompaniment to emaciation, obstruction of the superior or inferior vena cava, superficial venous obstruction or portal vein obstruction.

■ Tests for irritation resulting from appendicitis

Iliopsoas muscle test. An inflamed or perforated extrapelvic appendix may cause contact irritation of the lateral iliopsoas muscle. To elicit this tenderness, the client is placed in a supine position and asked to flex the lower extremity at the hip. The examiner simultaneously exerts a moderate downward pressure over the lower thigh (Fig. 15-32). With psoas muscle inflammation, the client will describe pain in the lower

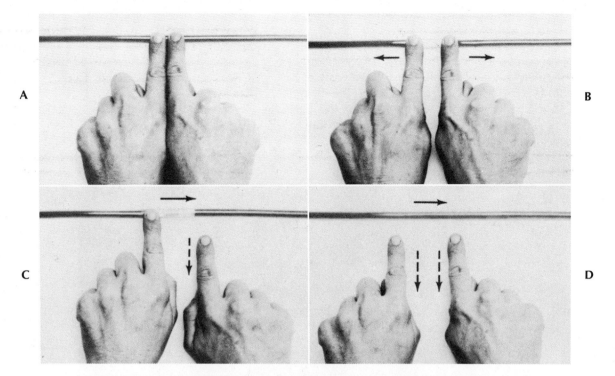

Fig. 15-31. Procedure for detecting the direction of venous flow. **A,** Press the blood from the vein with two index fingers in apposition. **B,** Slide the two index fingers apart, milking the blood from the intervening segment of vein. **C,** Release the pressure from one end of the segment to observe the time for refilling from that direction. **D,** Repeat the procedure, but release the other end to observe the time of filling. The flow of venous blood is in the direction of the faster filling. (From G. I. series; physical examination of the abdomen, part 2, Palpation, Richmond, Va., 1972, A. H. Robins Co.)

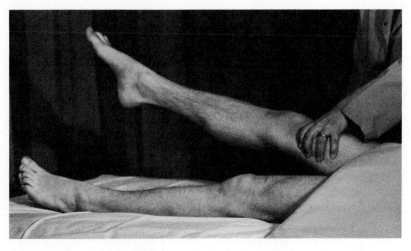

Fig. 15-32. Illiopsoas muscle test.

quadrant. A more sensitive test of psoas muscle irritation is performed with the client lying on his left side. Pain is elicited through full extension of the right lower limb at the hip.

Obturator muscle test. A perforated intrapelvic appendix may cause irritation of the obturator internus muscle. This pain is demonstrated with the client in the supine position. The client is asked to flex the right extremity at the hip and at the knee to 90°. The examiner grasps the ankle and rotates internally and externally (Fig. 15-33). A complaint of hypogastric pain denotes obturator muscle involvement.

■ Back

The final step in the abdominal examination is inspection of the back with the client in the sitting position (Fig. 15-34). The flanks in the normal individual will be symmetrical. Fullness or asymmetry may be due to renal disorders.

The costovertebral margin is percussed for tenderness.

Rectosigmoid region

The terminal gastrointestinal tract is accessible to methods of physical examination. This

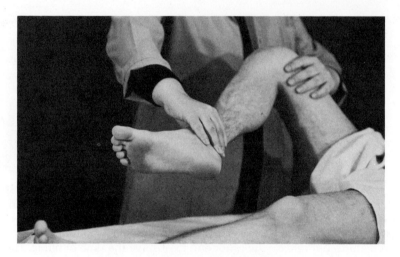

Fig. 15-33. Obturator muscle test.

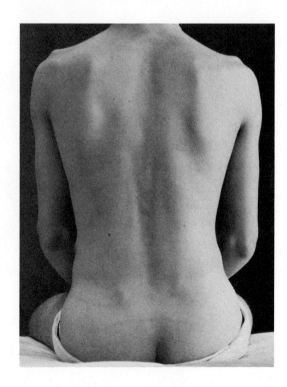

Fig. 15-34. Inspection of the back with the client in the sitting position is the final step in the abdominal examination.

distal section may be termed the rectosigmoid region and includes the anus, the rectum, and the caudal portion of the sigmoid colon.

ANATOMY

The anal canal is the final segment of the colon; it is 2.5 to 4 cm in length and opens into the perineum (Fig. 15-35). The tract is surrounded by the external and internal sphincters, which keep it closed except when flatus and feces are passed. These sphincters are laid down in concentric layers. The striated external muscular ring is under voluntary control, whereas the internal, smooth-muscle sphincter is under autonomic control. The internal sphincter is innervated from the pelvic plexus; sympathetic stimulation contracts the sphincter; parasympathetic stimulation relaxes it. The distal portion of the external sphincter extends past the internal sphincter and may be palpated by the examining finger. The stratified squamous epithelial lining of the anus is visible to inspection, since it extends beyond the sphincters, where it merges with the skin. The junction is characterized by pigmentation and the presence of hair. From an internal view of the anal canal, columns of mucosal tissue, which extend from the rectum and terminate in papillae, may be identified; these anal columns, or columns of Morgani, fuse to form the pectinate, or dentate, line. Spaces between these columns are called crypts. The anal columns are invested with cross channels of anastomosing veins, which form mucosal folds known as anal valves. These anastomosing veins form a ring known as the zona hemorrhoidalis. When dilated, these veins are called internal hemorrhoids. The lower section of the anal canal contains a venous plexus, which has only minor connection with the zona hemorrhoidalis and drains downward into the inferior rectal veins. Varicosed veins of this plexus are known as external hemorrhoids. Thus, internal hemorrhoids are encountered superior to the pectinate line and are characterized by the moist, red epithelium of the rectum, whereas external hemorrhoids are located inferior to the pectinate line and have the squamous epithelium of the anal canal or skin as their surface tissue.

The rectum is encountered as the portion of the gastrointestinal tract rostral to the anal canal. It is approximately 12 cm in length and is lined with columnar epithelium. Superiorly, the rec-

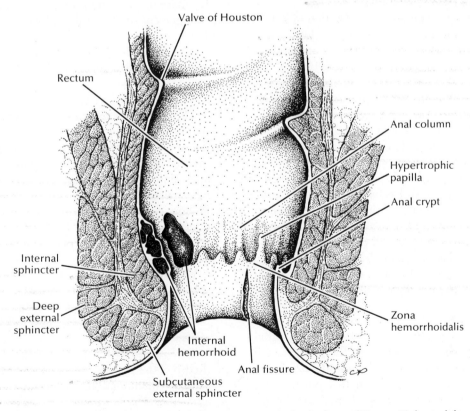

Fig. 15-35. Anorectal structures and common pathological conditions. (Adapted from Dunphy, J. E.: Arch. Surg. **57**:791, 1948.

tum has its origin at the third sacral vertebra and is continuous with the sigmoid colon. Its distal end dilates to form the rectal ampulla, which contains flatus and feces. Four semilunar transverse folds (Houston's valves) extend across half of the circumference of the rectal lumen. The purpose of the valves is not clear. It has been suggested that the valves serve to support feces while allowing flatus to pass. The rectum ends where the muscle coats are replaced by the sphincters of the anal canal.

The sigmoid colon has its origin at the iliac flexure of the descending colon and terminates in the rectum. It is approximately 40 cm in length. It is accessible to examination via the sigmoidoscope, and examination is limited by the length of the scope. Recently, flexible fiberoptic instruments have made possible inspection of the mucosal surfaces of the entire sigmoid colon as well as of the other portions of the colon.

EXAMINATION

The rectal examination is an important procedure in the physical examination; it is particularly significant when the client's chief complaint includes anal pain or spasm, itching or burning, and a history of black, tarry stools (melena).

The client may give some indication of a problem by his movements; for example, shifting from one buttock to the other often alleviates the discomfort of a thrombosed hemorrhoid.

The purposes of the rectal examination include assessment of anorectal status, assessment of the male prostate gland and seminal vessels (see Chapter 16, Assessment of the male genitalia and assessment of the inguinal area for hernias) and assessment of the accessible pelvic viscera.

Since most patients experience a good deal of embarrassment as well as fear of discomfort at the prospect of the rectal examination, the procedure should be preceded by an explanation and assurance that the examiner will proceed with gentleness. The client should be draped to avoid undue exposure and helped to assume the desired position. The client may be examined in several positions:

1. *Left lateral or Sims position:* The client lies on his left side with the superior thigh and knee flexed, bringing the knee close to the chest. The rectal ampulla is pushed down and posteriorly in this position and thus is advantageously aligned for the detection of rectal masses. However, the upper rectum and pelvic structure tend to fall

away in this position and a pathological condition of these structures may be overlooked.

2. *Knee-chest position:* The client is on his knees with his shoulders and head in contact with the examining table. The knees are positioned more widely apart than the hips. The angle at the hip is 75° to 80°. Assessment of the size of the prostate gland is best done in this position.

3. *Standing position:* The client's hips are flexed, and the trunk is resting on a bed or table. Prostate evaluation is facilitated in this position. This is the most commonly used position for examination of the prostate gland.

4. *Lithotomy position:* With the client supine, both knees are drawn up as far as possible toward the chest. It is convenient to perform the rectal examination in the female client immediately following the pelvic examination while her feet remain in stirrups.

5. *Squatting position:* Rectal prolapse may frequently be brought out in this position. Lesions of the rectosigmoid region and pelvis may be felt in this position only.

The equipment needed is a small penlight to facilitate inspection of the perianal and anal area, a finger cot or disposable glove, and lubricating jelly.

The methods of the rectal examination include inspection and palpation.

■ Inspection

The buttocks are carefully spread with both hands to examine the anus and the tissue immediately around the anus. This skis is more pigmented and coarser than the surrounding perianal skin. The examiner visually assesses the perianal region for skin lesions, scars or inflammation, fissures, external hemorrhoids, or fistula openings and tumors. The patient is asked to strain down, since this maneuver often accentuates hemorrhoids.

Valsalva's maneuver. The client is asked to strain downward as though defecating, so that with slight pressure on the skin, rectal fissures, rectal prolapse, polyps, or internal hemorrhoids might be identified.

The pilonidal area is inspected for dimples (at the tip of the coccyx), sinus openings, or the presence of inflammation. The pilonidal area is felt for tenderness, induration, or swelling.

The skin of the pilonidal sinus shows abundant hair growth. The accumulation of secretions often leads to infection, which is generally accompanied by a foul-smelling discharge and local tenderness. The sinus may be simply blocked up by secretion, so that a tumescence is observed, which is tender to palpation.

■ Palpation

While the patient strains downward, the pad of the lubricated, gloved index finger is gently placed against the anal verge; firm pressure is exerted until the sphincter begins to yield, and the finger is then slowly inserted in the direction of the umbilicus as the rectal sphincter relaxes (Fig. 15-36). The patient is asked to tighten the sphincter around the examining finger to provide a measurement of muscle strength of the anal sphinc-

ter. Hypertonicity of the external sphincter may occur with anxious, voluntary or involuntary contraction or as a result of an anal fissure or other local pathological condition. A relaxed or hypotonic sphincter is seen occasionally after rectal surgery or may be due to a neurological deficiency. The subcutaneous portion of the external sphincter is palpated on the inner aspect of the anal verge. The palpating finger is rotated to examine the entire muscular ring. The intersphincteric line is marked by a palpable indentation. Palpation of the deep external sphincter is performed through the lower part of the internal sphincter, which it surrounds. Assessment of the levator ani muscle is accomplished by palpating laterally and posteriorly where the muscle is at-

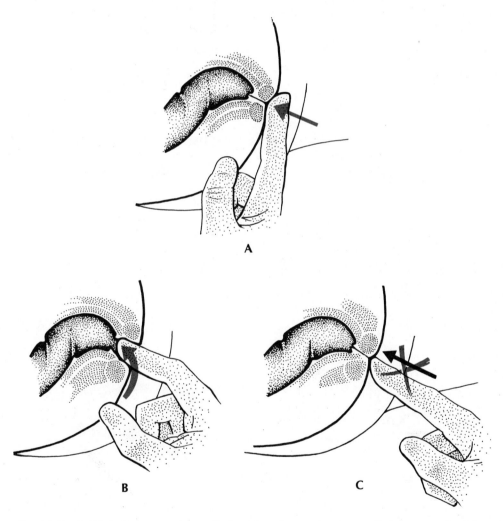

Fig. 15-36. A, Digital pressure is applied against the anal verge until the external sphincter is felt to yield. **B,** The gloved, lubricated finger is slowly introduced in the direction of the umbilicus. **C,** Avoid discomfort for the client by this approach at a right-angle to the sphincter and without promoting relaxation. (Adapted from Dunphy, J. E., and Botsford, T. W.: Physical examination of the surgical patient; an introduction to clinical surgery, ed. 4, Philadelphia, 1975, W. B. Saunders Co.)

tached to the rectal wall on one side and then the other (Fig. 15-37).

The posterior wall of the rectum follows the curve of the coccyx and sacrum and feels smooth to the palpating finger. The mucosa of the anal canal is palpated for tumor or polyps.

The examining finger is able to palpate a distance of 6 to 10 cm of the rectal canal. A bidigital palpation of the sphincter area may yield more information than would be obtained by probing with the index finger alone. This is accomplished by pressing the thumb of the examining hand against the perianal tissue and moving the examining index finger toward it. This is a useful technique for detecting a perianal abscess and for palpating the bulbourethral (Cowper's) glands.

Rectal valves may be misinterpreted as protruding intrarectal masses, especially when they are well developed.

The lateral walls of the rectum may be palpated by rotating the index finger along the sides of the rectum. The ischial spines and sacrotuberous ligaments may be identified through palpation.

The prostate gland is situated anterior to the rectum; therefore, palpation through the mucosa of the anterior wall of the rectum allows the examiner to assess the size, shape, and consistency of the prostate gland. The client is asked to bear down so that a mass not otherwise reached might be pushed downward into the range of the examining finger.

The prostate gland, a bilobed structure, has a normal diameter of approximately 4 cm. It should feel firm and smooth. The client should be asked to report tenderness to touch.

The normal cervix can be felt as a small round mass through the anterior wall of the rectum.

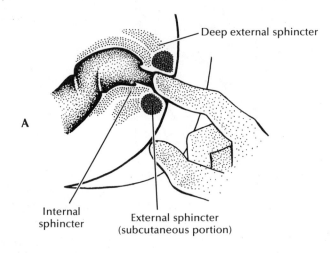

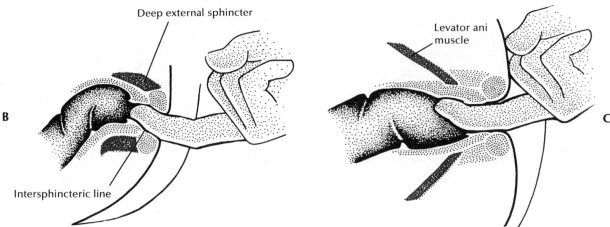

Fig. 15-37. The subcutaneous portion of the external sphincter is palpated, **A,** followed by digital exploration of the deep external sphincter, **B. C,** Palpation of the levator ani muscle. (Adapted from Dunphy, J. E., and Botsford, T. W.: Physical examination of the surgical patient; an introduction to clinical surgery, ed. 4, Philadelphia, 1975, W. B. Saunders Co.)

■ Examination of the stool

On withdrawal of the examining finger, the nature of any feces clinging to the glove should be examined (Table 15-3). The presence of pus or

Table 15-3. Characteristics of the stool related to the possible pathological conditions

Description of the stool	Possible pathological condition
Light tan, gray	Absence of bile pigments —obstructive jaundice
Greasy, pale, and yellow; increased fat content (steatorrhea, sprue)	Malabsorption syndromes
Tarry, black (melena)	Gastrointestinal tract bleeding; ingestion of iron compounds or bismuth preparations
Small flakes of jellylike mucus mixed with stool	Inflammation

blood is noted. Bright red blood in small or large amounts may be from the large intestine, the sigmoid colon, the rectum, or the anus. Colonic bleeding may be suspected when blood is mixed with the feces, whereas rectal bleeding is probably occurring when the blood is observed on the surface of the stool. The presence of a good deal of blood in the stool may be associated with marked malodor.

A black, tarry stool (melena) results from bleeding in the stomach or small intestine; the blood is partially digested during its passage to the rectum. On the other hand, the black color may result from ingested iron compounds and bismuth preparations.

A small quantity of the feces is subjected to a chemical test for the presence of occult blood. Minimal abrasions of the gastrointestinal tract are thought to be responsible for blood loss of 1 to 3 ml daily in the feces. The loss of more than 50 ml from the upper gastrointestinal tract

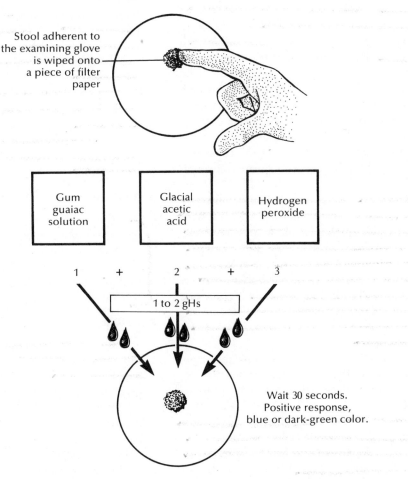

Fig. 15-38. Procedure for the guaiac assessment for occult blood. (Adapted from Dunphy, J. E., and Botsford, T. W.: Physical examination of the surgical patient; an introduction to clinical surgery, ed. 4, Philadelphia, 1975, W. B. Saunders Co.)

will produce melena. To detect quantities less than 50 ml or to determine whether black stools actually do contain blood, several reagents may be used.

The guaiac test is the most frequently used test for routine screening. The gum guaiac solution can identify 0.5% to 1% of hemoglobin in aqueous solution. The procedure involves wiping the gloved examining finger on a piece of filter paper and then adding 1 to 2 drops of guaiac solution, glacial acetic acid, and hydrogen peroxide. A positive reaction is denoted by the solution turning blue or dark green within 30 seconds (Fig. 15-38). Orthotoluidine is also useful in the detection of occult blood and is more sensitive than guaiac solution (it detects 0.01% to 0.1% of hemoglobin in aqueous solution).

Endoscopic procedures

The presence of a pathological condition detected by the digital examination is further explored by endoscopy.

Proctoscopy. Direct visualization of anal or lower rectal pathological conditions (or 9 to 15 cm of the lower gastrointestinal tract) is possible with a proctoscope. The position most frequently used for this procedure is the knee-chest position. The warmed and lubricated instrument is passed with the obturator in place to its full length. The obturator is removed, and the proctoscope is removed slowly while the examiner observes for ulcers, inflammation, strictures, or the cause of a palpable mass. Biopsy may be performed through the tube.

Sigmoidoscopy. Visual examination of the upper portion of the rectum that cannot be felt with the examining finger is possible with a sigmoidoscope; it allows direct visualization of the lower 24 cm of the gastrointestinal tract. This examination is particularly important since one half of all carcinomas occur in the rectum and colon. The early detection of polyps and malignant lesions may result in early and successful treatment of an otherwise fatal disease.

Careful explanation of the procedure and gentle manipulation of the client's tissue allow the examination to take place with little discomfort to the client.

The procedure is effective for the identification of proctitis, polyps, and carcinoma. Sigmoidoscopy is also helpful in the identification of diarrhea of colonic origin. The mucous membrane may be inspected, and scrapings may be taken for microscopic examination.

PATHOLOGY

Pruritus ani

Excoriated, thickened, and pigmented skin may result from chronic inflammation of pruritus ani. The itching and burning of the rectal area are most often traceable to pinworms in children and to fungal infections in adults. Diabetic clients are particularly vulnerable to fungal infections. A dull, grayish pink color of the perianal skin is a characteristic of fungal infections. The radiating folds of skin may appear enlarged, and the skin may be cracked or fissured. Pruritus ani characterized by dry and brittle skin is thought to be psychosomatic in origin.

Rectal tenesmus

Rectal tenesmus is the painful straining at stool associated with spasm of anal and rectal muscles; the client complains of a distressing feeling of urgency. The client is questioned concerning the nature of the stool. A hard, dry stool is indicative of constipation. A bloody, diarrheal stool might be indicative of ulcerative colitis. Rectal fissure may be the cause of tenesmus with normally constituted stools.

Tenesmus may also be a symptom experienced by the client with a perirectal inflammation, such as prostatitis.

The client who complains of constant rectal pain is examined carefully for thrombosed rectal hemorrhoids.

Anal fissure

A thin tear of the superficial anal mucosa, generally weeping, may be identified by asking the client to perform Valsalva's maneuver. The fissure is most commonly found in the posterior midline of the anal mucosa and less frequently in the anterior midline.

Fistula in ano

A tract from an anal fissure that terminates in the perianal skin or other tissue is termed an anorectal fistula; it usually has its origin from local crypt abscesses. The fistula is a chronically inflamed tube made up of fibrous tissue surrounding granulation tissue and may frequently be palpated.

The site from which drainage from an anal infection occurs can be identified by relating the location of the external opening of the fissure to the anus (Table 15-4 and Fig. 15-39).

Hemorrhoids

Hemorrhoids are dilated veins of the hemorrhoidal group. The swelling is associated with increased hydrostatic pressure in the portal venous system. The pressure associated with hemorrhoids correlates highly with pregnancy, straining at stool, chronic liver disease, and sudden increases in intra-abdominal pressure. Bowel habits also play a role in that hemorrhoids frequently occur with diarrhea or incomplete bowel emptying. Local factors such as abscess or tumor may also contribute to venous stasis.

Hemorrhoidal tags are ragged, flaccid, skin sacs located around the anus, which is the locus of resolved external hemorrhoids. Clients describe these tags as painless. Internal hemorrhoids occur proximal to the pectinate line, whereas external hemorrhoids are those that are seen distal to this boundary. External hemorrhoids are covered by skin or anal squamous tissue.

External hemorrhoids are often accompanied by pain, particularly if the skin is stretched by a sudden increase in mass; since the mass is located near the sphincter muscles, spasm is not uncommon. These dilated veins may appear as bluish, swollen areas at the anal verge.

Internal hemorrhoids generally do not contribute to pain sensation unless they are complicated by thrombosis, infection, or erosion of overlying mucosal surfaces. Discomfort is increased if the hemorrhoids prolapse through the anal opening. Proctoscopy is generally necessary for their identification.

Rectal polyps

Rectal polyps are encountered frequently. They may be pedunculated (on a stalk) or sessile (irregularly moundlike, growing from a relatively broad base, and closely adherent to the mucosal wall). Because of their soft consistency they may be difficult or impossible to identify by palpation. Proctoscopy is usually necessary for identification.

A pedunculated rectal polyp occasionally prolapses through the anal ring.

Rectal prolapse

Internal hemorrhoids are the type most commonly identified because of mucosal tissue prolapsing through the anal ring. The pink-colored mucosa is described as appearing like a doughnut or rosette. In the older client, however, protruding mucosa may herald eversion or prolapse of the rectum. Incomplete prolapse involves only mucosa, whereas complete rectal prolapse involves the sphincters.

The prolapse of tissue through the anal ring is described by the client as occurring on exercise or while straining at stool. Frequently, the client describes being able to push the mass back in with digital pressure. Inspection reveals a red, bulging mucosal mass protruding through the anal ring.

Abscesses or masses

Abscesses of the lower gastrointestinal tract that may be identified by physical examination (Fig. 15-40) include:

Table 15-4. Location of fissure site related to the external opening

	External opening	Location in the anus
Goodsell's rule	Posterior to a line between the ischial tuberosities	Posterior
	Radial from the drainage site	Anterior
Salmon's law	Posterior to the anus or more than 2.5 cm anterior	Posterior
	Less than 2.5 cm anteriorly	Anterior

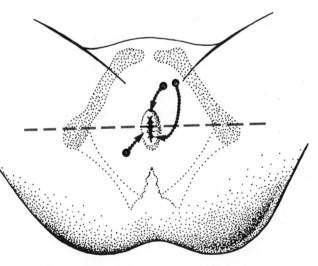

Fig. 15-39. Fissure location related to the aperture of the fistula. (Adapted from Dunphy, J. E., and Botsford, T. W.: Physical examination of the surgical patient; an introduction to clinical surgery, ed. 4, Philadelphia, 1975, W. B. Saunders Co.)

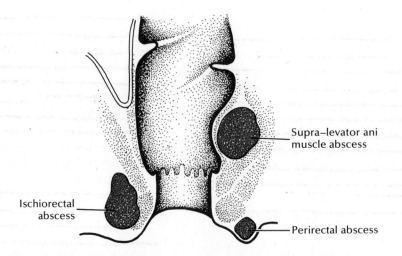

Fig. 15-40. Common sites of abscess formation of the lower gastrointestinal tract. (Adapted from Dunphy, J. E., and Botsford, T. W.: Physical examination of the surgical patient; an introduction to clinical surgery, ed. 4, Philadelphia, 1975, W. B. Saunders Co.)

1. *Perirectal abscess:* This abscess may be palpated as a tender mass adjacent to the anal canal. The increased temperature of the mass may be helpful in the identification of the inflammatory process.
2. *Ischiorectal abscess:* This abscess may be palpated as a tender mass protruding into the lateral wall of the anal canal.
3. *Supra–levator ani muscle abscess:* This abscess may be felt by the examining finger as a tender mass in the lateral rectal wall.

The presence of a mass in the rectum deserves special attention since nearly half of those discovered are malignant. The client frequently denies pain or other symptoms. Extension of metastatic carcinoma from the peritoneum to the pelvic floor is described as a rectal shelf. The consistency of the malignant mass is often stony hard, and the contour is irregular.

An ulcerated carcinoma may be identified through palpation by its firm, nodular, rolled edge.

BIBLIOGRAPHY

Brooks, F. P., editor: Gastrointestinal pathophysiology, New York, 1974, Oxford University Press, Inc.

Castell, D. O.: The spleen percussion sign; a useful diagnostic technique, Ann. Int. Med. **67:**1265, 1967.

Castell, D. O., O'Brien, K. D., Muench, H., and others: Estimation of liver size by percussion in normal individuals, Ann. Int. Med. **70:**1183, 1969.

Cope, Z.: The early diagnosis of acute abdomen, ed. 14, New York, 1972, Oxford University Press, Inc.

Dunphy, J., and Botsford, T.: Physical examination of the surgical patient; an introduction to clinical surgery, Philadelphia, 1975, W. B. Saunders Co.

Dworken, H. J.: The alimentary tract, Philadelphia, 1974, W. B. Saunders Co.

Gelin, L., Nyhus, L., and Condon, R.: Abdominal pain; a guide to rapid diagnosis, Philadelphia, 1969, J. B. Lippincott Co.

16

Assessment of the male genitalia and assessment of the inguinal area for hernias

Male genitalia

The examination of the genital organs of any client is usually perceived by both the client and the practitioner as being different from the examination of other body parts. Culturally, male gynecologists have been accepted and sometimes even preferred by female clients. This chapter discusses the approach of the female practitioner to the examination of the male client's genital system.

First, the female practitioner should feel emotionally comfortable with the examination. If she does not, she should routinely refer this part of the physical examination to a male practitioner. Next, if she is comfortable with the examination, she must accept the possibility of the male client's reluctance to having his genitalia examined by a woman. Cajoling a client into an uncomfortable procedure may destroy further rapport; his wishes in the situation should be respected. In most clinical settings, there is a male practitioner present who would be available for a few minutes to examine the male genitalia. Our experience has been that most male clients are agreeable to examination by a woman; if there is discomfort, it is usually on the part of the examiner. It is therefore recommended that the beginning female examiner critically analyze her own feelings, fears, and beliefs; attempt male genital examination under supervision and with several cooperative clients; and then reexamine her feelings.

The examination should be preceded by a thorough history of the urinary system and a history of sexual functioning. As with the female client, questioning about sexual activity or performance while the genitalia are being handled may be perceived by the client as evaluative or provocative.

ANATOMY

The following is a review of the anatomy of the male genitalia (Fig. 16-1).

The shaft of the penis is formed by three columns of erectile tissue bound together by heavy fibrous tissue to form a cylinder. The dorsolateral columns are called the corpora cavernosa; the ventromedial column is called the corpus spongiosum, and this column contains the urethra. Distally the penis terminates in a cone-shaped entity called the glans penis. The glans penis is formed by an extension and expansion of the corpus spongiosum penis, which fits over the blunt ends of the corpora cavernosa penis. The corona is the prominence formed where the glans joins the shaft. The urethra traverses the corpus spongiosum, and the external urethral orifice is a slit-like opening located slightly ventrally on the tip of the glans.

The skin of the penis is thin, hairless, dark, and only loosely connected to the internal parts of the organ. At the area of the corona, the skin forms a free fold, called the prepuce or foreskin. When allowed to remain, this flap covers the glans to a variable extent. Often the prepuce is surgically removed in circumcision (Fig. 16-2).

The scrotum is a deeply pigmented cutaneous pouch, containing the testes and parts of the spermatic cords (Fig. 16-3). The sac is formed by an outer layer of thin, rugous skin overlying a tight muscle layer. The left side of the scrotum is often lower than the right side because the left spermatic cord is usually longer. Internally the scrotum is divided into halves by a septum; each half contains a testis and its epididymis, and part of the spermatic cord. The testes are ovoid and are suspended vertically, slightly forward; they lean slightly laterally in the scrotum. The mediolateral

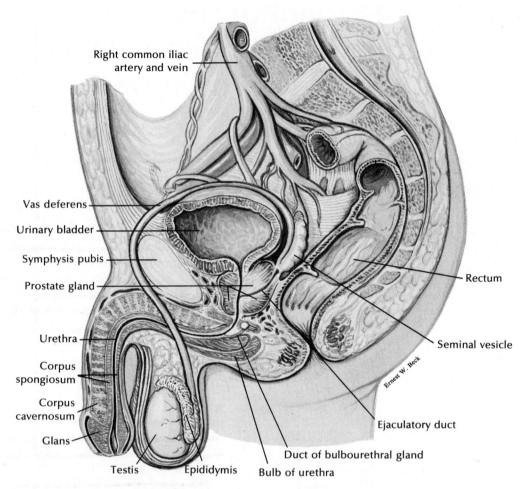

Fig. 16-1. Male pelvic organs. (From Anthony, C. P., and Kolthoff, N. J.: Anatomy and physiology, ed. 9, St. Louis, 1975, The C. V. Mosby Co.)

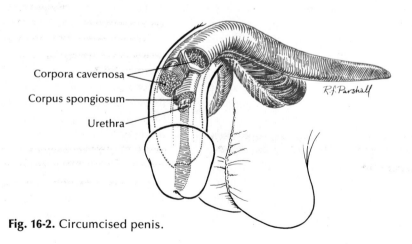

Fig. 16-2. Circumcised penis.

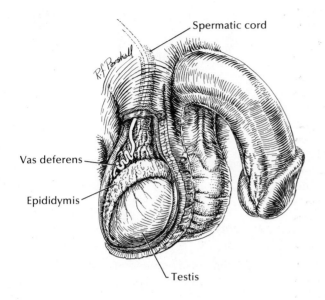

Fig. 16-3. Scrotum and scrotal contents.

Spermatic cord

Vas deferens

Epididymis

Testis

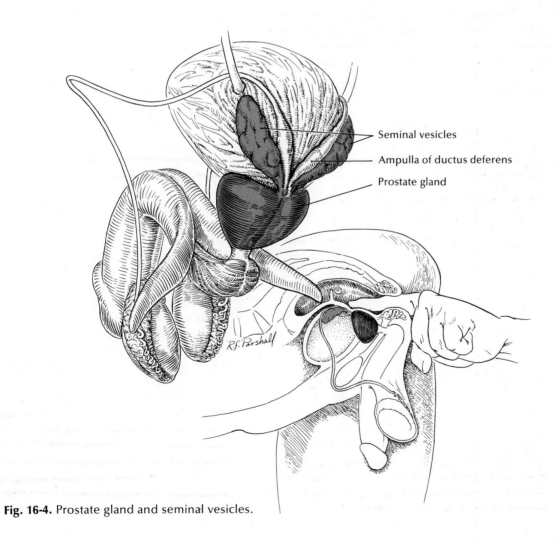

Seminal vesicles

Ampulla of ductus deferens

Prostate gland

Fig. 16-4. Prostate gland and seminal vesicles.

surfaces are flattened. Each is approximately 4 to 5 cm long, 3 cm wide, and 2 cm thick.

The epididymis is a comma-shaped structure that is curved over the posterolateral surface and upper end of the testis; it creates a visual bulge on the posterolateral surface of the testis. The ductus deferens begins at the tail of the epididymis, ascends the spermatic cord, travels through the inguinal canal, and eventually descends on the fundus of the bladder (Fig. 16-1).

The prostate, a slightly conical gland, lies under the bladder, surrounds the urethra, and measures approximately 4 cm at its base or uppermost part, 3 cm vertically, and 2 cm in its anteroposterior diameter. The prostate gland has been compared to the chestnut in size and shape. It has three lobes, left and right lateral lobes and a median lobe. These lobes are not well demarcated from each other. The median lobe is the part of the prostate that projects inward from the upper, posterior area toward the urethra. It is the enlargement of this lobe that causes urinary obstruction in benign prostatic hypertrophy.

The posterior surface of the prostate is in close contact with the rectal wall and is the only portion of the gland accessible to examination. Its posterior surface is slightly convex; a shallow median furrow divides all except the upper portions of the posterior surface into right and left lateral lobes.

The seminal vesicles are a pair of convoluted pouches, 5 to 10 cm long, which lie along the lower posterior surface of the bladder, anterior to the rectum (Fig. 16-4).

EXAMINATION

The techniques of inspection and palpation are used to examine the male genitalia. After the inguinal and genital areas are exposed, the skin, hair, and gross appearance of the penis and scrotum are inspected. Examination of the skin, nodes, and hair distribution are discussed elsewhere in this text. The size of the penis and the secondary sex characteristics are assessed in relationship to the client's age and general development. If inflammation or lesions are observed or suspected, gloves are used for the examination.

The onset of the appearance of adult sexual characteristics is extremely variable. Pubic hair appears and the testes enlarge between the ages of 12 and 16 years. Penile enlargement and the onset of seminal emission normally occurs between the ages of 13 and 17 years.

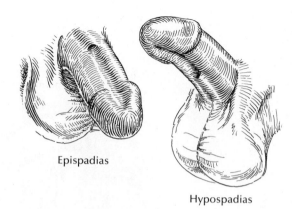

Fig. 16-5. Malpositioning of the urethral meatus.

■ Penis

The penis is observed for lesions, nodules, swelling, inflammation, and discharge. If the client is uncircumcised, he is requested to retract the prepuce from the glans and the glans and foreskin are examined carefully. The client is also asked to compress the glans anteroposteriorly. This opens the distal end of the urethra for inspection. If any discharge is present, a smear and culture for gonorrhea are obtained (see Chapter 17 on Assessment of the female genitalia and procedures for smears and cultures). If the client has reported a discharge, he is requested to milk the penis from the base to the urethra; if a discharge is present, it is cultured.

Among the more common penile lesions are syphilitic chancre, condylomata acuminata, and cancer. The syphilitic chancre is the primary lesion of syphilis. It begins as a single papule that eventually erodes into an oval or round red ulcer with an indurated base that discharges serous material. It is usually painless.

Condylomata acuminata are wart-appearing growths. They are caused by a venereal infection and may be seen occurring singly or in multiple, cauliflower like patches.

Carcinoma of the penis occurs most frequently on the glans and on the inner lip of the prepuce. It may appear dry and scaly, ulcerated, or nodular. It is usually painless.

The urethral meatus should be positioned rather centrally on the glans. When the distal urethral ostium occurs on the ventral corona or at a more proximal and ventral site on the penis or perineum, the condition is called hypospadias (Fig. 16-5). A similar malpositioning of the urethral meatus in the dorsal area is called epispadias.

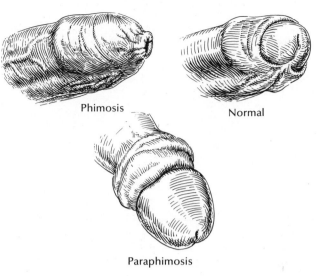

Phimosis

Normal

Paraphimosis

Fig. 16-6. Phimosis, normal retraction of the prepuce, and paraphimosis.

The prepuce should be easily retractable from the glans and returnable to its original position. Phimosis exists when retraction cannot occur (Fig. 16-6). This condition presents problems with cleanliness and prevents observation of the glans and interior surfaces of the prepuce. If the foreskin has been partially retracted but has impinged on the penis, so that it cannot be returned to its usual position, the condition is called paraphimosis.

The penile shaft should be carefully palpated. Occasionally, hard, nontender subcutaneous plaques are palpated on the dorsomedial surface. The client with this condition, called Peyronie's disease, may report penile bending with erection and painful intercourse.

■ **Scrotum**

The client is instructed to hold the penis out of the way, and the examiner observes the general size, superficial appearance, and symmetry of the scrotum. The scrotum may normally appear asymmetrical because the left testis is generally lower than the right testis. Also, the tone of the dartos muscle determines the size of the scrotum; it contracts when the area is cold and relaxes when the area is warm. In advanced age, the dartos muscle is somewhat atonic and the scrotum may appear pendulous.

When the scrotal skin is being observed, its rugated surface should be spread. Also, the examiner should remember to inspect the posterior and posterolateral as well as anterior and anterolateral skin areas. A common abnormality, occur-

ring as a single lesion or as multiple lesions, is that of sebaceous cysts. There are firm, yellow to white, nontender cutaneous lesions measuring up to 1 cm in diameter.

The scrotum may become edematous, and palpation may produce pitting. This may occur in any condition that causes edema in the lower trunk, for example, cardiovascular disease.

The contents of each half of the scrotal sac are palpated. Both testes should be present in the scrotum at birth; if not present, their location should be determined by retracing their course of descent back into the abdomen.

Both testes are palpated simultaneously between the thumb and the first two fingers. Their consistency, size, shape, and response to pressure are determined. They should be smooth, homogenous in consistency, regular, equal in size, freely movable, and slightly sensitive to compression.

Next, each epididymis is palpated. The epididymides are located in the posterolateral area of the testes in 93% of males. In approximately 7% of males they are in the anterolateral or anterior areas. They are palpated, and their size, shape, consistency, and tenderness are noted. Then each of the spermatic cords are palpated by bilaterally grasping each between the thumb and the forefinger. The vas deferentia feel like smooth cords and are movable; the arteries, veins, lymph vessels, and nerves feel like indefinite threads along the side of the vas.

If swelling, irregularity, or nodularity is noted in the scrotum, attempts are made to transilluminate it by darkening the room and placing a lit flashlight behind the scrotal contents. Transillumination is a red glow. Serous fluid will transilluminate; tissue and blood will not. The more commonly occurring abnormalities of the scrotum are described and illustrated in Table 16-1.

All scrotal masses should be described by their placement, size, shape, consistency, tenderness, and whether they transilluminate.

■ **Prostate gland**

With an ambulatory client it is most satisfactory to execute the rectal and prostate examination with the client standing, hips flexed, toes pointed toward each other, and upper body resting on the examining table. This position flattens the buttocks, deters gluteal contraction, and makes the anus and rectum more accessible to evaluation. A debilitated client may be examined in the left lateral or lithotomy position. In the left lateral position he is reminded to flex his right knee and

Table 16-1. Description of scrotal abnormalities

Abnormality	Illustration	Definition/causation	Basis for diagnosis
Hydrocele		An accumulation of serous fluid between the visceral and parietal layers of the tunica vaginalis	Transilluminates; fingers can get above the mass
Scrotal hernia		A hernia within the scrotum	Bowel sounds auscultated; does not transilluminate; fingers cannot get above the mass
Varicocele		Abnormal dilatation and tortuosity of the veins of the pampiniform plexus; often described as a "bag of worms" in the scrotum*	Complaints of a dragging sensation or dull pain in the scrotal area; feels like a soft bag of worms; collapses when the scrotum is elevated and increases when the scrotum is dependent; more commonly present on the left side; usually appears at puberty
Spermatocele		An epididymal cyst resulting from a partial obstruction of the spermatic tubules*	Transilluminates; round mass, feels like a third testis; painless
Epididymal mass or nodularity		May be due to benign or malignant neoplasms, syphilis, or tuberculosis	Nodules are not tender; in tuberculosis lesions, vas deferens often feels beaded

Table 16-1. Description of scrotal abnormalities—cont'd

Abnormality	Illustration	Definition/causation	Basis for diagnosis
Epididymitis		An inflammation of the epididymis, usually due to *Escherichia coli*, *Neisseria gonorrhea*, or *Mycobacterium tuberculosis* organisms*	Spermatic cord often thickened and indurated; pain relieved by elevation
Torsion of the spermatic cord		Axial rotation or volvulus of the spermatic cord, resulting in infarction of the testicle	Elevated mass; pain not relieved by further elevation; more common in childhood or adolescence; history of extreme pain and tenderness of the testis, followed by hyperemic swelling and hydrocele
Testicular tumor		Multiple causes	Usually not painful; hydroceles may develop secondary to tumor —if a testis cannot be palpated, fluid may need to be aspirated so that the testis can be accurately evaluated.

*Btesh, S., editor: Diseases of the urinary tract and male genital organs, Geneva, 1974, Council for Internal Organizations for Medical Sciences, pp. 86-90.

hip and to have his buttocks close to the edge of the examining table. The general procedure for the anal and rectal examination is described in Chapter 15 on Assessment of the abdomen and rectosigmoid region. The general rectal examination is performed first; then the prostate gland and seminal vesicles are palpated (Fig. 16-4). The pad of the index finger is used for palpation. The prostate gland is located on the anterior rectal wall but should not be protruding into the rectal lumen.

Prostatic enlargement is protrusion of the prostate gland into the rectal lumen and is commonly described in grades:

Grade I: Encroaches less than 1 cm into the rectal lumen.

Grade II: Encroaches 1 to 2 cm into the rectal lumen.

Grade III: Encroaches 2 to 3 cm into the rectal lumen.

Grade IV: Encroaches more than 3 cm into the rectal lumen.

The gland should be approximately 3 cm in length, symmetrical, movable, and of a rubbery consistency. Its median sulcus normally can be felt. The proximal portions of the seminal vesicles can sometimes be palpated as corrugated structures above the lateral to the midpoint of the gland. Normally they are too soft to be palpated. The examiner should attempt to examine all available surfaces of the prostate gland and seminal vesicles. Significant abnormalities of the prostate gland or seminal vesicles include protrusion into the rectal lumen; hard, nodular areas; bogginess; tenderness; and asymmetry.

The examiner should mentally consider the following questions about these structures:

Surface: Smooth or nodular?

Consistency: Rubbery, hard, boggy, soft, or fluctuant?

277

Shape: Rounded or flat?
Size: Normal, enlarged, or atrophied?
Sensitivity: Tender or not?
Movability: Movable or fixed?

A hard, single or multiple lesion on a firm and fixed prostate gland may be carcinoma or tuberculosis. The initial lesion of carcinoma is frequently on the posterior lobe and can be easily identified during the rectal examination. A soft, symmetrical, boggy, nontender prostate gland may indicate benign prostatic hypertrophy, a condition very common in men over 50 years of age. In the later stages of this condition, the median sulcus may be obliterated. A boggy, fluctuant, or tender prostate gland may indicate acute or chronic prostatitis. The prostate gland can be massaged centrally from its lateral edges to force secretions into the urethra. Secretion at the urethral opening can be examined and cultured.

Inguinal area: assessment for hernias

If a client has an inguinal or groin area hernia, he (or she) will probably complain of a swelling or bulging in that area, especially during abdominal straining. All clients should be screened for inguinal and femoral hernias, even if they do not complain of groin swelling, as part of the routine physical examination.

No special equipment is needed for the examination.

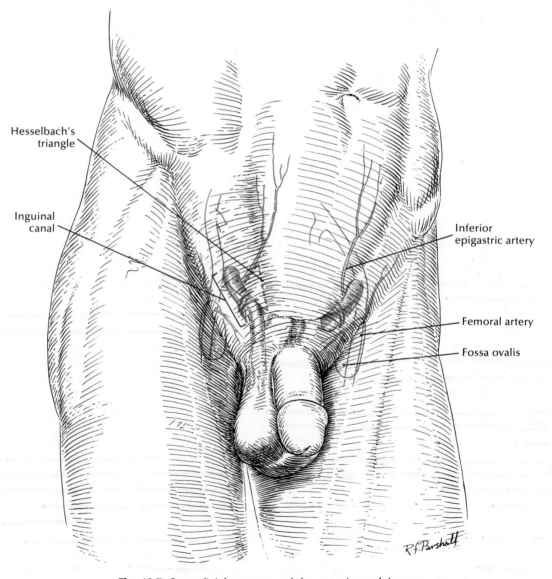

Fig. 16-7. Superficial anatomy of the anterior pelvic area.

ANATOMY

The following is a review of the anatomy of the inguinal area (Fig. 16-7).

The inguinal (Poupart's) ligament extends from the anterosuperior spine of the ilium to the pubic tubercle. The inguinal canal is a flattened tunnel between two layers of abdominal muscle, measuring approximately 4 to 6 cm in the adult. Its internal ring is located 1 to 2 cm above the midpoint of the inguinal ligament. The spermatic cord traverses through this internal ring, passes through the canal, exits the canal at its external (subcutaneous) ring, and then moves up and over the inguinal ligament and into the scrotum.

Hesselbach's triangle is the region superior to the inguinal canal, medial to the inferior epigastric artery, and lateral to the margin of the rectus muscle.

The femoral canal is a potential space just inferior to the inguinal ligament and 3 cm medial and parallel to the femoral artery. If the examiner's right hand is placed on the client's right anterior thigh with the index finger over the femoral artery, the femoral canal will be under the ring finger.

The three main types of pelvic area hernias are shown in Fig. 16-8. In the *indirect inguinal hernia*, the hernial sac enters the internal inguinal canal and its tip is located somewhere in the inguinal canal or beyond the canal. In males, indirect inguinal hernias may descend into the scrotum. The *direct inguinal hernia* emerges directly from behind and through the external inguinal ring. The *femoral hernia* emerges through the femoral ring, the femoral canal, and the fossa ovalis.

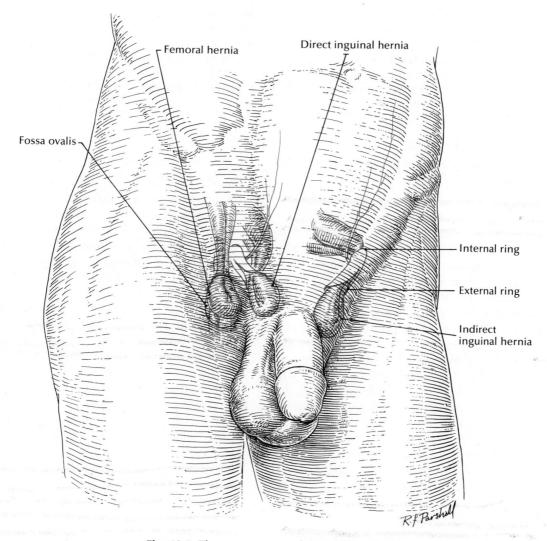

Fig. 16-8. Three common pelvic area hernias.

Table 16-2. Comparison of inguinal and femoral hernias

	Inguinal hernia		Femoral hernia
	Indirect	**Direct**	
Course	Sac emerges through the internal inguinal ring, lateral to the inferior epigastric artery; can remain in the canal, exit the external ring, or pass into the scrotum	Sac emerges directly from behind and through the external inguinal ring; located in the region of Hesselbach's triangle	Sac emerges through the femoral ring, the femoral canal, and the fossa ovalis; observed lateral to the femoral vein
Incidence	More common in infants under 1 year and in males 16 to 20 years; more common in males than in females at a ratio of approximately 4:1; 60% of all hernias	Most often observed in men over 40 years of age; rarer than the indirect hernia	Less common than inguinal hernias; seldom seen in children; more common in women; 4% of all hernias
Cause	Congenital or acquired	Congenital weakness exacerbated by (1) lifting, (2) atrophy of abdominal muscles, (3) ascites, (4) chronic cough, or (5) obesity	Acquired; may be caused by (1) stooping frequently, (2) increased abdominal pressure, or (3) loss of muscle substance
Clinical symptoms and signs	Soft swelling in the region of the internal inguinal ring—swelling increases when client stands or strains, is sometimes reduced when client reclines; pain during straining	Abdominal bulge in the area of Hesselbach's triangle, usually in the area of the internal ring; usually painless; easily reduced when client reclines; rarely enters scrotum	Right side more commonly affected; pain may be severe; strangulation frequent; sac may extend into the scrotum, into the labium, or along the saphenous vein

EXAMINATION

Inspection and palpation are the techniques used. Whenever possible, the examination for hernias is performed with the client standing. However, if the client is debilitated or especially tense, the examination may be performed while the client is lying down on a flat surface.

First, the areas of inguinal and femoral hernias are exposed and observed with the client at rest and while the client holds his breath and exerts abdominal pressure with the diaphragm. Straining is preferred to coughing because a more sustained pressure is elicited. Sometimes the impulse of coughing can be confused with the impulse of a hernia. Often, small hernias in women and children are more easily observed than felt because of the fatty tissue in the area.

The examiner palpates for a direct inguinal hernia by placing two fingers over each external inguinal ring and instructing the client to bear down. The presence of a hernia will produce a palpable bulge in the area.

To determine the presence of an indirect inguinal hernia, the client is asked to flex the ipsi-lateral knee slightly while the examiner attempts to direct his index or little finger into the path of the inguinal canal. When the finger has traversed as far as possible, the client is asked to strain. A hernia will be felt as a mass of tissue meeting the finger and then withdrawing. The left index or little finger, hand with palm side out, is used to examine the client's left side. The right hand in turn is used for the client's right side. In women, the canal is narrow and the finger cannot be inserted far, if at all. In men, the finger invaginates scrotal skin into the inguinal canal (Fig. 16-9).

In both men and women, each fossa ovalis area is palpated while the client is straining. The femoral hernia will be felt as a soft tumor at the fossa, below the inguinal ligament and lateral to the pubic tubercle.

Occasionally, the client may complain of the symptoms of hernia but none can be palpated. In such cases a load test is suggested. The client lifts a heavy object while the inguinal area is being observed. A previously unobserved bulge may become prominent.

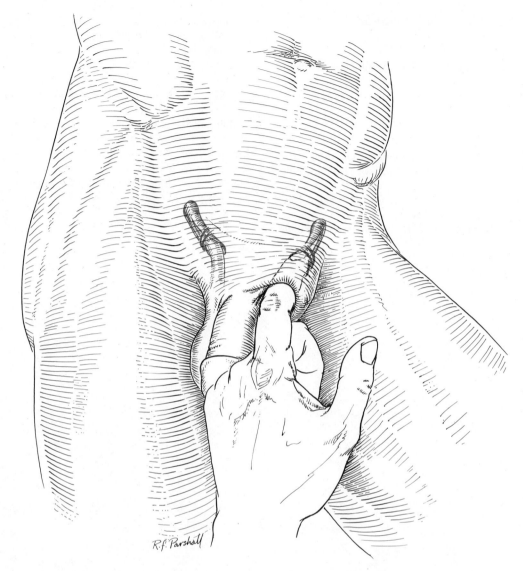

Fig. 16-9. Examination of a male client for indirect inguinal hernia.

Summary

The following outline summarizes the assessment of the male genitalia and the assessment of the inguinal area for hernias:

I. Male genitalia
   A. General inspection
      1. Skin
      2. Hair
         a. Distribution
         b. Parasites
      3. Inguinal area
         a. Swelling
         b. Inflammation
   B. Inspection of the penis
      1. Size relative to age and general development

2. Discharge
3. Skin
4. Urethral meatus
5. Prepuce
   C. Palpation of the penis
   D. Palpation of the inguinal nodes
   E. Inspection of the scrotum
      1. Skin
      2. Symmetry
      3. Size
   F. Palpation of the scrotum
      1. Testes
      2. Epididymides
      3. Spermatic cords
   G. Transillumination (if any swellings or masses are present)
   H. Observation and palpation of the rectal area

1. General rectal examination
2. Prostate gland
3. Seminal vesicles

II. Inguinal area: assessment for hernias (direct, inguinal, and femoral)
   A. Inspection
   B. Palpation

BIBLIOGRAPHY

Bodner, H.: Diagnostic and therapeutic aids in urology, Springfield, Ill., 1974, Charles C Thomas, Publishers.

Brandes, D., editor: Male accesory sex organs, New York, 1974, Academic Press, Inc.

Btesh, S., editor: Disease of the urinary tract and male genital organs, Geneva, Switzerland, 1974, Council for International Organizations for Medical Sciences.

Calman, C. H.: An atlas of hernia repair, St. Louis, 1966, The C. V. Mosby Co.

Johnson, D. E., editor: Testicular tumors, Flushing, N.Y., 1972, Medical Examination Publishing Co., Inc.

Maingot, R., editor: Abdominal operation, ed. 6, New York, 1974, Appleton-Century-Crofts.

Ravitch, M. M.: Repairs of hernias, Chicago, 1969, Yearbook Medical Publishers, Inc.

Scott, R., editor: Current controversies in urologic management, Philadelphia, 1972, W. B. Saunders Co.

17 Assessment of the female genitalia and procedures for smears and cultures

Female genitalia

Most female clients perceive the examination of their reproductive organs as being different from the examination of other body parts. Past admonitions of "do not touch" and "keep it covered" have created a population of anatomically unaware and sometimes inappropriately "modest" women who are often unnecessarily difficult to examine. Most practitioners believe that a great amount of information about a female client can be obtained by examining the genital area and performing screening tests; but because of their experience with the fearful and tense reactions of many clients, practitioners have sometimes routinely omitted the examination of the genital organs or have referred their clients to gynecological specialists for screening examinations.

One cause of the female client's tenseness during an examination of the genital area may be fear of discovery. During the history the practitioner investigates areas of anatomical and physiological function and dysfunction. The review of systems on all clients should include a sexual history. If this portion of the history is accomplished skillfully and if the client has been cooperative, she should not be apprehensive about the possible discovery of sexual "secrets."

Other causes of tenseness during the pelvic examination include fear of discovery of disease and the memory of previous, uncomfortable pelvic examinations.

Also, many clients are not knowledgeable regarding the anatomy of the pelvic area. The practitioner should determine the client's need for basic information regarding the structure of the genital organs and provide this instruction before the pelvic examination, along with a demonstra-tion of the instruments and an explanation of the procedure. If a relatively short amount of time were taken to inform and orient all female clients at the time of their first examination, practitioners and clients would reap the benefits of enhanced mutual cooperation.

Teaching the client a relaxation technique will often make an examination shorter or even possible. One relaxation technique that has been successful is the following: the client is instructed to place her hands on her chest at about the level of the diaphragm, breath deeply and slowly through her mouth, concentrate on the rhythm of breathing, and relax all body muscles with each exhalation. The tense client is apt to hold her breath and tighten. Even the coached client may forget and hold her breath; a gentle reminder, advising her to keep breathing, usually enables the client to maintain relaxation. This technique is particularly helpful in the adolescent or virginal client, whose introitus may be especially tight.

Another relaxation or, more specifically, distraction technique that has been used by some practitioners is the placement of a sign or mobile above the examining table. Clients appreciate having something to look at, and their attention is constructively diverted from the activities of the examiner.

For most clients it is distressing to attempt to converse while in a lithotomy position. Most clients appreciate an explanation and reassurance from the examiner but prefer not to have to respond to questions until they are again upright and at an equal posture with the examiner. Questioning a client during the pelvic examination is apt to make her tense.

Environmental conditions are also important in enhancing cooperation during the examination of the genital area. The environment and the client should be warm. The examining area should be private and safe from unexpected intrusion.

ANATOMY AND PHYSIOLOGY
External genitalia

The external female genitalia are termed the vulva or pudendum (Fig. 17-1). The symphysis pubis is covered by a pad of fat called the mons pubis or mons veneris. In the postpubertal female the mons is covered by a patch of coarse, curly hair that extends to the lower abdomen. The abdominal portion of the female escutcheon is flat and forms the base of an inverted triangle of hair.

The labia majora are two bilobate folds of adipose tissue extending from the mons to the perineum. After puberty, their outer surfaces are covered with hair and their inner surfaces are smooth and hairless. The labia minora are two folds of skin that are thinner and darker in color than the labia majora. The labia minora lie within the labia majora and extend from the clitoris to the fourchette. Anteriorly, each labium minus divides into a medial and a lateral part. The lateral parts join posteriorly to form the prepuce of the clitoris, and the medial parts join anterior to the clitoris to form the frenulum of the clitoris. The clitoris is composed of erectile tissue and is homologous to the corpora cavernosa of the penis. Its body is normally about 2.5 cm in total length; the length of its visible portion is 2 cm or less.

The vestibule is the boat-shaped anatomical region between the labia minora. It contains the urethral and vaginal orifices. The urethral orifice is located approximately 2.5 cm posterior to the clitoris and is visualized as an irregular, vertical slit. The vaginal orifice, or introitus, lies immediately behind the urethral orifice and can be observed as a thin vertical slit or as a large orifice with irregular skin edges, depending on the condition of the hymen. The hymen is a membranous, annular, or crescentic fold at the vaginal opening. When unperforated, it is usually a continuous membrane but on occasion may be cribriform. After perforation small rounded fragments of hymen attach to the introital margins; these are called hymenal caruncles.

The ducts of two pairs of glands open on the vulva. Skene's glands are multiple, tiny organs located in the paraurethral area. Their ducts, numbering approximately 6 to 31, lie inside and just outside of the urethral orifice and are usually not visible. These ducts open laterally and slightly posterior to the urethral orifice in approximately 5 and 7 o'clock positions; the urethral orifice is the center of the clock. Bartholin's glands are small, ovoid organs located lateral and slightly posterior to the vaginal orifice, partially behind the bulb of the vestibule. Their ducts are approximately 2 cm long and open in the groove between the labia minora and the hymen. These ducts are also usually not visible.

The perineum consists of the tissues between the introitus and the anus.

The pelvic floor consists of a group of muscles attached to points on the bony pelvis (Fig. 17-2). These muscles form a suspended sling that assists in holding the pelvic contents in place. The muscles are pierced by the urethral, vaginal, and rectal orifices and function both passively as a pelvic support and actively in voluntary contraction of the vaginal and anal orifices.

Internal genitalia

Fig. 17-3 illustrates the internal genitalia.

The vagina is a pink, transversely rugated, collapsed tube that in the adult is approximately 9 cm long posteriorly and 6 to 7 cm long anteriorly. It inclines posteriorly at approximately a 45° angle with the vertical plane of the body. The vagina is highly dilatable, especially in its superior portion and anteroposterior dimension. When collapsed, it is H shaped in transverse section. Superiorly and usually anteriorly, the vagina is pierced by the uterine cervix. The recess between the portion of the vagina adjacent to the cervix and the cervix is called the vaginal fornix. Although it is actually continuous, the fornix is anatomically divided into anterior, posterior, and lateral fornices.

The uterus is an inverted, pear-shaped, muscular organ that is flattened anteroposteriorly. It is usually found inclined forward 45° from the vertical plane of the erect body and is approximately 5.5 to 8 cm long, 3.5 to 4 cm wide, and 2 to 2.5 cm thick. The uterus of the parous client may be normally enlarged an additional 2 to 3 cm in any of the three dimensions. The uterus is divided into two main parts: the body and the cervix. The body in turn is composed of three parts: the fundus, the prominence above the insertion of the fallopian tubes; the body, or main portion, of the uterus; and the isthmus, the constricted lower portion of the uterus, which is adjacent to the cervix. The cervix extends from the isthmus and into the vagina.

The uterine cavity communicates with the vagina via an ostium, the cervical os. The os is a

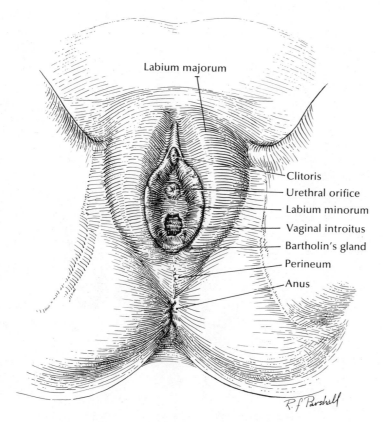

Fig. 17-1. External female genitalia.

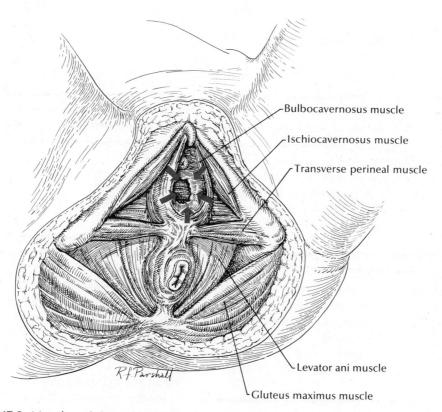

Fig. 17-2. Muscles of the pelvic floor. Arrows illustrate the direction of contraction of the bulbocavernosus muscle.

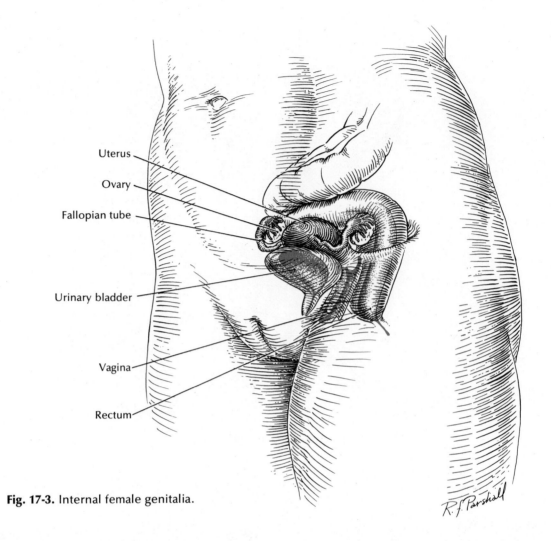

Fig. 17-3. Internal female genitalia.

Labels: Uterus, Ovary, Fallopian tube, Urinary bladder, Vagina, Rectum

small, depressed, circular opening in the nulliparous client. In women who have borne children the os is enlarged and irregularly shaped. The position of the uterus is not fixed; it is a relatively movable organ. The uterus may be anteverted, anteflexed, retroverted, or retroflexed in position; or it may be in midposition. In the normal adult with an empty bladder the uterus is usually anteverted and slightly anteflexed in position.

The ovaries are a pair of oval organs; each is approximately 3 cm long, 2 cm wide, and 1 cm thick. They are usually located near the lateral pelvic wall, at the level of the anterosuperior iliac spine. The two uterine tubes insert in the upper portion of the uterus, are supported loosely by the broad ligament, and run laterally to the ovaries. Each tube is approximately 10 cm long.

The uterus, ovaries, and tubes are supported by four pairs of ligaments: the cardinal, uterosacral, round, and broad ligaments (Fig. 17-4).

The rectouterine pouch, or Douglas' cul-de-sac, is a deep recess formed by the peritoneum as it passes over the intestinal surface of the rectum. It is the lowest point in the abdominal cavity.

EXAMINATION
■ Preparation

Clients should be advised not to douche during the 24 hours preceding the pelvic examination and reminded to empty their bladders immediately before the examination.

Some clients have difficulty assuming the lithotomy position, especially in moving their buttocks sufficiently downward to the edge of the table. The practitioner can assist the client by asking the client to raise her buttocks (while the client is lying on the table with heels in the stirrups) and by guiding the client's buttocks downward from a position at the client's side or from a position at the foot of the table. Clients usually

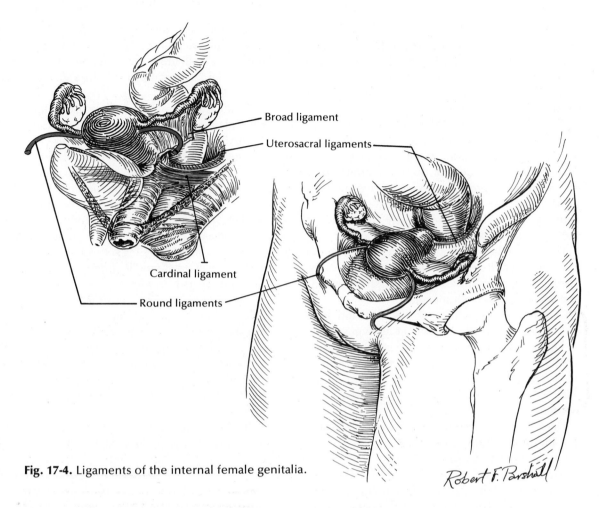

Broad ligament

Uterosacral ligaments

Cardinal ligament

Round ligaments

Robert F. Barshall

Fig. 17-4. Ligaments of the internal female genitalia.

feel more comfortable wearing shoes when their feet are in the stirrups, rather than supporting their weight with bare heels against the hard, cold stirrups.

Materials needed for the examination should be assembled and readily available before the client is put in the lithotomy position. Materials needed for the examination minimally include:

Rubber gloves
Speculums of various sizes
Culture plates for gonorrhea screening
Glass slides
Glass cover slides
Ayre spatula
Sterile cotton swabs
Lubricant on a piece of paper or gauze
Cotton balls
Sponge forceps
Cytology fixative
Source of light

■ **Components of the examination**

The regional examination of the female genital system consists of (1) the abdominal examination,

(2) inspection of the external genitalia, (3) palpation of the external genitalia, (4) the speculum examination, (5) the obtaining of specimens, (6) the bimanual vaginal examination, and (7) the rectovaginal examination.

The abdominal examination is discussed in Chapter 15 on Assessment of the abdomen and rectosigmoid region. The examination of the female genital system should be preceded by a thorough examination of the abdomen.

It is recommended that the examiner wear two gloves for the genital area examination. This will allow for a thorough external examination and complete spreading of the labia and also will protect subsequent clients from the possible transfer of infection.

Inspection of the external genitalia. First, the skin and hair distribution are observed. Hair distribution should be approximately shaped as an inverse triangle. Some abdominal hair is normal and may be hereditary. Male hair distribution patterns are abnormal. Growth of hair commences approximately 1 year before menarche. The total skin area is inspected for lesions and parasites. The gloved fingers should be used to spread the hair and labia so that all skin surfaces can be adequately visualized. The area of the clitoris particularly is a common site for chancres of syphilis in the younger client and for cancerous lesions in the older client.

The labia are flat in childhood and atrophic in old age. Estrogen influences fat deposition, which causes a round, full appearance of the labia. The labia majora of the nulliparous client will be in close approximation, covering the labia minora and the vestibule area. After a vaginal delivery, the labia may be slightly shriveled and gaping in appearance.

The skin of the vulvar area is of a slightly darker pigment than the skin of the rest of the body. The mucous membranes are normally dark pink in color and moist in appearance.

Common abnormalities of the skin and labia include parasites, skin lesions of all types, areas of leukoplakia, varicosities, hyperpigmentation, erythema, depigmentation, and swelling. Leukoplakia appears as white, adherent patches on the skin; it may be likened to spots of dried white paint.

The clitoris is examined for size; the visible portion of the clitoris should not exceed 2 cm in length and 1 cm in width.

The urethral orifice normally appears slitlike or stellate and is of the same color as the membranes surrounding it. The openings of the paraurethral (Skene's) glands are not usually visible. Erythema or a polyp located in this area or a discharge from the urethra or gland ducts is abnormal.

The examiner next observes the area of the Bartholin's glands and their ducts for swelling, erythema, duct enlargement, or discharge. The presence of any of these conditions is abnormal.

The perineum is inspected for evidence of an episiotomy and its healing. The anus is also inspected at this time (see Chapter 15 on Assessment of the abdomen and rectosigmoid region).

Palpation of the external genitalia. Any areas of observed abnormality are palpated to determine the size, shape, consistency, and tenderness of the mass or lesion. The labia are palpated. They should feel soft, and the texture should be homogenous.

The index finger and the middle finger are inserted into the vagina. First, the urethra and area of Skene's duct openings are gently milked from about the level of 4 cm in on the anterior vaginal wall down to the orifice (Fig. 17-5). This procedure should not normally cause pain or discharge. If a discharge is present, a specimen

inoculated onto a Thayer-Martin culture plate. Then the area of Bartholin's glands and their ducts are palpated for swelling or tenderness (Fig. 17-6). Normally Bartholin's glands are not palpable.

While the examiner's fingers are in the vagina, several maneuvers are performed to assess the integrity of the pelvic musculature. First, the perineal area is palpated between the fingers inside the vagina and the thumb of that same hand. In the nulliparous client the perineum is felt as a firm, muscular body. After an episiotomy has healed, the perineum feels thinner and more rigid because of scarring. If this area is very thin and if the palpating fingers can almost approximate, the client should be questioned again about bowel or sexual problems.

The client is then asked to constrict her vaginal orifice around the examiner's fingers while they are still placed in the vagina. Again, a nulliparous client will demonstrate a high degree of tone and a multiparous client, less tone. A client whose vaginal orifice has poor tone will probably admit to some dissatisfaction expressed by her sexual partner.

In the third maneuver the index and middle fingers remain in the vagina; they are spread laterally, and the client is asked to push down against them. The presence of urinary stress incontinence, cystocele, rectocele, enterocele, or uterine prolapse can be observed if present.

Cystocele is the prolapse into the vagina of the anterior vaginal wall and the bladder. Clinically, a pouching would be seen on the anterior wall as the client strains.

Rectocele is the prolapse into the vagina of the posterior vaginal wall and the rectum. Clinically, a pouching would be seen on the posterior wall as the client strains.

Enterocele is a hernia of the pouch of Douglas into the vagina. Clinically, a bulge would be seen emerging from the posterior fornix. If this is observed, the client should be additionally examined by assessing the effect of straining (1) during the speculum examination with the speculum inserted, half opened, three fourths of its length into the vagina; and (2) during the bimanual examination with the intravaginal fingers in the posterior fornix.

There are three degrees of *uterine prolapse*. In first-degree prolapse, the cervix appears at the introitus when the client strains. In second-degree prolapse, the cervix is outside of the introitus when the client strains. In third-degree prolapse, the whole uterus is outside the introitus and the

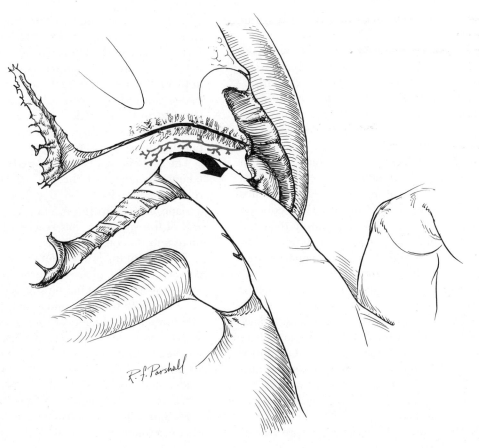

Fig. 17-5. Palpation of Skene's glands.

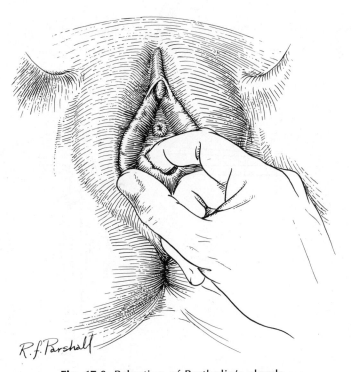

Fig. 17-6. Palpation of Bartholin's glands.

vagina is essentially turned inside out when the client strains.

Speculum examination. The examiner will have obtained clues regarding the most appropriate type and size of speculum to use in the speculum examination through the history and inspection of the external genitalia. There are two basic types of speculums, the Graves speculum and the Pederson speculum (Fig. 17-7). The Graves speculum is one of the most commonly used in the examination of the adult female client. It is available in lengths varying from 3½ to 5 inches and in widths from ¾ to 1½ inches. The Pederson speculum is both narrower and flatter than the Graves speculum and is used with virgins, nulliparous clients, or clients whose vaginal orifices have contracted postmenopausally.

A metal speculum needs to be warmed before insertion. An effective way to do this is by running warm water over it. Lubricant is bacteriostatic and also distorts cells on Papanicolaou (Pap) smears; thus, it cannot be used if a culture or smear is to be obtained. The warm water also assists in lubricating both the metal and plastic speculums and may be used if cultures and smears are to be taken.

The index finger and middle finger are placed 1 inch into the vagina. The fingers are then spread, and pressure is exerted toward the posterior vaginal wall. The client is advised that she will feel intravaginal pressure. The speculum is held in the opposite hand with the blades between the index and middle fingers. The client is asked to bear down. This maneuver helps to additionally open the vaginal orifice and to relax perineal muscles (Fig. 17-8, *A*).

The speculum blades are inserted obliquely, taking advantage of the H configuration of the relaxed vagina (Fig. 17-8, *B*). They are inserted at a plane parallel to the examining table until the end of the speculum has reached the tips of the fingers in the vagina.

The speculum is then rotated to a transverse position, and the plane is altered in adaptation to the plane of the vagina, approximately one of a 45° angle with the examining table (Fig. 17-8, *C*). The intravaginal fingers are simultaneously withdrawn, and the speculum is inserted until it touches the end of the vagina. The lever of the speculum is then depressed; this opens the blades and allows visualization. Hopefully, the cervix is seen between the blades (Fig. 17-8, *D*). Sometimes, however, especially for the beginning examiner, it is not. In such cases the specu-

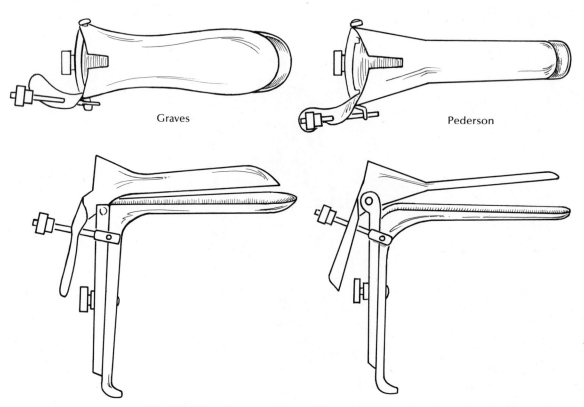

Graves

Pederson

Fig. 17-7. Graves speculum and Pederson speculum.

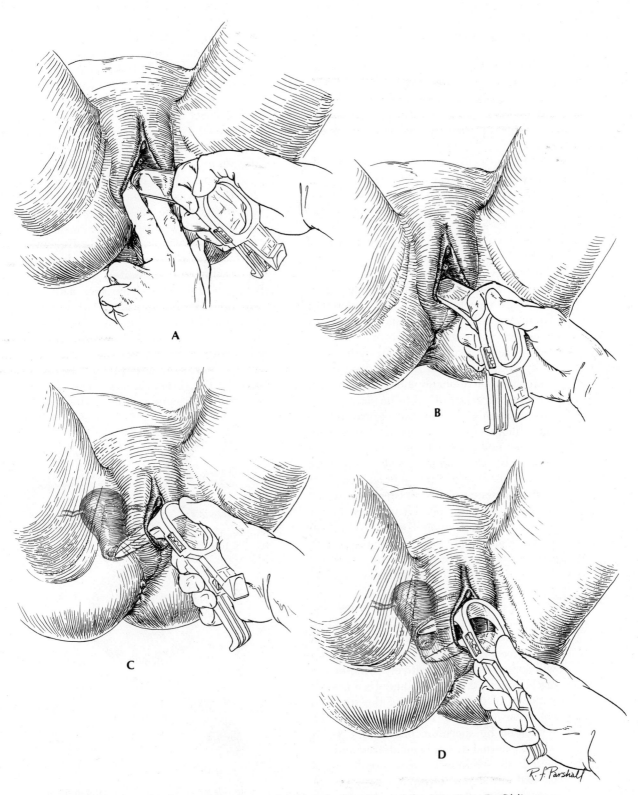

Fig. 17-8. Procedure for vaginal examination. **A,** Opening of the introitus. **B,** Oblique insertion of the speculum. **C,** Final insertion of the speculum. **D,** Opening of the speculum blades.

lum is either anterior (usually the situation) or posterior to the cervix. If this occurs, the speculum is withdrawn halfway and reinserted in a different plane. After the entire cervix is in view of the examiner, the depressed lever is fixed in an open position.

The appearance of the normal cervix has already been described. The cervix is observed for color, position, size, projection into the vaginal vault, shape, general symmetry, surface characteristics, shape and patency of the os, and discharge:

1. *Color:* The color of the cervix is normally pale after menopause and cyanotic in pregnancy. Cyanosis can occur with any condition that causes systemic hypoxia or regional venous congestion. Hyperemia may be an indication of inflammation. An additional cause of pallor is anemia.

2. *Position:* A cervix projecting more deeply than 3 cm into the vaginal vault may indicate uterine prolapse. A cervix situated on a lateral vaginal wall may indicate tumor or adhesion of a superior structure.

3. *Size:* A cervix larger than 4 cm in diameter is hypertrophied, and the presence of inflammation or tumor should be considered.

4. *Surface characteristics:* Lesions and polyps are commonly seen on the cervix and require more visual assessment. Any irregularity or nodularity of the cervical surface should be considered possibly abnormal (Fig. 17-9). One relatively benign condition is the presence of nabothian cysts, which appear as smooth, round, small (less than 1 cm in diameter) yellow lesions. Nabothian cysts are caused by obstruction of the cervical gland ducts. Because of the occasional presence of the squamocolumnar junction on the ectocervix, the differential assessment of normal cervix from abnormal cervix using inspection alone is impossible. When the squamocolumnar junction is on the ectocervix, the columnar epithelium will appear as a red, relatively symmetrical circle around the os. This may be a normal variation of the placement of the squamocolumnar junction or may be caused by the separation by speculum blades of a cervix whose external os has been altered and enlarged by childbirth; this condition is termed eversion or ectropion. Erosions appear similar to eversions. However, erosions are irregular, rough, and friable. They require further assessment and treatment.

Diffuse punctile hemorrhages, colloquially termed "strawberry spots" are occasionally observed in association with trichomonal infections.

5. *Discharge:* The character of the normal cervical mucus varies in the menstrual cycle. It is always odorless and nonirritating. Its color and consistency may vary from clear to white and from thin to thick and stringy. Colored or purulent discharges exuding from the os or present in the area of the cervix are probably abnormal.

6. *Shape of the os:* The cervical os of the nulliparous client is small and evenly round. The cervical os of a parous client shows the effects of the stretching and laceration of childbirth and is irregular in shape.

After the cervix is inspected, a Pap smear, culture for gonorrhea, and hanging drop specimen may be obtained if indicated. The procedures for these are described at the end of this chapter. The vagina is then inspected. This is done during speculum insertion, while the speculum is open, and during its removal. The color and condition of the vaginal mucosa and the color, odor, consistency, and appearance of vaginal secretions are noted. Pallor, cyanosis, and hyperemia may be present for the same reasons as described for the

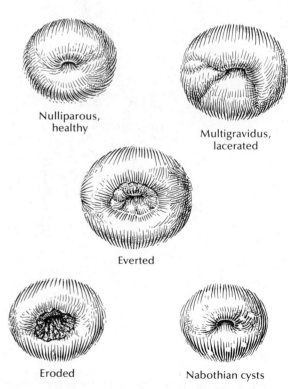

Nulliparous, healthy

Multigravidus, lacerated

Everted

Eroded

Nabothian cysts

Fig. 17-9. Common appearances and lesions of the cervix.

cervix. Leukoplakia may also occur on vaginal mucosa.

As with cervical discharge, vaginal discharge is normally odorless, nonirritating, thin or mucoid, and clear or cloudy. Also, the presence of some whitish, creamy material is normal. Any other vaginal discharge should be described according to its color, odor, consistency, amount, and appearance. Three basic types of vaginal infections produce observable discharge: monilial infections, characterized by thick, white, curdy, exudates that appear as adherent patches and free discharge; trichomonal infections, characterized by a profuse watery, gray or green, frothy, odorous discharge; and bacterial infections, characterized by an odorous, gray, homogenous discharge of moderate amount.

After the inspection of the vaginal area, the speculum is slowly withdrawn. As it is withdrawn, the nut, or catch, is loosened and the lever is again controlled by the thumb. The blades are slowly closed as they are removed, and the speculum is carefully rotated so that all areas of vaginal tissue are inspected. As the blades are closed, caution is taken to prevent pinching of tissue or the catching of hairs in the blades.

The speculum is inspected for odors and is either discarded or placed in a soaking solution.

Bimanual vaginal examination. The purpose of the bimanual examination is the palpation of the pelvic contents between the examiner's two hands (Figs. 17-10 and 17-11). Examiners vary in their preference of the placement of the dominant, more sensitive hand. The beginning examiner should attempt alternating hands for examinations and then decide on a routine that is most workable for him.

The client remains in the lithotomy position. The vaginal examining hand assumes the obstetrical position: index and middle fingers extended and together, thumb abducted, and fourth and little fingers folded on the palm of the hand. The vaginal examining fingers are lubricated. The labia are spread with the thumb and index finger

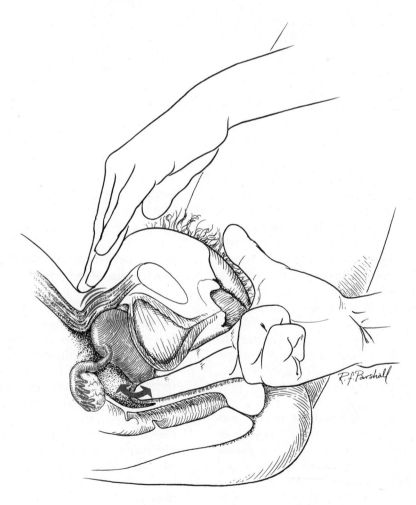

Fig. 17-10. Bimanual palpation of the uterus.

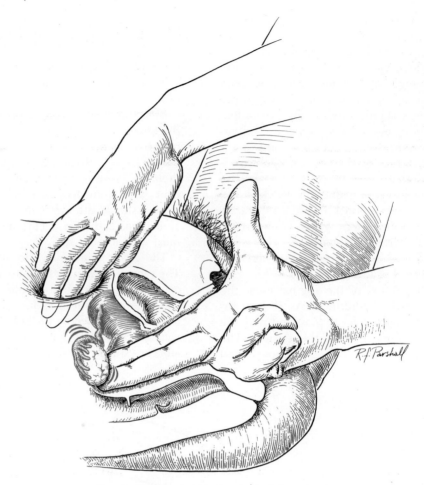

Fig. 17-11. Bimanual palpation of the adnexa.

of the opposite hand. The lubricated fingers are inserted into the vagina with the palmar surface of the hand directed toward the anterior vaginal wall. The examiner should always palpate with the palmar surface of the fingers rather than with the less sensitive tips or backs. The other hand is placed on the abdomen. This hand will be used to press the abdominal and pelvic contacts toward the intravaginal hand. Movement of both hands should be slow and firm. In order for the examiner to palpate adequately, the client must be relaxed. If the client becomes tense, the procedure is stopped, and the client is helped to relax; however, the examiner's hands remain in position.

The cervix is located and assessed for size, contour, surface characteristics, consistency, position, patency of the os, and mobility. The palmar surfaces of both fingers are used to completely palpate the cervix and the fornices. A finger is gently placed into the external os to assess its patency. It is determined on which vaginal wall

the cervix is placed and if the cervix is approximately midline. The fingers are placed in the lateral fornices, and the cervix is wagged, or moved back and forth, between the fingers for approximately 1 to 2 cm in each direction. The cervix and uterus should be freely movable and should move without tenderness. An immobile or tender cervix and uterus are abnormal.

The surface of the cervix is normally smooth. Nabothian cysts, tumors, or lesions will make it feel nodular or irregular. The consistency of the cervix is firm and slightly resilient and feels analogous to the tip of the nose. The cervix softens in pregnancy and hardens with tumors. The cervix is normally located on the anterior wall in the midline or on the posterior wall. A laterally displaced cervix may indicate tumor or adhesion. The external os in the nonpregnant client should admit a finger for about a quarter inch. It should be open and firm. A stenosed external os is abnormal.

The size, shape, surface characteristics, consis-

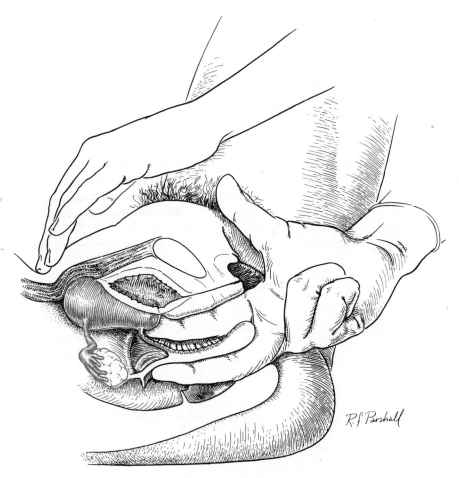

Fig. 17-12. Rectovaginal palpation.

tency, position, mobility, and tenderness of the uterine body and fundus are assessed. It is useful to first determine the position of the uterus, because techniques used to assess the uterine body and fundus will vary with the uterine position in the client (Fig. 17-12). The uterus is in one of the three basic positions: anteversion, mid-position, or retroversion. In the first and third positions the uterus may in addition be flexed, or bent on itself, to produce two additional variations of position: anteflexion and retroflexion. The position of the cervix and the direction of the os provide the examiner with clues of the uterine position. A cervix on the anterior wall may indicate an antepositioned or retroflexed uterus; a centrally located cervix probably indicates a uterus in mid-position; and a cervix on the posterior vaginal wall probably indicates a uterus in retroversion.

Approximately 85% of uteri are in anteposition, therefore, palpation is first attempted anteriorly. The intravaginal fingers are placed in the anterior fornix. The hand on the abdomen is placed flat on the midline and in a position approximately halfway between the symphysis pubis and the umbilicus. This hand acts as a resistance against which the pelvic organs are palpated by the intravaginal fingers. The fingers in the anterior fornix gently lift the tissues against the hand on the abdomen. If the uterus is in anteposition, it will be palpated between the hands. If the uterus is not palpated anteriorly, the fingers are placed in the posterior fornix and again raised forward toward the hand on the abdomen. If the uterus is in retroversion, only the isthmus will be felt between the hands and the corpus may be felt with the backs of the intravaginal fingers. A retroverted uterus is felt best during the rectovaginal examination.

If the uterus is identified as being in anteposition or midposition, an attempt is made to palpate all its anterior and posterior surfaces by maneuvering its position and by "walking up" its surface with the intravaginal fingers. After the uterus is palpated, the adnexal areas are examined. The structures in these areas are of a size, consistency, and position that they may not be specifically palpated. If the examiner has appropriately examined the area and no masses larger than the normal-size ovaries are identified, it is assumed that no masses are present.

Each of the adnexal areas, left and right, are palpated. The index and middle finger of the intravaginal hand are placed in one of the lateral fornices; the hand on the abdomen is placed on the ipsilateral iliac crest; and the hands are brought together and moved in an inferior and medial direction, allowing the tissues lying between the two hands to slip between them. The hand on the abdomen acts as resistance, and the intravaginal hand palpates the organs between the hands. Frequently, no specific organ is palpated in this maneuver. If normal ovaries are palpated, they are smooth, firm, slightly flattened, ovoid, and no larger than 4 to 6 cm in their largest dimension. Ovaries of prepubertal girls or postmenopausal women are normally smaller than 4 cm in their largest dimension. The ovaries are sensitive to touch but are not tender. They are highly movable and will easily slip between the palpating hands.

Normal fallopian tubes are not palpable. One clue to an ectopic pregnancy is the presence of arterial pulses in the adnexal areas.

Table 17-1. Findings in bimanual vaginal and rectovaginal examination

Position of uterus	Bimanual		
	Illustration	Direction of cervical os	Body and fundus
Anteverted		Posterior	Palpable by one hand on the abdomen and the fingers of the other in the vagina
Midposition		In the same plane as the vagina	May not be palpable

Cordlike structures that are sometimes palpable are round ligaments.

Rectovaginal examination. After the completion of the vaginal examination, the hands are withdrawn, the secretions are washed off of the gloved fingers, and the index and middle fingers are relubricated. The index finger is placed into the vagina and the middle finger is placed into the rectum. The intravaginal finger remains on the cervix, identifying it, lest it be mistaken for a mass by the intrarectal finger.

The uterine position is confirmed by the rectal examination. If the uterus is retroverted, its body and fundus are now palpated. In addition, the adnexal areas are reassessed. The procedure is the same as that described with the vaginal examination (Fig. 17-12).

The area of the rectovaginal septum and cul-de-sac are palpated. The rectovaginal septum should be palpated as a firm, thin, smooth, pliable structure. The posterior cul-de-sac is a potential space. The normal pelvic organs are palpated through it. Often, abnormal masses and normal ovaries are discovered in the cul-de-sac.

Uterosacral ligaments may be palpable.

The rectal examination is completed (see (Chapter 15 on Assessment of the abdomen and rectosigmoid region), and the client is helped up.

| Anterior and posterior portion of uterus | Rectovaginal | | |
	Illustration	Cervix	Body and fundus
Palpable as the uterus is rotated even more anteriorly		Palpable through the rectovaginal septum	Not palpable by fingers in the rectum
May not be palpable		Posterior portion felt through the rectovaginal septum	May not be palpable

Continued.

Table 17-1. Findings in bimanual vaginal and rectovaginal examination—cont'd

Position of uterus	Bimanual		
	Illustration	Direction of cervical os	Body and fundus
Retroverted		Anterior	Not palpable
Anteflexed		Anterior or midposition; the axis of the cervix is different from the axis of the body of the uterus; angulation of the isthmus may be felt in the anterior fornix	Easily palpable
Retroflexed		Anterior, midposition, or posterior	Not palpable

Anterior and posterior portion of uterus	Rectovaginal		
	Illustration	Cervix	Body and fundus
Posterior portion may be palpable by fingers in the posterior fornix		May not be palpable by fingers in the rectum	Body easily palpable by fingers in the rectum; fundus may not be palpable
Easily palpable		Same as anteverted	Same as anteverted
Not palpable		Palpable through the rectovaginal septum	Angulation palpable; body and fundus easily palpable

■ Examination of clients who are unable to assume the lithotomy position

The lithotomy position is the optimal one for a pelvic examination. However, it may be difficult for a very ill or debilitated client to assume and maintain a lithotomy position. An alternative position for the female genital examination is the left lateral or Sims position (Fig. 17-13). The client's buttocks should be as close to the edge of the examining table as safety allows. The knees are bent and abducted, and the left leg is positioned on top of or over the right leg. The examiner stands behind and at the side of the client. All of the examination procedures described previously in this chapter can be performed with the client in this position.

■ Pelvic assessment in the first trimester of pregnancy

Probably the first symptom of pregnancy is a "missed period" or amenorrhea. Clients with this complaint alert the examiner to be especially observant for the signs of early pregnancy.

In early pregnancy the uterus changes in form, size, consistency, and position. In the first 4 weeks of pregnancy there is an enlargement in the anteroposterior diameter of the uterus. In the fourth to sixth week of pregnancy the cervix (Goodell's sign) and the cervicouterine junction (Laden's sign) soften. This softening allows for a compressibility of the lower uterine segment at 6 weeks (Hegar's sign). At this time the uterine

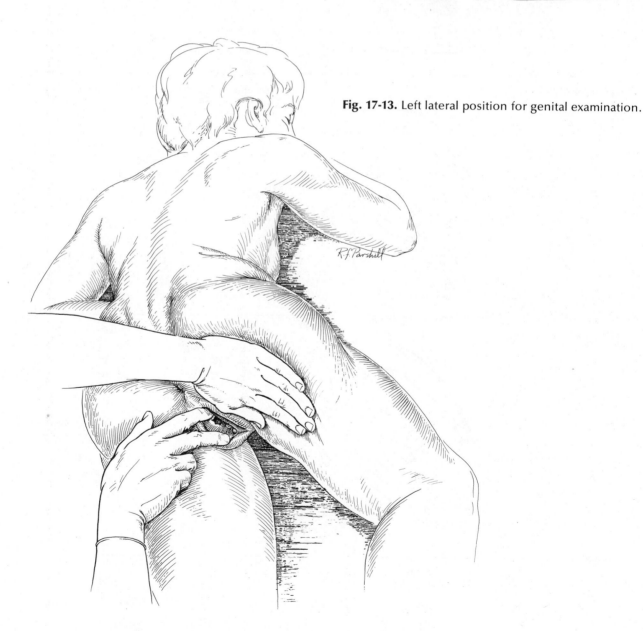

Fig. 17-13. Left lateral position for genital examination.

artery pulsations may be palpable in the lateral fornices (Oslander's sign). At 8 weeks the uterus is globular in shape and feels soft and spongy. In addition, it is in an exaggerated anteflexed position and lies on the bladder.

Inspection might also yield clues to early pregnancy. At 8 to 12 weeks the vagina and cervix may appear bluish violet in color (Jacquemier's or Chadwick's sign). At approximately this same time the breast veins dilate and become more prominent.

At 12 weeks the uterus begins to become an abdominal organ and is palpable above the symphysis pubis.

Procedures for smears and cultures

CERVICAL PAPANICOLAOU SMEAR

The client is in the lithotomy position, and the speculum has been inserted. All materials listed earlier in the chapter are assembled. If a cervical mucous plug is present, it can be removed with a cotton ball held with forceps. There are many variations among laboratories regarding the areas from which cell samples are to be obtained, the mixing of cells from two or more areas, and the fixing of cells. One procedure is described here. However, variations are acceptable and the prac-

titioner should consult with the cytopathologist from the laboratory reading the smears for locally recommended procedures.

Endocervical smear

Fig. 17-14 illustrates the procedure for an endocervical smear:

1. A sterile applicator is inserted approximately 0.5 cm into the cervical os. It is rotated 360° and left in 10 to 20 seconds to ensure saturation.
2. The endocervical smear is spread on the portion of the slide marked *E*. The swab is rotated so that all sampled areas are smeared on the slide. The smear should not contain thick areas that would be difficult to visualize microscopically.

Cervical smear

Fig. 17-15 illustrates the procedure for a cervical smear:

1. The larger humped end of the Ayre spatula is inserted into the cervical os, so that the cervix fits comfortably into the groove created by the two humps. With moderate pressure, the spatula is rotated 360°, scraping the entire cervical surface and the squamocolumnar junction.
2. The material from both sides of the spatula is spread on the portion of the slide marked *C*.

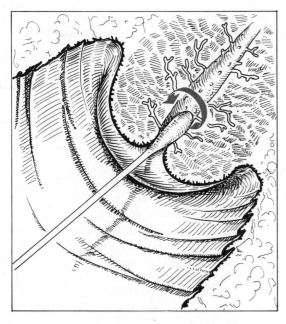

Fig. 17-14. Endocervical smear.

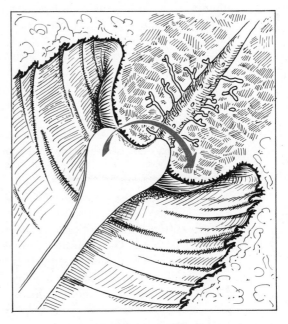

Fig. 17-15. Cervical smear.

■ **Vaginal pool smear**

1. With the paddle or handle end of the Ayre spatula, the area of the posterior fornix is scraped.
2. The material on the slide is spread in the area marked *V*.
3. The slide is fixed immediately by spraying or immersion into a fixative solution.

GONORRHEAL CULTURE

The female client is in the lithotomy position. The male client can be seated when a urethral specimen is to be taken. If a rectal culture is also to be taken, the male client may assume the Sims position or bend over an examining table with buttocks exposed, feet spread, and toes pointing inward. An oropharyngeal culture is sometimes indicated.

■ **Endocervical culture**

1. A specimen from the endocervical canal is obtained with a sterile cotton applicator. The technique is the same as that described for the Pap smear.
2. The Thayer-Martin culture plate is inoculated. With the medium at room temperature, the swab is rolled in a large **Z** pattern on the culture plate; the swab is simultaneously rotated as it is creating the **Z**, so that all swab surfaces will be inoculated (Fig. 17-16).
3. The culture plate is incubated within 15 minutes of its inoculation in a warm, anaerobic environment. The culture plate is placed medium side up in a candle jar; the candle is lit; the cover of the jar is tightly secured; and the jar is left in a warm area until specimens can be placed in an incubator. In some clinic situations, the inoculation is immediately cross streaked with a sterile wire loop. Usually however, this is done in the laboratory, not in the examining room.

■ **Anal culture: female or male client**

Fig. 17-17 illustrates the procedure for an anal culture:

1. A sterile cotton-tipped applicator is inserted into the anal canal. The applicator is rotated 360° and moved from side to side. It is left in for a total of 10 to 30 seconds to allow for absorption of secretion and organisms. If the swab contains feces, it is discarded and another specimen taken.
2. The culture plate is inoculated and incu-

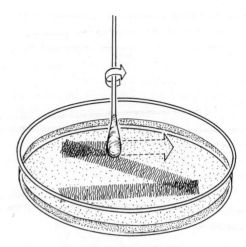

Fig. 17-16. Inoculation of the Thayer-Martin culture.

bated as described previously, using a separate culture plate.

■ **Urethral culture: male client**

1. A urethral culture is obtained. A sterile bacteriological loop is inserted into the urethra for 1 to 2 cm, and the mucosa is gently scraped.
2. The culture medium is inoculated and incubated.

■ **Oropharyngeal culture**

1. A specimen of secretion from the oropharynx is obtained with a sterile swab.
2. The medium is inoculated and incubated as described for endocervical specimens.

SMEARS FOR VAGINAL INFECTIONS

1. A specimen of vaginal secretions is obtained directly from the vagina or from material in the inferior speculum blade. For *Trichomonas vaginalis*, the secretions are mixed with a drop of normal saline solution on a glass slide. For *Candida albicans*, the secretions are mixed with a drop of 10% potassium hydroxide solution on a slide. For *Hemophilus vaginalis*, the secretions are not mixed with any solution.
2. A cover glass is placed on the slide.
3. The slide is immediately observed under a microscope (Fig. 17-18). If positive for *T. vaginalis*, trichomonads will be seen. These are single-cell flagellates about the size of a white blood cell. If positive for *C. albicans*, mycelia and spores are seen. If positive for *H. vaginalis*, characteristic "cue cells" are seen.

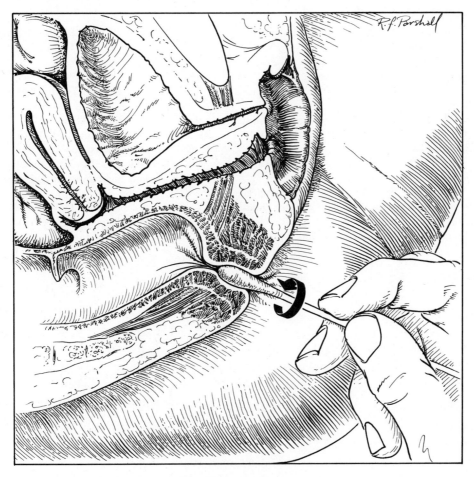

Fig. 17-17. Anal smear.

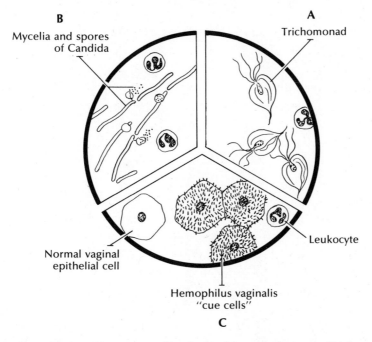

Fig. 17-18. Microscopic appearance of vaginal microorganisms. **A,** Trichomonads. **B,** Mycelia and spores. **C,** Epithelial cells stippled by *Hemophilus vaginalis* bacteria.

BIBLIOGRAPHY

Barr, W.: Clinical gynecology, Edinburgh, 1972, Churchill Livingstone.

Burghardt, E.: Early histological diagnosis of cervical cancer, Philadelphia, 1973, W. B. Saunders Co.

Frankfort, E.: Vaginal politics, New York, 1972, Quadrangle Books.

Garrey, M. M., Govan, A. D. T., Hodge, C., and others: Obstetrics illustrated, ed. 12, Edinburgh, 1974, Churchill Livingstone.

Greenhill, J. P.: Office gynecology, Chicago, 1971, Yearbook Medical Publishers, Inc.

Greenhill, J. P., and Friedman, E. A.: Biological principles and modern practices of obstetrics, Philadelphia, 1974, W. B. Saunders Co.

Howkins, J., and Bourne, G.: Shaw's textbook of gynecology, Edinburgh, 1971, Churchill Livingstone.

Hughes, E. C., editor: Obstetric-gynecologic terminology, Philadelphia, 1972, W. B. Saunders Co.

Kistner, R. W.: Gynecology; principles and practice, ed. 2, Chicago, 1971, Yearbook Medical Publishers, Inc.

Novak, E. R., Jones, G. S., and Jones, H. W., Jr.: Textbook of gynecology, ed. 9, Baltimore, 1975, The Williams & Wilkins Co.

U.S. Department of Health, Education, and Welfare: Criteria and techniques for the diagnosis of gonorrhea, Atlanta, 1974, U.S. Public Health Service.

Willson, J. R., Beecham, C. T., and Carrington, E. R.: Obstetrics and gynecology, ed. 5, St. Louis, 1975, The C. V. Mosby Co.

18 Musculoskeletal assessment

The skeletal system is made up of 206 bones and the joints by which they articulate. Bone, cartilage, connective and hematopoietic (myeloid) tissues make up this system. These structures (1) provide support for the body, (2) allow movement as those muscles attached to the bones shorten in contraction (thereby pulling the bones), and (3) provide for the formation of red blood cells.

The musculoskeletal system is comprised of more than 600 voluntary or striated muscles and constitutes the principal organ of movement as well as a repository for metabolites. The muscle mass accounts for as much as 40% of the weight of the adult man.

It is the partial contracture of skeletal muscle that makes all of the characteristic postures of man possible, including the upright position that distinguishes the anthropoid.

Seven types of joint motion have been defined. These movements are flexion, extension, abduction, adduction, internal rotation, external rotation, and circumduction (Figs. 18-1 to 18-4).

Flexion is the bending of the joint so as to approximate the bones it connects, thereby decreasing the joint angle. *Extension* is the straightening of a limb so that the joint angle is increased, the placement of the distal segment of a limb in such a position that its axis is continuous with that of the proximal segment, or the pulling or dragging force exerted on a limb in a direction away from the body.

Abduction is the movement of a limb away from the midline of the body or one of its parts. *Adduction* is the movement of a limb toward the central axis of the body or beyond it.

Internal rotation is the turning of the body part inward toward the central axis of the body. *External rotation* is the turning of the body part away from the midline.

Circumduction is the movement of a body part in a circular pattern. This is not a singular motion but a combination of the other motions.

Muscles are categorized according to the type of joint movement produced by their contraction. Muscles, thus, are flexors, extensors, adductors, abductors, internal rotators, external rotators, or circumflexors. Muscles shorten on contraction and in so doing exert pull on the bones to which they are attached to move them closer together. Most muscles attach to two bones that articulate at an intervening joint. Generally, one bone moves while the other is held stable. This is due to simultaneous shortening of other muscles. The body of the muscle that produces movement of an extremity generally lies proximal to the bone that is moved.

Thus, the joint, with its synovial membrane, capsule, ligaments, and the muscles that cross it, is considered to be the functional unit of the musculoskeletal system. This discussion of musculoskeletal assessment assumes that the practitioner has an understanding of the anatomy and physiology of the joints involved.

The examination of neuromuscular coordination begins as the practitioner first meets and observes the client, and it continues as the client advances into the room, sits, rises from a sitting position, climbs onto the examining table, lies down, and rolls over. The practitioner should note the speed, coordination, and strength of motion. He should particularly note clumsy, awkward, or involuntary movements, as well as tremor or fasciculation. During the interview the flamboyance or paucity of gesture may provide valuable clues to the client's personality and general mobility.

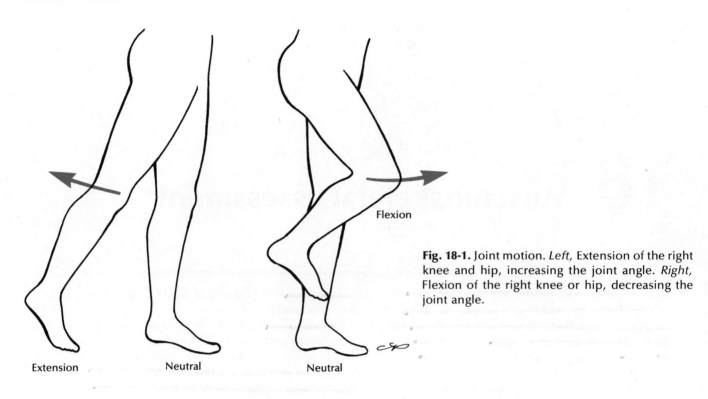

Fig. 18-1. Joint motion. *Left,* Extension of the right knee and hip, increasing the joint angle. *Right,* Flexion of the right knee or hip, decreasing the joint angle.

Extension Neutral Neutral Flexion

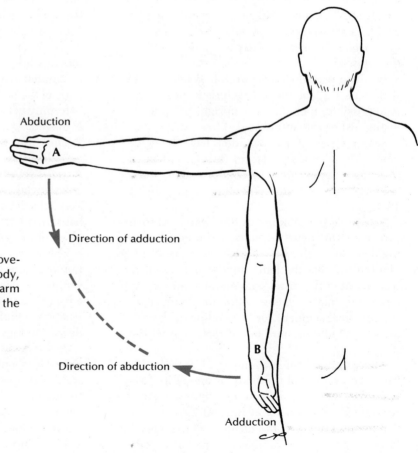

Fig. 18-2. Joint motion. Abduction is the movement of a limb away from the midline of the body, as seen in position A. Position B illustrates an arm in adduction, the movement of a limb toward the central axis of the body.

Abduction

A

Direction of adduction

Direction of abduction

B

Adduction

Fig. 18-3. Joint motion. Internal rotation is the turning of a body part inward toward the midline, as seen in position *A*. Position *B* illustrates external rotation, the turning of a body part away from the midline.

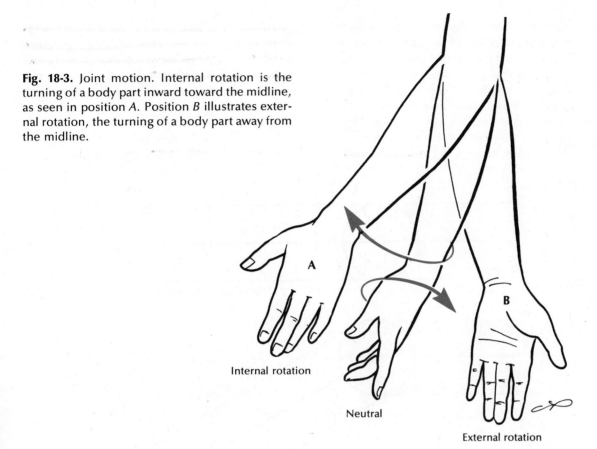

Internal rotation

Neutral

External rotation

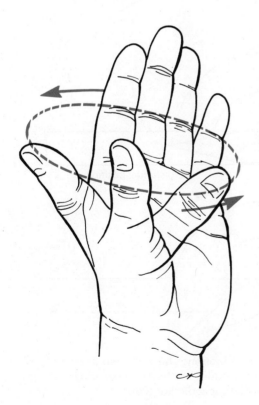

Fig. 18-4. Joint motion. Circumduction is the movement of a body part in a circular pattern.

The chief complaint of the client may indicate the direction for emphasis of the physical assessment. The individual with a chief problem of bodily deformity, paralysis, weakness, or pain associated with movement causes the examiner to focus attention on the bones, joints, and muscles as the possible sites of disorder. The structure and function of the body's equipment for movement are explored essentially through the techniques of inspection and palpation, assessment of the ranges of active and passive motion, and tests for muscle strength. A cloth or metal tape measure that will not stretch and a goniometer—a protractor with movable arms that is used to measure the range of joint motion—are necessary to this examination (Fig. 18-5).

As in previously described assessments, the cephalocaudal (head to toe) organization for exam-

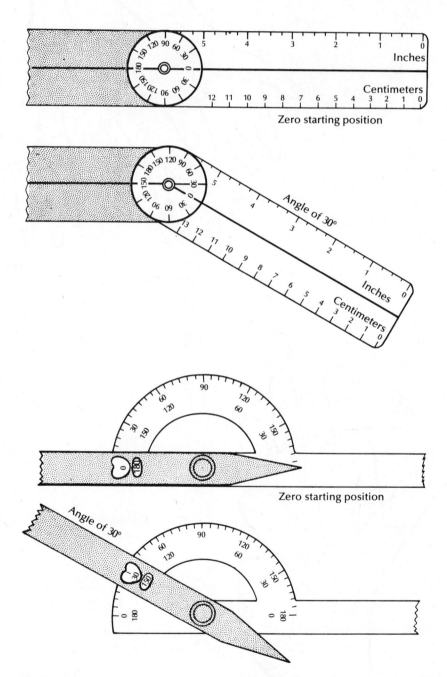

Fig. 18-5. Goniometers used to measure joint motion. The extended anatomical position is accepted as zero degrees. (From Joint motion; method of measuring and recording, Chicago, 1965, American Academy of Orthopaedic Surgeons.)

ination is used in the examination of the bones, joints, and muscles. This organization provides order and aids in avoiding omissions.

Thorough assessment of the musculoskeletal system can only be accomplished through the appropriate exposure of the client. The ambulatory individual can best be examined in shorts or swimming trunks. In this manner the extremities and spine are available for examination. Modesty may be protected for the female client by allow-

ing her to wear a brassiere or some other abbreviated form of chest cover. Although every effort is made to protect the modesty of the client, an honest examination cannot be made on a fully clothed client. Frequently the practitioner has anxiety about viewing the nude client; this must be worked through if the practitioner is to obtain an adequate data base.

For each examination the client should be in the position that provides the greatest stability.

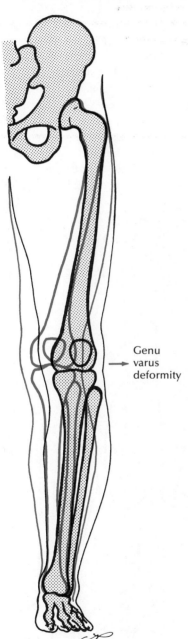

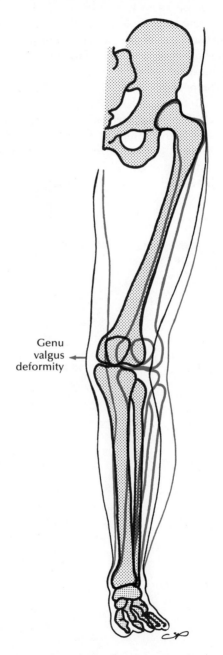

Fig. 18-6. Varus deformity of the leg: lateral deviation from the midline (bowleg). This condition was called valgus deformity in earlier times. Outline figure shows normal position.

Fig. 18-7. Valgus deformity of the leg: deviation of the leg toward the midline (knock-knee). This condition was called varus deformity in earlier times. Outline figure shows normal position.

Muscles are examined in symmetrical pairs, that is, first one and then the other for equivalence in size, contour, and strength. The contralateral, matching muscle pairs should be uniformly positioned while they are examined. They are examined both at rest and in a state of contraction.

INSPECTION

General inspection of the musculoskeletal system includes a visual scanning for symmetry, contour, and size of the two sides of the body, gross deformities, areas of swelling or edema, and ecchymoses or other discoloration.

The posture, or stance, and body alignment are viewed from both in front of and behind the client. The structural relationship of the feet to the legs and the hips to the pelvis are noted, as are those of the upper extremities, shoulder girdle, and upper trunk.

The shape of the spine is assessed, and its structural apposition to the shoulder girdle, thorax, and pelvis are ascertained.

A deformity is an abnormality in appearance. *Varus* and *valgus* are terms used to describe an angular deviation from the normal structure of an extremity. The reference point is the midline of the body. A varus deformity of the leg (bowlegs) is the lateral deviation of the leg from the midline (Fig. 18-6). A valgus deformity (knock-knees) is one wherein the deviation of the deformity is toward the midline (Fig. 18-7).

Scoliosis is a deformity of the spine seen as a lateral deviation (Fig. 18-8). This angling of the spine produces a downward slant of the thoracic cage on the affected side and an upward tilt of the pelvis on the contralateral side. A rotary deformity of the rib cage occurs as well. The ribs protrude posteriorly on the convex side of the spine. A hump or "razor back" may be observed. The protrusion may be made more obvious by asking the client to bend over to touch his toes. The deformity is best observed from behind (Fig. 18-9).

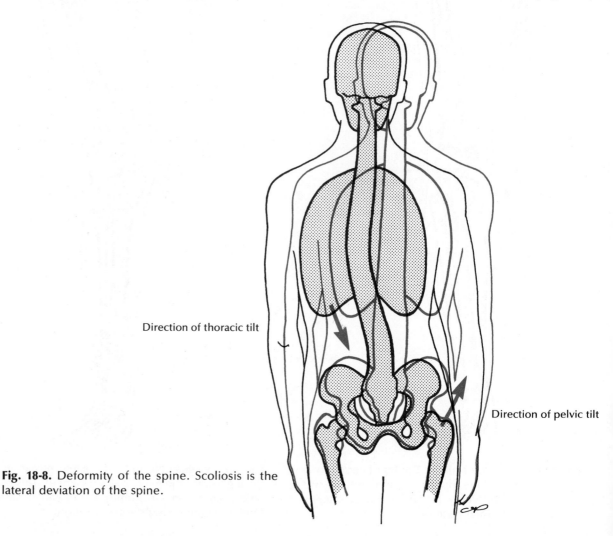

Direction of thoracic tilt

Direction of pelvic tilt

Fig. 18-8. Deformity of the spine. Scoliosis is the lateral deviation of the spine.

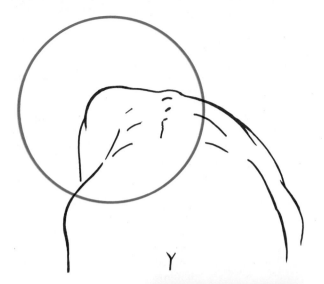

Fig. 18-9. The rotary deformity of scoliosis produces a hump or "razor back" deformity. This deviation is best demonstrated by asking the client to bend at the waist.

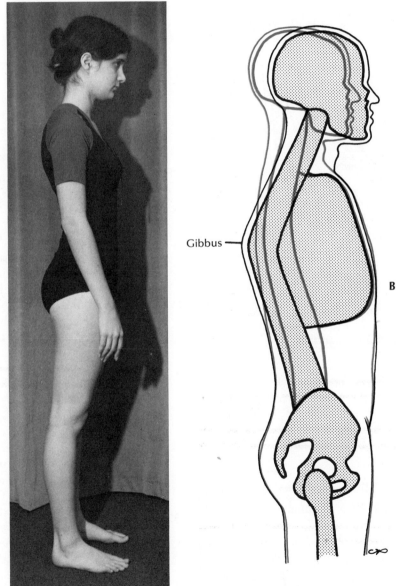

Gibbus

Fig. 18-10. A, Normal curvature of the spine. **B,** Deformity of the spine. Kyphosis is flexion of the spine. When the angle of the defect is sharp, the apex is called a gibbus.

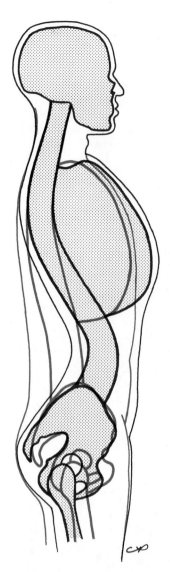

Fig. 18-11. Deformity of the spine. Lordosis (sway-back) is extension of the spine. It is most commonly found in the lumbar area.

Kyphosis is a flexion deformity (Fig. 18-10, *B*). When the angle of the defect is sharp, the apex is called a gibbus.

Lordosis (swayback) is an extension deviation of the spine commonly found in the lumbar area (Fig. 18-11).

■ Measurement of the extremities

The musculoskeletal examination frequently includes the measurement of the extremities for length and circumference. The measurements are made with the client lying relaxed on a hard surface (examining table) with the pelvis level and the hips and knees fully extended and with both hips equally adducted. Frequently, apparent discrepancies in limb size are due to position.

Table 18-1. Anatomical guideposts for measuring extremities

Area	From	To
Entire upper extremity	Tip of acromion process	Tip of middle finger
Upper arm	Tip of acromion process	Tip of olecranon process
Forearm	Tip of olecranon process	Styloid process of ulna
Entire lower extremity	Lower edge of anterosuperior iliac spine	Tibial malleolus
Thigh	Lower edge of anterosuperior iliac spine	Medial aspect of knee joint
Lower leg	Medial aspect of knee	Tibial malleolus

The length of the upper extremity is the distance from the tip of the acromion process to the tip of the middle finger; the shoulder is adducted and the other joints are at neutral zero. The length of the lower extremity is the distance from the lower edge of the anterosuperior iliac spine to the tibial malleolus.

■ Measurement of muscle mass

The muscles are examined for gross hypertrophy or atrophy. Only in the markedly obese client are changes in muscle mass difficult to assess. The difference in the firm, hypertrophic muscle of the athlete and the limp, atrophic muscle of the paralytic are obvious both on inspection and to the palpating finger. Although muscle size is largely a function of the use or disuse of the muscle fibers, changes in the size of muscles may be indicative of disease. Malnutrition and lipodystrophy tend to reduce muscle size as well as markedly weaken the strength of contraction. Lack of neural input due to lesions of the spinal cord or peripheral motor neuron may lead to a reduction in muscle size of as much as 75% of the normal volume; this may occur over as short a time as 3 months. Measurements taken of limbs at their maximum circumference may provide a baseline for comparison when swelling or atrophy are suspected or in subsequent routine examination. The limbs should be in the same position and the muscles in the same state of tension each time measurements are performed. Several corresponding points may be measured above and

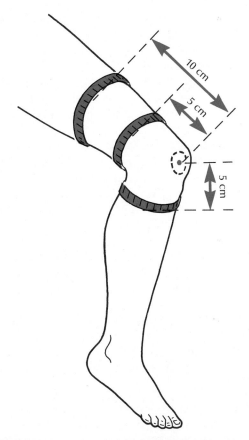

Fig. 18-12. The sites at which a limb is measured are carefully noted so that they may be accurately located for future comparative measurements.

below the patella and olecranon process. Some clinics routinely measure at 10 cm below and at points 10 and 20 cm above the midpatella in order to provide uniformity. At any rate, a small diagram showing the points measured (Fig. 18-12) will obviate ambiguity. Differences in symmetry or of limb size at different times of less than 1 cm are not significant.

PALPATION

Palpation is utilized in the examination of the musculoskeletal system to detect swelling, localized temperature changes, and marked changes in shape.

The consistency of the muscle on palpation is noted.

Muscle tone or tonus is the tension that is present in the resting muscle. This is the slight resistance that is felt when the relaxed limb is passively moved.

While palpating the muscle, the examiner should be alert to fasciculations, which are in-

voluntary contractions or twitchings of groups of muscle fibers.

The client should be requested to tell the examiner of any sensation he has while the muscles and tendons are being felt. The client's descriptions of pain or tenderness on palpation are recorded.

Tendon stretch reflexes are generally altered in diseased muscle, especially if the peripheral nerves are involved. For instance, the tendon reflexes are diminished in muscular dystrophy and polymyositis in proportion to the loss of muscle strength. A lengthened reflex cycle is characteristic of hypothyroidism, whereas a shortened period is indicative of the hypermetabolic state.

TESTING OF MUSCULOSKELETAL FUNCTION

Muscle strength is assessed throughout the full range of motion for each muscle or group of muscles. The usual method of testing is manual and subjective. Resistance is applied to the muscles; the client is placed in the position that best allows movement through the full range. The muscle contractions are graded according to the examiner's judgment of the client's responses.

The following criteria for recording the grading of muscle strength has been frequently used:

Functional level	Lovett scale	Grade	Percentage of normal
No evidence of contractility	Zero (0)	0	0
Evidence of slight contractility	Trace (T)	1	10
Complete range of motion with gravity eliminated	Poor (P)	2	25
Complete range of motion with gravity	Fair (F)	3	50
Complete range of motion against gravity with some resistance	Good (G)	4	75
Complete range of motion against gravity with full resistance	Normal (N)	5	100

Some examiners prefer simple descriptive words, such as *paralysis, severe weakness, moderate weakness, minimal weakness,* and *normal.* Disability is considered to exist if the muscle strength is less than grade 3; external support may be required to make the involved part functional, and activity of the part cannot be achieved in a gravity field.

There is an expectation that muscle strength will be greater in the dominant arm and leg.

■ Screening test for muscle weakness

Although muscle weakness in adults is generally mild and transitory, it may be the outcome of musculoskeletal, neurological, metabolic, or infectious problems. Therefore, an evaluation is necessary. A simple screening test has been suggested that can be performed in as short a time as 5 minutes and allows the examiner to find nearly any muscle or reflex abnormality. The test allows for a systematic testing of muscle groups from head to toe. As he walks into the examining room and undresses, the client is carefully observed for cues to neurological and motion deficit. He is carefully observed to ascertain that the chief complaint is verifiable by physical evidence. The following procedure may then be used:

1. The examiner assesses the ocular musculature by asking the client to close his eyes tightly as the examiner attempts to open the lids. The client is instructed to look up, down, right, and left as the examiner checks for lid lag and appropriate tracking of the eyes.

2. The examiner assesses the facial musculature by asking the client to blow out his cheeks while the examiner assesses the pressure against the fingers held against the resultant cheek bulge. The client is then asked to put his tongue into the cheek, and the tension created in this bulge is tested. The client is then asked to stick out his tongue and to move it to the right and left.

3. The examiner assesses the neck musculature by asking the client to extend his head backward while standing erect as the examiner attempts to break the extension (Fig. 18-13). The client is then asked to bend his chin toward his chest forcefully as far as he is able while the examiner attempts to bend the chin upward.

4. The examiner tests the deltoid muscles by asking the client to hold his arms upward while the examiner tries to push them down. The client is asked to extend his arms while the examiner attempts to press them down.

5. The examiner tests the biceps by asking the client to fully extend his arms and then to try to flex them while the examiner attempts to pull them into extension (Fig. 18-14).

6. The examiner tests the triceps by asking the client to flex his arms and then to extend them while the examiner attempts to push them into a flexed position (Fig. 18-15).

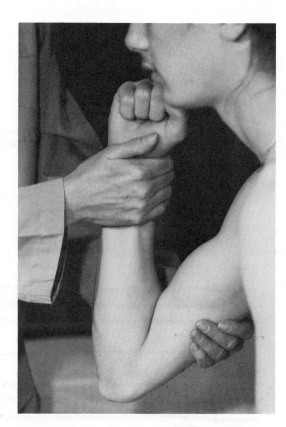

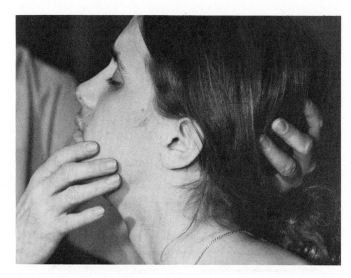

Fig. 18-13. Assessment of the neck musculature. The client flexes his head backward while the examiner attempts to break the extension.

Fig. 18-14. Assessment of biceps strength. The client flexes his arm while the examiner attempts to pull the arm into extension.

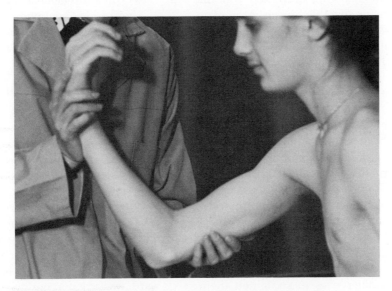

Fig. 18-15. Assessment of triceps strength. The client attempts to extend his arm while the examiner attempts to push the arm into a flexed position.

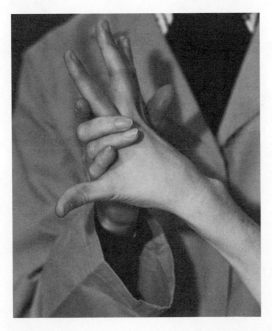

Fig. 18-16. Assessment of wrist strength. The client pushes against the examiner's hand in an attempt to extend the wrist.

7. The examiner assesses the wrist and finger musculature by asking the client to extend his hand and then to try to resist the examiner with the hand up, alternately with the fingers out or together, in an attempt to flex the wrist (Fig. 18-16).
8. The examiner assesses hip strength by asking the client to assume the supine position and then to raise the extended leg while the examiner attempts to hold it down.
9. The examiner assesses the hamstring, gluteal, abductor, and adductor muscles of the leg by asking the client to sit and perform alternate leg crossing (Fig. 18-17).
10. The examiner assesses quadriceps muscle strength by asking the client to extend the leg stiffly as the examiner tries to bend it (Fig. 18-18).
11. The examiner assesses the hamstring muscles by asking the client to bend his knees as the examiner tries to straighten them (Fig. 18-19).

12. The examiner assesses the ankle and foot musculature by asking the client to exert upward foot pressure and then big toe pressure against the examiner's hands.

Muscle fasciculations are checked for in the face, neck, torso, and extremities. A sharp tap to the muscle mass may induce this visible twitching.

■ Screening assessment of neurological adequacy

Neurological adequacy can be assessed by examining the pupillary reflex and the fundus. Pyramidal tract function is evaluated through the use of deep tendon reflex tests, including Babinski's test.

Cerebellar tract function may be elicited by asking the client to stand erect with his eyes closed and then checking Romberg's sign. The client is then asked to touch his finger to his nose and to rapidly rotate his hands inward and outward. Sensory perception is assessed by checking for pain, vibration, and temperature responses.

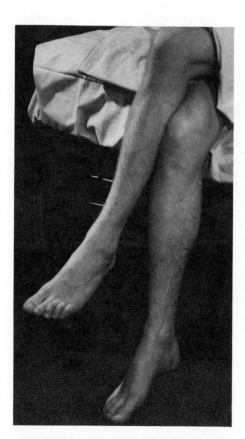

Fig. 18-17. Alternate leg crossing for assessment of hamstring, gluteal, abductor, and adductor muscle strength.

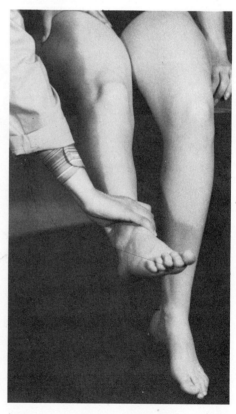

Fig. 18-18. Assessment of quadriceps muscle strength. The client attempts to straighten the leg while the examiner attempts to flex it.

(Neural function tests are described in Chapter 20 on Neurological assessment.)

■ Measurement of the range of joint motion

A standardized method for measuring and recording joint motion has been published by the American Academy of Orthopaedic Surgeons (1965). The range of motion is described in degrees of deviation from a defined neutral zero point for each joint. The position of neutral zero is that of the extended extremity or anatomical position.

Goniometry and arthrometry are the terms used to describe the measurement of joint motion. The practitioner should learn to use the goniometer to measure the range of motion and to communicate his findings to other health team professionals.

The two arms of the goniometer are a protractor and a pointer that are joined at the zero point of the protractor (Fig. 18-5). The hinge should provide sufficient friction that the instrument remains in position when picked up for reading after being set against the joint. The scale should be easily read from a distance of 18 inches. Some goniometers have full-circle scales, whereas

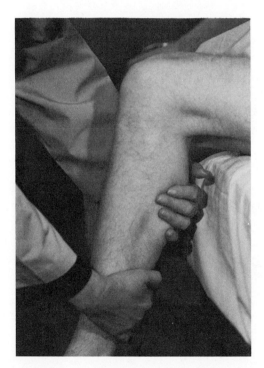

Fig. 18-19. Assessment of hamstring muscle strength. The client flexes his knees while the examiner tries to straighten them.

others have half-circle scales. The length of the arms is generally about 6 inches so that it can be easily carried.

Motion is described as active when the client moves the joint and passive when the examiner provides the motion. Active joint motion that is smooth and painless through its complete range generally indicates the absence of any advanced lesion.

Active motion. Less muscle tension and joint compression are produced by the voluntary movement of the joints through their range of motion than when the joints are moved against resistance as in the strength tests. Therefore, the range of active motion should be assessed before muscle strength since the more marked contraction may induce pain in the client and skew the test results.

Should the range of active motion of a given joint be less than the range of passive motion, further investigation should focus on true weakness, joint stability, pain, malingering, or hysterical weakness as possible causes.

Passive motion. The examiner moves the relaxed joint through the limits of its movement. When the range of motion is limited, the examiner explores further to determine whether there (1) is an excess of fluid within the joint; (2) are loose bodies in the joint; or (3) is joint surface irregularity or contracture of the muscles, ligaments, or capsule. Moving the joint through the range of its motion may also reveal hypermobility of the joint. In this case, further examination is directed toward differentiating between (1) a connective tissue disruption such as the relaxation of the ligaments that occurs in Marfan's syndrome, (2) a ligamentous tear, and (3) an intra-articular fracture. An example of how this information might aid in diagnosis would be seen in a joint that could be flexed to a smaller angle with passive movement than with active flexion. Such a finding would probably indicate a problem related to the musculature rather than a problem within the joint causing a block in the flexion.

■ Testing by functional group

The movement of the neck and the trunk are examined in functional groups for muscle strength and for the range of joint motion. The full range of motion is not assessed as part of the screening examination, unless the history or other parts of the physical examination indicate that muscular or neural dysfunction is a possible problem for the client.

Table 18-2. TESTING FOR MUSCLE STRENGTH AND RANGE OF JOINT MOTION

NECK

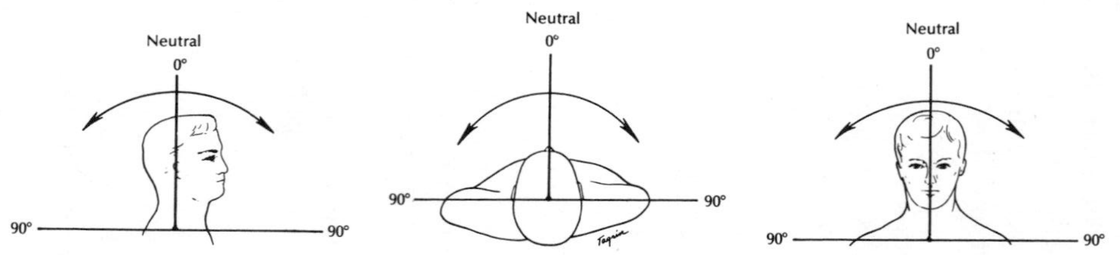

A   B   C

Fig. 1. Range of motion of the cervical spine.* **A,** Flexion and extension. These motions are usually designated by degrees, but the examiner may indicate the distance the chin lacks from touching the chest. **B,** Rotation. This is estimated in degrees from the neutral position or in percentages of motion, as compared to individuals of similar age and physical build. **C,** Lateral bend. This motion is also measured in degrees but can be indicated by the number of inches the ear lacks from reaching the shoulder.

Movement	Muscles	Motor nerves	Positions for testing	Instructions and tests for muscle strength
Flexion	Prime mover: sternocleido-mastoid (Fig. 2†)	Spinal accessory nerve (cranial XI) Cervical 2, 3	Standing, sitting, supine	"Bend your head to touch your chin to your chest." Resistance is applied to the forehead. Pressure is exerted over the tip of the xiphoid process to obviate the tendency to contract the abdominal muscles to raise the chest (Fig. 3).
	Accessory muscles Scalene anterior Scalene medius Scalene posterior Rectus capitis anterior Longus capitis Longus colli Infrahyoid group			

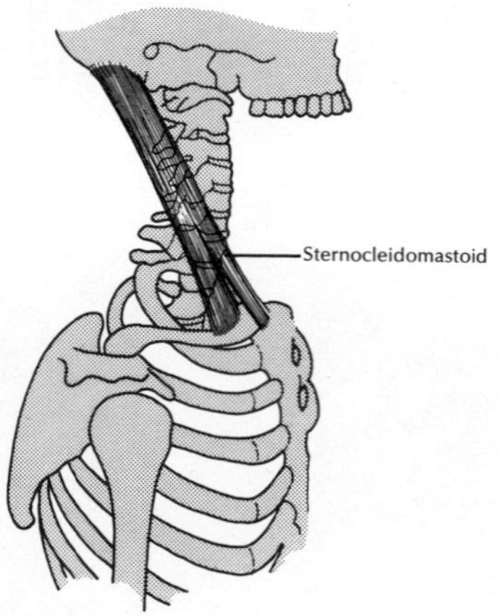

Sternocleidomastoid

Fig. 2

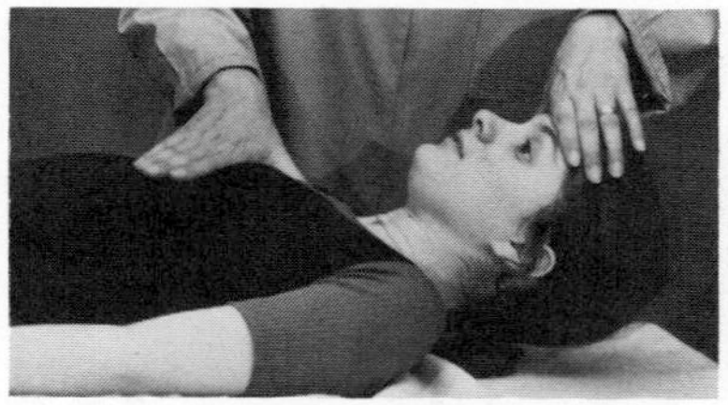

Fig. 3

Motion	Muscles	Innervation	Patient position	Instructions
Extension	Prime movers Trapezius (superior fibers)	Spinal accessory nerve (cranial XI) Cervical 3, 4	standing, sitting, prone	"... as far as possible." "Lift your head up as far as you can." Resistance is applied to the occipital prominence (Fig. 5).
	Semispinalis capitis	Dorsal rami of spinal nerves		
	Semispinalis cervicis	Dorsal rami of spinal nerves		
	Splenius capitis	Dorsal rami of middle and lower cervical nerves		
	Splenius cervicis	Dorsal rami of middle and lower cervical nerves		
	Spinalis capitis	Adjacent spinal nerves		
	Spinalis cervicis	Adjacent spinal nerves		
	Longissimus capitis	Adjacent spinal nerves		
	Longissimus cervicis	Adjacent spinal nerves		
	Accessory muscles Levator scapulae Multifidus Oblique capitis Rectus capitis posterior			
Rotation Anterolateral	Prime mover: sternocleidomastoid (Fig. 2)	Spinal accessory nerve (cranial XI) Cervical 2, 3	Standing, sitting, supine	"Bend your head forward and turn your head as far as you can to the right [left]." "Bend your head so that your ear is close to your chest." Resistance is applied to the right (left) temple.
	Accessory muscles Scalene anterior Scalene medius Scalene posterior Rectus capitis anterior Longus capitis Longus colli Infrahyoid group			
Posterolateral	Prime movers (Fig. 4) Trapezius (superior fibers)	Spinal accessory nerve (cranial XI) Cervical 3, 4	Standing, sitting, prone	"Bend your head back and turn your head to the right [left]." Resistance is applied to the right (left) occiput.
	Semispinalis capitis	Dorsal rami of spinal nerves		
	Semispinalis cervicis	Dorsal rami of spinal nerves		
	Splenius capitis	Dorsal rami of middle and lower cranial nerves		

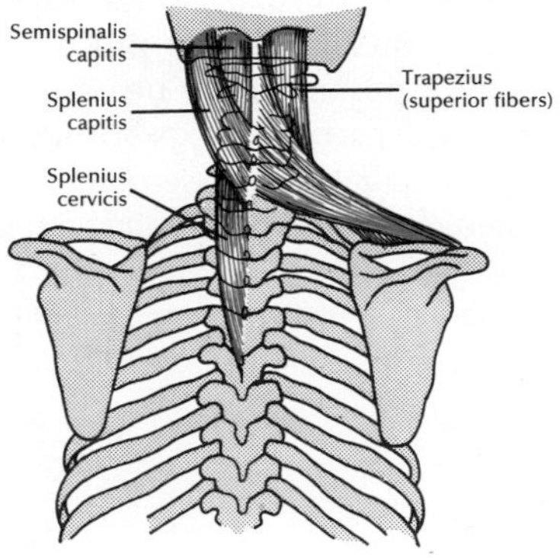

Fig. 5

Fig. 4

(Labels: Semispinalis capitis, Splenius capitis, Splenius cervicis, Trapezius (superior fibers))

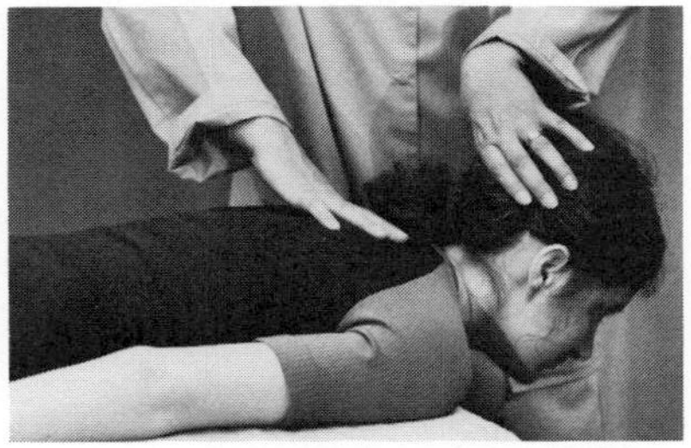

*From Joint motion; method of measuring and recording, Chicago, 1965, American Academy of Orthopaedic Surgeons.
†Adapted from Daniels, L., and Worthingham, C.: Muscle testing; techniques of manual examination, ed. 3, Philadelphia, 1972, W. B. Saunders Co.
‡From Francis, C. C., and Farrell, G. L.: Integrated anatomy and physiology, St. Louis, 1957, The C. V. Mosby Co.
§From Anthony, C. P., and Kolthoff, N. J.: Textbook of anatomy and physiology, ed. 9, St. Louis, 1975, The C. V. Mosby Co.

Continued.

Table 18-2. TESTING FOR MUSCLE STRENGTH AND RANGE OF JOINT MOTION—cont'd

Movement	Muscles	Motor nerves	Positions for testing	Instructions and tests for muscle strength
Posterolateral—cont'd	Splenius cervicis	Dorsal rami of middle and lower cranial nerves		
	Spinalis capitis	Adjacent spinal nerves		
	Spinalis cervicis	Adjacent spinal nerves		
	Longissimus capitis	Adjacent spinal nerves		
	Longissimus cervicis	Adjacent spinal nerves		
	Accessory muscles			
	Levator scapulae			
	Multifidus			
	Oblique capitis			
	Rectus capitis posterior			
Lateral bend	Prime mover: sternocleido-mastoid (Fig. 2)	Spinal accessory nerve (cranial XI)	Standing, sitting, supine	"Bend your head so that your right [left] ear touches your shoulder. Don't bring your shoulder up to meet your ear."
	Accessory muscles	Cervical 2, 3		
	Scalene anterior			Resistance is applied to the right (left) temporal bone.
	Scalene medius			
	Scalene posterior			
	Rectus capitis anterior			
	Longus capitis			
	Longus colli			
	Infrahyoid group			

TRUNK

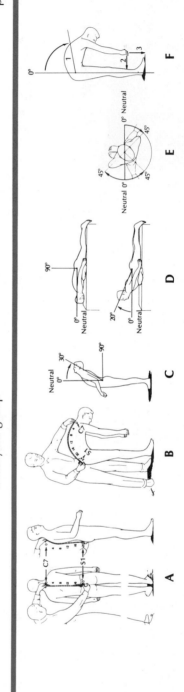

Fig. 6. Range of motion of the spine.* **A** and **B**, Steel tape measure method. This is perhaps the most accurate clinical method of measuring true motion of the spine in flexion. The flexible steel or plastic tape adjusts very accurately to the thoracic and lumbar contours of the spine. **A**, With the client standing, the 1-inch marker of the tape is held over the spinous process C7 and the distal tape over the spinous process S1. **B**, As the client bends forward, if the lumbar curve reverses and the spinous processes spread, this will be indicated by lengthening of the measured distance from C7 to S1. In the normal healthy adult there is, on the average, an increase of 4 inches in forward flexion. If the client bends forward with his back straight (as in rheumatoid spondylitis), the tape will not record motion. One is able to record motion of the thoracic spine per se by taping from the spinous process C7 to the spinous process T12. Likewise, motion of the lumbar spine can be measured from T12 to S1. Usually, if the total spine lengthening in flexion is 4 inches, the examiner will find that 1 inch occurs in the dorsal spine and 3 inches occur in the lumbar spine. **C**, Client standing (extension). **D**, Client lying prone (extension). **E**, Rotation of spine. **F**, Client bending forward (flexion). *1*, Degrees of inclination of trunk (note reversal of lumbar curve); *2*, level of fingertips to leg; *3*, distance between fingertips and floor.

Movement	Muscles	Motor nerves	Positions for testing	Instructions and tests for muscle strength
Flexion	Prime mover: rectus abdominis (Fig. 7‡) Accessory muscles Oblique internus abdominis Oblique externus abdominis	Intercostal nerves (thoracic 6-12, lumbar 1)	Standing Supine (knees not bent)	"Bend over; touch your toes" (Fig. 8). "Try to sit up without using your hands." Leg is stabilized (Fig. 9). Two important signs may be elicited in assessing abdominal muscle strength: 1. Beevor's sign, upward movement of the umbilicus on contraction of the abdominal muscles, is associated with comparative weakness of the lower abdominal muscles in relation to the upper abdominal muscles. 2. Hyperextension of the lumbar spine when the client tries to rise to a sitting position occurs when strong hip flexors are contracted in the presence of weak abdominal muscles.

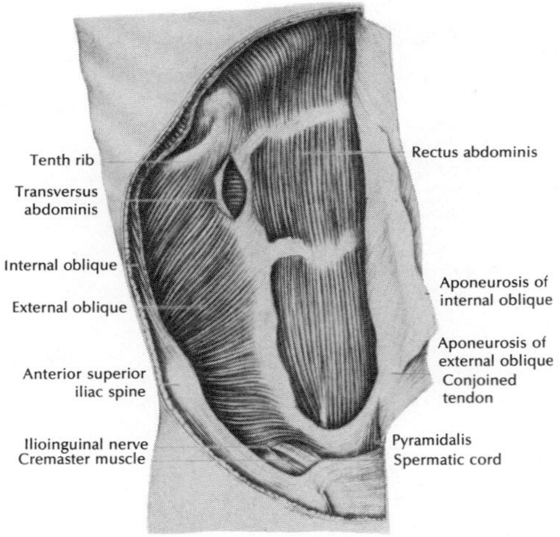

Continued.

Tenth rib
Transversus abdominis
Internal oblique
External oblique
Anterior superior iliac spine
Ilioinguinal nerve
Cremaster muscle
Rectus abdominis
Aponeurosis of internal oblique
Aponeurosis of external oblique
Conjoined tendon
Pyramidalis
Spermatic cord

Fig. 7

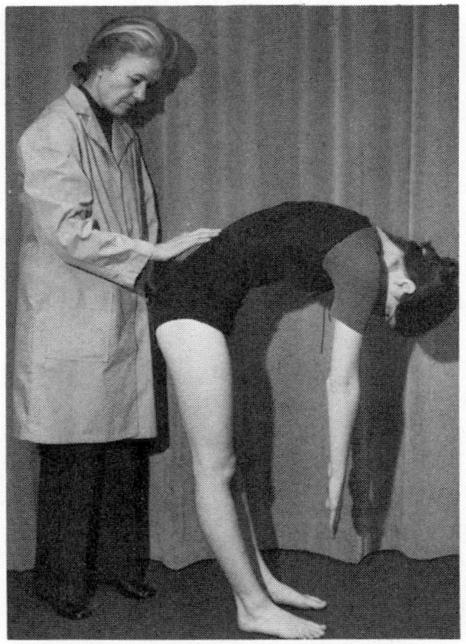

Fig. 8

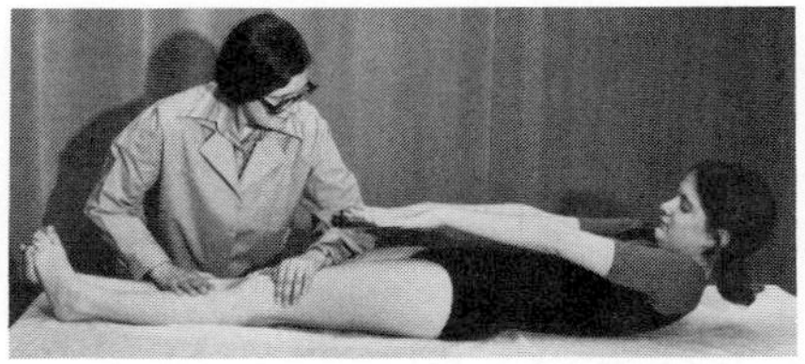

Fig. 9

Table 18-2. TESTING FOR MUSCLE STRENGTH AND RANGE OF JOINT MOTION—cont'd

Movement	Muscles	Motor nerves	Positions for testing	Instructions and tests for muscle strength
Extension	Prime movers (Fig. 10†) Longissimus thoracis Iliocostalis thoracis Spinalis thoracis Iliocostalis lumborum Quadratus lumborum Accessory muscles Rotators Multifidus Semispinalis	Adjacent spinal nerves Adjacent spinal nerves Adjacent spinal nerves Adjacent spinal nerves Thoracic 12, lumbar 1	Standing Prone	"Bend your head and shoulders back as far as you can." "Lift your head and shoulders up from the table without using your hands." Pelvis is stabilized. Resistance is applied between the scapulae (Fig. 11).
Rotation	Prime movers (Fig. 12†) Oblique externus abdominis Oblique internus abdominis Accessory muscles Rectus abdominis Latissimus dorsi Semispinalis Multifidus Rotators	Intercostal nerves (thoracic 8-12) Intercostal nerves (thoracic 8-12)	Sitting (hips flexed) Supine (hands behind head, legs stabilized)	"Twist your right [left] shoulder to the opposite knee." "Turn your right [left] shoulder to the opposite knee" (Fig. 13). Resistance may be applied against the right (left) anterior shoulder.

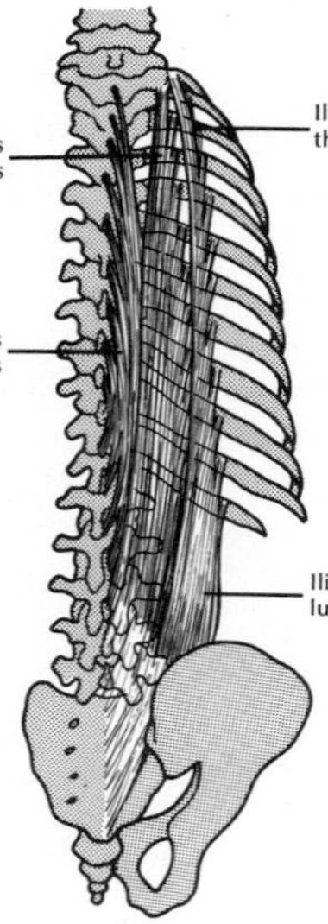

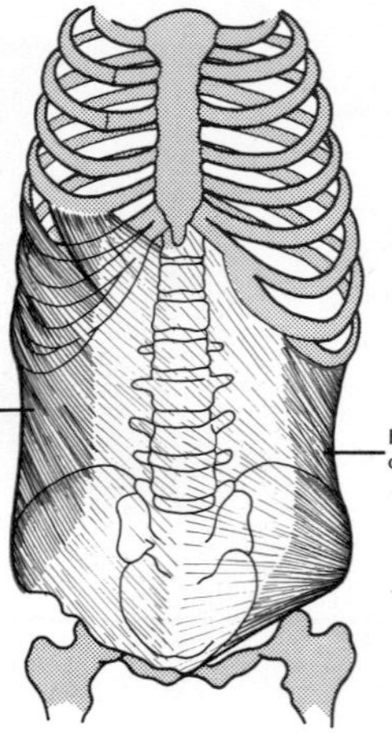

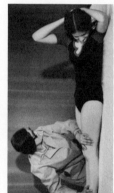

Fig. 11

Fig. 13

Iliocostalis thoracis

Longissimus thoracis

Spinalis thoracis

Iliocostalis lumborum

Fig. 10

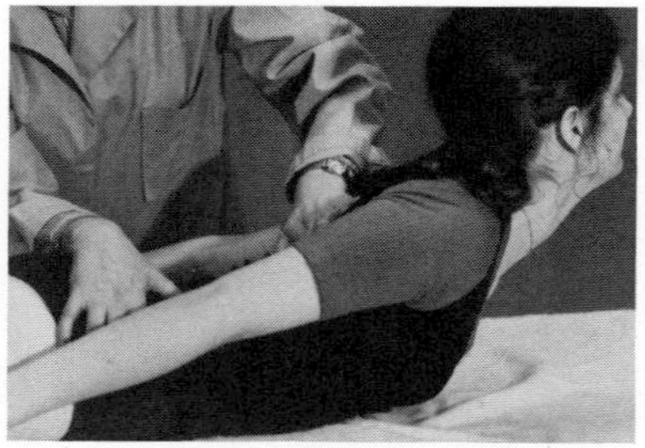

Internal oblique

External oblique

Fig. 12

Elevation

Prime movers (Fig. 14+)
  Quadratus lumborum
  Iliocostalis lumborum
Accessory muscles
  Oblique internus
    abdominis
  Oblique externus
    abdominis
  Latissimus dorsi
  Abductor muscles of hip

Thoracic 12; lumbar 1, 2
Adjacent spinal nerves

Supine (legs
  together)

"Try to lift your right
[left] hip toward your
shoulder."
Resistance is applied by
the examiner holding
the ankle (Fig. 15).

Standing

"Thrust your right [left]
hip forward and up."

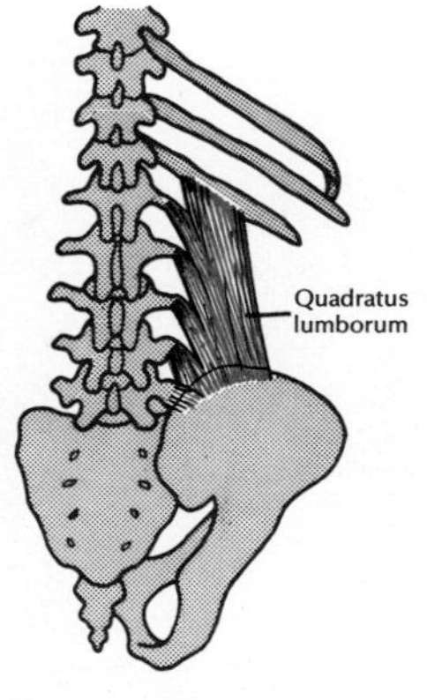

Fig. 14

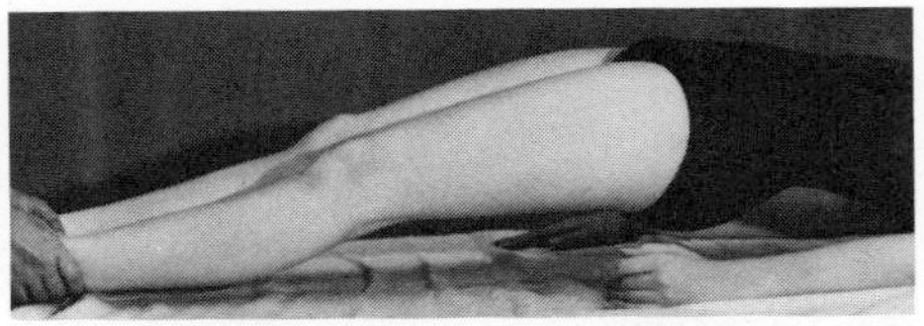

Fig. 15

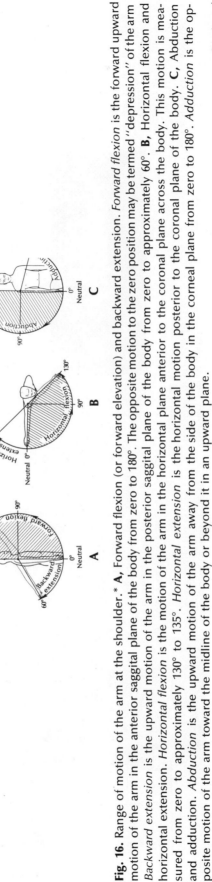

SHOULDER

Fig. 16. Range of motion of the arm at the shoulder.* **A,** Forward flexion (or forward elevation) and backward extension. *Forward flexion* is the forward upward motion of the arm in the anterior saggital plane of the body from zero to 180°. The opposite motion to the zero position may be termed "depression" of the arm. *Backward extension* is the upward motion of the arm in the posterior saggital plane of the body from zero to approximately 60°. **B,** Horizontal flexion and horizontal extension. *Horizontal flexion* is the motion of the arm in the horizontal plane anterior to the coronal plane across the body. This motion is measured from zero to approximately 130° to 135°. *Horizontal extension* is the horizontal motion posterior to the coronal plane of the body. **C,** Abduction and adduction. *Abduction* is the upward motion of the arm away from the side of the body in the corneal plane from zero to 180°. *Adduction* is the opposite motion of the arm toward the midline of the body or beyond it in an upward plane.

Continued.

Table 18-2. TESTING FOR MUSCLE STRENGTH AND RANGE OF JOINT MOTION—cont'd

Movement	Muscles	Motor nerves	Positions for testing	Instructions and tests for muscle strength
Forward flexion	Prime movers (Fig. 17†) Deltoid (anterior fibers) Coracobrachialis Accessory muscles Deltoid (middle fibers) Pectoralis major (clavicular fibers) Biceps brachii	Axillary nerve (cervical 5, 6) Musculocutaneous nerve (cervical 6, 7)	Standing, sitting, supine	"Move your arms forward and up." Resistance is applied at the level of the inferior angle of the scapula on the upper side of the arm (Fig. 18).
Backward extension	Prime movers (Fig. 19†) Latissimus dorsi Teres major Deltoid Accessory muscles Teres minor Triceps (long head)	Thoracodorsal nerve (cervical 6, 7, 8) Lowest subscapular nerve (cervical 5, 6) Axillary nerve (cervical 5, 6)	Standing, sitting, prone	"Move your arms downward and back." "Clasp your arms behind your back." Resistance is applied to the posterior aspect of the arm proximal to the elbow (Fig. 20).

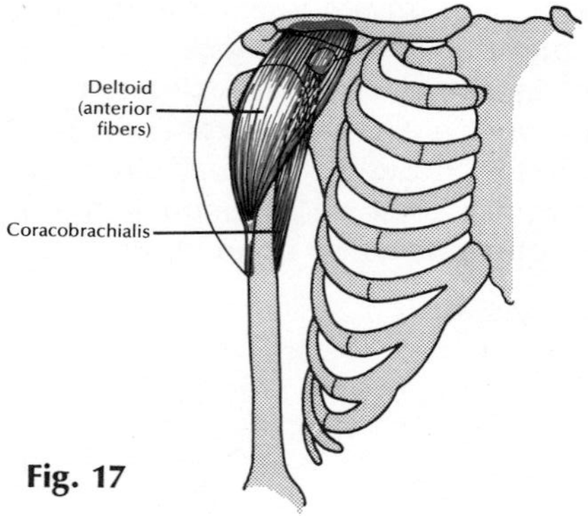

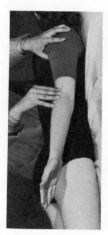

Fig. 18

Fig. 20

Deltoid (anterior fibers)

Coracobrachialis

Fig. 17

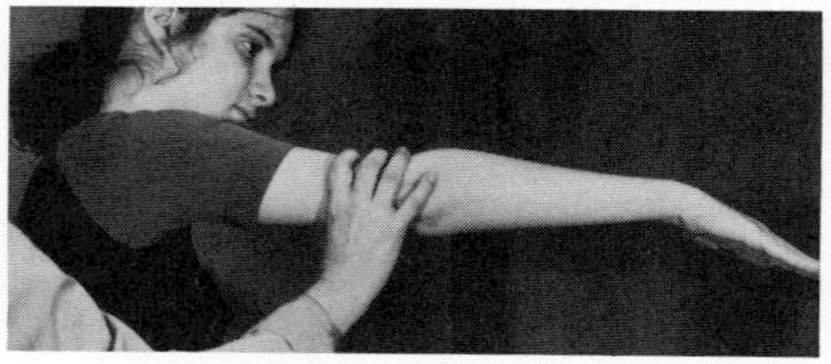

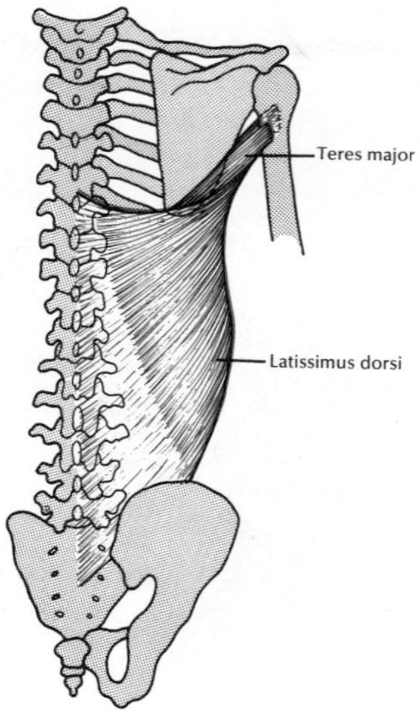

Teres major

Latissimus dorsi

Fig. 19

Abduction

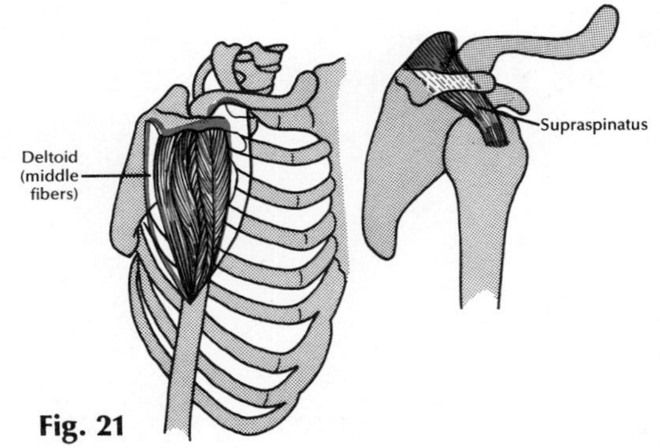

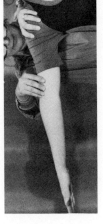

Deltoid (middle fibers)

Supraspinatus

Fig. 21

Prime movers (Fig. 21†)
Deltoid (middle fibers)
Supraspinatus

Accessory muscles
Deltoid (anterior and posterior fibers)
Serratus anterior

Axillary nerve (cervical 5, 6)
Suprascapular nerve (cervical 5)

Standing, sitting (scapula stabilized)

"Lift your arm straight out and to your side, away from your body."
Resistance is applied to the superior aspect of the arm proximal to the elbow (Fig. 22).

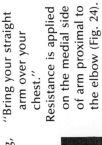

Fig. 22

Horizontal adduction

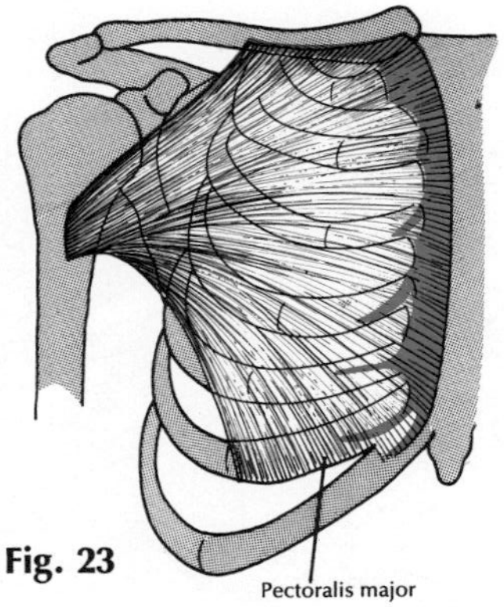

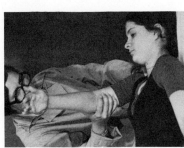

Pectoralis major

Fig. 23

Prime mover: pectoralis major (Fig. 23†)

Accessory muscle: deltoid (anterior fibers)

Medial and internal pectoral nerves (cervical 5, 6, 7, 8; thoracic 1)

Standing, sitting, supine (arm abducted)

"Bring your straight arm over your chest."
Resistance is applied on the medial side of arm proximal to the elbow (Fig. 24).

Fig. 24

Continued.

325

Table 18-2. TESTING FOR MUSCLE STRENGTH AND RANGE OF JOINT MOTION—cont'd

Movement	Muscles	Motor nerves	Positions for testing	Instructions and tests for muscle strength
Horizontal abduction	Prime mover: deltoid (posterior fibers) (Fig. 25†) Accessory muscles Teres minor Infraspinatus	Axillary nerve (cervical 5, 6)	Standing, sitting, prone (scapula stabilized, arm adducted)	"Keeping your arm at shoulder height, move it backward as far as you can." Resistance is applied on the posterior surface of the arm proximal to the elbow (Fig. 26).

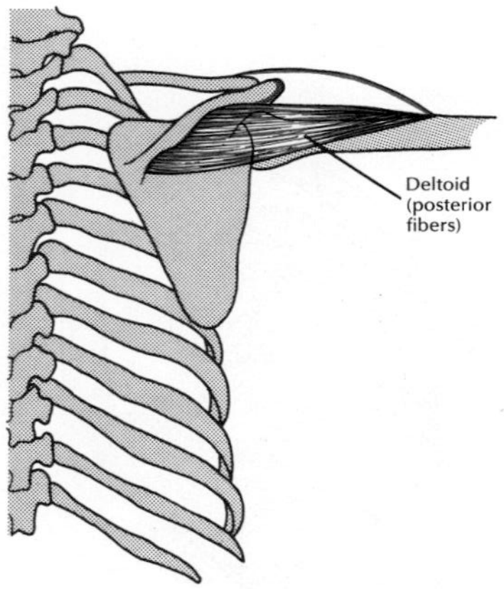

Deltoid (posterior fibers)

Fig. 25

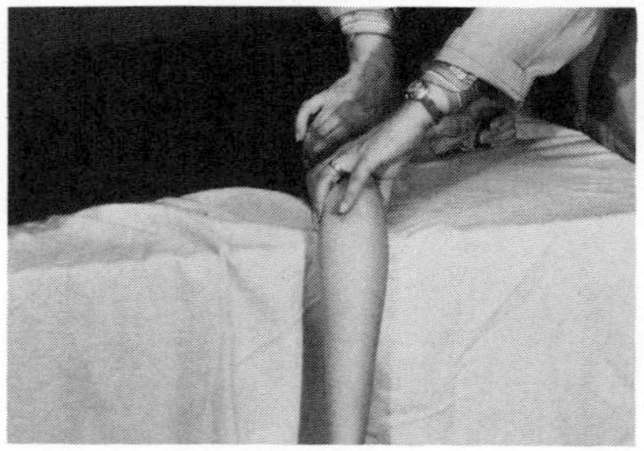

Fig. 26

SHOULDER—cont'd

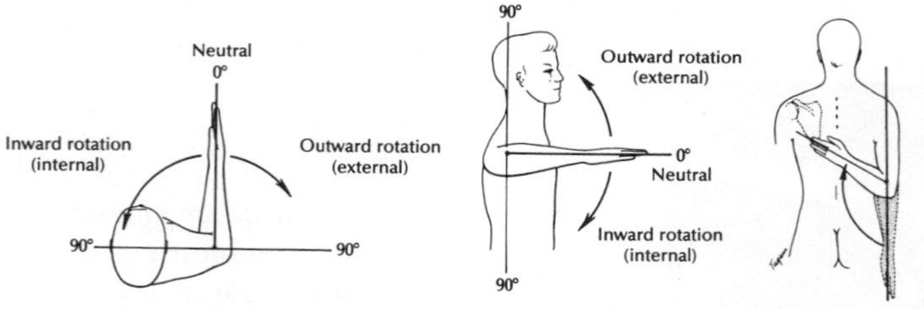

Outward rotation (external)

Inward rotation (internal)

Neutral 0°

90°

A

90°

Outward rotation (external)

0° Neutral

Inward rotation (internal)

90°

B

C

Fig. 27. Rotation of the shoulder.* **A,** Rotation with arm at side of body. Inward and outward rotation is recorded in degrees of motion from the neutral starting point. **B,** Rotation in abduction. Rotation in this position is less than with the arm at the side of the body. It is recorded in degrees of motion from the zero starting point. **C,** Internal rotation posteriorly. A clinical method of estimating function is the distance the fingertips reach in relation to the scapula or the base of the neck.

Movement	Muscles	Motor nerves	Positions for testing	Instructions and tests for muscle strength
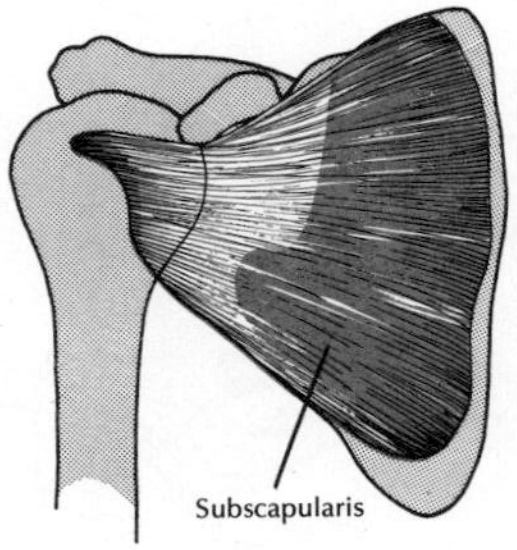 Rotation Internal	Prime movers (Fig. 28†) Subscapularis	Upper and lower subscapular nerves (cervical 5, 6) 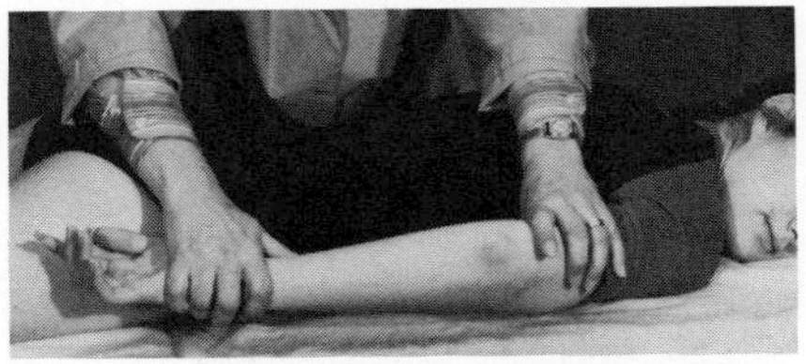	Standing, sitting, prone (scapula stabilized)	"Rotate your shoulder inward, swing your arm backward with your palm upward, and point your fingers toward the ceiling." Resistance is applied to the volar surface of the wrist (Fig. 29).
	Pectoralis major	Medial and lateral pectoral nerves (cervical 5, 6, 7, 8; thoracic 1)		
	Latissimus dorsi	Thoracodorsal nerve (cervical 6, 7, 8)		
	Teres major	Lowest subscapular nerve (cervical 5, 6)		
	Accessory muscle: deltoid (anterior fibers)			
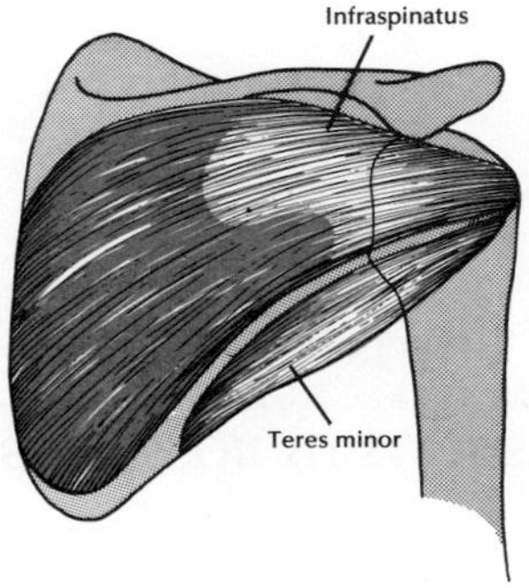 External	Prime movers (Fig. 30†) Infraspinatus	Suprascapular nerve (cervical 5, 6)	Standing, sitting, prone (scapula stabilized)	"Rotate your shoulder outward with your palm facing you posteriorly; bring your arm upward as if throwing a ball behind you." Resistance is applied to the dorsum of the wrist (Fig. 31).
	Teres minor Accessory muscle: deltoid	Axillary nerve (cervical 5) 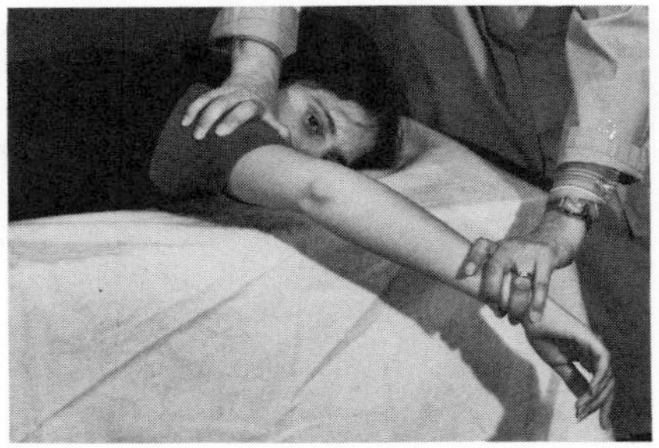		

Subscapularis

Fig. 28

Fig. 29

Infraspinatus

Teres minor

Fig. 30

Fig. 31

Continued.

Table 18-2. TESTING FOR MUSCLE STRENGTH AND RANGE OF JOINT MOTION—cont'd

SHOULDER—cont'd

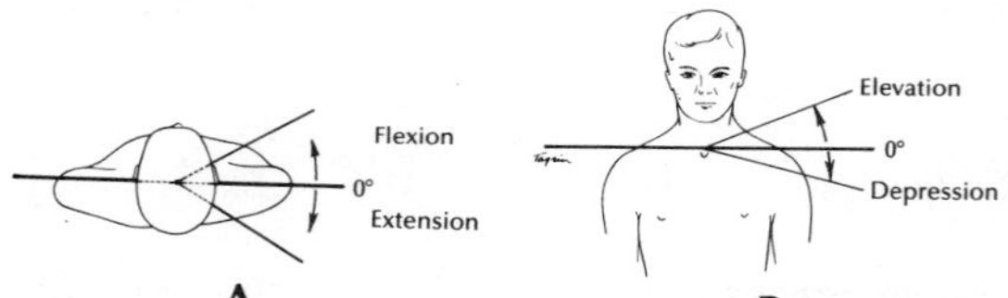

Fig. 32. Range of motion of the shoulder girdle.* **A,** Flexion and extension. Forward flexion and backward extension of the shoulder girdle are measured in degrees from the neutral starting position. This is primary motion of the scapula and the clavicle. **B,** Elevation and depression. Upward motion of the shoulder girdle in elevation is measured in degrees. The opposite downward motion may be described as "depression" of the shoulder. Rotatory motion in the shoulder girdle is possible but cannot be accurately measured. It can be estimated in percentage of motion as compared to individuals of similar age and physique.

A — Flexion, Extension, 0°

B — Elevation, Depression, 0°

Movement	Muscles	Motor nerves	Positions for testing	Instructions and tests for muscle strength
Scapular abduction and upward rotation	Prime mover: serratus anterior (Fig. 33†)	Long thoracic nerve (cervical 5, 6, 7)	Standing, sitting	"Push your arm upward and forward as if pushing open a door." Resistance is applied with a hand at the wrist and elbow, making pressure toward the chest (Fig. 34).

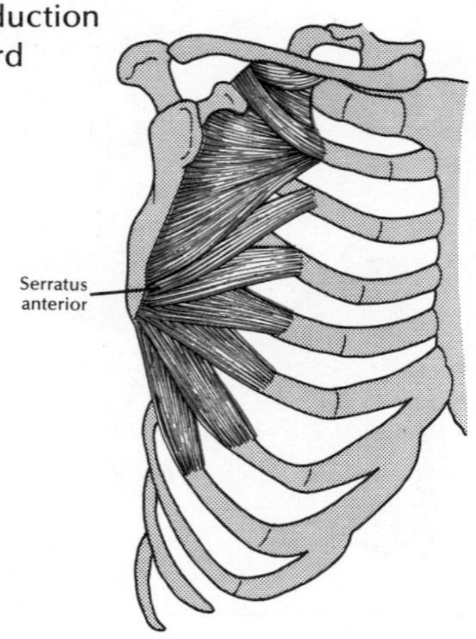

Serratus anterior

Fig. 33

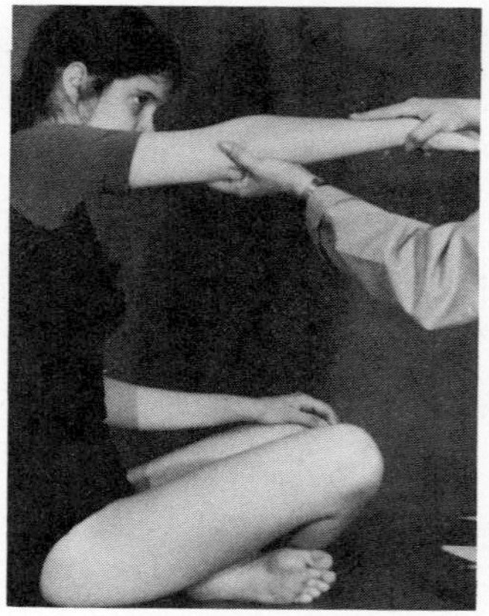

Fig. 34

Scapular adduction

Fig. 35

Prime movers (Fig. 35+)
Trapezius (middle fibers)

Rhomboid major

Rhomboid minor

Accessory muscle: trapezius (upper and lower fibers)

Spinal accessory nerve (cranial XI)
Cervical 3, 4
Dorsal scapular nerve (cervical 5)
Dorsal scapular nerve (cervical 5)

Standing, sitting, prone

"Try to bring your shoulder blades together in back." Resistance is applied over the posterior shoulder (Fig. 36).

Fig. 36

Scapular elevation

Fig. 37

Prime movers (Fig. 37+)
Trapezius (superior fibers)

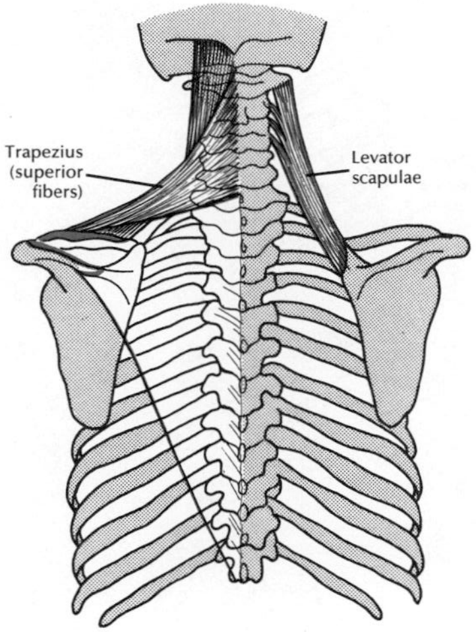

Levator scapulae
Accessory muscles
Rhomboid major
Rhomboid minor

Spinal accessory nerve (cranial XI)
Cervical 3, 4

Standing, sitting, lying

"Shrug your shoulders." "Hunch your shoulders against my hand." Resistance is applied to the superior aspect of the shoulder centered over the trapezius muscle (Fig. 38).

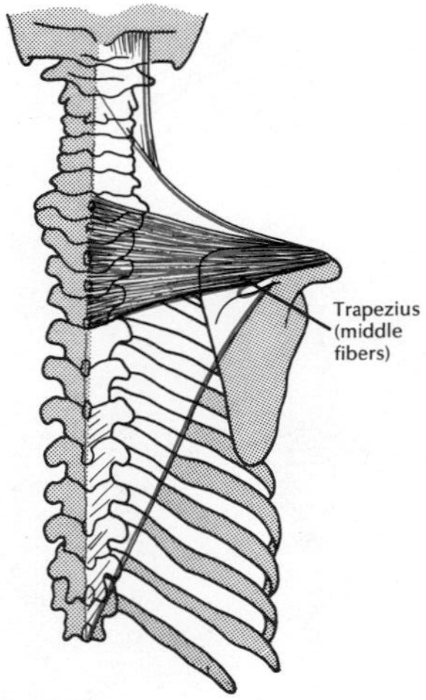

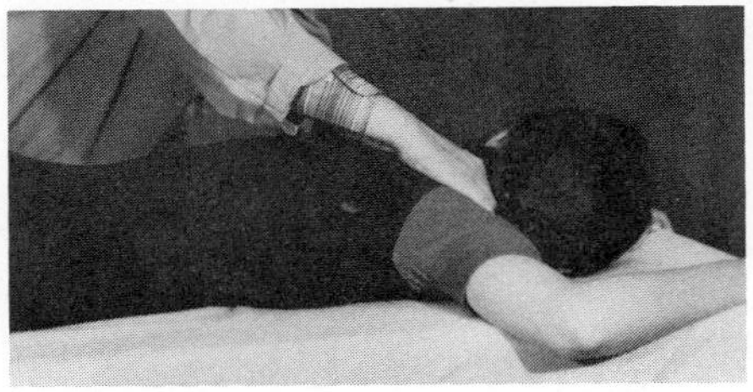

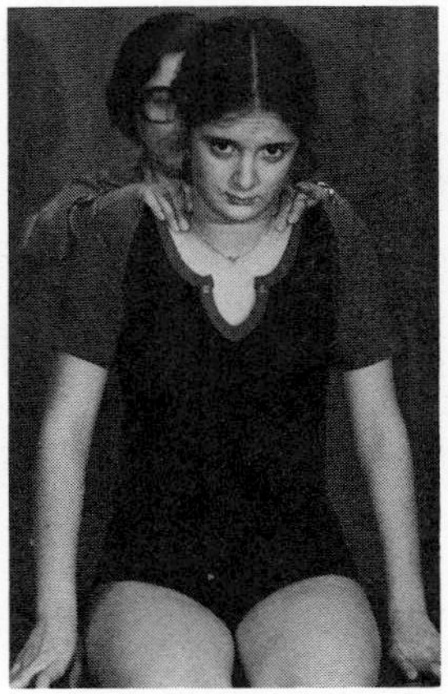

Fig. 38

Continued.

Table 18-2. TESTING FOR MUSCLE STRENGTH AND RANGE OF JOINT MOTION—cont'd

Movement	Muscles	Motor nerve	Positions for testing	Instructions and tests for muscle strength
Scapular depression and adduction	Prime mover: trapezius (inferior fibers) (Fig. 39†)	Spinal accessory nerve (cranial XI) Cervical 3, 4	Standing, sitting, prone	"Lift your arm and bring your shoulder blade down and close against your back chest wall. Bring the shoulder blade down against the chest." Upward pressure is applied against the deltoid muscle (Fig. 40).
Adduction and downward rotation	Prime movers (Fig. 41†) Rhomboid major Rhomboid minor	Dorsal scapular nerve (cervical 5) Dorsal scapular nerve (cervical 5)	Standing, sitting, prone (arm adducted over back in medial rotation)	"Lift up your arm. Concentrate on your elbow." Resistance is applied over the scapula (Fig. 42).

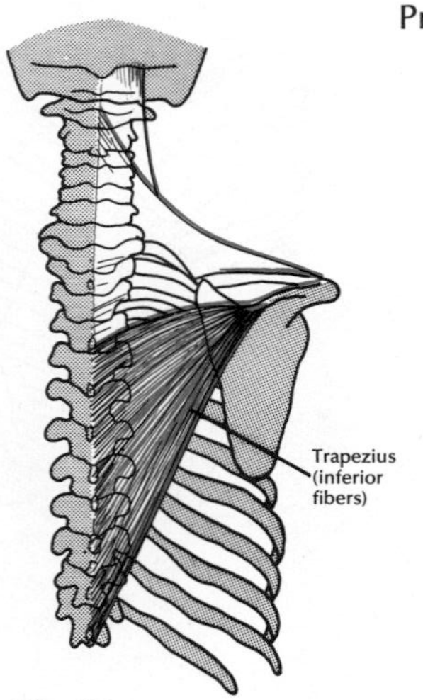

Fig. 40

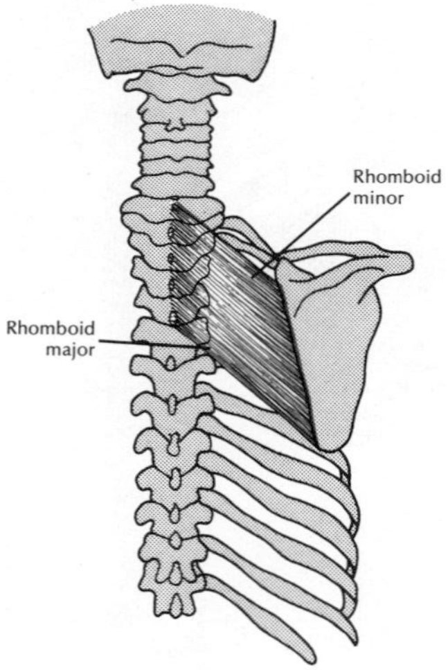

Fig. 42

Fig. 39

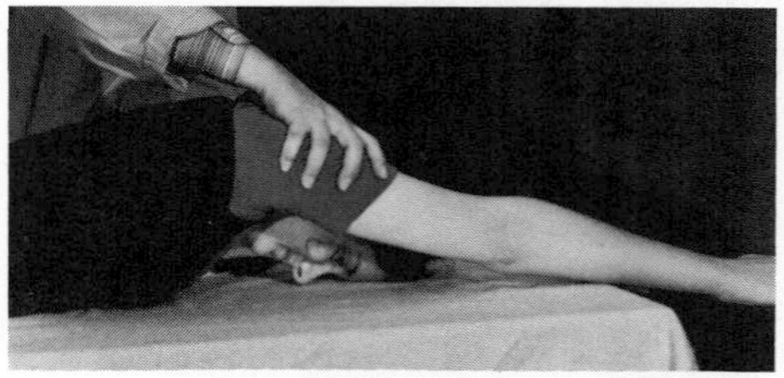

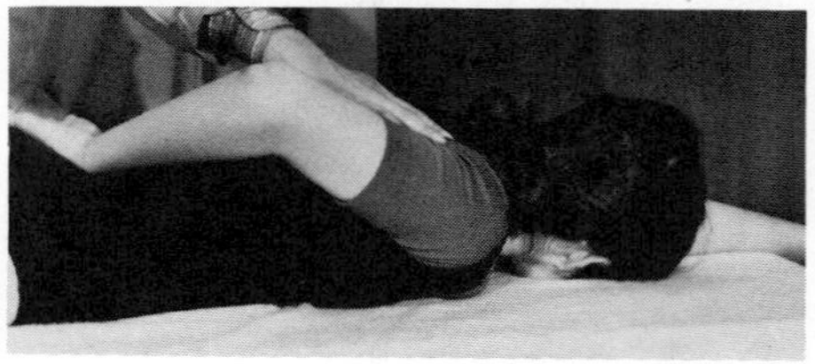

Fig. 41

ELBOW

Fig. 43. Range of motion of the elbow.* **A,** Flexion and hyperextension. *Flexion:* zero to 150°. *Extension:* 150° to zero (from the angle of greatest flexion to the zero position). *Hyperextension:* measured in degrees beyond the zero starting point. This motion is not present in all individuals. When it is present, it may vary from 5° to 15°. **B,** Measurement of limited motion. (The unshaded area indicates the range of limited motion.) Limited motion may be expressed in the following ways: (1) the elbow flexes from 30° to 90° (30° → 90°); (2) the elbow has a flexion deformity of 30° with further flexion to 90°.

Movement	Muscles	Motor nerves	Positions for testing	Instructions and tests for muscle strength
Flexion	Prime movers (Fig. 44§) Biceps brachii	Musculocutaneous nerve (cervical 5, 6)	Standing, sitting, supine (arm extended)	"Move your right [left] hand to your right [left] shoulder."
	Brachialis	Musculocutaneous nerve (cervical 5, 6)		"Make a fist; try to bring your fist to your shoulder."
	Brachioradialis	Radial nerve (cervical 5, 6)		Resistance is applied to the lower arm (Fig. 45).
	Accessory muscles: flexor muscles of forearm			

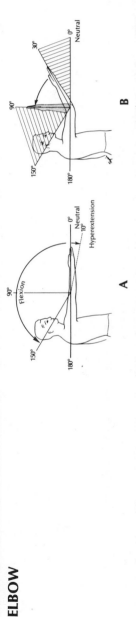

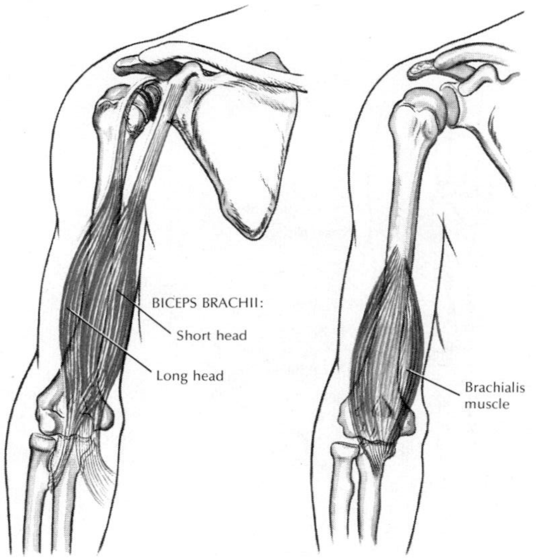

Fig. 44

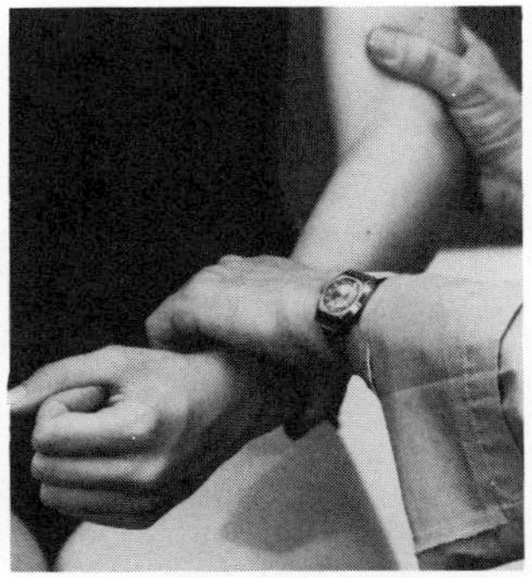

Fig. 45

Continued.

Table 18-2. TESTING FOR MUSCLE STRENGTH AND RANGE OF JOINT MOTION—cont'd

Movement	Muscles	Motor nerves	Positions for testing	Instructions and tests for muscle strength
Extension	Prime mover: triceps brachii (Fig. 46§) Accessory muscles Anconeus Extensor muscles of fore-arm	Radial nerve (cervical 7, 8)	Standing, sitting, supine (arm flexed)	"Straighten out your right [left] arm." Resistance is applied to the dorsal surface of the arm (Fig. 47).

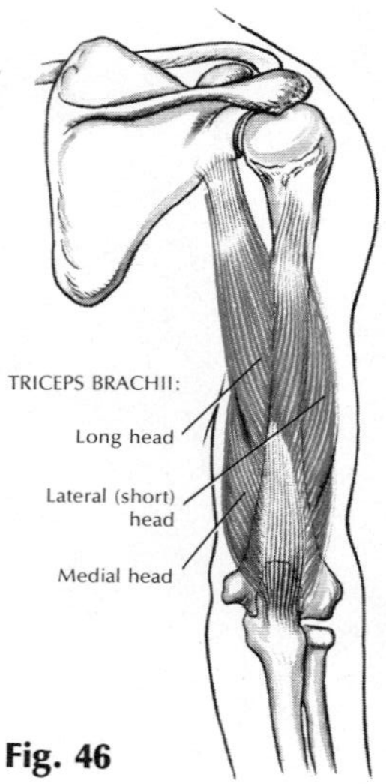

TRICEPS BRACHII:
Long head
Lateral (short) head
Medial head

Fig. 46

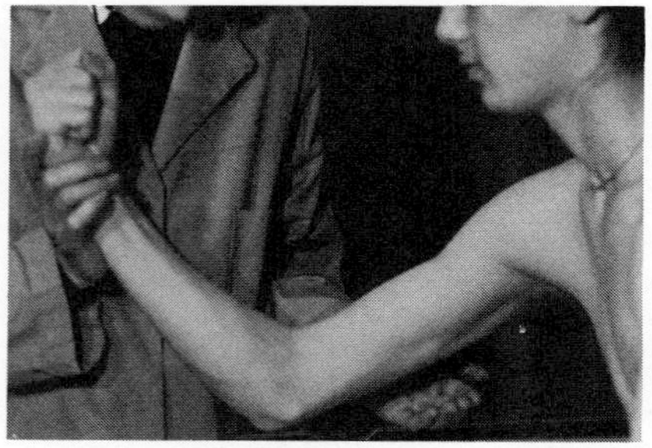

Fig. 47

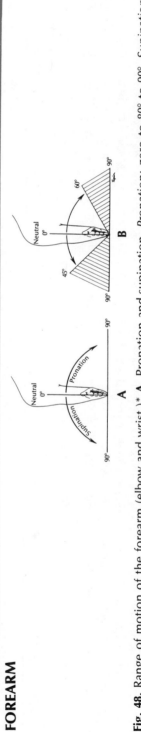

FOREARM

Fig. 48. Range of motion of the forearm (elbow and wrist.)* **A,** Pronation and supination. *Pronation:* zero to 80° to 90°. *Supination:* zero to 80° to 90°. *Total forearm motion:* 160° to 180°. Individuals may vary in the range of supination and pronation. Some individuals may reach the 90° arc, whereas others may have only 70° plus. **B,** Limited motion. *Supination:* 45° (0 → 45°). *Pronation:* 60° (0 → 60°). *Total joint motion:* 105°.

Movement	Muscles	Motor nerves	Positions for testing	Instructions and tests for muscle strength
Pronation	Prime movers (Fig. 49§) Pronator teres Pronator quadratus Accessory muscle: flexor carpi radialis	Median nerve (cervical 6, 7) Median nerve (cervical 8, thoracic 1)	Standing, sitting, supine (elbow flexed, hands extended, palms up)	"Rotate your right [left] hand inward so that your palm is downward." Resistance is applied at the base of the thumb on the volar surface (Fig. 50).
Supination	Prime movers (Fig. 51†) Biceps brachii Supinator Accessory muscle: brachioradialis	Musculocutaneous nerve (cervical 5, 6) Radial nerve (cervical 6)	Standing, sitting, supine	"Rotate your right [left] hand outward so that the palm is upward." Resistance is applied on the base of the thumb or over the surface of the hand on the dorsal surface (Fig. 52).

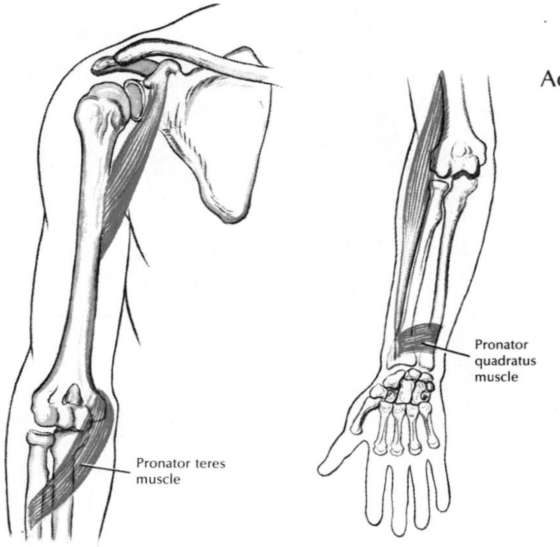

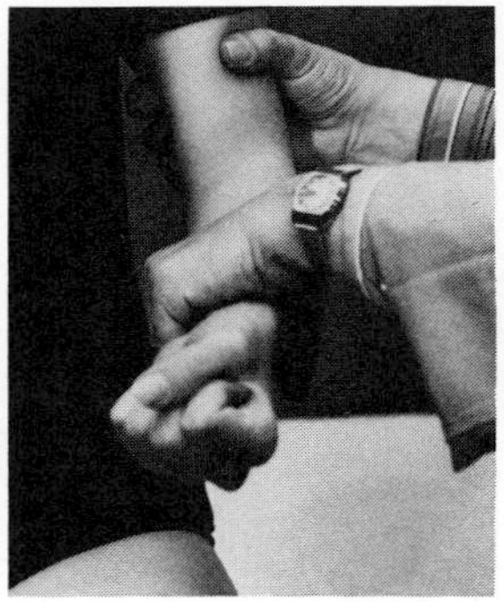

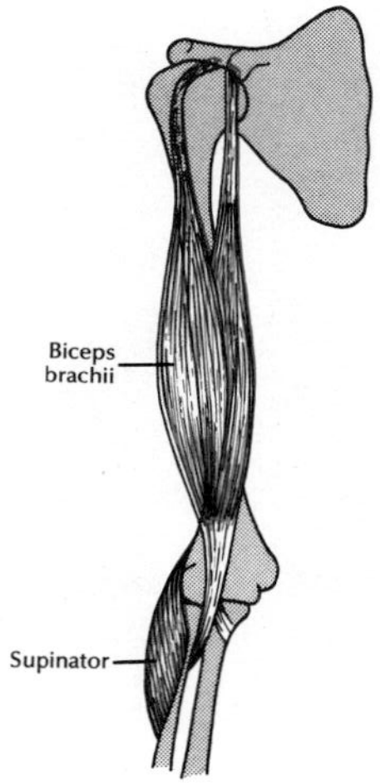

Fig. 50

Fig. 52

Continued.

Pronator quadratus muscle

Pronator teres muscle

Fig. 49

Biceps brachii

Supinator

Fig. 51

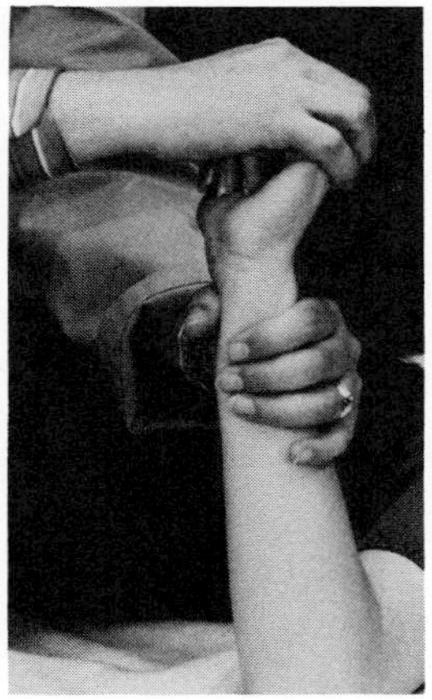

Table 18-2. TESTING FOR MUSCLE STRENGTH AND RANGE OF JOINT MOTION—cont'd

WRIST

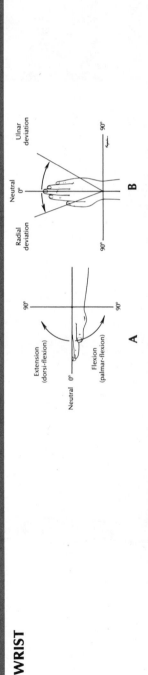

Fig. 53. Range of motion of the wrist.* **A,** Flexion and extension. *Flexion* (palmar flexion): zero to ±80°. *Extension* (dorsiflexion): zero to ±70°. **B,** Radial and ulnar deviation. *Radial deviation:* zero to 20°. *Ulnar deviation:* zero to 30°. Ulnar deviation is usually measured with the wrist in pronation. When measured in supination, ulnar deviation will be somewhat increased.

Movement	Muscles	Motor nerves	Positions for testing	Instructions and tests for muscle strength
Flexion	Prime movers (Fig. 54§) Flexor carpi radialis Flexor carpi ulnaris Accessory muscle: palmaris longus	Medial nerve (cervical 6, 7) Ulnar nerve (cervical 8, thoracic 1)	Standing, sitting, supine (un-extended)	"Bend your right [left] hand down toward you." Resistance is applied to the volar surface of the hand (Fig. 55).

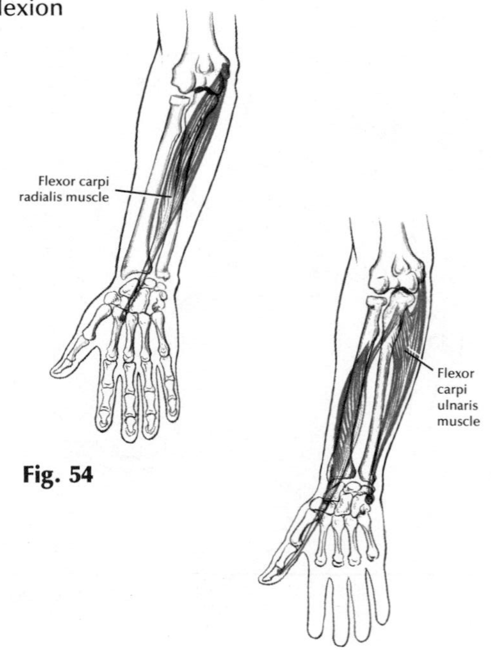

Fig. 55

Flexor carpi radialis muscle

Flexor carpi ulnaris muscle

Fig. 54

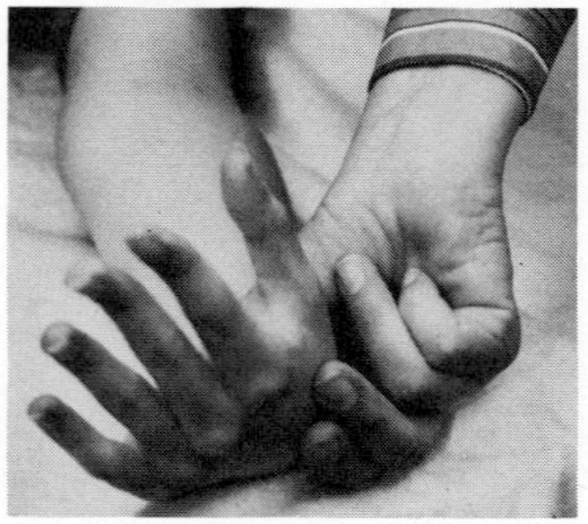

334

Extension

Prime movers (Fig. 56+)
Extensor carpi radialis longus
Extensor carpi radialis brevis
Extensor carpi ulnaris

Radial nerve (cervical 6, 7)
Radial nerve (cervical 6, 7)
Radial nerve (cervical 6, 7, 8)

Standing, sitting, supine (wrist flexed)

"Bend your right [left] hand back on itself."
Resistance is applied on the dorsal surface of the hand (Fig. 57).

Continued.

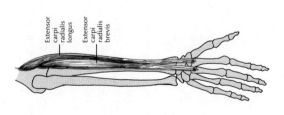

Extensor carpi radialis longus
Extensor carpi radialis brevis

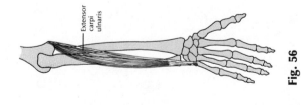

Extensor carpi ulnaris

Fig. 56

Fig. 57

Table 18-2. TESTING FOR MUSCLE STRENGTH AND RANGE OF JOINT MOTION—cont'd

THUMB

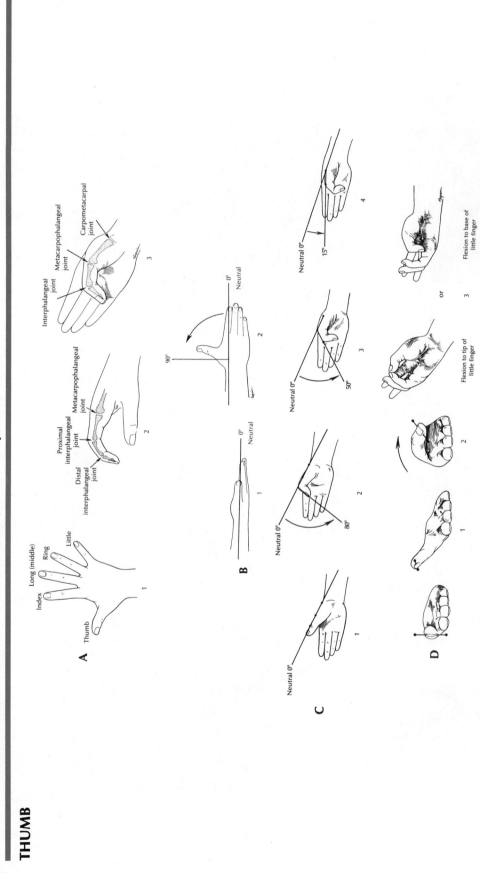

Fig. 58. Hand and range of motion of the thumb.* **A,** Hand. *1,* Nomenclature: In order to avoid mistaken identity, the fingers and thumb are referred to by name rather than by number. Anatomical nomenclature is used for joints of the fingers and thumbs. *2,* Joints of the fingers. *3,* Joints of the thumb. **B,** Abduction. *1,* Zero starting position: the extended thumb alongside the index finger, which is in line with the radius. *Abduction* is the angle created between the metacarpal bones of the thumb and index finger. This motion may take place in two planes. *2,* Abduction parallel to the plane of the palm (extension). **C,** Flexion. *1,* Zero starting position: the extended thumb. *2,* Flexion of the interphalangeal joint: zero to ±80°. *3,* Flexion of the metacarpophalangeal joint: zero to ±50°. *4,* Flexion of the carpometacarpal joint: zero to ±15°. **D,** Opposition. Zero starting position *(far left):* the extended thumb in line with the index fingers. *Opposition* is a composite motion consisting of three elements: *1,* abduction, *2,* rotation, and *3,* flexion. This motion is usually considered complete when the tip, or pulp, of the thumb touches the tip of the fifth finger. Some surgeons, however, consider the arc of opposition complete when the tip of the thumb touches the base of the fifth finger. Both methods are illustrated.

Movement	Muscles	Motor nerves	Positions for testing	Instructions and tests for muscle strength
Flexion of joints Metacarpophalangeal Interphalangeal	Prime movers (Fig. 59†) Flexor pollicis brevis Flexor pollicis longus	Median nerve (cervical 6, 7) Ulnar nerve (cervical 8, thoracic 1)	Standing, sitting, supine (thumb extended)	"Bend your right [left] thumb to touch your palm." Resistance is applied to the thenar eminence —the dorsal surface of the distal phalanx (Fig. 60).
Extension of joints Metacarpophalangeal Interphalangeal	Prime movers (Fig. 61†) Extensor pollicis brevis Extensor pollicis longus	Radial nerve (cervical 6, 7) Radial nerve (cervical 6, 7, 8)	Standing, sitting, supine (thumb flexed)	"Straighten out your thumb as if thumbing a ride." "Thumb your nose." Resistance is applied to the dorsal surface of the distal phalanx (Fig. 62).

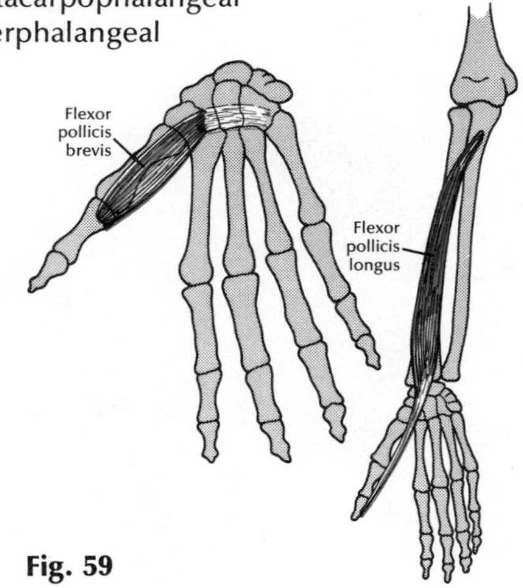

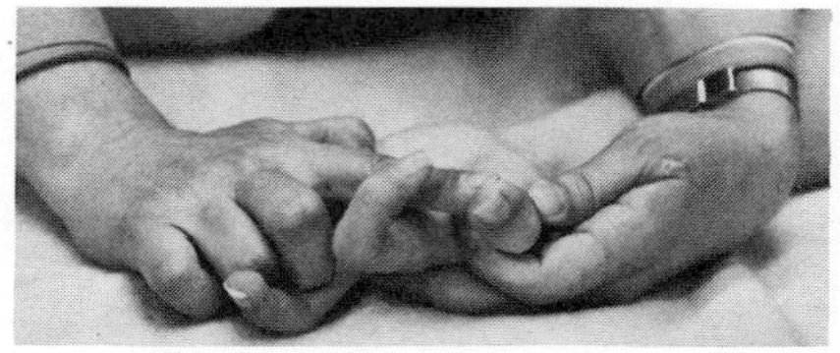

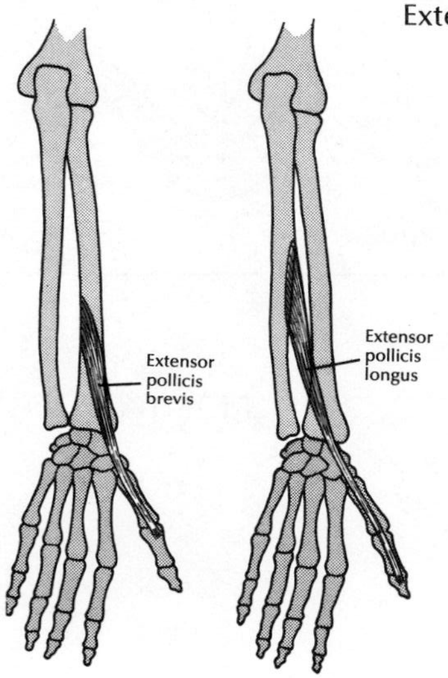

Fig. 60

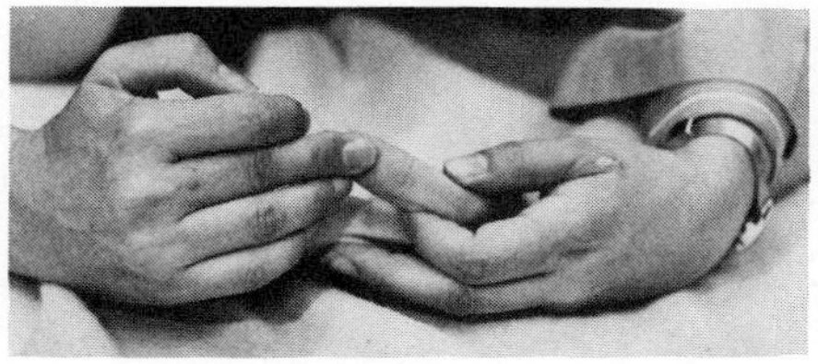

Fig. 62

Flexor pollicis longus

Flexor pollicis brevis

Fig. 59

Extensor pollicis longus

Extensor pollicis brevis

Fig. 61

Continued.

Table 18-2. TESTING FOR MUSCLE STRENGTH AND RANGE OF JOINT MOTION—cont'd

Movement	Muscles	Motor nerves	Positions for testing	Instructions and tests for muscle strength
Abduction	Prime movers (Fig. 63†) Abductor pollicis longus Abductor pollicis brevis Accessory muscle: palmaris longus	Radial nerve (cervical 6, 7) Median nerve (cervical 6, 7)	Standing, sitting, supine (arms extended, may have hands in clapping position)	"Raise your right [left] thumb to the ceiling." Resistance is applied to the dorsal surface of the thumb (Fig. 64).
Adduction	Prime movers (Fig. 65†) Adductor pollicis oblique Adductor pollicis transverse	Ulnar nerve (cervical 8, thoracic 1) Ulnar nerve (cervical 8, thoracic 1)	Standing, sitting, supine	"Bring your thumb down against the index finger." Resistance is applied against the terminal phalanx.

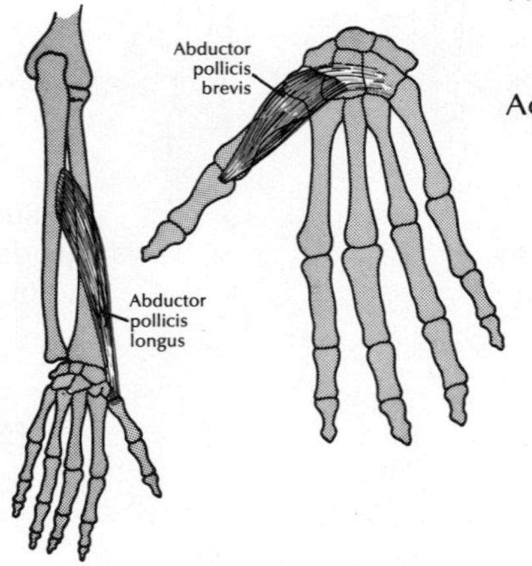

Fig. 64

Abductor pollicis brevis

Abductor pollicis longus

Fig. 63

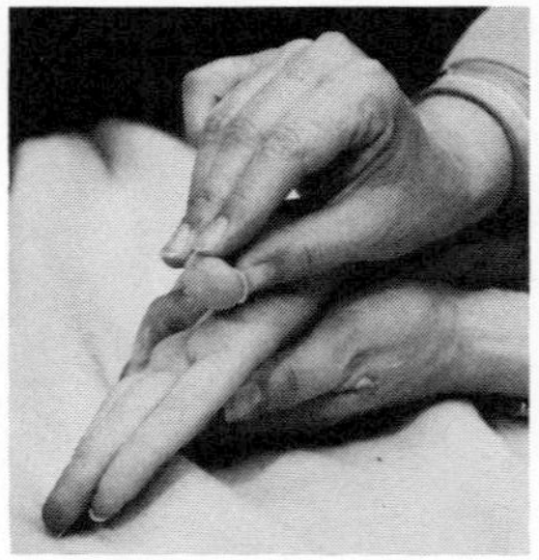

Adductor pollicis

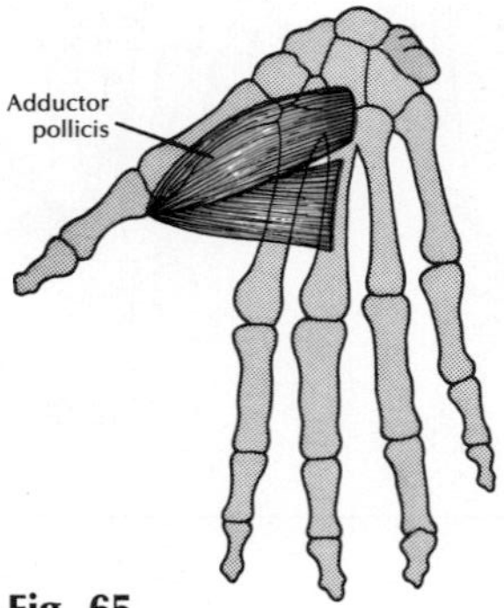

Fig. 65

Opposition

Prime movers (Fig. 66†)
Opponens pollicis
Opponens digiti minimi

Median nerve (cervical 6, 7)
Ulnar nerve (cervical 8, thoracic 1)

Standing, sitting, supine

"Touch the top of the right [left] thumb to the tip and then to the base of the little, ring, middle, and index fingers."
Resistance is applied to the palmar surfaces of the thumb and fingers. (Fig. 67).

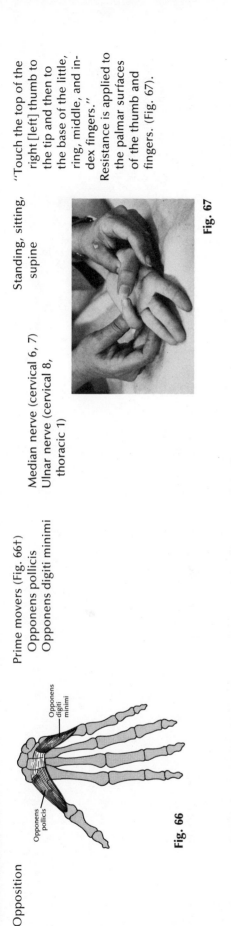

Fig. 66

Opponens digiti minimi

Opponens pollicis

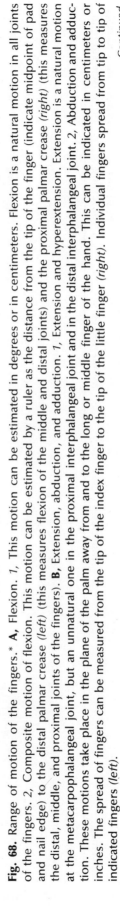

Fig. 67

FINGERS

Fig. 68. Range of motion of the fingers.* **A,** Flexion. *1,* This motion can be estimated in degrees or in centimeters. Flexion is a natural motion in all joints of the fingers. *2,* Composite motion of flexion. This motion can be estimated by a ruler as the distance from the tip of the finger (indicate midpoint of pad and nail edge) to the distal palmar crease (*left*) (this measures flexion of the middle and distal joints) and the proximal palmar crease (*right*) (this measures the distal, middle, and proximal joints of the fingers). **B,** Extension, abduction, and adduction. *1,* Extension and hyperextension. Extension is a natural motion at the metacarpophalangeal joint, but an unnatural one in the proximal interphalangeal joint and in the distal interphalangeal joint. *2,* Abduction and adduction. These motions take place in the plane of the palm away from and to the long or middle finger of the hand. This can be indicated in centimeters or inches. The spread of fingers can be measured from the tip of the index finger to the tip of the little finger (*right*). Individual fingers spread from tip to tip of indicated fingers (*left*).

Continued.

339

Table 18-2. TESTING FOR MUSCLE STRENGTH AND RANGE OF JOINT MOTION—cont'd

Movement	Muscles	Motor nerves	Positions for testing	Instructions and tests for muscle strength
Flexion of joints Metacarpophalangeal	Prime movers (Fig. 69†) Lumbricales Dorsal interossei Palmar interossei	Ulnar nerve (cervical 8) Ulnar nerve (cervical 8) Ulnar nerve (cervical 8, thoracic 1)	Standing, sitting, supine	"Bend your fingers at the first [proximal] joint." Resistance is applied to the palmar surface of the proximal phalanges (Fig. 70).
	Accessory muscles Flexor digiti minimi brevis Flexor digitorum superficialis Flexor digitorum profundus			
Proximal interphalangeal	Prime mover: flexor digitorum superficialis	Median nerve (cervical 7, 8; thoracic 1)	Standing, sitting, supine	"Bend your fingers at the middle joint." "Crook your fingers." Resistance is applied to the palmar surface of the middle phalanges.
Distal interphalangeal	Prime mover: flexor digitorum profundus	Ulnar nerve (cervical 8, thoracic 1)	Standing, sitting, supine	"Bend your distal finger joint." "Crook your finger." Resistance is applied to the pad of the finger (Fig. 71).

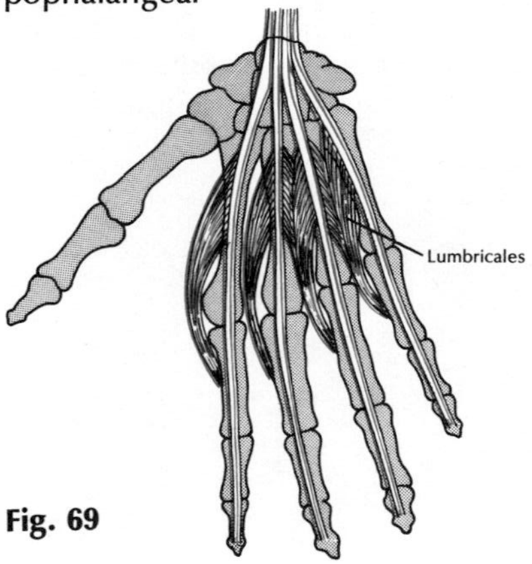

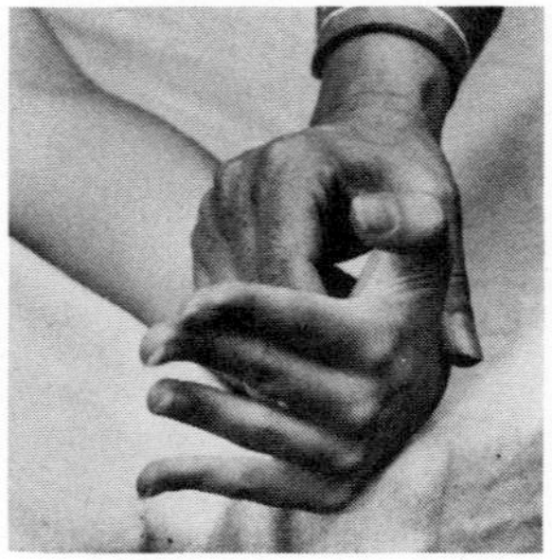

Fig. 70

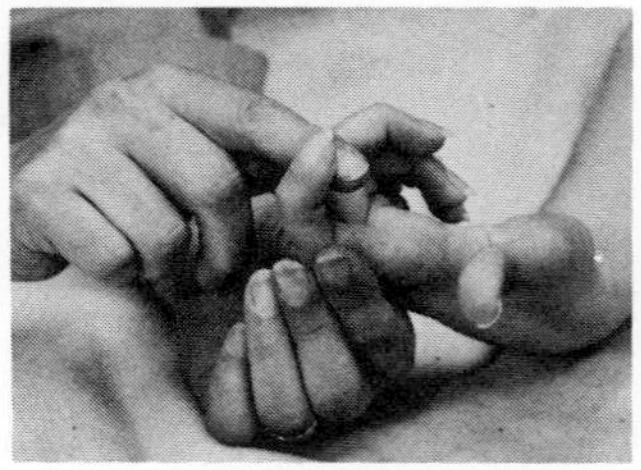

Fig. 71

Lumbricales

Fig. 69

metacarpophalangeal joints

Extensor digitorum communis
Extensor indicis proprius
Extensor digiti minimi

Radial nerve (cervical 6, 7, 8)
Radial nerve (cervical 6, 7, 8)
Radial nerve (cervical 7)

Standing, sitting, supine (fingers flexed)

Resistance is applied to the dorsal surface of the proximal and distal phalanges (Fig. 57).

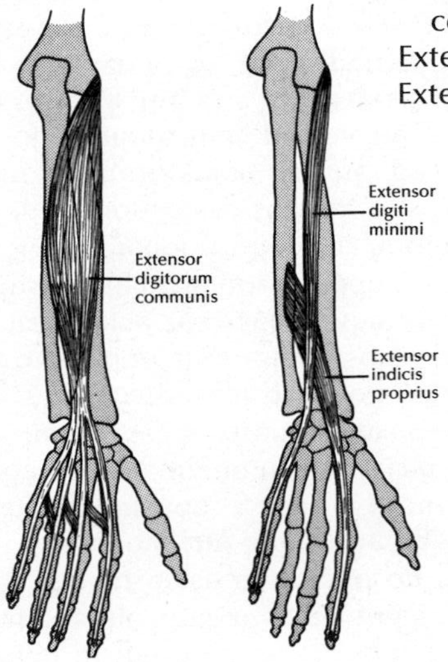

Fig. 72

Abduction

Prime movers (Fig. 73†)
Dorsal interossei
Abductor digiti minimi

Ulnar nerve (cervical 8, thoracic 1)
Ulnar nerve (cervical 8)

Standing, sitting, supine (fingers together)

"Spread your fingers as far apart as possible." Pressure is exerted against the outside surfaces of the fingers being tested to resist spread of the fingers (Fig. 74).

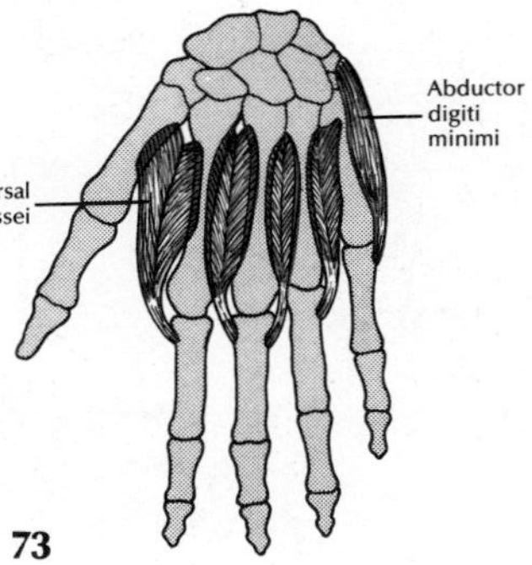

Fig. 73

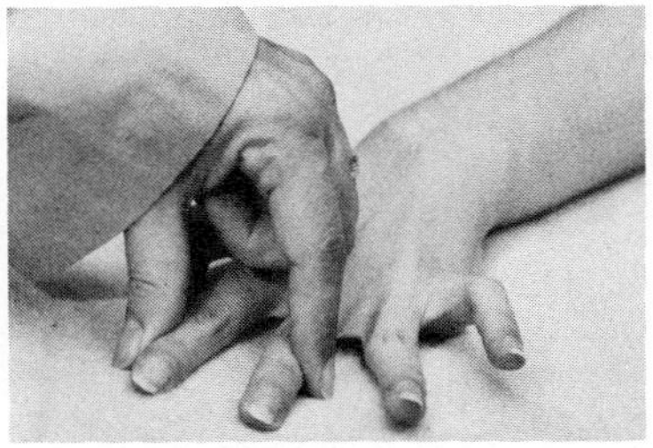

Fig. 74

Adduction

Prime movers: palmar interossei (Fig. 75†)

Ulnar nerve (cervical 8, thoracic 1)

Standing, sitting, supine (fingers apart)

"Put your fingers together. Press them hard against each other." An attempt is made to pull them apart (Fig. 76).

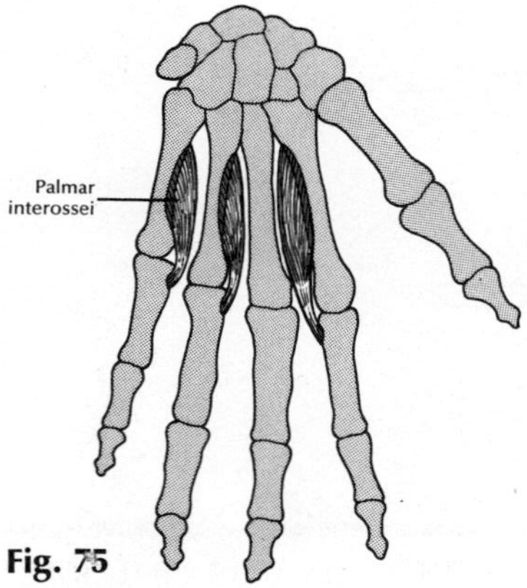

Fig. 75

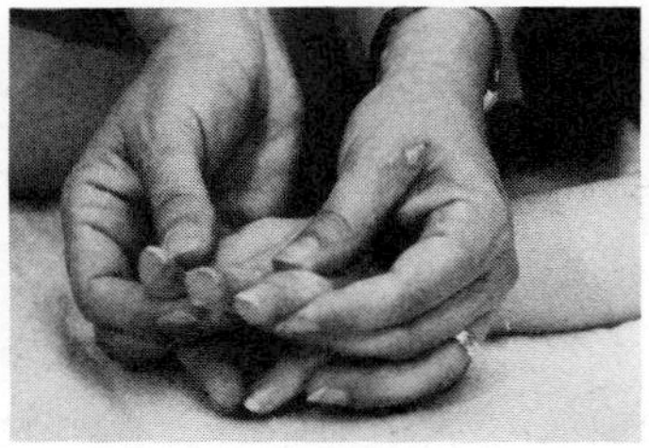

Fig. 76

Continued.

341

Table 18-2. TESTING FOR MUSCLE STRENGTH AND RANGE OF JOINT MOTION—cont'd

HIP

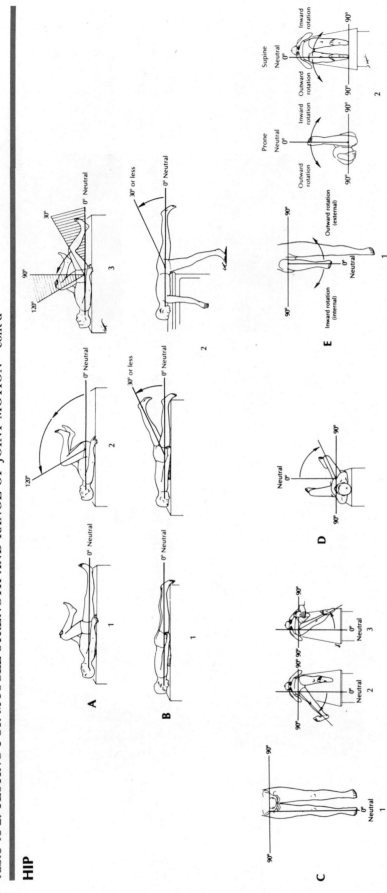

Fig. 77. Range of motion of the hip.* **A,** Flexion. *1,* Zero starting position of the right hip: client is supine on a firm, flat surface with the opposite hip held in full flexion. This flattens the lumbar spine and demonstrates a flexion deformity of the hip if present. *2,* Flexion. The motion is recorded from zero to 110° or 120°. The examiner should place one hand on the iliac crest to note the point at which the pelvis begins to rotate. *3,* Limited motion in flexion. Limited motion is noted as in the elbow and knee: the hip flexes from 30° to 90° (30° → 90°); the hip has a flexion deformity of 30° with further flexion to 90°. **B,** Extension. *1,* Zero starting position: Client is prone on a firm, level surface. *2,* The upward motion of the hip is measured in degrees from the zero starting position. Two methods are commonly used. *Left,* With the client prone and a small pillow under the abdomen, the leg is extended with the knee straight or flexed. *Right,* With the opposite extremity flexed over the end of the examining table, the hip is extended. This method is a more accurate method of measuring extension. There is an anatomical question whether extension is present in the hip at all. Extension as seen from examination is that deviation of the extremity past the zero position and reflects some back motion. **C,** Abduction and adduction. *1,* Zero starting position: client is supine with the legs extended at right angles to a transverse line across the anterosuperior spine of the pelvis. *2,* Abduction. The outward motion of the extremity is measured in degrees from the zero starting position. *3,* Adduction. In measuring adduction the examiner should elevate the opposite extremity a few degrees to allow the leg to pass under it. **D,** Abduction in flexion. Abduction can be measured in degrees at any level of flexion. Usually, this is carried out in 90° of flexion. **E,** Rotation. *1,* Rotation in flexion. Zero starting position: Client is supine with the hip and knee flexed 90° each and the thigh perpendicular to the transverse line across the anterosuperior spine of the pelvis. *Inward (internal) rotation* is measured by rotating the leg away from the midline of the trunk with the thigh as the axis of rotation, thus producing inward rotation of the hip. *Outward (external) rotation* is measured by rotating the leg toward the midline of the trunk with the thigh as the axis of rotation, thus producing outward rotation of the hip. *2,* Rotation in extension. Zero starting position: With client prone *(left),* the knee is flexed to 90° and is perpendicular to the transverse line across the anterosuperior spine of the pelvis. *Inward rotation* is measured by rotating the leg inward. *Outward rotation* is measured by rotating the leg outward. *Outward rotation* in extension can also be measured with the client supine *(right).*

Movement	Muscles	Motor nerves	Positions for testing	Instructions and tests for muscle strength
Flexion	Prime movers (Fig. 78†) Psoas major Iliacus Accessory muscles Sartorius Rectus femoris Tensor fasciae latae Pectineus Adductor brevis Adductor longus Adductor magnus (oblique fibers)	Femoral nerve (lumbar 2, 3) Femoral nerve (lumbar 2, 3)	Supine Sitting	"Draw your knees up to your chest." "Bend your right [left] knee up to your chest." Resistance is applied to the anterior surface of the leg proximal to the knee (Fig. 79).
Extension	Prime movers (Fig. 80§) Gluteus maximus Semitendinosus Semimembranosus Biceps femoris (long head)	Inferior gluteal nerve (lumbar 5; sacral 1, 2) Sciatic nerve (lumbar 4, 5; sacral 1, 2) Sciatic nerve (lumbar 5; sacral 1, 2) Sciatic nerve (sacral 1, 2, 3)	Prone	"Lift your right [left] leg toward the ceiling." Resistance is applied to the dorsal surface of the leg proximal to the knee (Fig. 81).

Fig. 79

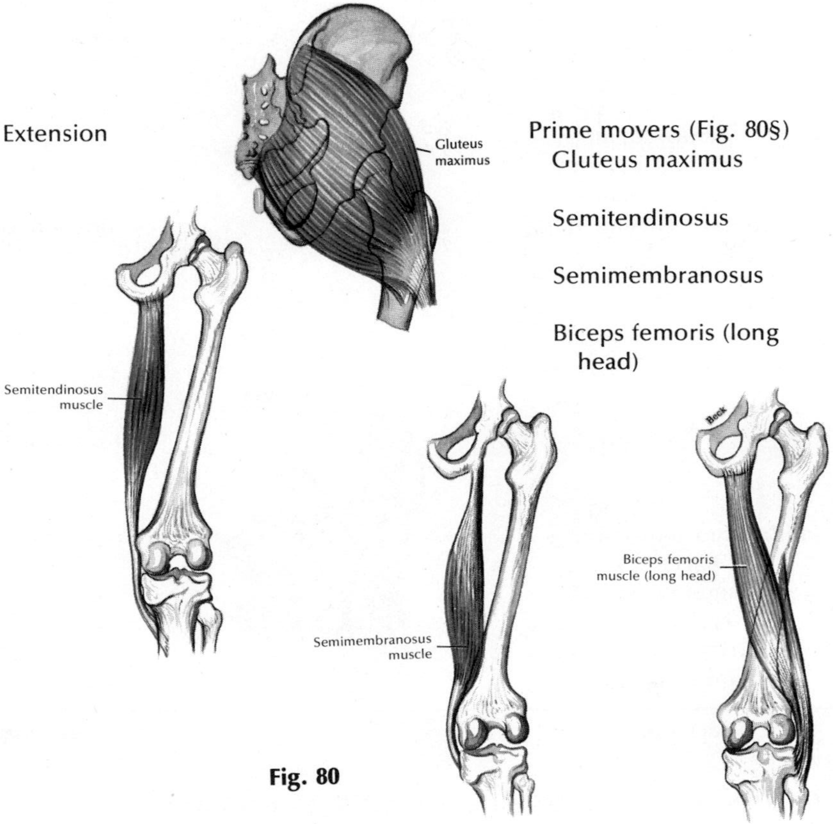

Fig. 81

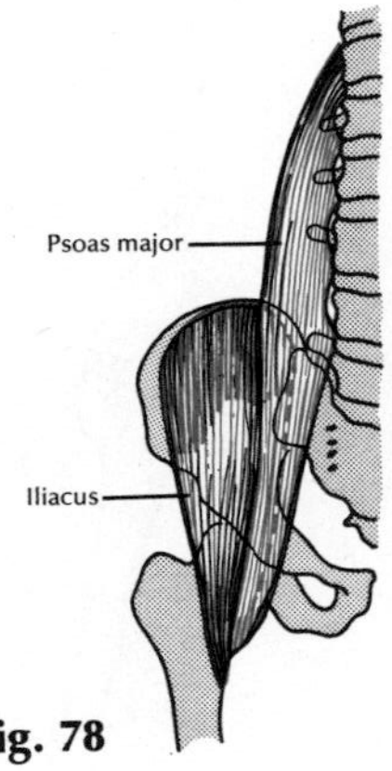

Psoas major

Iliacus

Fig. 78

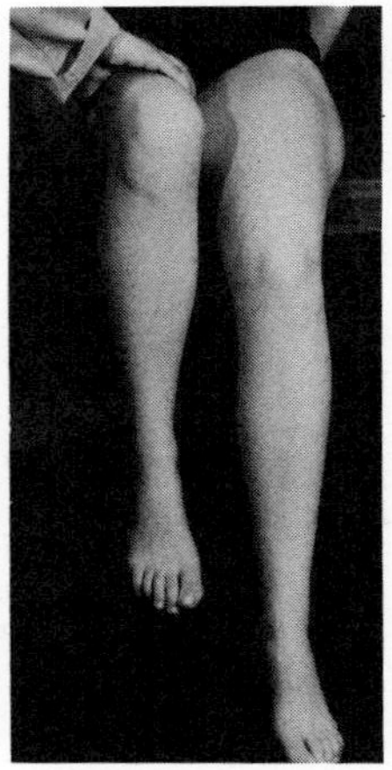

Gluteus maximus

Semitendinosus muscle

Biceps femoris muscle (long head)

Semimembranosus muscle

Fig. 80

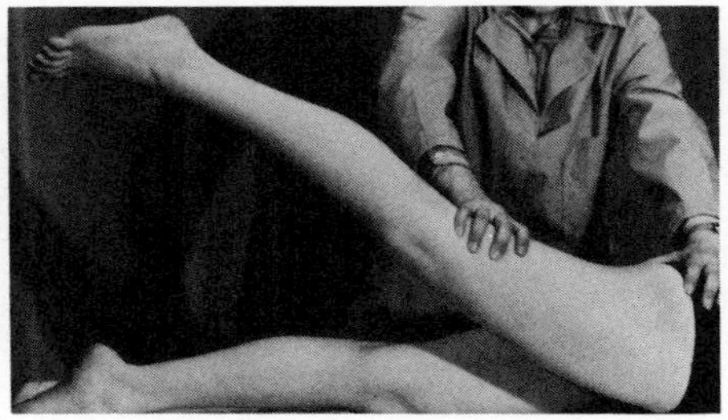

Continued.

343

Table 18-2. TESTING FOR MUSCLE STRENGTH AND RANGE OF JOINT MOTION—cont'd

Movement	Muscles	Motor nerves	Positions for testing	Instructions and tests for muscle strength
Abduction	Prime mover: gluteus medius (Fig. 82§) Accessory muscles Gluteus minimus Tensor fasciae latae Gluteus maximus (upper fibers)	Superior gluteal nerve (lumbar 4, 5; sacral 1)	Lateral lie	"Move your upper leg toward the ceiling." Resistance is applied to the lateral surface of the upper leg (Fig. 83).
Adduction	Prime movers (Fig. 84§) Adductor magnus Adductor brevis Adductor longus Pectineus Gracilis	Obturator nerve (lumbar 3, 4) Obturator nerve (lumbar 3, 4) Obturator nerve (lumbar 3, 4) Obturator nerve (lumbar 2, 3, 4) Obturator nerve (lumbar 3, 4)	Lateral lie, legs apart	"Try to bring your legs together." Resistance is applied to the medial surface of the thighs proximal to the knees (Fig. 85).

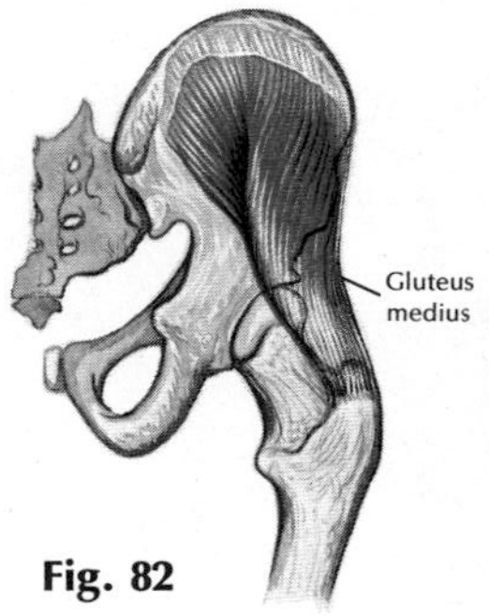

Fig. 82

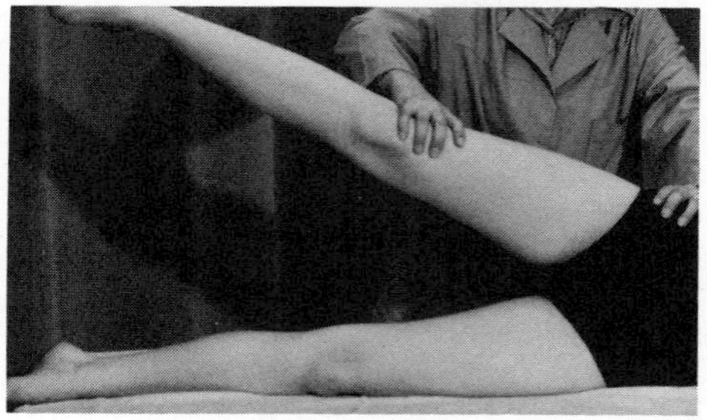

Gluteus medius

Fig. 83

Pectineus muscle

Adductor longus muscle

Gracilis muscle

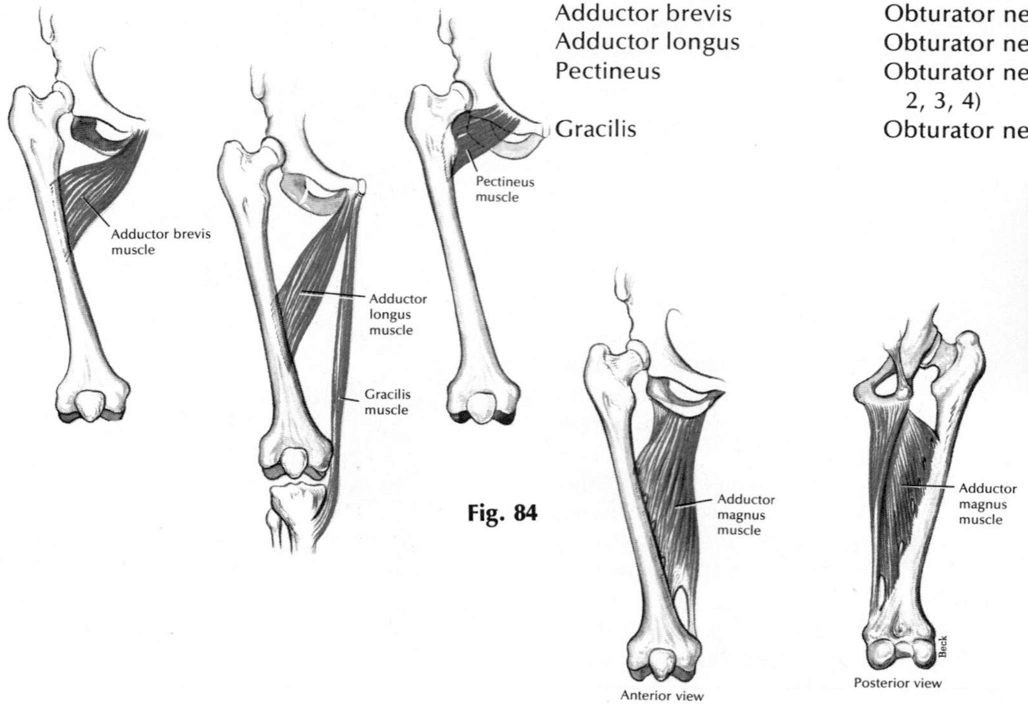

Adductor brevis muscle

Fig. 84

Adductor magnus muscle

Anterior view

Adductor magnus muscle

Posterior view

Beck

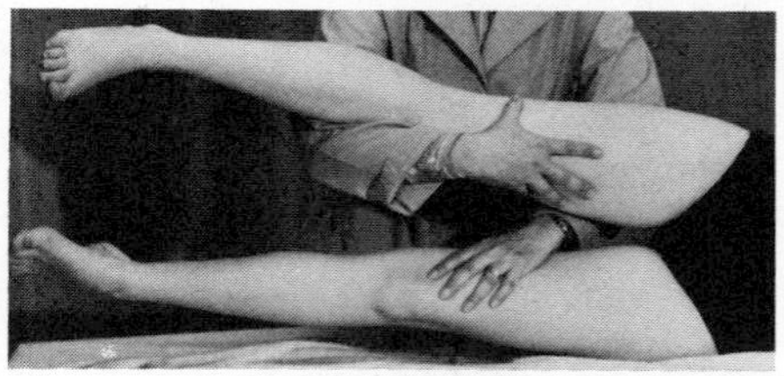

Fig. 85

Rotation (knees extended)

Internal

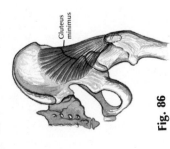

Fig. 86

Prime movers (Fig. 86§)
Gluteus minimus   Superior gluteal nerve (lumbar 4, 5; sacral 1)

Tensor fasciae latae   Superior gluteal nerve (lumbar 4, 5; sacral 1)

Accessory muscles
Gluteus medius (anterior fibers)
Semitendinosus
Semimembranosus

Sitting, supine, (legs about a foot apart at ankle)

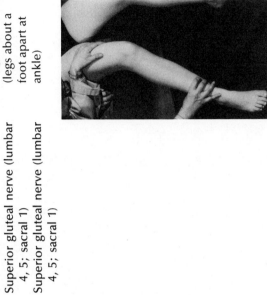

"Pivot your right hip inward—your foot will move away from your body." Resistance is applied toward the midline at the lateral surface of the ankle (Fig. 87).

Fig. 87

External

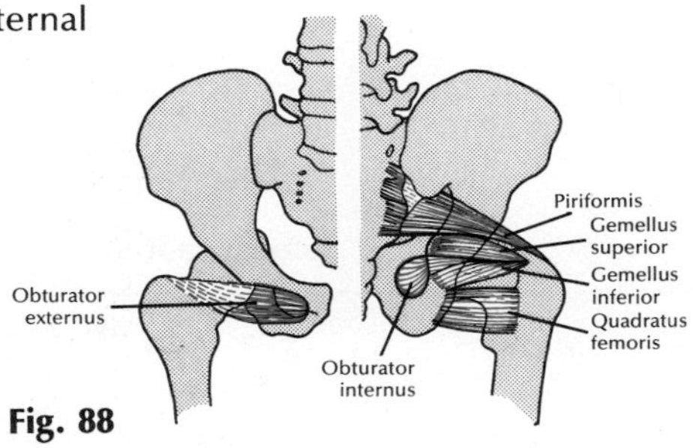

Fig. 88

Prime movers (Fig. 88†)
Obturator externus   Obturator nerve (lumbar 3, 4)
Obturator internus   Obturator nerve (lumbar 5; sacral 2, 3)

Quadratus femoris   Obturator nerve (lumbar 5; sacral 1)

Piriformis   Obturator nerve (sacral 1, 2)
Gemellus superior   Obturator nerve (lumbar 5; sacral 1, 2, 3)

Gemellus inferior   Obturator nerve (lumbar 5; sacral 1)

Gluteus maximus   Obturator nerve (lumbar 5; sacral 1)

Accessory muscles
Sartorius   Obturator nerve (lumbar 5; sacral 1, 2)
Biceps femoris (long head)

Sitting, supine

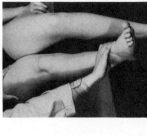

"Rotate your hip outward; your foot will turn in." Resistance is applied to the medial aspect of the ankle (Fig. 89).

Fig. 89

Continued.

Table 18-2. TESTING FOR MUSCLE STRENGTH AND RANGE OF JOINT MOTION—cont'd

Movement	Muscles	Motor nerves	Positions for testing	Instructions and tests for muscle strength
Rotation (knees flexed)	Prime mover: sartorius Accessory muscles External rotators of hip Flexors of hip, knee	Femoral nerve (lumbar 2, 3, 4)	Supine (knees flexed)	"Rotate your knees outward. Bend them toward the table. Bring them as close as you can to the table." Resistance is applied to the lateral aspects of the knees.
Abduction	Prime mover: tensor fasciae latae Accessory muscles Gluteus medius Gluteus minimus	Superior gluteal nerve (lumbar 4, 5; sacral 1)	Supine	"Bend your knees out." Resistance is applied to the upper outer aspect of each leg.

KNEE

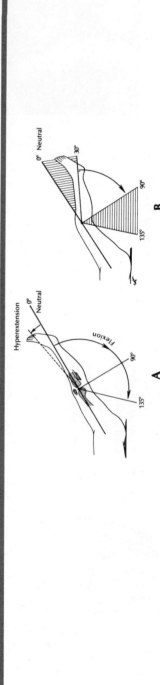

Fig. 90. Range of motion of the knee.* **A,** Flexion. Zero starting position: the extended straight knee with client either supine or prone. *Flexion* is measured in degrees from the zero starting point. *Hyperextension* is measured in degrees opposite to flexion at the zero starting point. **B,** Measurement of Limited motion of the knee. The terminology for recording limited motion of the knee is similar to that of the elbow and hip: (1) the knee flexes from 30° to 90° (30° → 90°); (2) the knee has a flexion deformity of 30° with further flexion to 90°.

Movement	Muscles	Motor nerves	Positions for testing	Instructions and tests for muscle strength
Flexion	Prime movers (Fig. 91§) Biceps femoris (long head)	Sciatic nerve (sacral 1, 2, 3)	Prone	"Bend your right [left] leg. Try to touch your heel to the back of your leg." Resistance is applied to the dorsal aspect of the ankle (Fig. 92).
	Biceps femoris (short head)	Sciatic nerve (lumbar 4, 5; sacral 1, 2)		
	Semitendinosus	Sciatic nerve (lumbar 4, 5; sacral 1, 2, 3)		
	Semimembranosus	Sciatic nerve (lumbar 4, 5; sacral 1, 2, 3)		
	Accessory muscles Popliteus Sartorius Gracilis Gastrocnemius			

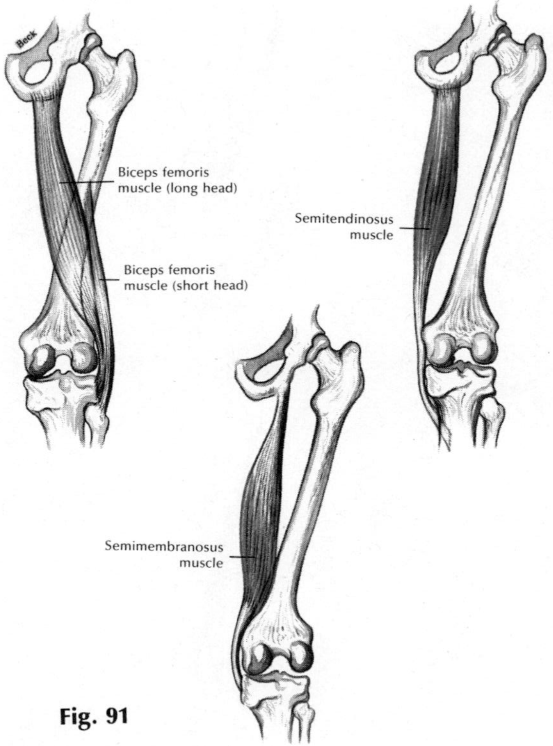

Fig. 91

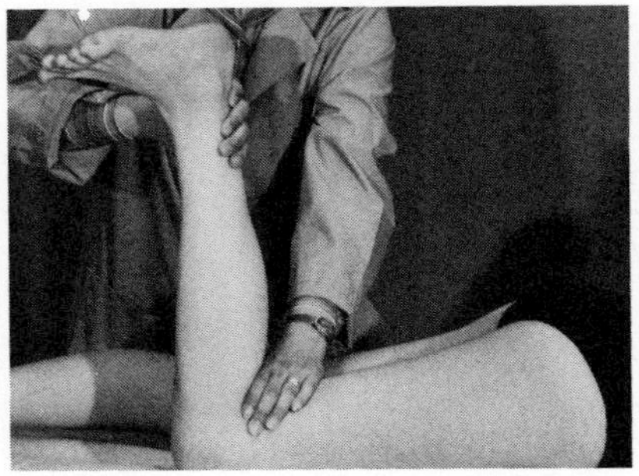

Fig. 92

Continued.

347

Table 18-2. TESTING FOR MUSCLE STRENGTH AND RANGE OF JOINT MOTION—cont'd

Movement	Muscles	Motor nerves	Positions for testing	Instructions and tests for muscle strength
Extension	Prime movers (Fig. 93§)		Sitting	"Straighten out your right [left] leg." Resistance is applied against the anterior aspect of the ankle.
	Rectus femoris	Femoral nerve (lumbar 2, 3, 4)		
	Vastus intermedius	Femoral nerve (lumbar 2, 3, 4)		
	Vastus medialis	Femoral nerve (lumbar 2, 3, 4)		
	Vastus lateralis	Femoral nerve (lumbar 2, 3, 4)		

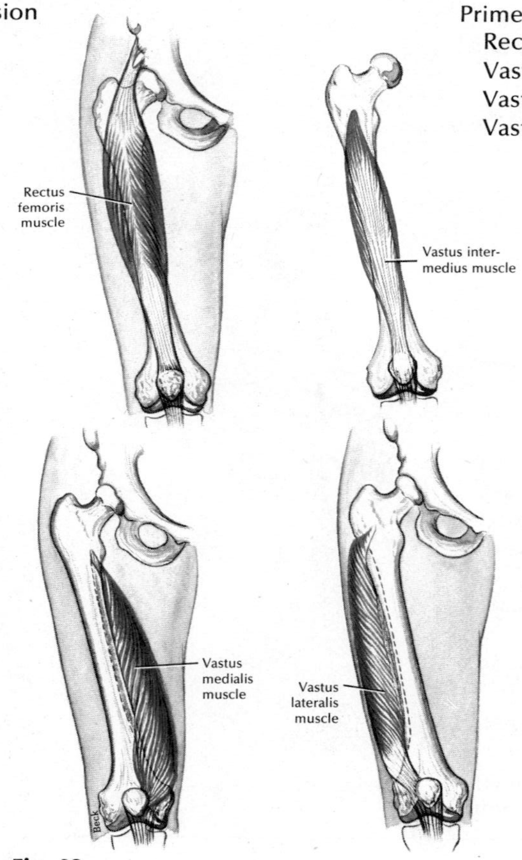

Fig. 93

ANKLE

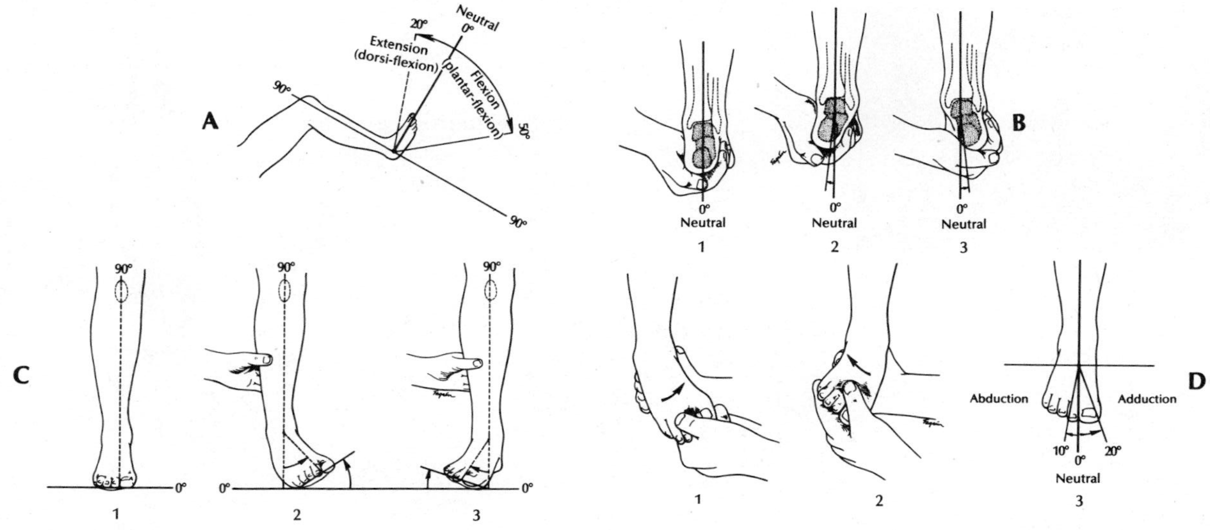

Fig. 94. Range of motion of the ankle and foot.* **A,** Extension (dorsiflexion) and flexion (plantar flexion). These motions are measured in degrees from the right-angle neutral position or in percentages of motion as compared to the opposite ankle. **B,** Motions of the hind part of the foot (passive motion). *1,* Zero starting position: the heel in line with the midline of the tibia. *2,* Inversion. The heel is grasped firmly in the cup of the examiner's hand. Passive motion is estimated in degrees or percentages of motion by turning the heel inward. *3,* Eversion. This motion is estimated by turning the heel outward. **C,** Motions of the fore part of the foot (active motion). *1,* Zero starting position: The foot in line with the tibia in the long axis from the ankle to the knee. The axis of the fore part of the foot is the second toe. *2,* Active inversion. The foot is directed medially. This motion includes supination, adduction, and some degree of plantar flexion. This motion can be estimated in degrees or expressed in percentages as compared to the opposite foot. *3,* Active eversion. The sole of the foot is turned to face laterally. This motion includes pronation, abduction, and dorsiflexion. *NOTE:* Problems exist when the foot motions are divided into forefoot and hindfoot descriptions. Care must be made to record motions pertaining to that part of the foot described or to the whole foot, as the case may be. **D,** Motions of the fore part of the foot (passive motion). *1,* Inversion. The examiner carries the foot passively through the motions of active inversion. The heel must be held firmly by the examiner's hand, with the other hand turning the foot inward. *2,* Eversion. The examiner passively turns the foot outward in pronation, abduction, and slight dorsiflexion. *3,* Adduction and abduction. These passive motions are obtained by grasping the heel and moving the fore part of the foot inward or outward. This motion must take place in the plane of the sole of the foot.

Continued.

349

Table 18-2. TESTING FOR MUSCLE STRENGTH AND RANGE OF JOINT MOTION—cont'd

Movement	Muscles	Motor nerves	Positions for testing	Instructions and tests for muscle strength
Dorsiflexion	Prime mover: tibialis anterior (Fig. 95†)	Deep peroneal nerve (lumbar 4, 5; sacral 1)	Sitting, supine	"Bend your toes toward your knees." Resistance is applied to the dorsal aspect of the foot.
Internal rotation and dorsiflexion	Prime mover: tibialis posterior (Fig. 95)	Deep peroneal nerve (lumbar 5; sacral 1)	Sitting, supine	"Rotate your right [left] foot toward the left [right] foot. Turn it as far as you can." Resistance is applied to the medial aspect of the foot at the first metatarsal joint.
Plantar flexion	Prime movers (Fig. 96†) Gastrocnemius Soleus Accessory muscles Tibialis posterior Peroneus longus Peroneus brevis Flexor hallucis longus Flexor digitorum longus Plantaris	Tibial nerve (sacral 1, 2) Tibial nerve (sacral 1, 2)	Sitting, supine	"Point your toes away from you [downward] as far as you can." Resistance is applied to the ball of the foot (Fig. 97).

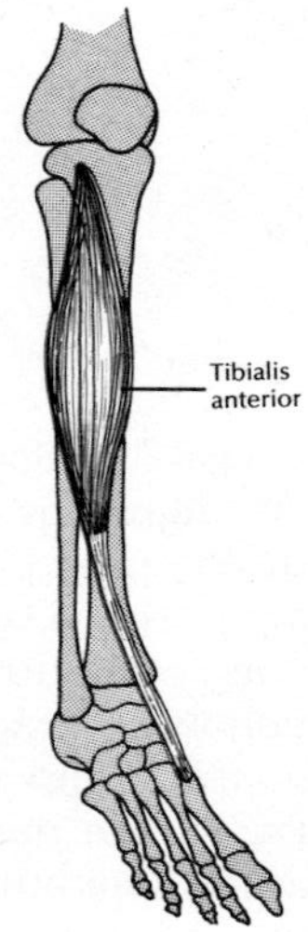

Tibialis anterior

Fig. 95

Soleus

Gastrocnemius

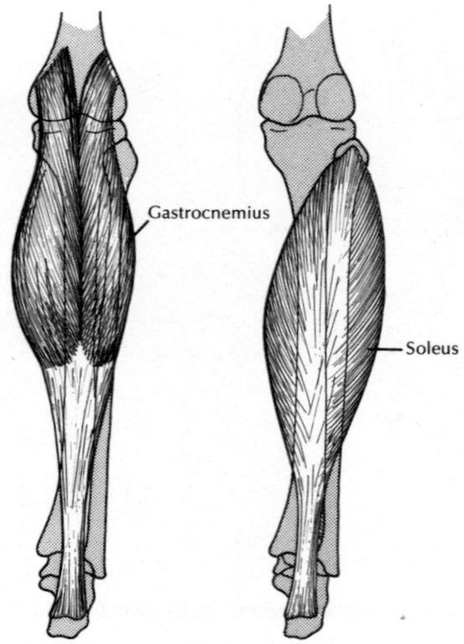

Fig. 96

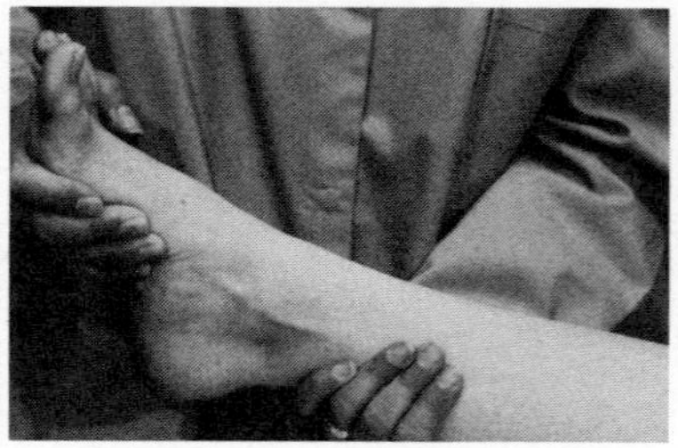

Fig. 97

FOOT

Movement	Muscles	Motor nerves	Positions for testing	Instructions and tests for muscle strength
Inversion	Prime mover: tibialis posterior (Fig. 98†) Accessory muscles Flexor digitorum longus Flexor hallucis longus Gastrocnemius (medial head)	Tibial nerve (lumbar 5, sacral 1)	Sitting, supine	"Point your toes; then rotate them inward." Resistance is applied against the medial aspect of the first metatarsal bone (Fig. 99).
Eversion	Prime movers (Fig. 100†) Peroneus longus Peroneus brevis Accessory muscles Extensor digitorum longus Peroneus tertius	Superficial peroneal nerve (lumbar 4, 5; sacral 1) Superficial peroneal nerve (lumbar 4, 5; sacral 1)	Sitting, supine	"Point your toes and rotate them outward." Resistance is applied against the lateral aspect of the fifth metatarsal bone.

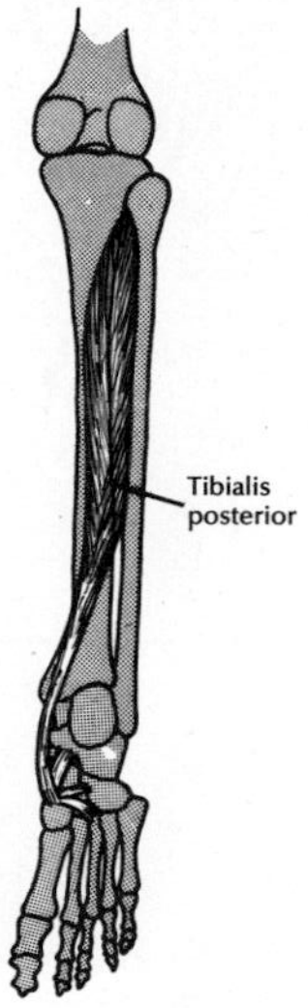

Fig. 99

Tibialis posterior

Fig. 98

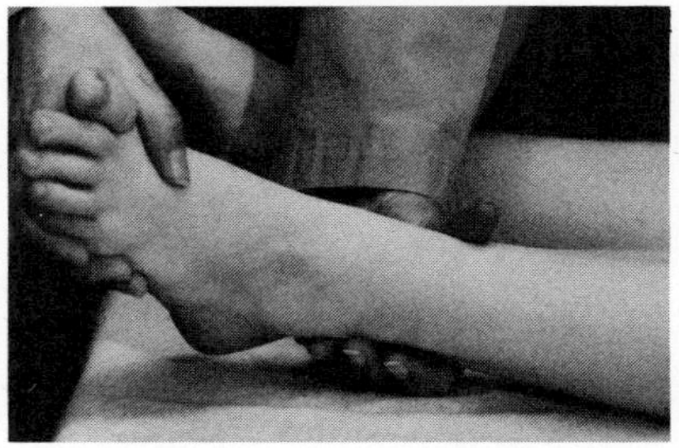

Peroneus brevis

Peroneus longus

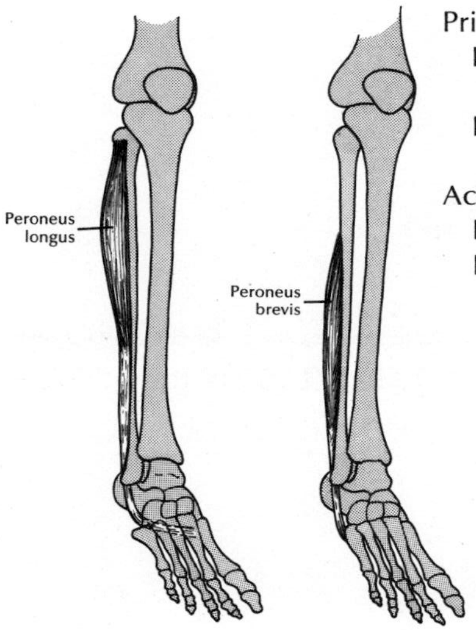

Fig. 100

Continued.

Table 18-2. TESTING FOR MUSCLE STRENGTH AND RANGE OF JOINT MOTION—cont'd

GREAT TOE

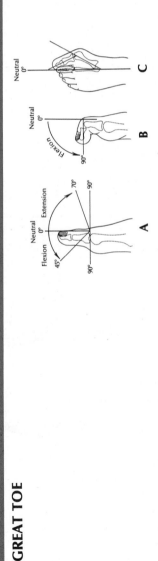

Fig. 101. Range of motion of the great toe.* **A,** Flexion and extension of the great toe. Zero starting position: the extended great toe in line with the first metatarsal bone. **B,** Flexion and extension are present at the metatarsophalangeal joint, and flexion only is present at the interphalangeal joint. **C,** The degree of deformity of the great toe in this instance, hallux valgus, may be measured in degrees of abduction of the metatarsal bone and in degrees of adduction of the proximal and distal phalanges.

Movement	Muscles	Motor nerves	Positions for testing	Instructions and tests for muscle strength
Flexion of joints Metatarsophalangeal	Prime mover: flexor hallucis brevis (Fig. 102†) Accessory muscle: flexor hallucis longus	Medial plantar nerve (lumbar 4, 5; sacral 1)	Sitting, supine	"Bend your right [left] big toe down." "Curl your toe." Resistance is applied to the plantar side of the toe (Fig. 103).

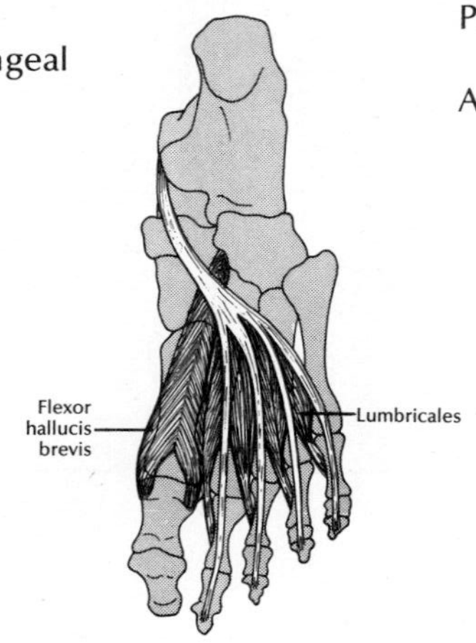

Fig. 102

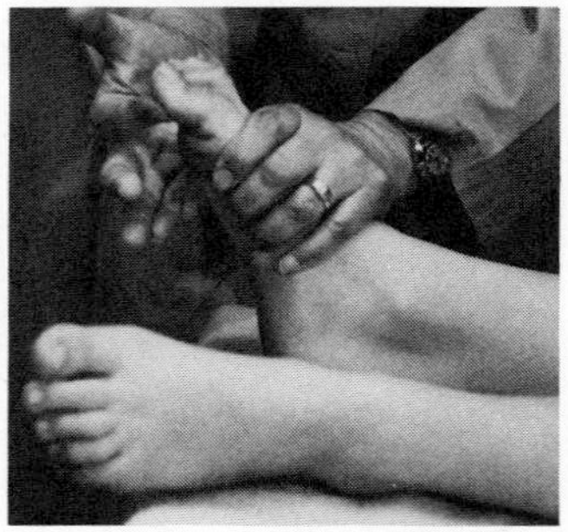

Fig. 103

Interphalangeal

Prime mover: flexor hallucis longus (Fig. 104†)

Tibial nerve (lumbar 5; sacral 1, 2)

Sitting, supine

"Bend your right [left] big toe down."
"Curl your toe."
Resistance is applied to the plantar surface of the distal phalanges.

Flexor hallucis longus

Flexor hallucis longus

Flexor digitorum brevis

Fig. 104

Extension of metatarsophalangeal joint

Prime movers (Fig. 105†)
Extensor digitorum longus

Extensor digitorum brevis

Deep peroneal nerve (lumbar 4, 5; sacral 1)
Deep peroneal nerve (lumbar 5; sacral 1)

Sitting, supine

"Bend your big toe upward."
Resistance is applied to the dorsum of the toe (Fig. 106).

Extensor digitorum longus

Extensor hallucis longus

Extensor digitorum brevis

Fig. 105

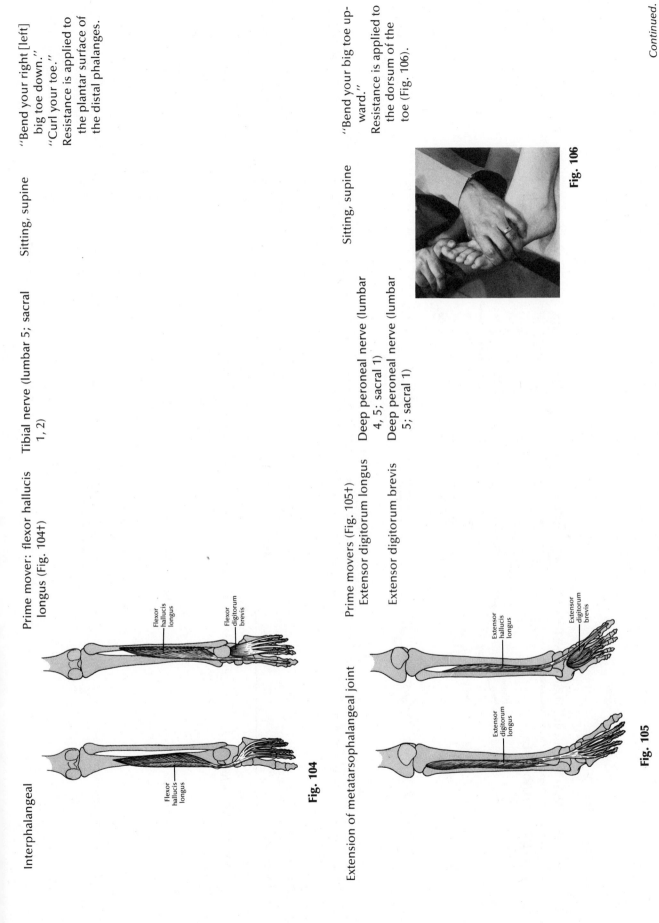

Fig. 106

Continued.

Table 18-2. TESTING FOR MUSCLE STRENGTH AND RANGE OF JOINT MOTION—cont'd

LATERAL FOUR TOES

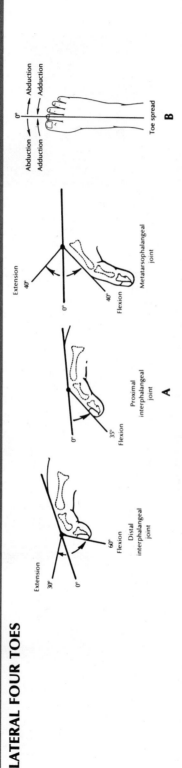

Fig. 107. Range of motion of the lateral four toes.* **A,** Second to fifth toes. Motion in flexion is present in the distal, middle, and proximal joints of the toes. Extension is present at the metatarsophalangeal joint. These motions can be simply expressed in degrees. **B,** Abduction and adduction (toe spread). This can be measured in relation to the second toe, which is the midline axis of the foot.

Movement	Muscles	Motor nerves	Positions for testing	Instructions and tests for muscle strength
Flexion of toe joints Metatarsophalangeal	Prime mover: lumbricales (Fig. 102)	Medial plantar nerve (lumbar 4, 5) Lateral plantar nerve (sacral 1, 2)	Sitting, supine	"Bend all your toes downward." Resistance is applied to the plantar surface of the proximal phalanges.
	Accessory muscles Dorsal and plantar interossei Flexor digiti quinti brevis Flexor digitorum longus Flexor digitorum brevis			
Proximal interphalangeal	Prime mover: flexor digitorum brevis (Fig. 104)	Medial plantar nerve (lumbar 4, 5)	Sitting, supine	"Bend your toes downward." Resistance is applied to the plantar surface of the medial phalanges.

Distal interphalangeal

Prime mover: flexor digi-
torum longus (Fig. 104)

Tibial nerve (lumbar 5, sacral 1)

Sitting, supine

"Bend your toes
downward."
Pressure is applied to
the plantar surface
of the distal pha-
langes (Fig. 108).

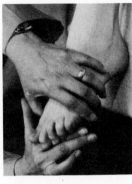

Fig. 108

Extension of metatarsophalangeal joint

Prime movers (Fig. 105)
Extensor digitorum longus

Extensor digitorum brevis

Deep peroneal nerve (lumbar
4, 5; sacral 1)

Deep peroneal nerve (lumbar
5; sacral 1)

Sitting, supine

"Straighten out your
toes. Point your toes
upward."
Resistance is applied to
the dorsum of the
proximal phalanges.

■ Recording of data

The following chart provides a listing of clinically testable muscles.* Although the methodical recording of data for each muscle is painstaking, it serves as a baseline for subsequent changes and does indicate that the muscle was actually tested.

■ Special tests of musculoskeletal function

Although the following tests are described separately, they may be incorporated into the systematic evaluation of the client, which progresses in a cephalocaudal direction.

Range of motion	Tone	Fasciculation	Strength				Range of motion	Tone	Fasciculation	Strength
					Face:					
				Neck:	Flexor	Sternocleidomastoid				
					Extensor group					
				Trunk:	Flexor	Rectus abdominis				

					Rotators
					  Right oblique internal abductor
					  Left oblique internal abductor
					  Left oblique external abductor
					  Right oblique external abductor					

					Extensors	Thoracic group Lumbar group				
					Pelvic elevator	Quadratus lumbar				
				Scapula:	Abductor	Serratus anterior				
					Elevator	Trapezius (superior)				
					Depressor	Trapezius (inferior)				
					Adductors	Trapezius (middle) Rhomboid major and minor				
				Shoulder:	Flexor	Deltoid (anterior)				
					Extensors	Latissimus dorsi Teres major				
					Abductor (to 90°)	Deltoid (middle)				
					Horizontal abductor	Deltoid (posterior)				
					Horizontal adductor	Pectoralis major				

					Rotators
					  Lateral rotator group
					  Medial rotator group					

				Elbow:	Flexors	Biceps brachii Brachialis				
					Extensor	Triceps brachii				

*Adapted from Daniels, L., and Worthingham, C.: Muscle testing; techniques of manual examination, ed. 3, Philadelphia, 1972, W. B. Saunders Co.

Range of motion	Tone	Fasciculation	Strength				Range of motion	Tone	Fasciculation	Strength
				Forearm:	Extensors Supinator group					
					Pronator group					
				Wrist:	Flexors	Flex. carpi radialis Flex. carpi ulnaris				
					Extensors	Ext. carpi rad. longus and brevis Ext. carpi ulnaris				
				Fingers:	MP flexors	Lumbricales				
					IP flexors (first)	Flex. digit. superficialis				
					IP flexors (second)	Flex. digit. profundus				
					MP extensors	Ext. digit. communis				
					Adductors	Interossei palmates Interossei dorsales				
					Abductors	Abductor digit minimi Opponens digit minimi				
				Thumb:	MP flexor	Flex. poll. brevis				
					IP flexor	Flex. poll. longus				
					MP extensor	Ext. poll. brevis				
					IP extensor	Ext. poll. longus				
					Abductors	Abd. poll. brevis Abd. poll. longus				
					Adductors	Adductor pollicis Opponens pollicis				
				Hip:	Flexor	Iliopsoas				
					Extensor	Gluteus maximus				
					Abductor	Gluteus medius				
					Adductor group					
					Rotators Lateral rotator group Medial rotator group					
				Knee:	Flexors	Biceps femoris Inner hamstrings				
					Extensor	Quadriceps femoris				
				Ankle:	Plantar flexors	Gastrocnemius Soleus				

Continued.

357

Range of motion	Tone	Fasciculation	Strength				Range of motion	Tone	Fasciculation	Strength
				Foot:	Invertors	Tibialis anterior Tibialis posterior				
					Evertors	Peroneus brevis Peroneus longus				
				Toes:	MP flexors	Lumbricales				
					IP flexors (first)	Flex. digit. brevis				
					IP flexors (second)	Flex. digit. longus				
					MP extensors	Ext. digit. longus Ext. digit. brevis				
				Hallux:	MP flexor	Flex. hall. brevis				
					IP flexor	Flex. hall. longus				
					MP extensor	Ext. hall. brevis				
					IP extensor	Ext. hall. longus				

Gait:

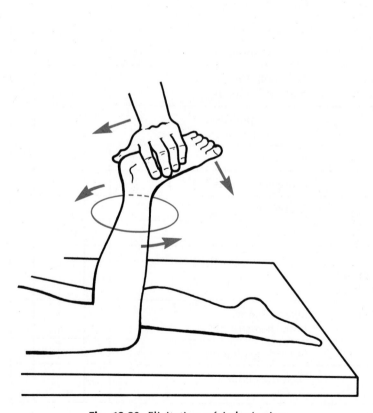

Fig. 18-20. Elicitation of Apley's sign.

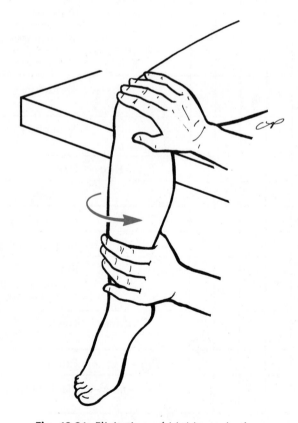

Fig. 18-21. Elicitation of McMurray's sign.

Tests for a foreign body in the knee

Apley's sign. An attempt is made to elicit Apley's sign (Fig. 18-20) in the client who is suspected of having a loose object in the knee joint or who has given a history of knee joint locking. The client assumes the prone position with the suspected knee flexed to 90°. The tibia is firmly opposed to the femur by exerting downward pressure on the foot. The leg is rotated externally and internally. Locking of the knee (positive sign) or the sound of clicks may indicate that a loose body, such as torn cartilage, is trapped in the articulation. Clicks or popping sounds are generated as the object escapes.

McMurray's sign. An attempt is made to elicit McMurray's sign (Fig. 18-21) in the individual who says he "feels something in the knee joint" or complains that "sometimes it just won't bend." The test may be performed with the client in the sitting position and while obtaining as much flexion of the suspected knee as possible. The leg is internally rotated while it is slowly being extended with one hand. The other hand is used to provide resistance at the medial aspect of the knee. Extension of the knee may not be possible (positive sign) if a loose body impedes its movement. The procedure may be repeated employing external rotation and resistance applied to the lateral aspect of the knee.

Straight leg–raising test. The straight leg–raising test (Fig. 18-22) is useful in defining herniated lumbar disc as the cause of sciatic nerve pain. The test is indicated for those individuals who complain of low back pain or of pain that radiates down the leg. The test is performed with the client lying on his back on a firm surface. The extended leg is raised until the client complains of pain. The foot is then dorsiflexed. Pain induced in this manner is caused by pressure on the dorsal roots of the lumbosacral nerves and is characteristic of herniated disc.

In flexion of the hip in the normal individual, the lumbar spine is not flexed. The individual with an immobile hip demonstrates flexion of the lumbar spine when the leg is raised.

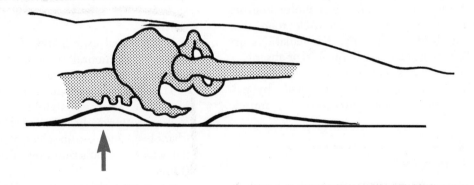

Fig. 18-22. Straight leg–raising test.

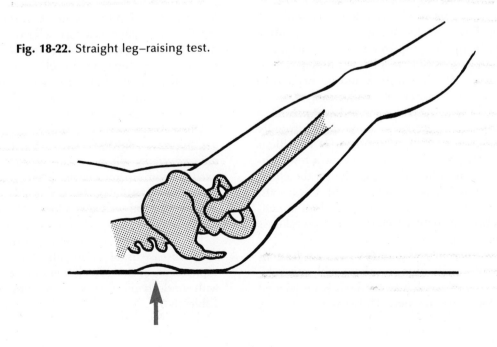

DISTINCTION BETWEEN UPPER AND LOWER MOTOR NEURON INVOLVEMENT

A concept of clinical importance in the examination of the musculoskeletal system is the distinction between upper and lower motor neuron involvement. The cells of the upper motor neurons are in the cortex and terminate in the brainstem (corticobulbar) tract or cross over in the anterior gray horn of the medulla and end in the spinal cord (corticospinal tract). The corticobulbar fibers terminate in cranial nerve nuclei.

The corticospinal axons passing through the medullary pyramids are known as the pyramidal tracts. The lower motor neurons include the cranial nerve nuclei and their axons as well as anterior horn cells of the cord and their axons.

Lesions of the upper motor neuron produce a spasticity or hypertonicity of the affected muscles, and muscle strength is diminished. Tendon stretch reflexes are brisk and Babinski's sign is present if the lesion is in the corticospinal tract. Atrophy occurs only with disuse of the muscles. By contrast, lesions of the lower motor neurons produce flaccidity or loss of muscle tone. The hypotonus leads to atrophy. Fasciculations are seen. Tendon reflexes are depressed or absent.

The distinctions between the two types of nerve involvement can often be made by palpation of the muscle and tests for muscle strength.

MUSCLE WEAKNESS

The client who has difficulty in getting up from the sitting position, who is able to rise only by pushing off with his hands and arms or by pulling himself up by grasping some nearby furniture, may have a problem involving the hip girdle musculature. Further tests would be needed to ascertain the presence of muscular dystrophy, myasthenia gravis, parkinsonism, or polymyositis. Myasthenia gravis may be more strongly suspected if the following are true: (1) The client is instructed to sit back and relax for a few minutes, after which he can rise easily; (2) the client is a woman in her 20s or a man in his 50s or 60s; (3) muscle atrophy is not present; and (4) the client has a ptosis or extraocular muscle weakness resulting in diplopia.

The presence of myasthenia gravis may be conclusively determined in the client with ptosis by the use of the Tensilon test, which is performed in the following manner. The examiner injects

edrophonium (Tensilon) chloride 2 mg while watching the client's eyelids. If there is no change after a minute, the examiner injects another 8 mg. In 90% of clients who have myasthenia gravis the ptosis is markedly improved as muscle strength increases following the injection.

The client who has polymyositis may have pain, muscle atrophy, or a rash, particularly around the eyelids, as well as a low-grade fever.

Parkinsonism may be the underlying cause when the aging client has difficulty rising from a chair. This impression may be substantiated if the client gives stiffness as one of his problems. The examiner should be alert in this case for signs of flexion posture, slow and intermittent movement, frequent tremor, masked facies, or movement of several joint units at one time; since these signs are also characteristic of the victim of Parkinson's disease.

Viral, upper respiratory tract infections may be suspected in the individual who has a mild elevation in temperature and whose chief complaint revealed that he had no symptoms only a day or so before but now feels weak, almost unable to move.

If the initial examination fails to demonstrate muscular or neural disease, the possibility of fatigue should be entertained.

The client who complains of intermittent bouts of muscle weakness should be investigated for ischemic attacks, disorders of glucose metabolism (diabetes), and serum electrolyte disturbances, particularly of potassium or calcium ion concentrations.

Transient ischemic attacks (TIAs) may cause a focal episode of motor dysfunction related to vascular disease, such as arteriosclerosis or essential hypertension. It is particularly important to listen for bruits over the neck vessels in the elderly client with muscle weakness, since these bruits might strengthen the impressions of vascular disease.

Clinical correlation of signs of muscle weakness and disease entities have shown that each neuromuscular disease has a predilection for a particular group of muscles. A given pattern of weakness, then, intimates the possibility of a certain disease and excludes others. An example lies in the adage that peripheral muscle involvement in the extremities is of muscular origin, whereas distal disease is of neuropathic origin. Further explanation of the correlation of assessment data with underlying disease processes appears in Table 18-3.

Table 18-3. Topographical patterns of muscle palsy

Muscle weakness of paralysis	Signs	Possible etiology
Ocular	Diplopia Ptosis Strabismus	Myasthenia gravis Thyroid disease Ocular dystrophy and botulism
Bifacial	Inability to smile Inability to expose teeth Inability to close eyes	Myasthenia gravis Facioscapulohumeral dystrophy Guillain-Barré syndrome
Bulbar	Dysphonia Dysarthnia Dysphagia Hanging jaw facial weakness (may or may not be present)	Myasthenia gravis Myotonic dystrophy Botulism Diphtheria Poliomyelitis Early polymyositis
Cervical	Inability to lift head from pillow (hanging head syndrome) Weakness of posterior neck muscles	Polymyositis Dermatomyositis Progressive muscular dystrophy
Bibrachial	Weakness, atrophy, and fasciculations of hands, arms, and shoulders (hanging arm syndrome)	Amyotrophic lateral sclerosis
Bicrural	Lower leg weakness Floppy feet Inability to walk on heels and toes	Diabetic polyneuropathy
Limb-girdle	Inability to raise arms Inability to rise from sitting position Difficulty in climbing stairs without use of arms Waddling gait	Polymyositis Dermatomyositis Progressive muscular dystrophy
Distal limb	Foot drop with steppage gain Weakness of all leg muscles Wrist drop—weakness of handgrips ("claw hand") (later sign)	Familial polyneuropathy
Generalized or universal	Limb and cranial muscle weakness (acute in onset and periodic) Slow onset and progressive paralysis Atrophy Fasciculations of limb and trunk muscles No sensory loss Paralysis developing over several days Mild degree of generalized weakness	Electrolyte imbalance Hypokalemia Hypocalcemia Hypomagnesemia Motor system disease Guillian-Barré syndrome Glycogen storage diseases Vitamin D deficiency
Single muscles or groups of muscles	Inability to contract affected muscles	Thyrotoxic myopathy (almost always neuropathic)

■ Hypokalemia

Since the ratio of the concentrations of potassium ion of the intracellular milieu to the extracellular fluid determines the rate of cell firing, a deficit of this ion is accompanied by disorders of structure and function in muscular and neural tissues. Both skeletal and smooth muscles are affected by hypokalemia. The client complains of varying degrees of weakness and lassitude. Extreme hypokalemia may be accompanied by muscular paralysis. Some other signs that will help to confirm the cause of muscle weakness as due to hypokalemia are abnormalities in motor and secretory activities of the gastrointestinal tract, changes in electrocardiograms, and dilute urine. Some of the conditions known to be correlated with a deficiency of this ion are diarrhea, excessive losses in the urine due to the use of chlorothiazide or mercurial diuretics or steroid hormones; Cushing's syndrome; and primary aldosteronism.

■ Age-related muscle weakness

Wasting of muscles and a decrease in muscle strength has been traditionally attributed to the aging process. Histologically, the muscle tissue shows increased amounts of collagen initially, followed by fibrosis of connective tissue.

INVOLUNTARY CONTRACTION OF SKELETAL MUSCLES
■ Fasciculations

Fasciculations are the visible, spontaneous contraction of a number of muscle fibers supplied by a single motor nerve filament. Visible dimpling or twitching may be seen, although there is usually insufficient power generated to move the joint.

Twitching. Fasciculations during muscular contraction occur in conditions of irritability that result in poorly coordinated contraction of small and large motor units. Benign fasciculation occurs in the normal individual and is characterized by normal muscle strength and size. Rarely, myokymia, a rippling appearance of the muscle occasioned by numerous fasciculations, is noted in a normal individual.

Fascicular twitches that occur during rest in a client with exaggerated muscular weakness and atrophy are characteristic of a peripheral motor neuron disorder. Generalized fasicular twitching occurring in a progressive, wavelike pattern over an entire muscle and progressing to complete paralysis is characteristic of certain types of poisoning (organic phosphate) and of poliomyelitis.

■ Cramps, spasm

Muscular spasm may occur at rest or with movement and may occur in the normal individual with metabolic and electrolyte alterations. Cramping is commonly noted following excessive sweating and with hyponatremia, hypocalcemia, hypomagnesemia, and hyperuricemia. Diseases that magnify these alterations are correlated with the presence of muscle spasm. A continuous spasm that is heightened by attempts to move the affected muscles is seen in tetanus and following the bite of the black widow spider.

Paravertebral muscle spasm is often responsible for low back pain.

Table 18-4. Tremor classification

Etiology	Type and rate of movement	Description
Anxiety	Fine, rapid, 10 to 12 per second	Irregular, variable
		Increased by attempts to move part; decreased by relaxation of part
Parkinsonism	Fine, regular, or coarse, 2 to 5 per second	Occurs at rest
		May be inhibited by movement
		Involves flexion of finger and thumb "pill rolling"
		Accompanied by rigidity, "cogwheel" phenomena, bradykinesia
Cerebellar tremor	Variable rate	Evident only on movement (most prominent on finger-to-nose test)
		Dysmetria (seen when client is asked to pat rapidly—pats are of unequal force and do not all arrive at same point)
Essential or senile	Coarse, 3 to 7 per second	Involves the jaw, sometimes the tongue, and sometimes the entire head
Metabolic		Disappears on complete relaxation or in response to alcohol
		Variable
		Client is obviously ill; if illness is due to hepatic failure, client will have other signs, such as palpable liver, spider nevi

Tetany. Hypocalcemia, as well as hypomagnesemia, may cause the involuntary spasms of skeletal muscle that resemble cramping. The calcium deficit causes depolarization of the distal segments of the motor nerve; furthermore, there is a change within the muscle fibers themselves since nerve section or block does not prevent these tetanic contractions. Tetanic cramps can be elicited by percussing the motor nerve leading to a muscle group at frequencies of 15 to 20 per second. Chvostek's sign is the spasm of the facial muscles produced by tapping over the facial nerve near its foramen of exit. The instability of the neuromuscular unit is heightened by hyperventilation (alkalosis) and hypoxia (ischemia). Trousseau's sign is the production of tetany of the carpal muscles following occlusion of the blood supply to the arms by a tourniquet. The client may also describe tingling and prickling paresthesia due to the stimulation of sensory nerve fibers. Electromyographic tracings show fast-frequency doublets and triplets of motor unit potentials. Tetany in its mildest form affects the distal musculature in the form of carpopedal spasm but may involve all the muscles of the body except those of the eye.

Muscle cramp. Muscle cramp frequently occurs after a day of vigorous exercise. As the feet cool, a sudden movement may trigger a strong contraction of the foot and leg. The musculature is visible, and the muscle is hard to palpation. The spasm will cease in response to stretch of the fibers. In the case of the gastrocnemius muscle, the stretch can be achieved by dorsiflexion of the foot. Occasionally massage is helpful in relaxing the spasm. Fasciculations may frequently be observed before and after the cramp and are further evidence of the hyperexcitability of the neuromuscular unit. Electromyogram recordings show high-frequency action potentials during the cramp. These muscle spasms have greater frequency when the client is dehydrated or sweating and in the pregnant client.

The cause of the pain associated with muscle cramp has not been determined but is thought by some to be due to the increased metabolic needs of the hyperactive muscles and to the collection of the metabolic waste products such as lactic acid within the muscle.

MUSCLE ENZYME LEVELS

Destructive diseases of striated muscle fibers result in the loss of enzymes from the intracellular compartment of the muscle. The enzymes enter the blood and can be measured. The usual laboratory analysis of serum enzymes includes alkaline phosphatase (alk. phos.), lactic dehydrogenase (LDH), serum glutamic oxaloacetic transaminase (SGOT), and creatine phosphokinase (CPK). Enzymes are found in all tissues. Since high concentrations of these enzymes are found in the heart and liver, elevated serum level values may be due to myocardial infarction or hepatitis. However, CPK, though present in the heart and brain, is most concentrated in the striated muscle. The level may rise from a normal level of 0 to 65 international units (IU) to more than 1,000 IU in clients with destructive lesions of the striated muscles.

MYALGIA

"I hurt all over" is frequently the chief complaint for the diffuse muscle pain that accompanies many types of systemic infection, for example, influenza, measles, rheumatic fever, brucellosis, dengue fever, or salmonellosis. Soreness and aching are other descriptive terms for this type of involvement. Little is known of the cause. Fibromyositis (myogelosis) is the term used to describe the inflammation of the fibrous tissue in muscle, fascia, and nerves. The client may complain of pain and tenderness in a muscle after exposure to cold, dampness, or minor trauma.

Firm, tender zones occasionally several centimeters in diameter are found on palpation. Palpation, active contraction, or passive stretching increases the pain. Intense pain localized to a smaller group of muscles may be due to epidemic myalgia, also called pleurodynia, "painful neck," or "devil's grip." Intense pain at the beginning of neurological involvement has been seen in poliomyelitis and herpes zoster.

The pain of poliomyelitis is described as marked during the initial involvement of the nerve, whereas the later sensation of the paralyzed muscle is said to be one of aching. The segmental pattern of the intense pain of herpes zoster is caused by the inflammation of spinal nerves and dorsal root ganglia that occurs 3 to 4 days prior to the skin eruption.

The initial symptoms of rheumatoid arthritis may be diffuse muscular soreness and aching, which may antedate the joint involvement by weeks or months. The muscles are tender, and the client describes the pain as occurring not at the time of activity but hours later. An increased sedimentation rate or a positive latex fixation test may support the conclusion of rheumatoid involvement.

ELECTROMYOGRAPHY

The electromyogram is the graph generated from the electrical potential of individual muscles. The test is accomplished by inserting needles directly into the muscle being studied and recording the potential with the muscle at rest, with slight voluntary contractions, and at maximal flexion. Whereas the heart can be sampled from a number of surface electrode positions, the skeletal muscles are variable in size, widely separated, and numerous. Therefore, no small number of leads can give an adequate picture of their activity. Furthermore, surface electrodes yield only a summation of the underlying activity. To ascertain the bursts of individual muscle units, sterile needle electrodes must be used to register the activity.

Thus, the electromyogram must be done for one muscle at a time. Information obtained from the tracing is useful in determining neural adequacy of the muscle and the presence of intrinsic muscle disease.

MUSCLE BIOPSY

Muscle biopsy was first used by Cachenne in 1868. Currently the use of muscle biopsy is felt to be indicated for five clinical problems: (1) atrophy of the muscle that is progressive (when doubt exists as to whether the disease is myogenic or neurogenic); (2) localized inflammatory disease of the muscle wherein biopsy may contribute to isolating the causative agent, thus allowing institution of the appropriate therapeutic regimen; (3) certain metabolic diseases wherein the histological or biological data, or both, thus provided may help to identify the disease; (4) fever associated with many visceral and cutaneous lesions wherein biopsy of the muscle may reveal further connective tissue and vascular involvement to support the conclusions of a generalized involvement; and (5) trauma wherein the biopsy may further define the degree of nerve and muscle injury.

ASSESSMENT OF GAIT

Gait is evaluated in both phases, the stance and the swing, for rhythm and smoothness. *Stance* is considered to consist of three processes: (1) heel strike—the heel contacts the floor or ground; (2)

midstance—body weight is transferred from the heel to the ball of the foot; and (3) push-off—the heel leaves the ground.

The *swing* phase also consists of three processes: (1) acceleration; (2) swing through—the lifted foot travels ahead of the weight-bearing foot; and (3) deceleration—the foot slows in preparation for heel strike.

The description of the observation of the client's gait should include: *phase* (conformity); *cadence* (symmetry, regular rhythm); *stride length* (symmetry, length of swing); *trunk posture* (related to phases); *pelvic posture* (related to phases); and *arm swing* (symmetry, length of swing).

If pain is present, it should be described in relationship to the phases of gait.

EXAMINATION OF THE BONE AND JOINTS
■ Bone

The bone is examined for deformity or tumors. The bone is also examined for integrity by testing its resistance to a deforming force. Palpation of the bone is performed to assess the presence of pain or tenderness. Tenderness of a bone may indicate tumor, inflammation, or the aftermath of a trauma. Frequently, traumatic injuries are associated with damage to both bone and nerve. Paralysis of the ulnar and median nerve in the hand is frequently the result of a hand injury and may result in a clawlike posture of the hand.

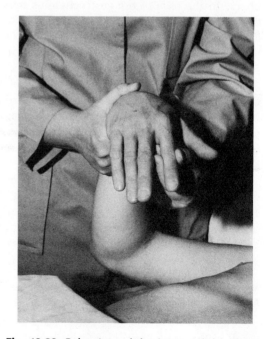

Fig. 18-23. Palpation of the joints of the finger.

■ Joints

Joints are inspected for gross deformity and swelling. The joint is palpated for crepitus, masses, and tenderness. The ranges of both active and passive motion are determined. This may be assessed during the muscle examination.

While determining the extent of joint motion, the examiner should ascertain the presence of any muscle spasm by palpation and carefully listen for crepitus.

The medial and lateral aspects of each interphalangeal joint are palpated with the thumb and index finger for bogginess, swelling, tenderness, or neoplasm.

The thumbs are used to palpate the metacarpophalangeal joints and the wrists (Fig. 18-23.)

The elbow is examined with the elbow flexed. The tissues of the joint are palpated between the thumb and the index finger (Fig. 18-24).

The joints of the foot are examined between the thumb and the index finger for bogginess, swelling, and tenderness.

The suprapatellar pouch is a part of the knee joint that is not surrounded by bones, ligaments, or tendons. Thus, joint effusion may be most readily palpated in the region superior to the patella (Fig. 18-25). Manual pressure is exerted over the dorsal aspect of the leg just superior to the patellar pouch in order to displace fluid into the space behind the patella (Fig. 18-26). A milking movement to the tissue immediately below the knee may also be effective. Ballottement of the patella may be performed when joint effusion is present. Since the fluid pushes the patella away from the femur, when the patella is tapped, a click is heard over the region as it strikes the femur.

Inflammation of joints. A red, swollen, warm, and painful area around a joint suggests the classic picture of inflammation. A red and swollen area around a joint suggests acute synovitis such as rheumatoid arthritis, gouty arthritis, or infectious arthritis. Swelling alone may indicate fluid or a thickened synovial membrane.

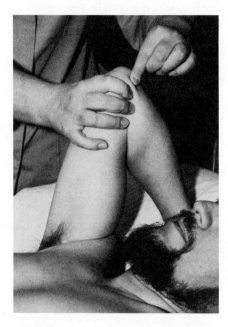

Fig. 18-24. Palpation of the extensor surface of the elbow.

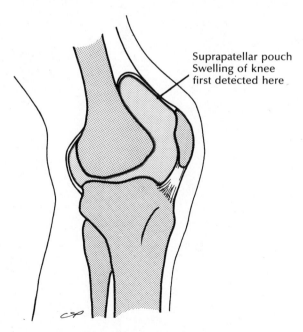

Suprapatellar pouch
Swelling of knee
first detected here

Fig. 18-25. Knee effusion.

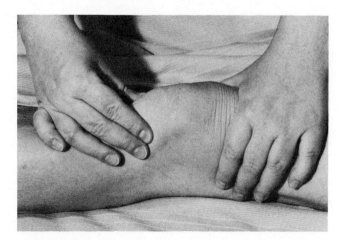

Fig. 18-26. Examination of the knee joint for effusion.

BIBLIOGRAPHY

Adams, R.: Diseases of the muscle, New York, 1975, Harper and Row, Publishers.

Beetham, W., Polley, H., Slocumb, C., and others: Physical examination of the joints, Philadelphia, 1965, W. B. Saunders Co.

Daniels, L., and Worthingham, C.: Muscle testing; techniques of manual examination, ed. 3, Philadelphia, 1972, W. B. Saunders Co.

Enneking, W. F., and Sherrard, M. G.: Physical diagnosis of the musculoskeletal system, Gainesville, Fla., 1969, Storter Printing Co., Inc.

Goodgold, J., and Eberstein, A.: Electrodiagnosis of neuromuscular diseases, Baltimore, 1972, The Williams and & Wilkins Co.

Joint motion; method of measuring and recording, Chicago, 1965, American Academy of Orthopaedic Surgeons.

Knapp, M. E.: Electromyography, Postgrad. Med. 47:213, 1970.

Layzer, R. B., and Rowland, L. P.: Cramps, N. Engl. J. Med. 285:31, 1971.

Moosa, A.: Paediatric electrodiagnosis, Arch. Dis. Child 46(6):149, 1972.

Rosse, C., and Clawson, D.: Introduction to the musculoskeletal system, New York, 1970, Harper and Row, Publishers.

Walton, J. N.: Disorders of voluntary muscle, ed. 3, Baltimore, 1974, The Williams & Wilkins Co.

Yates, D. A.: The electrodiagnosis of muscle disorders, Proc. R. Soc. Med. 65:617, 1972.

19 Assessment of the skin

The skin is an organ system readily accessible to examination. As a membrane barrier between the individual and his external environment, the skin responds to changes in the external environment and also reflects changes in the internal environment. A careful examination of the skin may yield valuable information about the client and his general health, which is reflected by the condition of the skin, as well as specific information that will aid in the identification of a systemic disease or a specific problem of the skin. It is important to describe the skin of the healthy client, as well as the skin of the client with a health problem, paying special attention to any deviation from normal.

The examination of the skin requires some understanding of the structure and function of the system and familiarity with the appearance of the skin, hair, nails, and mucous membranes in health and disease. This chapter includes a brief discussion of the anatomy and function of the skin, methods for conducting a systematic examination of the skin and appendages, and an approach to the description and classification of skin lesions.

ANATOMY AND FUNCTION

The skin has many important functions, including (1) assistance in maintaining an internal environment by providing a barrier to loss of water and electrolytes, (2) protection from external agents injurious to the internal environment, (3) regulation of body heat, and (4) function as a sense organ for touch, temperature, and pain.

The skin is divided into three layers: the epidermis, the dermis, and the subcutaneous tissues (Fig. 19-1).

The epidermis is an avascular, cornified, cellular structure. It is stratified into several layers and is composed chiefly of keratinocytes, cells that produce keratin. Keratin makes up much of the horny material in the outermost epidermal layer of dead cells and is the principal constituent of the harder, keratinized structures of nails and hair. The innermost layer of the epidermis contains melanocytes, the source of melanin, the pigment that gives color to the skin and hair.

Epidermal appendages include the hair, nails, eccrine sweat glands, apocrine sweat glands, and sebaceous glands. These are formed by invagination of the epidermis into the underlying dermis. The hair and nails are keratinized appendages and have no significant function in man. The eccrine, sebaceous, and apocrine appendages are glandular. The sebaceous glands usually arise from the hair follicles and produce sebum, which has a lubricating effect on the horny outer layer of the epidermis. The eccrine sweat glands are widely distributed and have an important function in the dissipation of body heat as sweat is produced and evaporated. The apocrine sweat glands are found in the axillary and genital areas and usually open into the hair follicles. The sweat produced by the apocrine glands decomposes when contaminated by bacteria, resulting in the characteristic body odor.

The dermis underlying the epidermis constitutes the bulk of the skin. It is a tough connective tissue that contains lymphatics and nerves and is highly vascular. It supports and nourishes the epidermis.

The subcutaneous layer beneath the dermis is distinguished by the storage of fat and is important in temperature insulation.

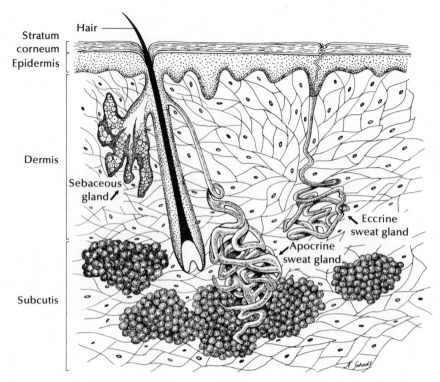

Fig. 19-1. Anatomy of the skin and its appendages. (From Prior, J. A., and Silberstein, J. S.: Physical diagnosis; the history and examination of the patient, ed. 5, St. Louis, 1977, The C. V. Mosby Co.)

EXAMINATION

The examination of the skin and appendages begins with a general inspection, which is followed by a detailed examination including palpation. A good source of illumination is necessary; indirect natural daylight is preferred.

■ Inspection

The examination may begin with an observation of the entire integument with the client disrobed; or a more simple approach may be taken: the skin that is exposed may be surveyed, followed by inspection of the skin, mucous membranes, and epidermal appendages of each body part as it is examined. Comparison of symmetrical anatomical areas is made throughout the examination.

The skin is inspected for color and vascularity and for evidence of perspiration, edema, injuries, or skin lesions. During the examination the practitioner should think about the underlying structures, the thinness of the skin, and the particular kind of exposure of a body part. It is also helpful to note those changes in the skin that are indicative of past injuries and habits by observing for calluses, stains, scars, needle marks, and insect bites and to note the grooming of the hair and nails.

Skin color varies from person to person and from one part of the body to another but is normally a whitish pink or a brown shade, depending on race. The exposed areas of the body, including the face, ears, back of the neck, and backs of the hands and arms, are noticeably different and may be more damaged after long exposure to the sun and weather. The vascular flush areas are the cheeks, the bridge of the nose, the neck, the upper chest, the flexor surfaces of the extremities, and the genital area. These areas may be involved in a vascular disturbance or may demonstrate increased color due to blushing or temperature elevation. They should be compared with areas of less vascularity. The pigment labile areas are the face, the backs of the hands, the flexors of the wrists, the axillae, the mammary areolae, the midline of the abdomen, and the genital area. These areas may demonstrate normal systemic pigmentary changes, such as occur during pregnancy.

There are other changes in skin color that

should be noted as evidence of systemic disease. Cyanosis, a dusky blue color, may be observed in the nailbeds and in the lips and the mouth area. It results from lowered hemoglobin levels, or decreased oxygenation of the blood, and can be caused by pulmonary or heart disease or by abnormalities of hemoglobin or occur as a result of cold. The yellow or greenish hue of jaundice occurs when tissue bilirubin is increased and may be noted first in the sclerae and then in the mucous membranes and the skin. Pallor, or decreased color in the skin, results from decreased blood flow to the superficial vessels or from decreased amounts of hemoglobin in the blood and is most evident in the face, conjunctiva, mouth, and nails. Localized changes in color may indicate specific skin lesions or a problem such as edema, which tends to blanch skin color.

■ Palpation

Palpation of the skin is used to amplify the findings observed on inspection and is usually carried out simultaneously as each body part is examined. Changes in temperature, moisture, texture, and turgor are detected by palpation.

Temperature of the skin is increased when blood flow through the dermis is increased. Localized areas of skin hyperthermia are noted in the presence of a burn or localized infection. Generalized skin hyperthermia involving all of the integument may occur when there is fever associated with a localized or systemic disease. Temperature of the skin is reduced when there is a decrease in blood flow in the dermis. Generalized skin hypothermia occurs when the client is in shock, whereas localized hypothermia occurs in conditions such as arteriosclerosis.

The moisture found on the skin will vary from one body area to another. It is normal to find the soles of the feet, the palms of the hands, and the intertriginous areas—where two surfaces are close together—containing more moisture than other parts. The amount of moisture found over the entire integument also varies with changes in the environmental temperature, with muscular activity, and with the body temperature. The skin functions in the regulation of body temperature and produces perspiration that evaporates and cools the body when the temperature is increased. The skin is normally drier during the winter months, when environmental temperatures and humidity are decreased, and with the increase in age of the individual. Abnormal dryness of the skin occurs with dehydration; the skin will feel dry even when the temperature is in-

creased. Dryness of the skin is also found in conditions such as myxedema and chronic nephritis.

Texture refers to the fineness or coarseness of the skin, and changes may indicate local irritation or trauma to defined skin areas or may be associated with problems of other systems. The skin becomes soft and smooth in hyperthyroidism and rough and dry in hypothyroidism.

Turgor refers to the elasticity of the skin and is most easily determined by picking up a fold of skin over the abdomen and observing how quickly it returns to its normal shape. There is a loss of turgor associated with dehydration, and the skin demonstrates a laxness and loss of normal mobility. It returns into place slowly. Loss of turgor is associated with aging; the skin becomes wrinkled and lax. Increased turgor is associated with an increase in tension, which causes the skin to return into place quickly.

■ Examination of appendages

The epidermal appendages, including the hair, nails, and sebaceous glands, are structures of the skin that demonstrate characteristics associated with health and changes associated with disease of the skin and other organ systems.

The hair over the entire body is examined to determine the distribution, quantity, and quality. There is a normal male or female hair pattern that evolves after puberty, and a deviation may be indicative of an endocrine problem. Changes in the quantity of the hair are of importance. Hirsutism, increased hair growth, is found in conditions such as Cushing's syndrome and acromegaly. Decreased hair growth or loss of hair may be

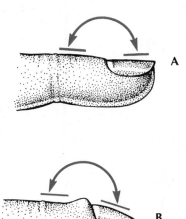

Fig. 19-2. A, Normal angle of the nail. **B,** Abnormal angle of the nail seen in late clubbing.

associated with hypopituitarism or a pyogenic infection. The quality of the hair is determined by the color and texture. Changes in color such as graying occur normally with aging, but patchy gray hair may develop following nerve injuries. Changes in texture of hair associated with hypothyroidism include dryness and coarseness, and changes associated with hyperthyroidism include increased silkiness and fineness.

The nails are examined for quantitative and qualitative changes. Quantitative changes of the nails include decreased or increased thickness, which may be hereditary or occur as a manifestation of other problems. Thickened nails may occur as the result of trauma or as a manifestation of acromegaly. Nails may become thinner in hyperthyroidism. Qualitative characteristics that should be noted in the examination of the nails include color, contour, consistency, and adherence to the nail bed. The hippocratic or clubbed nails associated with lung and heart disorders demonstrate qualitative and quantitative changes that are apparently due to prolonged anoxemia (Fig. 19-2, B). These nails demonstrate a chronic thickening and enlargement with bulbous enlargement of the ends of the fingers or toes. The nails show an exaggeration of their natural curves, and the obtuse angle between the distal portion of the digit and the nail becomes obliterated.

Pressure over the nail root gives a spongy or soft sensation.

The sebaceous glands, which are more numerous over the face and scalp areas, normally become more active during adolescence, resulting in increased oiliness of the skin. A sudden increase in the oil of the skin at other ages would not be normal and may be suggestive of an endocrine problem.

SKIN LESIONS: DESCRIPTION AND CLASSIFICATION

The initial examination of any skin lesions should be carried out at a distance of 3 or more feet in order to determine the general characteristics of the eruption. This first observation should provide the opportunity to determine the body areas affected and the configuration of the lesions. Next, a closer examination is required to determine the particular characteristics of the individual lesions. The examiner should then be able to give a concise description of a lesion or lesions in terms of the location and distribution, configuration, and morphological structure.

It is not possible to discuss the particular manifestations of the many skin problems that the examiner may find in practice. The discussion is limited to a few examples that demonstrate some

Text continued on p. 375.

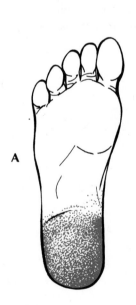
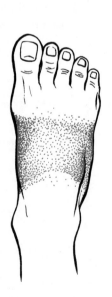
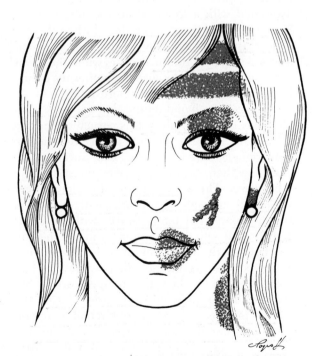

Fig. 19-3. Distribution of lesions in selected problems of the skin. **A,** Contact dermatitis (shoes). **B,** Contact dermatitis (cosmetics, perfumes, earrings).

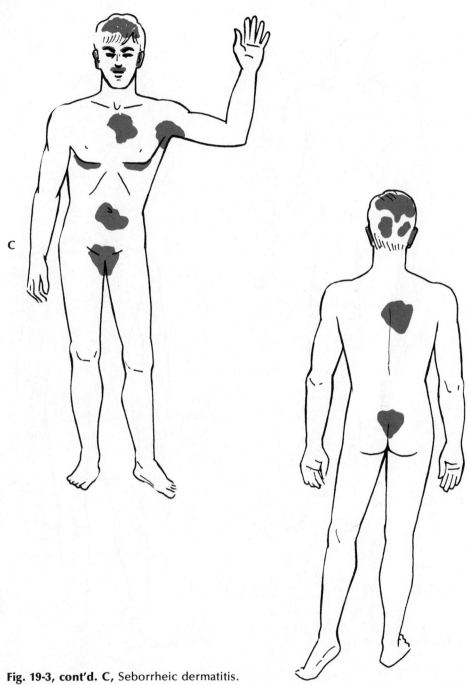

C

Fig. 19-3, cont'd. C, Seborrheic dermatitis.

Continued.

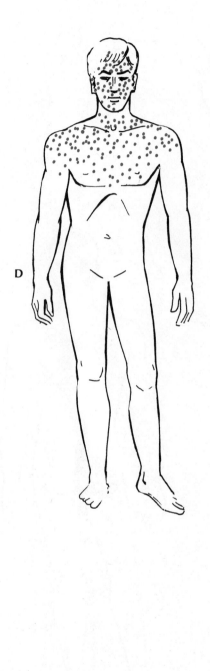

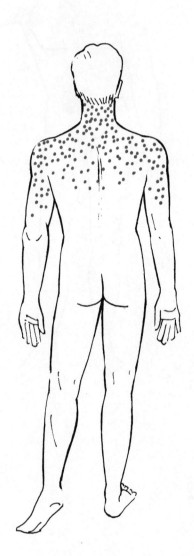

Fig. 19-3, cont'd. D, Acne.

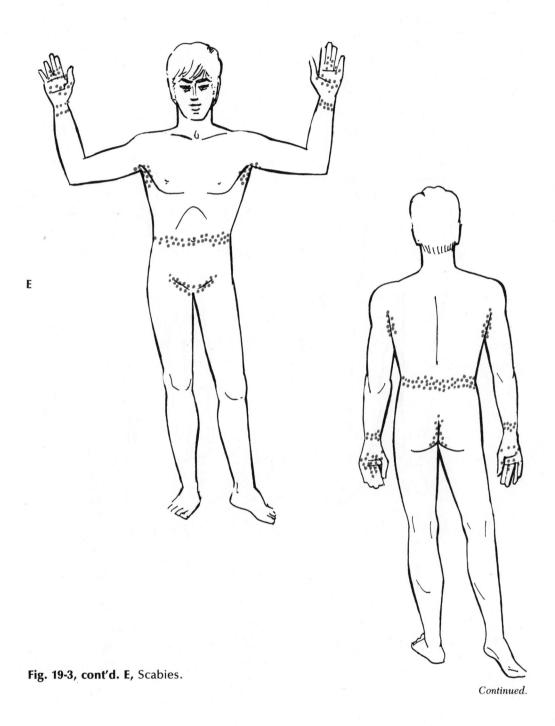

E

Fig. 19-3, cont'd. E, Scabies.

Continued.

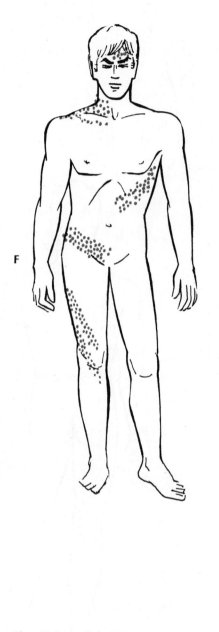

F

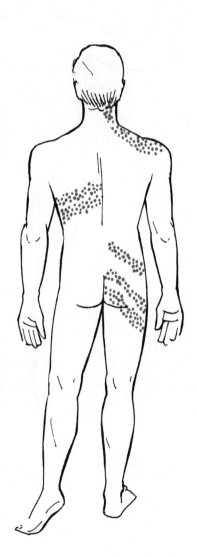

Fig. 19-3, cont'd. F, Herpes zoster.

of the different characteristics of skin lesions that will assist the examiner in describing the problem when consulting with a dermatologist or a textbook on dermatology.

The distribution of skin lesions is fairly simple to describe according to the location or body region affected and the symmetry or asymmetry of findings in comparable body parts. The examiner must keep in mind that there are characteristic patterns that provide the major clue in the diagnosis of a specific skin problem. Fig. 19-3 illustrates a few distribution patterns manifested by specific problems.

The configuration of skin lesions is equally important in defining the problem. Configuration refers to the arrangement or position of several lesions in relation to each other. For example, the skin lesions of tinea corporis, ringworm of the body, have an annular configuration that is circular. Fig. 19-4 illustrates some of the different configurations that occur.

Finally, there is a morphological classification of skin lesions that classifies lesions in terms of structure. It is important to identify the morphological structure of the individual lesion in order to identify the specific problem. Lesions are classified as primary or secondary. *Primary lesions* are those that appear initially in response to some change in the external or internal environment of the skin. *Secondary lesions* do not appear initially but result from modifications in the primary lesion. For instance, the primary lesion may

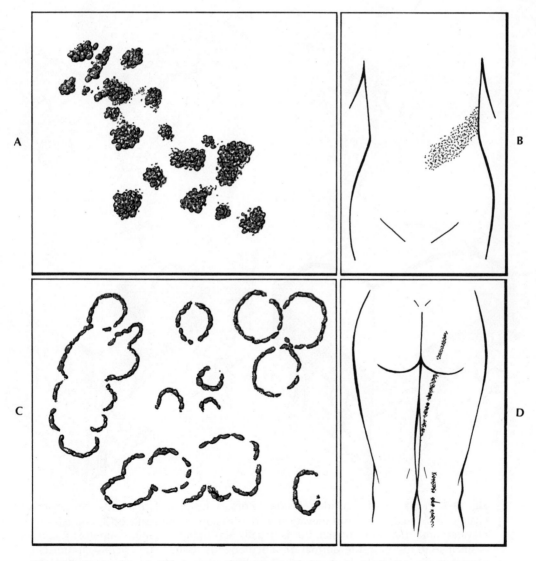

Fig. 19-4. Examples of different configurations of skin lesions. **A,** Grouped. **B,** Zosteriform. **C,** Annular and polycyclic. **D,** Linear.

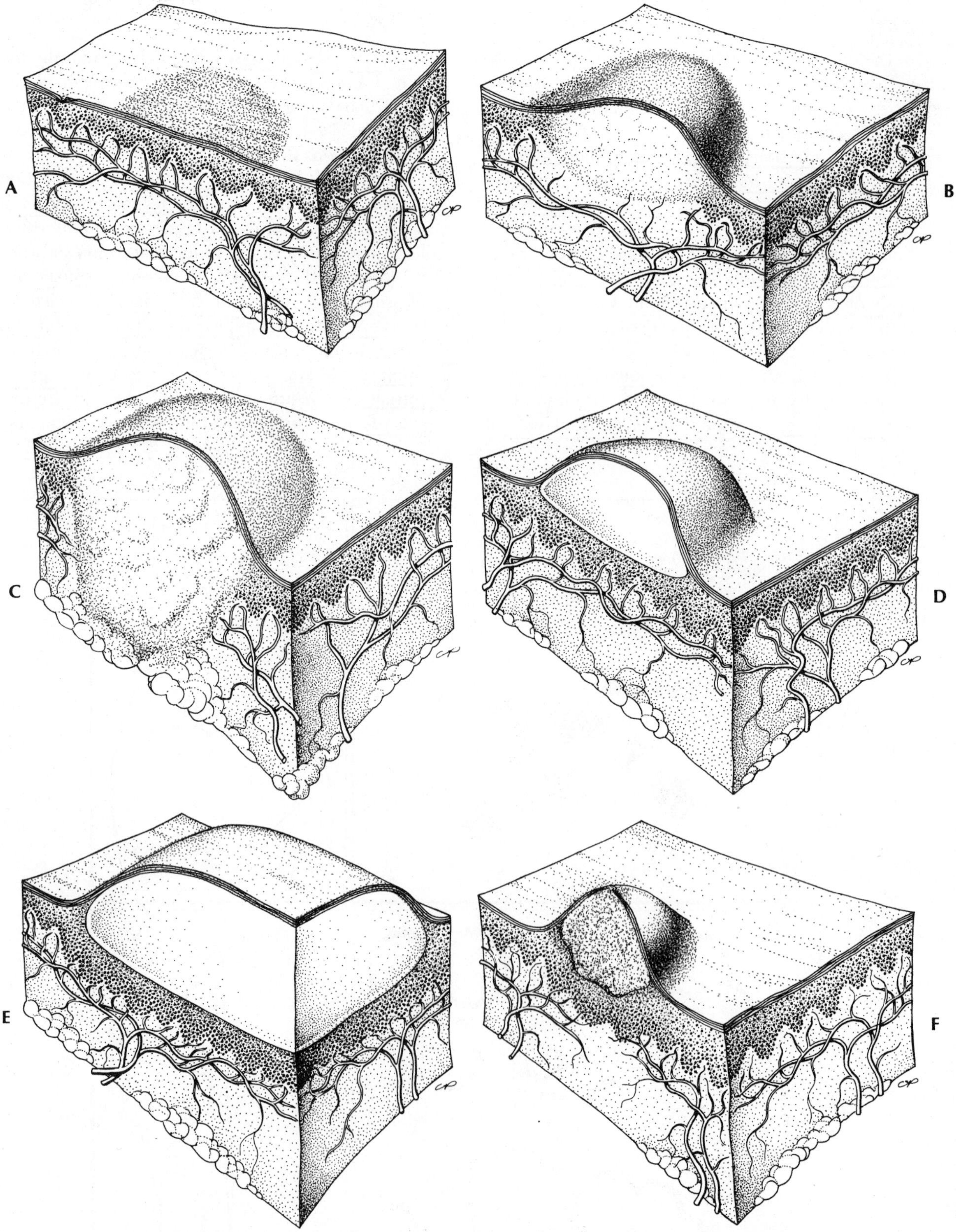

Fig. 19-5. Primary and secondary lesions. Primary lesions: **A,** *macule*—circumscribed change in skin color without elevation or depression of the surface; **B,** *papule*—solid, elevated area that varies in size but is usually less than 0.5 cm in diameter; **C,** *nodule* —small solid lesion in the dermal or subcutaneous tissue; **D,** *vesicle*—circumscribed elevated lesion containing serous fluid and less than 5 mm in diameter; **E,** *bullae*— vesicle larger than 5 mm in diameter; **F,** *pustule*—vesicle containing purulent exudate.

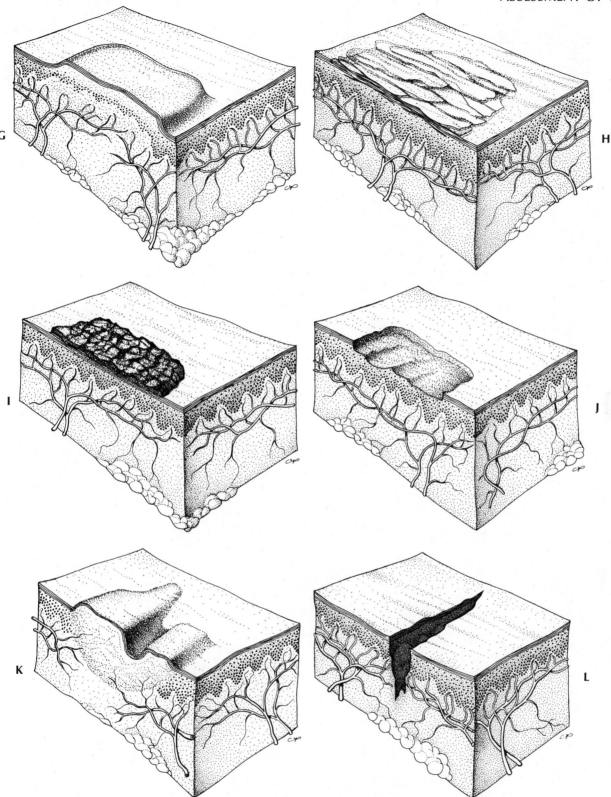

Fig. 19-5, cont'd. G, *Wheal*—circumscribed flat-topped, firm elevation of the skin with a well-defined palpable margin. Secondary lesions: **H,** *scale*—desiccated thin plates of cornified epithelial cells; **I,** *crust*—formed when serum, blood, or purulent exudate dries on the skin; **J,** *erosion*—moist, circumscribed, often depressed lesion; **K,** *scar*—area of replacement fibrosis of the dermis, resulting from destruction of the dermis or subcutaneous layers; **L,** *fissure*—deep linear cleavage of the skin that extends into the dermis.

be a vesicle, which is a small, circumscribed, elevated lesion containing clear fluid. The vesicle will rupture, leaving a small moist area, which is classified as a secondary lesion called an erosion. Fig. 19-5 illustrates some of the primary and secondary lesions.

BIBLIOGRAPHY

Fitzpatrick, T. B.: Dermatology in general practice, New York, 1971, McGraw-Hill Book Co.

Lewis, G. M., and Wheeler, C. E.: Practical dermatology, ed. 3, Philadelphia, 1967, W. B. Saunders Co.

Rook, A., and Wilkerson, D. S.: Textbook of dermatology, vol. 1, ed. 2, Oxford, 1972, Blackwell Scientific Publications Ltd.

Saver, G. C.: Manual of skin diseases, ed. 3, Philadelphia, 1973, J. B. Lippincott Co.

20 Neurological assessment

The neural system provides integration for all of the functions of the body. Even those cells such as beta cells of the pancreas, which show no direct neural response, are in fact dependent on such things as an adequate blood supply, which is subject to neural control. On the other hand, the neural system derives its homeostatic balance from the appropriate functioning of the peripheral organs. For instance, the cells of the central nervous system depend on an adequate supply of glucose for their metabolic processes, and this supply can be possible only if the pancreas functions well. This balance makes neurological assessment a part of all the components of the history and the physical examination.

ASSESSMENT OF MENTAL STATUS

The method of interviewing most frequently observed, that is, eliciting feelings and facts for the history, is a combination of asking questions and waiting, appearing alert and interested as the client provides the answers in his own language. This method allows for an observation of awareness, cognitive function, and affect. The questions asked the client are aimed at obtaining more data about symptoms, family and medical history, the parameters of the client's life situation, and an evaluation of his support systems.

The record should be kept as simple and direct as possible; hazy terminology should be avoided. Words such as *anxious*, *cheerful*, and *suspicious* are loaded words, fraught with connotation. They mean different things to different readers. A more meaningful record describes those observations of appearance and behavior indicating that a given condition exists.

The appraisal of mental status is a process that may be built into the interview and the physical examination. However, the client who demonstrates dysfunction in affect or thought processes may indicate further exploration.

In assessing the mental status of the client, the examiner usually deals with symptoms—the thought processes or behavior and how the client feels about them. Some signs may be available, such as behavior that is disturbing to others. The examiner elicits the evolutionary history of the client's complaints and makes his own observations. Because what the client reports may change with each examination and because the client's words may have different connotations for different examiners, it is difficult to obtain agreement in the assessment of symptoms. The most helpful record is one that describes the client's behaviors and words accurately and succinctly.

■ Appearance and general behavior

The examiner carefully observes the client's physical appearance, manner of dress, facial expression, and body posture as a measure of mental function. In essence, assessment of neural status will be the composite of the way the client looks, acts, and feels. (See also Chapter 7 on General assessment.)

Posture and behavior

The posture is important in providing clues to the client's feelings. The client who walks slowly into the room, barely lifting his feet, and who slumps in the chair while avoiding the examiner's glance may be eloquently describing a lack of affect or depression. On the other hand, the person who bounds into the room, energetically shaking the examiner's hand while rapidly glancing around the room may be demonstrating significant overreaction. The tense muscles and furrowed forehead or the furtive, darting eyes, coupled with the wet handshake of the individual with anxiety should alert the examiner to look for further symptoms to corroborate this impression. With each interchange the speed and appropriateness of reaction are evaluated.

General coordination of movement may be assessed through observation of the gait. To assess the complex acts of coordination, the examiner may give the client simple phrases to write and simple geometric figures to draw.

Grooming and apparel

Failure of the client to give attention to personal cleanliness is a clue to underlying emotional problems. Thus, dirty hair or a dirty body, uncombed hair, unkempt nails, an unshaven face (in men) or unshaven underarms (in occidental women) warrant further exploration. The nails are examined for evidence of nail biting by the client. The female client with no makeup or with carelessly or bizarrely applied cosmetics should also be examined further. (On the other hand, lack of makeup may have no significance, since the client may have an allergy to the chemicals in cosmetics or her makeup may look so natural that it is not detected by the examiner. What is looked for in the behaviors is a pattern.) The clothing is examined to determine its appropriateness to the occasion (place, time) and the client's position in life. Bright yellow and red are associated with euphoria, whereas drab olive green and black are associated with depression. Attention is given to the amount and type of jewelry worn by the client. The sexual impression conveyed by the clothing may also have diagnostic value. The female client who appears dressed in masculine clothing with closely cropped hair may be giving a message of her sexual identity (or may just be exhibiting the unisex nature of dress popular in the mid 70s).

Speech

The manner of speech may give clues of the status of thought processes.

The nature of responses to the examiner's questions is important. The normal individual answers questions frankly. Failure to answer a question, circumlocution, or other evasive replies should be noted. Criticism given to the examiner by the client and whether the client talks up or down to the examiner may be recorded. The client, just as the professional, chooses the words he feels best suited to his companion of the moment. In addition, the words chosen by the client

usually give a good idea of his general intelligence, educational level, social level, and level of functioning.

Disorders of the structures responsible for speech may be evident during conversation with the client. These include:

1. *Dysphonia*: Difficulty or discomfort in making laryngeal speech sounds, such as hoarseness. *Dysphonia puberum* is difficulty in controlling laryngeal speech sounds that occur as the larynx enlarges in puberty.
2. *Dysphasia*: Disturbance in the understanding or expressing of words.
3. *Dysprosody*: Difficulty in speech such that inflection, pronunciation, pitch, and rhythm are impaired.
4. *Dysarthria*: Difficulty in articulating single sounds or phonemes of speech; individual letters (*f, g, r*); labials—sounds produced with the lips (*b, m, w,* rounded vowels) (cranial nerve [CN] III); gutterals—sounds produced in the throat (CN X); and linguals—sounds produced with the tongue (*l, t, n*) (CN XII). Dysarthria may be demonstrated by asking the client to repeat a phrase such as "Methodist Episcopal."

Rapid-fire conversation should be noted as well as slow and halting delivery. The client who monopolizes the interview should also be noted.

■ Sensorium

The sensorium is assessed for consciousness, orientation, attention span, recent and remote memory, insight, and judgment.

State of consciousness, awareness

The first step in the evaluation of the client's sensorium is the determination of the state of consciousness, that is, the individual's awareness and responsiveness to his life's experiences.

Consciousness may be regarded as the individual's awareness of the stimuli from his environment and within himself. Clinical appraisal is more reliable for assessing the awareness of the client to external variables, since these can be checked against the examiner's impressions. However, the client may give a very informative discussion of his internal feelings.

The levels of conscious perception are thought to be a function of the conscious ego. The awareness of self and environment, which is called consciousness, may be affected by the nature and the amplitude of the stimuli received by the individual. Thus, the awareness of feelings and reactions have been described to be different for those excluded from external stimuli and reacting to signals from the self only; that is, for those individuals with perceptual deprivation. Consciousness may also be impaired by internal stimuli (fear, rage) and by some pathophysiological changes (fever, pain). The unconscious ego may also interfere with the client's level of consciousness. Clients with hysteria neurosis may dissociate or fail to perceive both internal and external stimuli.

More precise description of consciousness is obtained by differentiating between field of consciousness and clarity of consciousness. *Field of consciousness* is the range or area of stimuli perceived. *Clarity of consciousness* is the intensity or clarity of perception. An example of the differences in these two aspects is seen in the depressed individual. Although the depressed individual may not attend to all of the events in his milieu, he is clear in his perceptions of those he does describe. Thus, his field of consciousness is narrowed, but his clarity of consciousness remains intact.

A disturbance in consciousness results in lack of clarity or in confusion of the client's awareness of self or the environment. The examination of consciousness may focus on four areas of awareness: awareness of one's internal state, subject-object differentiation, clarity of ego boundaries, and body awareness.

The normal client is able to describe how he is feeling—his *internal state*—in words that are clear and logical to the examiner. His awareness of inner life experience is considered intact.

The client who is confused concerning time and place may have poor *subject-object differentiation,* frequently confusing one object for another or persons for inanimate objects.

Disruption of *ego boundaries* implies that the individual involved is hazy about his perception of the origin of stimuli—whether they are of an external, subconscious, or conscious origin. This is normal in the developing child. This lack of clarity of ego boundaries is also typical of some religious rituals practiced by adults.

The normal person is alert to the *parameters of his body* and its performance. Although there is considerable variation from one individual to another, the normal client can distinguish himself from the environment. The nursing infant is not always able to make this distinction, regarding the mother's breast as an extension of his own body.

Orientation

Orientation is assessed as the client's awareness of person, place, and time.

A typical kind of protocol used in obtaining this information is:

Person
   "What is your name? Address? Telephone number?"
   "Do you know who I am?"
   "Do you know what my job is?"
Place
   "Tell me where you are. What is the name of this place?"
   "Do you know the name of the town you are in?"
   "Who brought you here?"
Time
   "Do you know what day this is? Month? Year?"

The degree of disorientation is recorded. Descriptions should include enough data to allow the reader to know if the client has no awareness of a particular parameter, limited or dysfunctional awareness, or exact perception.

Attention span

The attention span is one of the first functions of the sensorium to suffer disturbance. Allowing the client to talk over a short period of time gives evidence of his stream of consciousness. The continuity of ideas is evaluated. The client's response to questions and directives will provide evidence of his attentiveness to external conditions. When a new idea is introduced in the interview, the normal client processes this alteration and responds appropriately. The client may be given two or three sentences that he is asked to memorize and repeat.

Attentiveness may be altered in the otherwise normal individual in toxic, drugged, or sleepy states.

Memory

Impairment of memory occurs in both neurological and psychiatric disorders. Some questions that may help the examiner establish a disorder in memory are:

   "How well do you remember what you are told? What has happened to you?"
   "Do you remember those things that happened years ago best or those that happened today or yesterday?"

Recent memory. Examples of questions and exercises for assessing recent memory are:

   "How long have you been here?"
   "Why did you come here?"

"What were you doing before you came here?"

"What time did you get up today?"

"How many meals have you eaten today?"

"What did you eat for breakfast today?"

"Please allow me to test your memory skills. I'd like you to repeat these numbers after me:
7, 4
9, 6, 5, 3
8, 9, 4, 1, 5
3, 8, 7, 4, 1, 6."

"I will say some numbers; you say them backward. For instance, I say 8, 2; you say 2, 8:
3, 8
7, 2, 0
5, 9, 2, 7."

The normal individual can generally repeat five to eight digits forward and four to six digits backward.

Recent memory may be impaired in senile dementia and Korsakoff's psychosis.

Remote memory. Examples of questions for assessing remote memory are:

"Where were you born?"

"Tell me the name of the high school you attended."

"What was your mother's maiden name?"

Remote memory may be dysfunctional in schizophrenic illnesses.

Cognitive skills

Abstraction ability. To assess abstraction ability, the examiner may ask the client to give the meaning of familiar proverbs:

"Tell me what this means: a bird in the hand is worth two in the bush."

Other proverbs might include:

"When the cat's away, the mice will play."

"Don't count your chickens before they are hatched."

"A rolling stone gathers no moss."

Similarities. The following exercises may be used to assess the client's ability to determine similarities:

"Tell me how the following are like each other: bird and butterfly; dog and goldfish; fish and plankton; window and door; German person and Swiss person; pencil and typewriter."

"Try to finish these comparisons for me: beer is to glass as coffee is to _____; engine is to airplane as pedal is to _____."

Ability to learn. The ability to learn includes abilities in retention, association, and recent memory. The client is given an address or a sen-

tence that does not contain familiar associations. The material may be presented in writing or may be spoken. The client is asked to remember the content verbatim:

"Listen to me carefully, I am going to give you an address that I want you to remember. Later on, I will ask you to repeat it for me: Apartment 13, Dover Hill Building."

Or the client might be given a sentence:

"One thing a nation must have in order to become rich and great is a large and secure stock of wood."

An approximate 5-minute interval is allowed before the client is asked to repeat the material.

Computation. The following exercise may be used to assess the client's computational abilities:

"Subtract 7 from 100. Continue on subtracting 7 from the resulting sum."

Ability to read. A copy of a current newspaper or popular periodical is generally available and may be used to determine the client's reading skills. The examiner should be certain that the client is wearing corrective lenses if they are needed for reading.

Impairment of the ability to read is called dyslexia.

Emotional status, affect

An interview protocol to help the examiner bring out the feelings of the client when he does not offer spontaneous data might contain the following:

"How do you feel inside?"

"How have your spirits been?"

"Do you feel this way most of the time?"

"Are you in good spirits, happy [unhappy] most of the time?"

"Do you let people know how you feel?" *If no,* "Are you afraid to let people see how you feel?"

"Can you control how you feel?"

"When do you feel the best, in the morning or in the evening?"

"How do you feel life has treated you?"

"Do you enjoy your life?"

"Is life worth living for you?"

"What does the future look like?" *If a negative reply,* "Does everything look hopeless? Do you think you will see tomorrow?"

"What plans have you made for your future?"

"Have you ever considered hurting yourself?" *If yes,* "Did you follow through and actually hurt yourself?"

"Do you think about dying?"

The appraisal of emotional status includes an investigation of the client's life situation and personality (general coping behavior). An interview protocol to elicit this information might be similar to the one below.

Queries	Frequently recorded responses
Present complaint	
"Tell me why you are here."	
Present illness	
"When did you last feel well?"	
"What changes have you noted in yourself?"	
"When did you first notice the problem?"	
"How long did it last?"	
"What do you feel is causing the problem?"	
"Have you had any other troubling bodily or psychological feelings (symptoms)?"	
"How are you sleeping? Eating?"	
"Do you feel better in the morning or in the evening?"	
"Have you gained or lost any weight?"	
Family history	
"How old is your father? Is he employed?"	
"What does [did] he do for a living?"	
"How old is your mother? Is [was] she employed?"	
"Did either your father or your mother have any other marriages?"	
"How well did they get along?"	
"Tell me about their personality [temperament]?"	Affectionate, warm, easy going, strict, cold, always worried, always in debt, drunk all the time
"How did you feel about your parents?"	
"Was your home a comfortable place?"	
"Did any of your family have any emotional problems? Ever need to see a doctor because of a nervous problem?"	
Childhood and premorbid personality	
"What were you like as a child?"	Friendly; happy; nervous; jumpy; shy; self-conscious; delicate; enuresis; nail biting; fears—of the dark, small rooms, open spaces, high places, crowds; depressed; loner; read all the time; hated sports; successful; unsure of self
"How did your parents [brothers, sisters] describe you to others?"	
"What did your teachers think of you?"	
"Did you like to be with people?"	
"Tell me how you would describe yourself."	

Queries	Frequently recorded responses
Medical history	
"Have you ever been diagnosed as having a disease?" *If yes,* "Explain this to me."	
Psychological history	
"Have you ever been in counseling or treatment for an emotional problem?"	
Recent stress	
"Have you had any recent cause for grief?"	
"Have you been bereaved over the loss of a loved person?"	
"Are all of your relatives and friends in good health?"	
"Are there any problems with your job?"	
"Is money a problem for you?"	
"Are there problems in your marriage? Love life?"	
Education	
"Where did you go to school?"	
"What was the highest grade you attended?"	
"How did you feel about school?"	
"How well did you do in school?"	Overachievement, truancy, suspension
Employment	
"What kind of work do you do?"	
"Tell me where you have worked and how long you worked at each job?"	Long periods of unemployment, frequent job turnover
"Have you ever served in a military service?"	
"Do you enjoy working?"	
"How do you get along with your boss? People who work for you?"	
Delinquency	
"Have you ever been in trouble with school? The police?"	
Drug history	
"Have you ever been given a prescription for medicine by a doctor?" *If yes,* "Tell me about it."	
"Have you ever used drugs available in the street?" *If yes,* "How much? How long? Are you taking drugs now?"	Grass (marijuana), uppers, downers, hash, tic (phencyclidine [PCP]), horse (heroin)
"Do you drink beer? Wine? Whiskey? How much? How long?" *or* "How much and what are you drinking these days?"	
Marital history	
"How old is your wife [husband]?"	
"How long have you been married?"	

Continued.

383

Queries	Frequently recorded responses
"How do you feel about your marriage?"	Hate to go home, often go out with the guys
"How many children do you have?"	
"Were there any other pregnancies?"	
"How do you get along with your children?"	
"What kinds of things do you do as a family?"	
"How many times were you engaged?"	
"Were you ever married before?" *If yes,* "Tell me about it."	
"Is your sexual relationship satisfactory to you?" *If no,* "How do you manage?"	Masturbation, homosexuality, extramarital intercourse
"Do you have any extramarital relationships?"	

Social milieu

"Tell me about your friends."

Support systems

"Who would you turn to if you were in trouble?"

Insight

"Do you consider yourself different now than before your problem began?"

"What do you think about your problem?"

"Do you think you are sick?" *If yes,* "Do you think you will get over it?"

"Do you think you need help?"

"In what way would you change if you had a choice?"

"Do you think the same way now that you always have?"

"Do your thoughts come slower [faster] than they used to?"

Self-drawings made by the client on blank pieces of paper may help the examiner in his examination of body image. ("Draw yourself for me.") The drawing is inspected with special reference to size of image, the facial expression (affect), the activity of the figure, the amount and nature of detail, and the diminution or exaggeration of body parts. Another useful device is that of asking the client to fill in an outline of the human body. ("Draw your insides.") The heart, lungs, and intestines are the structures most frequently added. The placement and size of the organs drawn by the client may provide clues of their meaning to him.

■ Mental dysfunction

Mental dysfunction or psychiatric symptoms are referred if some relief of symptoms can be anticipated. The symptoms that are most worthy of attention are those that are uselessly repetitive in nature, uncomfortable for the client, and disabling.

The common disorders of emotion and thought processes are defined here. Familiarity with this symptomatology may help the examiner to focus his questioning and to recognize a cluster of symptoms. As with the physical examination, the examiner is looking for a pattern.

DEFINITIONS

delusion A belief of great magnitude, not influenced by experience and improbable in nature.

eidetic imagery Vivid recall of past event, present in some artists; original experience more intense, however.

hallucination Perception for which no external stimuli can be ascertained. An endogenous experience in an individual whose sensorium is clear. *Simple hallucination:* simple perception, such as seeing light. *Complex hallucination:* more detailed experiences, such as seeing figure of a person.

illusion Perception based on an actual external stimulus with misinterpretation or distortion of the event.

Organic brain syndrome

Organic brain syndrome is a diagnostic term used to describe those individuals with signs indicating medical or neurological dysfunction causing an impairment of orientation, memory, or other mental functions. Affective symptoms, delusions, hallucinations, and obsessions may be present as well. An acute brain syndrome (delirium) is one of short duration that is usually reversible. A chronic brain syndrome (dementia) is long standing and often progressive in nature; its prognosis is less favorable.

Table 20-1. Organic brain syndrome: characteristic symptoms and signs

Acute delirium	Dementia
Impairment of consciousness	May be disoriented
Delusions possible	Attention span impaired
Hallucinations possible	Judgment impaired
May be disoriented	Recent memory impaired
Attention span impaired	Mood swings
Judgment impaired	Irritability
Mood swings	
Recent memory impaired	
Restlessness	
Anxiety	
Fear	

Affective disorders

The client with an affective disorder runs the gamut from depression to exaggerated euphoria or mania. The highs and lows show little correlation with the life situation.

During the down mood period the client evidences such symptoms as anorexia, insomnia, sense of worthlessness, sense of being a burden, and thoughts of self-destruction. On the high mood cusp the client may describe flights of ideas or hyperactivity.

Primary affective disorders are those observed in a client who has had no previous psychiatric disorders. *Secondary affective disorders* are those seen in a client who has been previously diagnosed as having psychiatric illness.

A *bipolar affective disorder* is diagnosed when mania is present whether or not depression occurs. Depression occurring in the absence of mania is known as a *unipolar affective disorder*.

The client with an affective disorder often tells the examiner that "something is wrong with my mind."

Paranoid ideations have been reported in clients with affective disorders. These thoughts appear to be augmented ideas of reference related to the feeling of worthlessness.

The periods of illness may last from a few days to several years, and the client appears to function well in the interim.

Primary affective disorders are most frequently first diagnosed when the client is about 40, whereas the client with a bipolar affective disorder may be in his 30s.

Clients being treated with tricyclic antidepressant drugs may have complaints of side effects, such as tremor, dry mouth, or orthostatic hypotension. Thus, a precise record of the client's drug history is important.

Schizophrenic disorders

Hallucinations and delusions are the diagnostic signposts of schizophrenia. These symptoms are the criteria by which mental disorders are classified as schizophrenic disorders. By this scale, primary affective disorders, organic brain syn-

Table 20-2. Affective disorders: characteristic symptoms and signs

Mania

Euphoria	*Somatic*
Irritability (sometimes)	Hyperactivity
Flight of ideas—generally comprehensible	Rapid speech rate
	Rhyming
Distractibility	Punning
Delusions possible (may be of grandeur)	Decreased sleep
Passivity—sensation that body is under external control	
Depersonalization	

Depression

Dejection	*Somatic*
Discouragement	Pain
Despondency	Tachycardia
Depression	Dyspnea
Feeling of being down in the dumps, blue	Gastrointestinal dysfunction
Irritability	Anorexia
Fearfulness	Constipation
Loss of interest in daily activities	Sleep disorders
Social withdrawal	Insomnia
Guilt	Hypersomnia
Inability to focus thoughts	Lack of energy
Indecisiveness	Psychomotor retardation
Recurring preoccupation with suicide, death	Frequent crying
Thoughts of self-destruction	Impotence (in men)
Hopelessness	Restlessness
Feeling of gloomy future, impending doom	Pacing, wringing of hands
Loss of interest in sexual activity	
Delusions possible (frequently involving self-deprecation)	

Table 20-3. Schizophrenia: characteristic symptoms and signs

Poor prognosis	Good prognosis
Delusions	Delusions
Hallucinations (most common of persecution) auditory	Hallucinations
	Clear sensorium
	Symptoms transitory
Clear sensorium	Symptoms develop abruptly
Chronic disorder	More likely to show affective responses, usually depression
Blunted, shallow (flat), or inappropriate affect	Recovery is usual
Catatonic motor behavior	
Waxy flexibility; periods of immobility	
Repeated grimacing, posturing	
Disordered thought processes	

dromes, alcoholism, and drug dependency may be classified under this category. Two classifications of these disorders are described in the literature related to prognosis. Schizophrenic disorders with a poor prognosis include *chronic schizophrenia*, *nuclear schizophrenia*, and *process schizophrenia*. Schizophrenic disorders with a good prognosis include *schizophreniform* and *schizoaffective disorders* and *acute, reactive, or remitting schizophrenia*.

The development of schizophrenia may occur over a long period of time.

A schizoid personality is said to exist in the client who is markedly shy, who withdraws from social relationships, and who is unable to establish close personal relationships. This behavior is generally noted in adolescence, though delusions and hallucinations generally start in the 20s.

The schizophreniform disorders are abrupt in onset and occur without a psychiatric history prior to the present illness.

Neuroses

Anxiety neurosis. The client with an anxiety neurosis has recurrent periods of abrupt onset anxiety that terminate without intervention. The client complains of fright. The autonomic nervous system is activated.

Characteristic symptoms and signs include:

Palpitations	Headache
Breathlessness, smothering	Fatigue, weakness
	Paresthesias
Dyspnea	Tremors, shakiness
Nervousness	Sighing
Dizziness	Nausea and vomiting
Faintness	Abdominal cramps
Feeling of impending doom	Diarrhea
	Flatus

The age of onset extends from mid adolescence through the early 30s.

Hysteria. Hysteria is a disorder characterized by multiple somatic symptoms. Examples of such complaints include gastrointestinal disturbances, pains (dysmenorrhea, headaches, back pain), anxiety, sexual problems, and conversion symptoms. The symptoms often defy the boundaries of what is commonly known about pathophysiology. The descriptions are often vividly portrayed or markedly exaggerated, or both, so that these clients often spend a good deal of time in hospitals and undergo many surgical procedures. Because there are often many vague symptoms, the history may be difficult to complete and to organize for the record. The examiner would do well to

record the complaints verbatim. Conversion symptoms are idiopathic symptoms that indicate neurological disorder. These might include amnesia, unconsciousness, paralysis, anesthesias, or blindness.

Hysteria is most commonly first seen in the teens. The incidence is higher in men than in women.

Compulsional or obsessional neurosis. *Obsessions* are long-lasting, upsetting thoughts or impulses that usually do not interest the individual and serve no purpose but cannot be ignored. *Compulsions* are the behaviors that are the result of obsessions. Thus, an obsessional neurosis is said to exist in the presence of obsessions and compulsions when no other disorder is evident. Other terms for this neurosis include psychasthenia, phobic-ruminative state, and obsessional state.

DEFINITIONS

obsessional convictions Magical formulations. ("If I have my purse here, nothing can happen to me.")

obsessional fears Repeated feelings of fright, particularly of disease, filth, sharp instruments.

obsessional ideas Words, phrases, or rhymes that recur in the thought processes of the individual, frequently interrupting other thought sequences.

obsessional images Recurrent imagined scenes, often dealing with sexual acts or excreta.

obsessional impulses Irresistible thoughts related to self-injury, to injury of others, or to some other embarrassing behavior.

obsessional rituals Recurrent, stylized actions; protocols for washing or combing hair, eating.

obsessional rumination Prolonged reflection on a subject without reaching a decision.

phobia A highly disturbing, recurring, and unrealistic fear; may relate to any situation or object.

Sociopathic, antisocial personality

The sociopathic personality is a synonym for the antisocial personality of an individual who has displayed a pattern of antisocial, delinquent, or criminal behavior. The disorder has its inception in adolescence. Early symptoms include restlessness, a short attention span, and defiance of discipline. A history of poor school and work adjustment is the rule. Promiscuous sexual behavior is a frequent observation. Conversion symptoms are frequently observed in the sociopathic personality.

Sample protocol for eliciting psychiatric symptoms

Questions leading to the elucidation of psychiatric symptoms might include the following:

Disturbing events
"How did you feel at the time?"

Hallucinations
"Have you heard [sounds, voices, messages], seen [lights, figures], smelled [strange, bad, good odors], tasted [strange, bad, good tastes], or felt [touching, warm, cold sensation] anything that others who were present did not? If no one was present, would I have been able to have the same impressions from the experience?"

Delusions
"Do you feel that someone or something outside you is controlling you in some way? Are you able to control other people?"
"Do you feel that you are being watched? Followed?"
"Are people talking about you?" *If yes*, "Explain to me how you know."
"Do you have anything to feel guilty about?"
"Do you feel you are a bad person?"

Obsessions
"Do you have some thoughts that keep coming back again and again?" *If yes*, "Tell me about them. How often? Are they pleasant [frightening] thoughts? Can you make them stop?"

Compulsions
"Are there some things you find yourself doing over and over?" *If yes*, "Tell me about them. How often? Can you stop doing these things?"
"Do you have someone or something outside you that is forcing you to do these things?"
"Do you find yourself checking and rechecking to make sure water is turned off? Gas? To make sure the doors are locked?"

Somatic symptoms
"Do you ever feel a lump in your throat?"
"Do you have difficulty swallowing? Speaking?"
"Have you ever been paralyzed?"
"How do your bowels function?"
"How is your appetite?"
"Do you have headaches?"
"Do you have enough energy to do all the things you would like to do?"

PHYSICAL EXAMINATION

The neurological physical examination may be performed as five areas of investigation: (1) assessment of cranial nerve function, (2) assessment of proprioception and cerebellar function, (3) musculoskeletal assessment (see Chapter 18 on Musculoskeletal assessment), (4) assessment of sensory function, and (5) assessment of reflexes.

■ Cranial nerve function

CN I: olfactory nerve

The olfactory nerve is sensory in function and makes possible the sense of smell, or olfaction.

The client is asked to close his eyes, occlude one nostril, and attempt to identify familiar substances. The substances should be mildly aromatic and unambiguous. Some odors that have been used are coffee, cigarettes, soap, peanut butter, toothpaste, oranges, vanilla, onions, and oil of cloves. Strongly aromatic compounds such as ammonia should be avoided in determining olfactory function since the vapors may prevent the perception of weaker substances.

The substances are housed in test tubes that are kept closed until the examiner is prepared to present them to the client.

The client is asked whether he smells anything and to identify the substance if he can. The process is repeated for each nostril.

Both the number of substances used as stimuli and the number of correct responses should be recorded. Differences in sensitivity from one nostril to the other are recorded.

If the client has difficulty identifying substances, he should be asked whether he is able to smell anything at all.

Anosmia is the loss of the sense of smell or the inability to discriminate vapors. Diminution of the ability to smell is termed hyposmia.

A pathophysiological condition of the nasal mucosa or olfactory bulb or tract can interfere with the sensation of smell. The client is not always aware of a deficit in olfaction.

The mucosal surfaces are examined when the client has difficulty in smelling, since an inflammation of the mucous membranes (viral, bacterial) decreases the sense of smell. Allergic rhinitis and excessive cigarette smoking are common causes of anosmia or hyposmia.

Lesions of the sinuses may result in distortion or hallucinations of smell but do not result in a loss of olfactory sensation. Unilateral loss of smell may be an early indication of a neoplasm involving the olfactory bulb or tract.

CN II: optic nerve

The optic nerve is described in Chapter 10 on Assessment of the eyes (note the sections on examination of visual acuity, visual fields, and the pupils—tests of pupillary constriction).

CN III: oculomotor nerve,
CN IV: trochlear nerve,
CN VI: abducens nerve

The oculomotor, trochlear, and abducens nerves are also described in Chapter 10 (note the sections on neuromuscular and extraocular muscle function—tests of eye movement).

CN V: trigeminal nerve

The trigeminal nerve has both a motor and a sensory component.

The motor fibers innervate the masseter, temporal, pterygoid, and digastric muscles.

The muscles of mastication are evaluated by asking the client to bite down with as much force as possible. The masseter muscles (Fig. 20-1) are

evaluated by palpation, as are the temporal muscles (Fig. 20-2).

The pterygoid muscles may be examined by asking the client to press his jaw laterally against the examiner's hand with the mouth slightly open.

Atrophy of the muscle is recorded. Deviation of the jaw to one side indicates that the muscles of

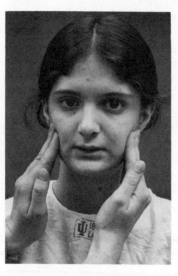

Fig. 20-1. Palpation of the masseter muscles for size, strength, and symmetry to test CN V.

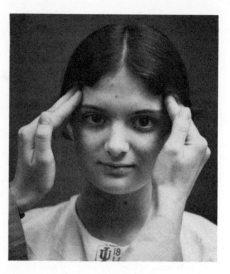

Fig. 20-2. Palpation of the temporal muscles for size, shape, and symmetry to test CN V.

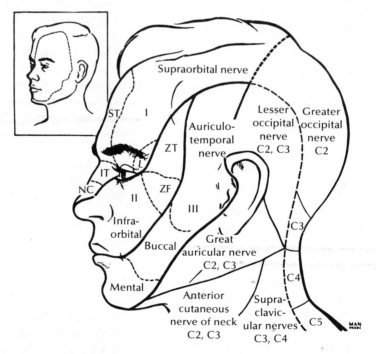

Fig. 20-3. Cutaneous fields of the head and upper part of the neck. Inset shows the area of sensory loss in the face following resection of the trigeminal nerve. The cutaneous fields of the three branches of the trigeminal nerve are identified as *I,* ophthalmic; *II,* maxillary; and *III,* mandibular. (From Haymaker, W., and Woodhall, B.: Peripheral nerve injuries, ed. 2, Philadelphia, 1959, W. B. Saunders Co.)

the side to which it is pulled are stronger than those of the opposite side. An idea of the extent of weakness of the muscle might be gained by asking the client to move his jaw toward the weak side.

The trigeminal nerve mediates sensation of pain, temperature, vibration, and touch from the cranial cavity above the tentorium, the skin structures of the anterior half of the scalp to the vertex, the paranasal sinuses, and the nasal and oral mucosa. The sensory division of the trigeminal nerve has three sections, ophthalmic, maxillary, and mandibular (Fig. 20-3).

The usual tests of sensation are employed on both sides of the face, taking care that each division of the nerve is tested. A wooden applicator may be used to touch various areas of the mucosa inside the mouth to test sensitivity to touch. The trigeminal nerve contains the afferent fiber for the corneal reflex (see Chapter 10 on Assessment of the eyes), and both the afferent and efferent fibers for the jaw closure reflex (described later in this chapter under Reflexes).

Motor pathophysiology

Myasthenia gravis. The weakness and ready fatigability of muscles that occur in myasthenia gravis may involve the muscles of mastication, making chewing difficult or impossible.

Amyotrophic lateral sclerosis. Degeneration of the motor nucleus of the trigeminal nerve may occur in amyotrophic lateral sclerosis, resulting in weakness and atrophy of the muscles of mastication. The client may be unable to chew or close his mouth.

Tetanus. Rigidly spastic muscles are frequently observed in tetanus infections. Spasm of the muscles of mastication is called lockjaw.

Sensory pathophysiology

Trigeminal neuralgia (tic douloureux). Trigeminal neuralgia is characterized by pain of the lips, gums, or chin. The regions of pain may map out one of the divisions of the trigeminal nerve. These zones are supraorbital, infraorbital, and inferior to the labial fold midway to the angle of the jaw. Sharp pain may be elicited by applying pressure at the point where the trigeminal nerve emerges from the bone.

Herpes zoster (shingles). The gasserian ganglia, just as any ganglion of the body, may be affected by the herpes virus. A characteristic papulovesicular rash generally involving the ophthalmic division may be observed. A neuralgia may remain after the rash has disappeared, and sensation may be lost from the involved area.

CN VII: facial nerve

The facial nerve also has both a motor and a sensory component.

The motor component controls most of the muscles of the facial expression. The client's face is inspected for indications of facial muscle weakness, such as drooping of one side of the mouth, flattening of the nasolabial fold, and laxity of the lower eyelid.

The client is asked to perform the following facial movements: elevate his eyebrows, wrinkle his forehead, frown (Fig. 20-4), smile or show his teeth (in this test, in addition to the facial muscles, the platysma muscle of the neck is noted)

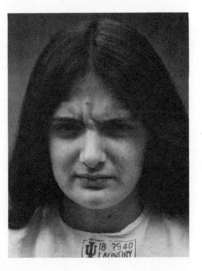

Fig. 20-4. Test of CN VII. Client's ability to frown is inspected as a function of the facial muscles.

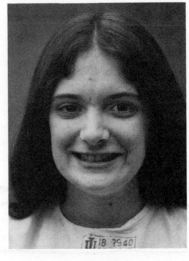

Fig. 20-5. Test of CN VII. Client's ability to expose the teeth is inspected as a function of the facial muscles and platysma muscle of the neck.

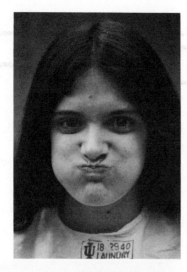

Fig. 20-6. Test of CN VII. Client's ability to puff out the cheeks is inspected as a function of the facial muscles.

(Fig. 20-5), puff out his cheeks (Fig. 20-6), or whistle. The examiner evaluates the movements for muscle strength and symmetry. The client is told to close his eyes and keep them closed while the examiner tries to open them.

Taste sensation for the anterior two thirds of the tongue is mediated through the sensory component of the facial nerve.

To test taste sensation, solutions of the following substances are applied to the lateral aspect of the tongue: sweet, salty, sour (vinegar, lemon juice), and bitter (quinine). A different applicator is used for each substance, and the client is allowed a sip of water in between testing to avoid mixing tastes. In addition, the tongue should remain protruded throughout the test. Each substance is used twice.

Both sides of the tongue must be assessed. The number of tests and the number of correct responses are recorded.

The facial nerve also innervates the submandibular, submaxillary, and lacrimal glands. However, the functions of salivation and lacrimation are generally not tested as a part of the routine physical examination.

Motor pathophysiology: Bell's palsy. Peripheral facial palsy of acute onset and unknown cause is called Bell's palsy. Evidence of this lower motor neuron disorder is seen when only one eye closes as the client attempts to close both eyes. Observation of a flat nasolabial fold may add to this suspicion. When the client attempts to raise his eyebrows, the eyebrow on the

affected side will not raise and the forehead does not wrinkle. Upper motor neuron paralysis (hemiparesis) is a possibility if the nasolabial folds appear flat when the client closes his eyes. In this case, both eyebrows raise and the forehead wrinkles. In upper motor neuron pathology, involuntary contractions of the facial muscle, as in smiling and frowning, may show normal strength, whereas voluntary contractions of these muscles prove to be weak.

Sensory pathophysiology: ageusia. Ageusia is the loss of taste and the lack of ability to discriminate sweet, sour, salty, and bitter tastes. The nature of the loss of taste sensation may aid in making a diagnosis. For example:

1. Unilateral loss of taste may be caused by lesions of the tractus solitarius and its nucleus.
2. Bilateral ageusia may be caused by pathophysiological phenomena occurring near the midline of the pons.
3. Hallucinations or perversions of taste may be caused by lesions of the uncus.

CN VIII: acoustic nerve

The acoustic nerve has two divisions: the vestibular and the cochlear.

Vestibular function. Tests for vestibular function are not done routinely in the physical examination. However, 5 to 10 ml of ice water may be put in the ear canal to reveal vertigo or nystagmus.

Cochlear function. Tests for cochlear function are described in Chapter 8 on Assessment of the ears, nose, and throat (note testing of auditory function—audiogram, Weber, and Rinne tests).

CN IX: glossopharyngeal nerve,
CN X: vagus nerve

The glossopharyngeal and vagus nerves are closely related both anatomically and physiologically. These nerves are tested clinically as a unit.

The glossopharyngeal nerve is sensory for taste for the posterior one third of the tongue and conveys general sensation from the tonsillar and pharyngeal mucosa. The same tests for taste sensation are conducted for the posterior tongue as are done for the anterior tongue (see CN VII: facial nerve).

In addition, the glossopharyngeal nerve has afferent sensory fibers for the carotid sinus and body. It is also the motor nerve for part of the pharyngeal musculature.

The vagus nerve is sensory for the walls of the

gastrointestinal viscera (to the transverse colon), the heart, lungs, and aortic bodies. The vagus is a motor nerve to the palate, pharynx, larynx, and the thoracic and abdominal visceral organs.

The clinical examination focuses on the examination of the musculature of the palate, pharynx, and larynx. The soft palate is inspected for symmetry. The median raphe is identified, and any deviation from the midline is recorded. Unilateral weakness is characterized by the drooping of the affected side and the absence of the arch on that side.

The client is asked to say, "Ah." The palate should rise symmetrically. The palatal reflex is elicited by stroking the mucous membrane of the soft palate with an applicator. The side touched retracts upward.

The gag reflex is obtained by touching the posterior wall of the pharynx with an applicator or a tongue blade. The response includes elevation of the palate and contraction of the pharyngeal muscles.

Swallowing is evaluated by giving the client a small quantity of water to drink and observing him while he swallows it. Retrograde passage of water through the nose while drinking indicates a weakness of the soft palate wherein the nasopharynx is not closed off during the swallow.

In the presence of a lesion of the vagus nerve, the uvula and soft palate deviate to the unaffected side since the muscles on the intact side are unopposed.

Vagus nerve alone. The client who is hoarse or who complains of a problem with vocalization is examined by indirect laryngoscopy. A laryngeal mirror and head light allow visualization of the vocal cords.

CN XI: spinal accessory nerve

The spinal accessory nerve provides motor innervation to the trapezius and sternocleidomastoid muscles. To test this nerve the symmetry, size, and strength of these muscles are evaluated.

For assessment of the sternocleidomastoid muscle, the client is asked to turn his head to one side and push the chin in the same direction against the resistance of the examiner's hand. The contralateral sternocleidomastoid muscle will stand out and may be inspected and palpated (Fig. 20-7).

For assessment of the trapezius muscles, the client is asked to shrug his shoulders while the examiner exerts downward pressure against the muscles. As the muscles contract, they may be

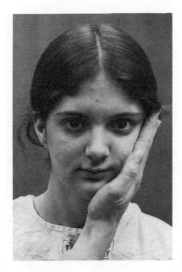

Fig. 20-7. Assessment of the symmetry, size, and strength of the sternocleidomastoid muscle in test of CN XI. The client is asked to turn the head to one side to push the chin against the resistance of the examiner's hand. The contralateral sternocleidomastoid muscle will stand out as it contracts.

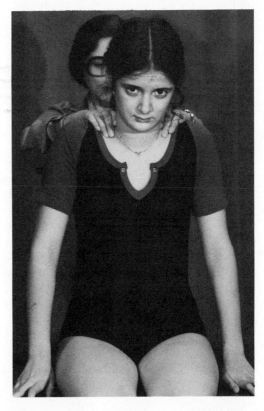

Fig. 20-8. Assessment of the symmetry, size, and shape of the trapezius muscles in test of CN XI. The client shrugs the shoulders against the resistance of the examiner's hand.

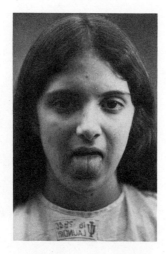

Fig. 20-9. Assessment of the symmetry, size, and shape of the muscles of the protruded tongue in test of CN XII.

evaluated for strength and symmetry (Fig. 20-8).

The trapezius muscles may be further tested by asking the client to raise his arms to a vertical position. Weakness of the trapezius muscles makes this position difficult to achieve.

Neck trauma is the most frequent cause of dysfunction of the spinal accessory nerve.

Torticollis is a condition of intermittent or constant contraction of the sternocleidomastoid muscle wherein the head is flexed forward and the chin is rotated away from the affected side.

CN XII: hypoglossal nerve

The hypoglossal nerve provides motor innervation to the muscles of the tongue, making possible articulation of lingual speech sounds and swallowing. The tongue is inspected for size and symmetry. Deviation to the affected side is characteristic of unilateral nerve damage.

The client is asked to stick out his tongue as far as he can. The examiner notes the ability of the client to stick the tongue straight out, the strength of the movement, and how far out the client sticks the tongue (Fig. 20-9).

The examiner tests lingual speech sounds by giving the client a phrase for repetition that includes a number of words containing *l*, *t*, *d*, or *n*.

Summary

Table 20-4 is a summary of the cranial nerves, including their functions, assessment, makeup, and components.

Table 20-4. The cranial nerves

Nerve	Function	Clinical test	Cells of origin	Major components	Afferent	Efferent
I Olfactory	Smell	Odor applied to one nostril	Olfactory epithelium	Olfactory filaments	Visceral special Smell	
II Optic	Vision	Visual acuity: Snellen chart Visual fields: confrontation, tangent screen, perimeter	Retinal ganglion cells	Optic nerves Optic chiasm Optic tracts	Somatic special Vision	
III Oculomotor	Upward, downward, medial eye movement	Eye movement	Nucleus 3	Oculomotor nerve		Somatic Extraocular muscles Levator palpebrae Superior rectus Medial rectus Inferior rectus Inferior oblique
	Lid elevation	Lid movement				
	Pupil constriction	Pupillary response to light and accommodation	Edinger-Westphal nucleus	Oculomotor nerve Ciliary ganglion Ciliary nerves		Visceral general Intrinsic eye muscles, iris,

Cranial Nerve	Function	Assessment	Nucleus	Nerve/Branch	Component	Type
IV Trochlear	Downward, medial eye movement	Eye movement	Nucleus 4	Trochlear nerve		Somatic — Superior oblique muscle
V Trigeminal	Sensory: Face, Scalp	Corneal reflex, Sensation of face	Gasserian ganglion	Opthalmic nerve, Maxillary nerve, Mandibular nerve	Somatic general — Sensory: Anterior half of scalp, Face, Buccal mucosa, Anterior two thirds of tongue, Dura, anterior, and middle fossa; Proprioception: Muscles of mastication	
	Jaw muscles		Mesencephalic Nucleus 5	Motor root		
	Motor: Masseter muscle, Temporal muscle, Diagastric muscle	Muscle strength of masseter and temporal muscles; muscles palpated with jaw clenched	Motor nucleus 5	Motor root		Visceral special — Muscles for mastication
VI Abducens	Lateral eye movement	Eye movement	Nucleus 6	Abducens nerve		Somatic — Lateral rectus
VII Facial	Sensory: External ear	Sensation	Geniculate ganglion	Intermediate nerve, Ramus of vagus nerve	Somatic general	
	Taste: anterior two thirds of tongue	Taste: sweet, salty, sour	Geniculate ganglion	Intermediate nerve, Chorda tympani nerve, Lingual nerve	Visceral special	
	Deep facial	Sensation, deep facial		Intermediate nerve	Visceral general	
	Motor: Facial movement, Scalp muscle, Auricular muscle, Stylohyoid muscle, Digastric posterior belly	Corneal reflex, Facial movement: client frowns, wrinkles forehead, shows teeth	Motor nucleus 7	Temporofacial branch, Cervicofacial branch	Visceral special	
	Salivation: submaxillary glands, sublingual glands		Superior salivary nucleus	Intermediate nerve, Chorda tympani nerve, Lingual nerve	Visceral general	

Continued.

Table 20-4. The cranial nerves—cont'd

Nerve	Function	Clinical test	Cells of origin	Major components	Afferent	Efferent
	Lacrimation: lacrimal glands, Mucous membrane, Nasopharynx		Superior salivary nucleus	Submaxillary ganglion, Intermediate nerve, Petrossal nerve, Sphenopalatine ganglion		Visceral general
VIII Acoustic	Vestibular		Vestibular ganglion	Vestibular nerve	Somatic special	
	Hearing	Audiometry	Spiral ganglion of cochlea	Cochlear nerve	Somatic special	
IX Glossopharyngeal	Sensory, External ear (part)		Superior ganglion	Ramus of vagus nerve	Somatic general	
	Taste: posterior one third of tongue	Taste: sweet, salty, sour	Petrosal ganglion		Visceral special	
	Carotid: reflexes, baroreceptors and chemoreceptors, sinus, body			Carotid sinus nerve	Visceral special	
	Motor					
	Pharynx: gag reflex, swallowing, pharyngeal muscles	Gag test: give drink; watch swallow	Petrosal ganglion, Nucleus ambiguus	Pharyngeal branch, Lingual branch, Pharyngeal plexus		Visceral special, Visceral special
	Parotid gland: salivation		Inferior salivatory nucleus	Tympanic nerve, Petrossal nerve		Visceral general
X Vagus	Sensory, External ear (part), Pharynx, Thoracic and abdominal viscera, Aortic arch, Chemoreceptors, Baroreceptors		Jugular ganglion, Nodose ganglion		Somatic general, Visceral general	
				Carotid sinus nerve	Visceral special	
	Motor					
	Swallowing, gag reflex		Nucleus ambiguus	Pharyngeal plexus		Visceral special
	Phonation	Observe speech		Laryngeal nerves		Visceral special
	Cardiac slowing		Dorsal motor nucleus 10			Visceral general

	Type	Function	Assessment	Nucleus/Origin	Root
	Visceral general	Bronchioconstriction			
	Visceral general	Gastric secretion			
	Visceral general	Peristalsis			
		Motor			
	Visceral special	Swallowing: pharyngeal muscles	Give drink; watch swallow	Nucleus ambiguus	Cranial root
XI Accessory	Visceral special	Turning of head: stenocleidomastoid muscles	Client turns head against resistance	Ventral horn C2	Spinal root
	Visceral special	Elevation of shoulders: trapezius muscles	Client shrugs shoulders against resistance	Ventral horn C3, 4	Ventral root branch / Ventral root branch
		Motor			
XII Hypoglossal	Somatic	Muscles that move tongue: hypoglossus, genioglossus, styloglossus	Client sticks out tongue, moves tongue from side to side; Observe speech	Nucleus 12	Hypoglossal nerve

■ Proprioception and cerebellar function

The proprioceptive system of the nervous system maintains posture, balance, and other acts of coordination. The neural structures that are involved in proprioception are the posterior columns (gracilis and cuneatus) of the spinal cord, the cerebellum, and the vestibular apparatus. The posterior columns carry stimuli from the proprioceptors in muscle tendons and joints. The posterior columns also carry fibers for touch sensation and two-point discrimination. Deficit of function of the posterior column results in impairment of muscle and position sense. Clients with such an impairment are often observed to be watching their own arm and leg movements so as to know the position of the limbs from these visual cues.

The cerebellum functions primarily in the integration of muscle contractions for the maintenance of posture. Loss of cerebellar function results in dyssynergia (impairment of muscle coordination or of the ability to perform movements smoothly), intention tremor, or hypotonia.

Abnormalities of muscle tone, gait, speech, and nystagmus in lateral gaze may also indicate cerebellar dysfunction.

The vestibular system is concerned with righting movements. Vestibular disease is characterized by vertigo. A subjective phenomenon, vertigo is the illusion of movement of the individual or his environment. Nausea and vomiting frequently accompany vertigo. Nystagmus is also frequently associated with vertigo and may be vertical, horizontal, or rotary.

Ataxia is the impairment of position sense. Ataxia is more severe if visual images are excluded in posterior column disease but not in cerebellar dysfunction.

The client with a *cerebellar gait* walks with a wide base; the trunk and head are held rigidly; the legs bend at the hips; arm movements are not coordinated with the stride; the client lurches and reels, frequently falling.

The client with *cerebellar speech* has slow, hesitant, or dysarthric verbalization.

Jerking movements are noted in the client with a *cerebellar sitting posture* as the client attempts to maintain balance.

The client with proprioceptive or cerebellar dysfunction may experience difficulty with the following tests of posture maintenance or coordination.

The client is asked to pat his knees with the palms of the hands followed by the backs of the hands at an ever increasing rate. The client with cerebellar disease has difficulty with rapid patting as well as supination-pronation changes. Clumsiness of movement and irregular timing are characteristic of affected individuals.

The client is asked to touch his nose with the index finger of first one hand and then the other with the eyes closed (Fig. 20-10). The client is then asked to repeat this activity several times while alternating hands and gradually increasing the speed with which he does it.

The client may be asked to touch his nose and then the examiner's finger at a distance of about 18 inches (Fig. 20-11). This maneuver is also repeated with increasing speed.

The client is asked to touch each finger of one hand to the thumb of the same hand as rapidly as possible (Fig. 20-12).

The client is asked to run the heel of each foot down the opposite shin (Fig. 20-13).

The client may be asked to draw a figure eight in the air while lying on his back.

While lying on his back, the client is asked to

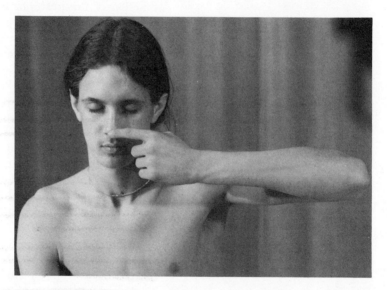

Fig. 20-10. Test of the proprioceptive system. The client is asked to alternately touch his nose with the tip of the index finger of each hand, repeating the motion with increasing speed.

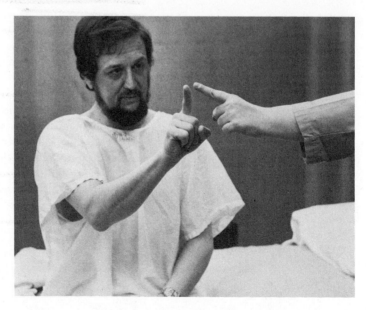

Fig. 20-11. Test of the proprioceptive system. The client is asked to touch his nose with an index finger and then to touch the examiner's index finger (at a distance of about 18 inches), repeating the motion with increasing speed.

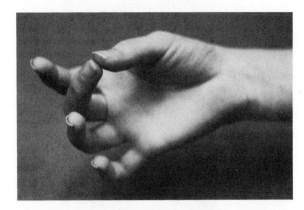

Fig. 20-12. Test of the proprioceptive system. The client is asked to touch each finger of one hand to the thumb of the same hand as rapidly as possible.

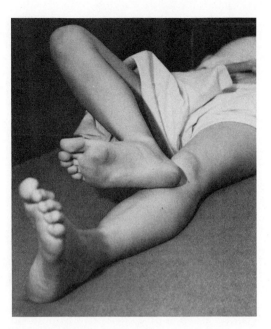

Fig. 20-13. Test of the proprioceptive system. The client is asked to run the heel of each foot down the opposite shin.

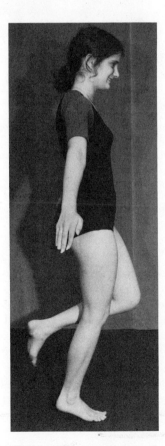

Fig. 20-14. Test of the proprioceptive system. The client who has demonstrated Romberg's sign is asked to hop in place on one foot and then the other.

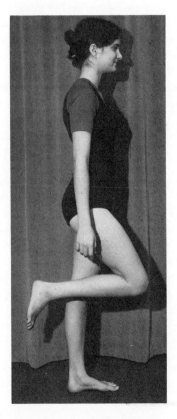

Fig. 20-15. Test of the proprioceptive system. The client is asked to stand on one foot and then the other. The normal individual is able to do this for about 5 seconds with the eyes closed.

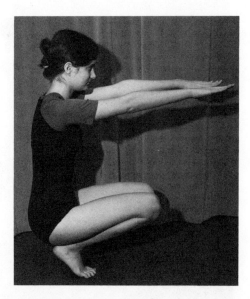

Fig. 20-16. Test of the proprioceptive system. The client is asked to do a knee bend without support.

touch the ball of each foot to the examiner's hand.

Romberg test. The client is asked to stand with his feet together, first with his eyes closed and then with them open, and is evaluated for swaying movement. Some swaying is normal. The client who demonstrates Romberg's sign is asked to hop in place on one foot and then the other (Fig. 20-14).

Gait is assessed as the client walks with his eyes closed and then with them open.

The client is asked to stand on one foot and then the other. The normal client is able to do this for about 5 seconds with his eyes closed (Fig. 20-15).

The client who is reasonably steady may be asked to do a knee bend from a standing position without support (Fig. 20-16).

The client is asked to walk a straight line, placing the heel of the leading foot against the toe of the other foot (Fig. 20-17).

The client is asked to pull against the resistance of the examiner's hands, and the client's hands are released without warning. The client with cerebellar disease may have difficulty in starting and stopping movement. Thus, there may be excessive after movement or rebound, so that the client hits himself.

DEFINITIONS

decomposition of movement Movements smoothly coordinated in the normal individual are performed in several parts.

dysdiadochokinesia Disturbance in the ability to stop

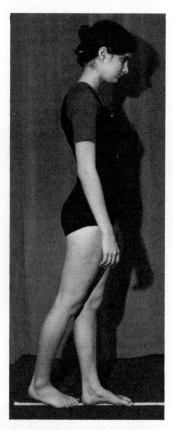

Fig. 20-17. Test of the proprioceptive system. The client is asked to walk a straight line.

one movement and follow it by the opposite action, such as supination and pronation of hands.

dysmetria Disturbance in the ability to stop a movement.

These definitions may be helpful in recording signs observed in cerebellar or proprioceptive dysfunction.

■ Sensory function

The equipment needed for sensory testing includes a cotton wisp or soft brush, a safety pin, test tubes for cold and warm water, a tuning fork, and calipers or a compass with dull points.

Although it is not necessary to evaluate sensation over the entire skin surface, stimuli should be applied strategically so that the dermatomes and major peripheral nerves are tested. A minimal number of test sites would include areas on the forehead, cheek, hand, lower arm, abdomen, foot, and lower leg.

As a general rule, the more distal area of the limb is checked first. In the screening examination the nerve may be assumed to be intact if sensation is normal at its most peripheral extent.

Table 20-5. Proprioceptive dysfunction: signs and symptoms

Cerebellar dysfunction	
Ataxia not made worse in darkness or with eyes closed	Dysmetria
	Dysdiadochokinesia
	Scanning speech
Clumsiness	Hypotonia
Poor coordination	Asthenia
Decomposition of movement	Tremor
	Nystagmus

Posterior column dysfunction	
Ataxia made worse in darkness or with eyes closed	Astereognosis
	Loss of two-point discrimination
Positive Romberg's sign	
Inability to recognize limb position	Loss of vibratory sensation

Vestibular dysfunction	
Nystagmus; may cause deviation of eyes to one side	Nausea
	Vomiting
	Ataxia

If evidence of dysfunction is found, the site of the dysfunction must be localized and mapped. This means determining the boundaries of the loss of sensation. A lucid method of recording would include a sketch of the region involved and a description of the sensory change.

The intensity of the stimulus is kept to a minimal level on initial application. Gradual increases in magnitude may be made until the client is aware of the stimulus.

Variation in sensitivity of skin areas is seen in the normal client, so that a stronger stimulus is required over the back, the buttocks, and areas where the skin is heavily cornified. Symmetry of sensation is established by checking first one spot and then its mirror image area.

The client's eyes should be closed during evaluation of sensory modalities. The visual cuing that occurs when the client is able to see the examiner apply the stimulus may lead to false positive responses in the client who is highly sensitive to suggestion.

Spurious results to sensory testing are risked when either the client or the examiner is fatigued. Inattention to instruction or lack of motivation may lead to an impression of sensory loss.

The examiner should avoid predictable patterns in applying the stimulus. That is, the examiner should vary testing sites and timing so that the client cannot predict the response he is expected to give.

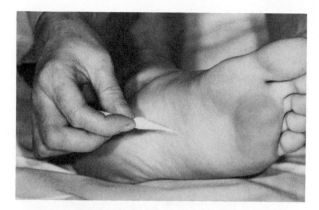

Fig. 20-18. Test of sensation of light touch using a wisp of cotton applied firmly enough to stimulate the sensory nerve endings but not so much that the skin is indented.

DEFINITIONS

anesthesia Absence of touch sensation.
hyperesthesia Greater than normal sensation to touch stimuli.
hypoesthesia Less than normal sensation to touch stimuli.
paresthesia Abnormal or perverted sensation; may include burning, itching, pain, or the feel of an electric shock.

The above definitions may be helpful in recording sensory dysfunction.

Light touch sensation

Light touch and deep touch are mediated by different nerve endings. Sensory fibers for simple touch enter the cord and travel upward before crossing to enter the anterior spinothalamic tract to the thalamus. Light touch is the sensory system that is least often obtunded. Both anterior spinothalamic tracts must suffer destruction before light touch is lost.

Light touch is tested by touching the skin with a wisp of cotton (Fig. 20-18) or a soft brush (Fig. 20-19). Pressure is applied in such a way that sensation is stimulated but not enough to perceptibly depress the skin. The client is instructed to say, "Yes," or "Now," when he feels his skin being touched. The hair of the skin should be avoided when testing for touch sensation in the skin. The follicles are innervated with sensory fibers that are stimulated by movement of the hair. Instances of distortion of sensation or anesthesia are recorded.

Tactile localization (point localization). The client is asked to point to the spot where he was touched.

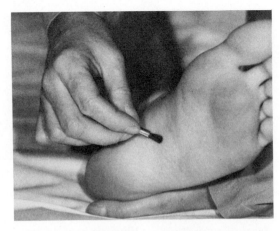

Fig. 20-19. Test of light touch sensation using a soft brush.

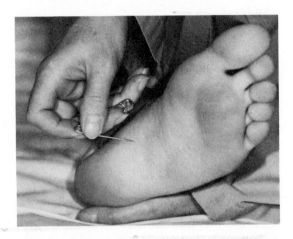

Fig. 20-20. Evaluation for superficial pain using the sharp point of a safety pin.

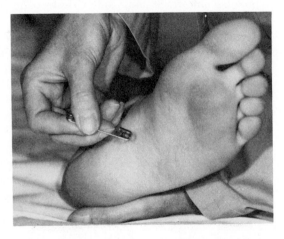

Fig. 20-21. Alternate use of the dull end of the pin for evaluation of pain.

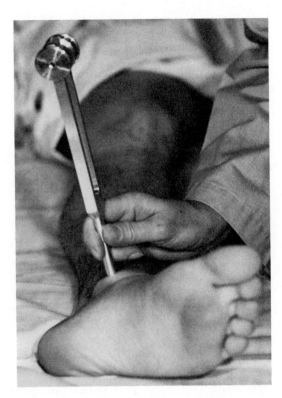

Fig. 20-22. Test of sensitivity to vibration. The base of the vibrating tuning fork is applied to bony prominences such as the sternum, elbow, or ankle.

Pain sensation

Pain and temperature fibers both travel in the dorsolateral fasciculus for a short distance, after which they cross and continue to the thalamus in the lateral spinothalamic tract.

Superficial pain. The evaluation of the sensory perception of superficial pain is conducted through the use of the sharp and dull points of a safety pin (Figs. 20-20 and 20-21). The client is asked to say, "Sharp," "Dull," or "Can't tell," when he feels the pin touch his skin. At least 2 seconds should be allowed between successive tests to avoid summation effects (several successive stimuli perceived as one). Pain sensation may be lost in the presence of lesions of the tegmentum of the brain stem.

Deep pressure. Deep pressure is tested over the eyeball, Achilles tendon, forearm, and calf muscles.

Temperature

In the screening examination, temperature assessment is not done when pain sensation is found to be within normal limits. When it is done, the stimuli are tubes filled with warm and

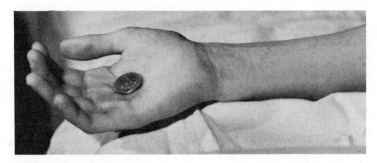

Fig. 20-23. Test for stereognosis. The normal client can discriminate a familiar object (coin, key) by touching and manipulating it.

cold water that are rolled against the skin sites to be tested. The client is asked to say, "Hot," "Cold," or "Can't tell." The tubes are applied to a sufficient number of areas to ascertain that all dermatomes are included.

Vibration

The normal client is able to distinguish vibration when the base of a vibrating tuning fork is applied to a bony prominence such as the sternum, elbow, or ankle. The client perceives the vibration as a buzzing or tingling sensation.

The greatest sensitivity to vibration is seen when the tuning fork is vibrating between 200 and 400 cycles per second. A large tuning fork is suggested since the decay of vibration occurs more slowly in the larger instrument.

The vibrating tuning fork may be applied to the clavicles, spinous processes, elbows, finger joints, knees, ankles, and toes (Fig. 20-22). The client is asked to say, "Yes," or "Now" (1) when he first feels the vibrations and (2) when the vibrations stop.

Vibratory sensation is diminished in the older client (after 65 years of age), particularly in the extremities.

Tactile discrimination

Tactile discrimination requires cortical integration. Three types of tactile discrimination that are tested clinically include: (1) stereognosis, (2) two-point discrimination, and (3) extinction. Afferent fibers for vibration, proprioception, and stereognosis are found to take one of three courses after entering the spinal cord: they (1) synapse immediately with motor cells to form a reflex arc, (2) run superiorly in the dorsal column to the cerebellum, or (3) travel in dorsal columns to the medulla and cross-run to the thalamus.

Stereognosis. Stereognosis is the act of recognizing objects on the basis of touching and ma-

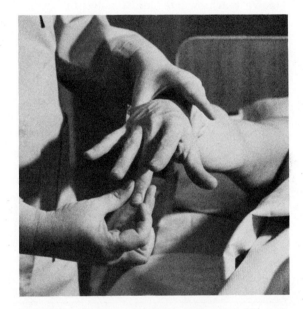

Fig. 20-24. Test of kinesthetic sensation. The normal client can discriminate the position of his body parts. With the client's eyes closed, the examiner changes the position of a finger. The client describes how the position was changed.

nipulating them. This is a function of the parietal lobes of the cerebral cortex. Objects used to test stereognosis should be universally familiar items, such as a key or coin. (Fig. 20-23).

Two-point discrimination. Two-point discrimination is defined as the ability to sense whether one or two areas of the skin are being stimulated by pressure. This may be done with pins. One pin is held in each hand and applied to the skin simultaneously. The client is asked to say if he feels one or two pin pricks. This determination may also be accomplished using calipers or a compass with dull points.

In the adult client there is considerable variability of perceptual ability over the different parts of the body. The following are exemplary of normal adult values:

Tongue: 1 mm
Fingertips: 2.8 mm
Palms of hand: 8 to 12 mm
Chest, forearms: 40 mm
Back: 40 to 70 mm
Upper arms, thighs: 75 mm
Toes: 3 to 8 mm

Extinction. The normal client, when touched in corresponding areas on both sides of the body, perceives touch in both areas. The failure to perceive touch on one side is called the extinction phenomenon. Impairment of the extinction phenomenon is frequently noted in lesions of the sensory cortex.

Kinesthetic sensation

Kinesthetic sensation is that facilitated by proprioceptive receptors in the muscles, tendons, and joints. Perception of the position, orientation, and motion of limbs and body parts is obtained from kinesthetic sensations.

With the client's eyes closed, the examiner changes the position of one finger of the client's hand. The client is asked to describe how the position of the finger was changed. The finger is always moved to a neutral position before it is moved again (Fig. 20-24). This procedure may be done for any joint.

Graphesthesia

The normal client can discern the identity of letters or numbers inscribed on the palm of the hand, back, or other areas with a blunt object.

Patterns of sensory loss

Loss of discriminatory sensation may indicate a lesion of the posterior columns or sensory cortex. Bilateral sensory loss in both lower extremities suggests a peripheral neuropathy, such as diabetic neuropathy. Frequently the pattern of sensory loss is useful in establishing a diagnosis. Some common patterns of sensory deficit are described in Table 20-6.

Sensory loss resulting from disease in a single peripheral nerve may be mapped over the skin surface distribution of that nerve. The nerves most commonly involved in disease include the medial, radial, ulnar, sciatic, femoral, and peroneal nerves. The examiner should be knowledgeable of the sensory, motor, and reflex distribution of these and other major nerves (Fig. 20-25). Body surface projections of the major nerves are seen in Fig. 20-26.

Pathophysiological conditions involving the dorsal root may result in sensory loss distributed

Table 20-6. Patterns of sensory loss

Pathological involvement	Common etiology	Characteristics
Peripheral nerve	Metabolic disorders, such as diabetes or nutritional deficiencies	Peripheral structures more frequently involved—"glove and stocking" involvement—may involve all sensory modalities
Specific peripheral nerve or root	Trauma Vascular occlusion	May map area of sensory loss specific to area innervated by the nerve and distal to the pathological lesion
Dorsal root		Loss of sensation in the segmented distribution (dermatome)
Spinal cord—hemisection (Brown-Séquard syndrome)	Trauma Medullary lesion Extramedullary lesion	Loss of pain and temperature perception on contralateral side, one or two segments below the lesion Loss of position sense, two-point discrimination, and vibratory sensation on ipsilateral side below the lesion
Brain stem	Trauma Neoplasm Vascular occlusion	Loss of pain and temperature sensation on contralateral side of body, ipsilateral side of face
Thalamus	Trauma Neoplasm Vascular occlusion	Loss of sensory modalities on contralateral side of body
Cortex—lesions of post-cortical cortex	Trauma Neoplasm Vascular occlusion	Loss of discriminatory sensation on contralateral side of body Loss of position sense, two-point discrimination, or stereognosis

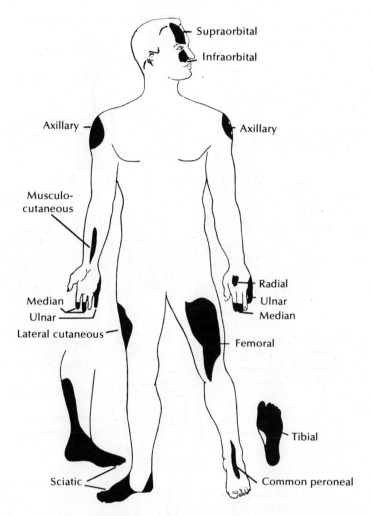

Fig. 20-25. Areas of sensory loss from peripheral nerve lesions. (From Prior, J. A., and Silberstein, J. S.: Physical diagnosis; the history and examination of the patient, ed. 4, St. Louis, 1973, The C. V. Mosby Co.)

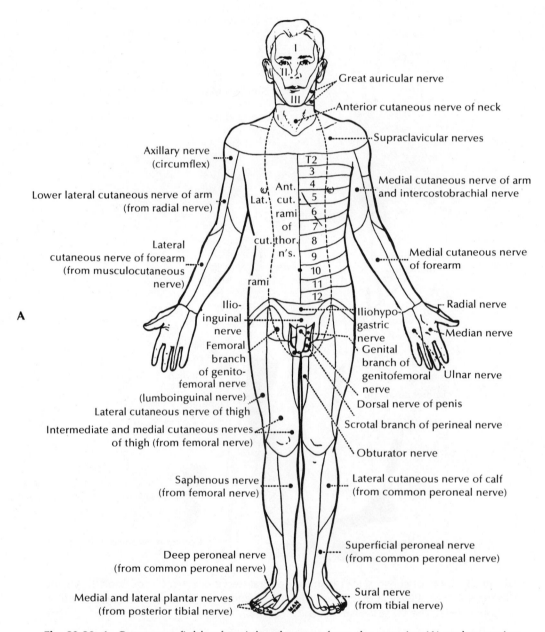

Great auricular nerve

Anterior cutaneous nerve of neck

Supraclavicular nerves

Axillary nerve
(circumflex)

Medial cutaneous nerve of arm
and intercostobrachial nerve

Lower lateral cutaneous nerve of arm
(from radial nerve)

Lateral
cutaneous nerve of forearm
(from musculocutaneous
nerve)

Medial cutaneous nerve
of forearm

Ilio-
inguinal
nerve

Iliohypo-
gastric
nerve

Radial nerve

Median nerve

Femoral
branch
of genito-
femoral nerve
(lumboinguinal nerve)

Genital
branch of
genitofemoral
nerve

Ulnar nerve

Lateral cutaneous nerve of thigh

Dorsal nerve of penis

Intermediate and medial cutaneous nerves
of thigh (from femoral nerve)

Scrotal branch of perineal nerve

Obturator nerve

Saphenous nerve
(from femoral nerve)

Lateral cutaneous nerve of calf
(from common peroneal nerve)

Superficial peroneal nerve
(from common peroneal nerve)

Deep peroneal nerve
(from common peroneal nerve)

Sural nerve
(from tibial nerve)

Medial and lateral plantar nerves
(from posterior tibial nerve)

Ant.
Lat. cut.
rami
of
cut. thor.
n's.

rami

T2
3
4
5
6
7
8
9
10
11
12

I
II
III

A

Fig. 20-26. A, Cutaneous fields of peripheral nerves from the anterior **(A)** and posterior **(B)** aspects. (From Haymaker, W., and Woodhall, B.: Peripheral nerve injuries, ed. 2, Philadelphia, 1959, W. B. Saunders Co.)

404

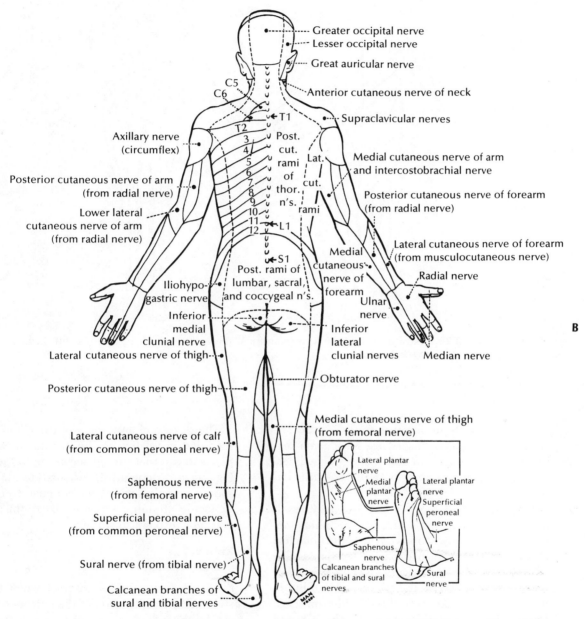

Greater occipital nerve
Lesser occipital nerve
Great auricular nerve
Anterior cutaneous nerve of neck
Supraclavicular nerves

C5
C6
T1
T2
3
4
5
6
7
8
9
10
11
12
L1
S1

Post. cut. rami of thor. n's.

Lat. cut. rami

Axillary nerve (circumflex)

Medial cutaneous nerve of arm and intercostobrachial nerve

Posterior cutaneous nerve of arm (from radial nerve)

Posterior cutaneous nerve of forearm (from radial nerve)

Lower lateral cutaneous nerve of arm (from radial nerve)

Lateral cutaneous nerve of forearm (from musculocutaneous nerve)

Medial cutaneous nerve of forearm

Radial nerve

Post. rami of lumbar, sacral, and coccygeal n's.

Iliohypogastric nerve

Ulnar nerve

Inferior medial clunial nerve

Inferior lateral clunial nerves

Lateral cutaneous nerve of thigh

Median nerve

Obturator nerve

Posterior cutaneous nerve of thigh

Medial cutaneous nerve of thigh (from femoral nerve)

Lateral cutaneous nerve of calf (from common peroneal nerve)

Lateral plantar nerve
Medial plantar nerve

Lateral plantar nerve
Superficial peroneal nerve

Saphenous nerve (from femoral nerve)

Superficial peroneal nerve (from common peroneal nerve)

Sural nerve (from tibial nerve)

Saphenous nerve
Calcanean branches of tibial and sural nerves

Sural nerve

Calcanean branches of sural and tibial nerves

B

Fig. 20-26, cont'd. For legend see opposite page.

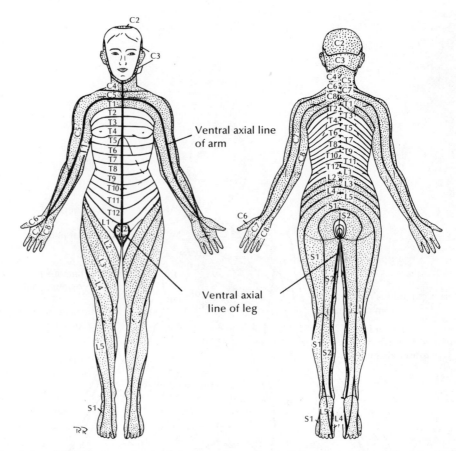

Fig. 20-27. Distribution of spinal dermatomes. (From Keegan, J. J., and Garrett, F. D.: Anat. Rec. **102**:411, 1948.)

over the dermatome for that root (Fig. 20-27). Clear description of sensory loss for a given segment may be difficult to obtain since a good deal of sensory overlap occurs between the distribution of one root and another.

Both nerve and root sensory loss may result from disease involving a plexus. This phenomenon is frequently observed for the brachial plexus. Superior brachial plexus lesions involve C5 and 6, resulting in sensory loss in the shoulder and in the lateral arm and forearm. In addition, there may be weakness of the shoulder muscles. Inferior brachial plexus lesions involve C8 and T1, resulting in sensory loss of the medial surface of the arm and in weakness of the arm muscles.

Pathophysiological conditions of the thalamo-cortical fibers on the cortex result in a loss of those cortical integrating functions (kinesthesis, two-point discrimination, stereognosis). Cortical mapping of the brain is seen in Fig. 20-28. Gross perceptions of vibration, pain, temperature, and crude touch may be retained.

The degree of awareness of the client is often recorded in relation to the manner in which he reacts to external stimuli according to the following: alert, cooperative, orientation intact, responds to spoken words and commands, responds to tactile stimuli, responds to painful stimuli, does not respond to stimuli.

■ **Reflexes**

Deep tendon reflex

The skeletal muscles contract when they are stretched by contraction of the antagonistic muscle, by the pull of gravity, or by external manipulation. The muscles will also contract when their tendons are stretched. These principles form the basis for an understanding of the deep tendon reflex (DTR). Afferent fibers for the reflex arise from both the muscle itself and the tendon.

Muscle spindles or fusiform capsules have been identified in abundance in skeletal muscles, particularly in antigravity muscles. The spindles are capsules surrounding two to ten specialized mus-

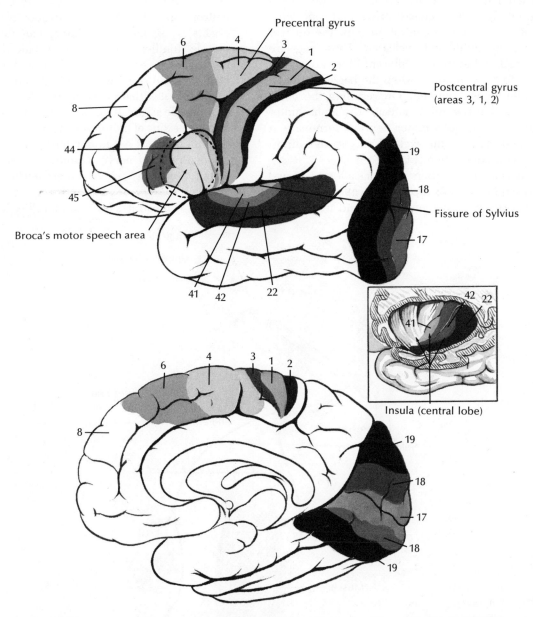

Fig. 20-28. Map of the human cortex. Identity of each numbered area is determined by structural differences in the neurons that compose it. Some areas whose functions are best understood are the following: areas *3, 1,* and *2,* somatic sensory areas; area *4,* primary motor area; area *6,* secondary motor area; area *17,* primary visual area; areas *18* and *19,* secondary visual areas; areas *41* and *42,* primary auditory areas; area *22,* secondary auditory area. Area *44* and the posterior part of area *45* constitute the approximate location of Broca's motor speech area. (From Anthony, C. P., and Kolthoff, N. J., Textbook of anatomy and physiology, ed. 9, St. Louis, 1975, The C. V. Mosby Co. Modified from Brodmann, K.: Feinere Anatomie des Grosshirns. In Handbuch der Neurologie, Berlin, 1910, Springer-Verlag.)

cle cells known as intrafusal fibers; these spindles are parallel with surrounding muscles and are attached to them by connective tissue. Both ends of the intrafusal fiber consist of striated contractile tissue, whereas the central portion, the nuclear bag, is expanded and nucleated. These bags are innervated, but primary afferent fibers are stimulated to carry impulses when the bag is stretched or otherwise deformed. On reaching the cord, these action potentials activate the alpha motor neurons. The alpha motor neurons terminate at the end-plates of the skeletal muscle and stimulate their contraction (Fig. 20-29).

Afferent nerve fibers (gamma afferent fibers) encased in a fibrous capsule are called Golgi tendon organs or tendon end-organs and are found in the tendons of skeletal muscles. Stretching of the muscle deforms and activates these afferent nerves, which end on and inhibit the alpha motor neurons. The threshold for activation of the Golgi organs is significantly greater than that of the muscle spindles, and these organs are thought to modulate excessive stretching through inhibition of the muscle spindle (autoinhibition).

Another cell that may inhibit reflex contraction of a muscle is the Renshaw cell, an interneuron between axons of motor nerves. The full nature of this inhibition is not understood.

Golgi efferent nerves terminate in the muscle spindles and may regulate their sensitivity.

Using patellar tendon reflex as an example, Fig. 20-30 illustrates the tendon reflex. The patel-

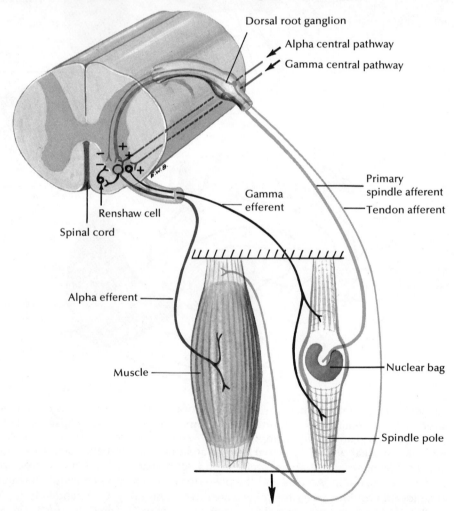

Fig. 20-29. Neural basis for the stretch reflex. Afferent fibers from muscle spindle and tendon organs and efferent fibers to muscle and spindle (gamma fibers) are shown. Excitation is indicated by plus signs, inhibition by minus signs. The Renshaw cell is an interneuron that provides recurrent inhibition to the active motoneuron pool. Muscle rigidly is fixed at the upper end and subject to stretch in the direction of the arrow at the lower end. (From Schottelius, B. A., and Schottelius, D. D.: Textbook of physiology, ed. 17, St. Louis, 1973, The C. V. Mosby Co.)

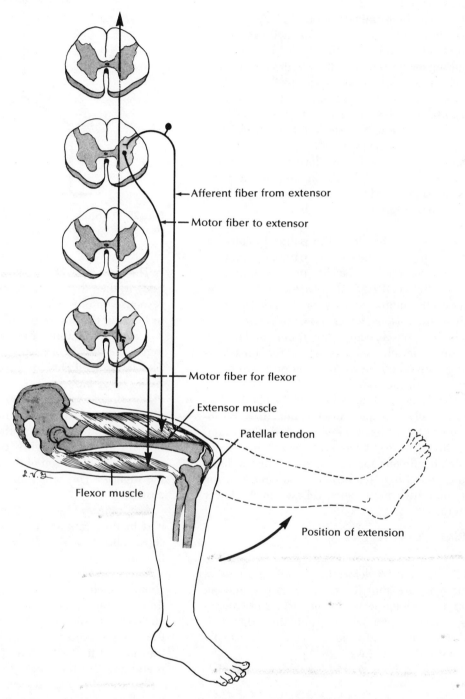

Afferent fiber from extensor

Motor fiber to extensor

Motor fiber for flexor

Extensor muscle

Patellar tendon

Flexor muscle

Position of extension

Fig. 20-30. Tendon reflex (knee jerk or patellar tendon reflex). Note that the patellar tendon of the extensor muscle is attached to the tibia below the knee. (From Schottelius, B. A., and Schottelius, D. D.: Textbook of physiology, ed. 17, St. Louis, 1973, The C. V. Mosby Co.)

lar tendon of the quadriceps muscle, an extensor muscle of the upper leg, is attached to the tibia. Deforming this tendon with a reflex hammer causes the muscle to be stretched, activating the muscle spindles, and thereby the primary afferent nerve, in terminating on the alpha motor nerve in the cord segment (L3 and 4). The action potential thus stimulates the alpha efferent fibers, resulting in shortening of the quadriceps muscle, which pulls up the tibia to extend the leg. Dysfunction of the tendon reflex, then, could be attributable to lesions of the afferent or efferent arc of the nerve or to lesions of the muscle, tendon, or spinal segment involved.

Assessment of the DTRs allows the examiner to obtain information about the function of the reflex arcs and spinal cord segments without implicating other cord segments or higher neural structures.

Reflexes may be altered in pathophysiological changes involving the sensory pathways from the tendons and muscles or the motor component, that is, the corticospinal or corticobulbar pathways (upper motor neuron), or the anterior horn cells or their axons (lower motor neuron).

The best muscle contraction is obtained in testing deep muscle tendons when the muscle is slightly stretched before the tendon is stretched (tapped with the reflex hammer).

Augmentation of the reflex may be obtained by isometrically tensing muscles not directly involved in the reflex arc being tested. For example, the client may be asked to clench his fists or to lock his fingers together and to pull one hand against the other (Jendrassik's maneuver) as the examiner attempts to elicit reflexes in the lower extremity.

Elicitation of reflexes

Three categories of reflexes are described: (1) DTRs, elicited by deforming (tapping) a tendon (synonyms are muscle stretch reflexes, muscle jerks, and tendon jerks); (2) superficial or cutaneous reflexes, obtained by stimulating the skin; and (3) pathological reflexes, which are usually present only in disease.

Reflexes may be graded for the record as follows:

4⁺ or ++++	Brisk, hyperactive, clonus
3⁺ or +++	More brisk than normal, not necessarily indicative of disease
2⁺ or ++	Normal
1⁺ or +	Low normal, slightly diminished response
0	No response

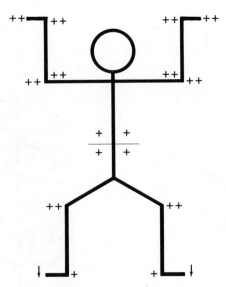

Fig. 20-31. Stick figure drawing for recording reflexes.

The symmetry of the reflex from one side of the body to the other is also recorded. Differences in response on one side of the body may be helpful in locating the site of the lesions.

A succinct method of recording the reflex findings is the stick figure representation (Fig. 20-31). This lends itself well to expression of both amplitude and symmetry.

Jaw closure reflex. The maxillary reflex, or jaw jerk, is elicited by tapping; the examiner's thumb is placed on the midline of the chin but below the lip with the mouth slightly open. The normal response is an elevation of the mandible (closure of the mouth). The reflex may be difficult to demonstrate.

Arm reflexes. Reflexes that are frequently elicited in the arms are the pectoralis, biceps, triceps, and brachioradialis reflexes and finger flexon.

Pectoralis reflex. The arm is held in a position about 6 inches from the body. The examiner's thumb is placed over the tendon while the hand encircles the shoulder. The thumb is struck with the reflex hammer in such a way that the blow is transmitted to the tendon. The normal response is adduction of the arm.

Biceps reflex (Fig. 20-33). The arm is flexed at the elbow. The examiner's thumb is placed over the biceps tendon. The thumb is struck with the reflex hammer with a slight downward thrust in order to augment the tendon stretch. The normal response is flexion of the arm at the elbow.

Triceps reflex (Fig. 20-34). The arm is flexed at the elbow. The triceps tendon is tapped with the

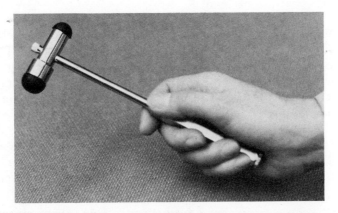

Fig. 20-32. The percussion hammer is held between the thumb and index finger.

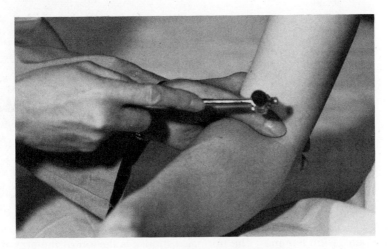

Fig. 20-33. Elicitation of the biceps reflex. A downward blow is struck over the thumb, which is situated over the biceps tendon. The normal response is flexion of the arm at the elbow.

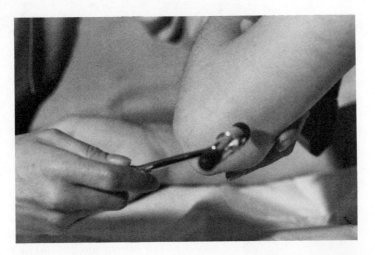

Fig. 20-34. Elicitation of the triceps reflex. With the arm flexed at the elbow, the triceps tendon is tapped with the percussion hammer. The normal response is straightening or extension of the arm.

reflex hammer. The normal response is extension of the arm or straightening.

Brachioradialis reflex (Fig. 20-35). The arm is placed in a relaxed position. The styloid process (body prominence on the thumb side of the wrist) or the radius is dealt a blow with the percussion hammer after palpation for the tendon (may best be elicited 3 to 5 cm above the wrist). The normal response is flexion of the arm at the elbow (pronation, supination) and at the forearm. The fingers of the hand may also flex.

Lower limb reflexes. Reflexes commonly elicited in the lower limb are the patellar, Achilles tendon, and plantar reflexes.

Patellar reflex (Fig. 20-36). The tendon is located directly inferior to the patellar bone or knee cap. With the legs of the client hanging freely over the side of the bed or chair or with the client in a supine position, the tendon is dealt a blow with the percussion hammer. The normal response is extension or kicking out of the leg as the quadraceps muscle contracts.

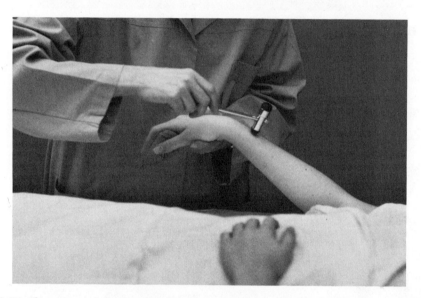

Fig. 20-35. Elicitation of the brachioradialis reflex. The styloid process is dealt a blow with the percussion hammer. The normal response is flexion of the arm at the elbow and slight flexion of the fingers.

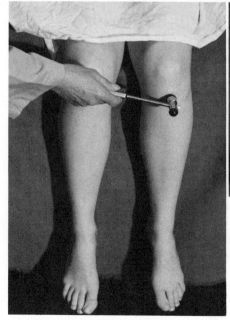

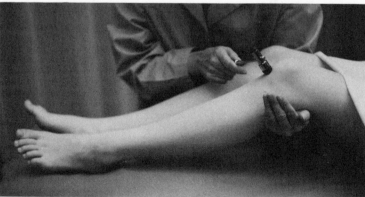

Fig. 20-36. Elicitation of the patellar reflex. With the legs hanging freely over the side of the bed **(A)** or with the client in a supine position **(B)**, a blow with the percussion hammer is dealt directly inferior to the patella. The normal response is extension of the leg or kicking out of the leg.

Achilles tendon reflex (Fig. 20-37). The foot is held in the hand in a slightly dorsiflexed position. The Achilles tendon is delivered a blow with the percussion hammer. The normal response is plantar flexion of the foot.

Plantar reflex (Fig. 20-38). A key, pin, half a tongue blade, an applicator stick, or the handle portion of the reflex hammer may be used to elicit the reflex. The stimulus is applied to the lateral border of the sole, starting at the heel and continuing to the ball of the foot and then proceeding at a right angle over the ball of the foot toward the great toe. The normal response is flexion of all of the toes (Fig. 20-39).

Before the child can walk, fanning and extension of the toes is the normal response.

Babinski's reflex is dorsiflexion of the great toe and fanning of the other toes (Fig. 20-40). Lesions of the pyramidal tract or motor nerves may be present in the client when Babinski's reflex is found.

If the examiner has difficulty in obtaining the plantar response, a similar reflex may be elicited by stimulating the lateral aspect of the dorsum of the foot. *Chaddock's sign* is the name given to a positive response (dorsiflexion of the great toe and fanning of the other toes) to this stimulus.

Other tests for eliciting the plantar response are *Gordon's reflex* (elicited by squeezing the calf muscles), *Oppenheim's reflex* (elicited by moving the thumb and index finger simultaneously and firmly over the tibial surface in a caudal direction) (Fig. 20-41), and *Schäffer's reflex* (elicited by squeezing the Achilles tendon).

Abdominal reflexes. See Chapter 15 on Assessment of the abdomen and rectosigmoid region.

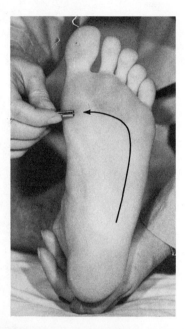

Fig. 20-38. Elicitation of the plantar reflex. A hard object is applied to the lateral surface of the sole, starting at the heel and going over the ball of the foot, ending beneath the great toe.

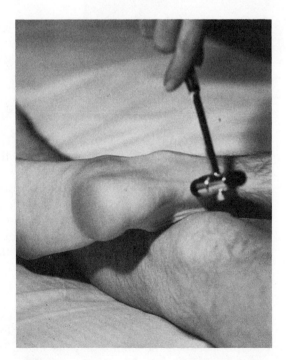

Fig. 20-37. Elicitation of the Achilles tendon reflex. The Achilles tendon is struck with the percussion hammer while the foot is slightly dorsiflexed. The normal response is plantar flexion of the foot.

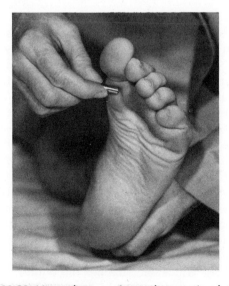

Fig. 20-39. Normal response to plantar stimulation: flexion of all the toes.

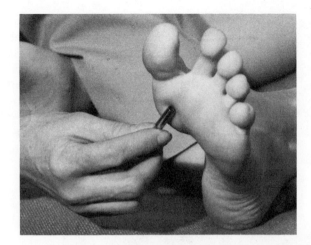

Fig. 20-40. Elicitation of Babinski's reflex: dorsiflexion of the great toe and fanning of the other toes.

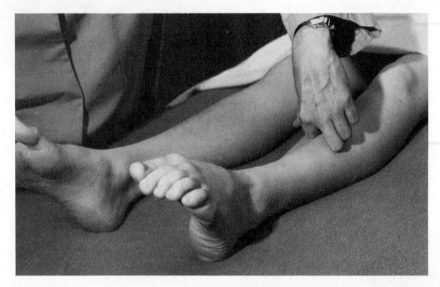

Fig. 20-41. Elicitation of Oppenheim's reflex. Plantar flexion of the toes is obtained by running the index finger and thumb firmly down the tibial surface in a caudal direction.

Cremasteric reflex. The inner thigh is stimulated with a sharp object, such as a key or the stick end of an applicator, or with cold or hot water. The expected response is retraction (elevation) of the testis on the same side, as the cremaster muscle contracts.

Gluteal reflex. The buttocks are spread, and the perianal area is stimulated. The normal response is contraction of the anal sphincter.

Reflexes elicited in disease states

Wartenberg's reflex. The examiner grasps the flexed fingers of the client with his own flexed fingers. Both individuals pull against the other; in doing so, the normal client will extend the thumbs. The individual with upper motor neuron disease will adduct and flex the thumb.

Finger flexor reflex. In *Trommer's method*, the metacarpophalangeal joint of the middle finger is extended (to stretch the flexor tendons). The palmar side of the distal phalanx is flicked by the examiner.

In *Hoffmann's method,* the examiner depresses the distal phalanx and allows it to flip up sharply. A positive response is recorded if flexion of the thumb and other finger is observed. This reflex is normally not elicited. Hoffmann's sign is the name given to the reflex when it is elicited. The presence of a pyramidal lesion may be suspected.

Grasp reflex (Fig. 20-42). The examiner places the index and middle finger in the client's palm, entering between the thumb and the index finger. The examiner's fingers are gently withdrawn, pulling the fingers across the skin of the client's palm. A positive response consists of the client grasping the examiner's fingers. Present in

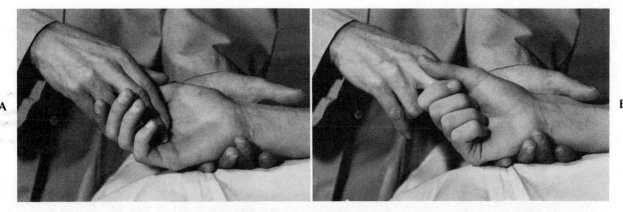

Fig. 20-42. Elicitation of the grasp reflex. **A,** The examiner places the index and middle finger in the client's palm and gently withdraws them. **B,** A positive response consists of the client grasping the examiner's fingers.

Table 20-7. Deep tendon reflex and muscle changes in upper and lower motor neuron lesions

Lesion	Common etiology	Characteristics
Upper motor neuron lesion (corticospinal tract)	Cerebrovascular occlusion	Brisk reflexes
	Neoplasm—cerebral hemispheres	Contralateral arm and leg muscles spasticity—more marked in the flexors in arm and leg extensions
	Amyotrophic lateral sclerosis	Muscle weakness—disuse atrophy
	Deficiency diseases, pernicious anemia	Babinski's sign present; clonus frequently seen
	Trauma	
Lower motor neuron lesion (anterior horn cell, somatic motor part of cranial nerves)	Poliomyelitis	Diminution or absence of deep tendon reflexes
	Amyotrophic lateral sclerosis	Muscle atrophy
	Neoplasm	Muscle weakness, fasciculation of muscle
	Trauma	Babinski's sign—diminished or absent

individuals with widespread brain damage, the grasp reflex is normal in infants less than 4 months of age.

Loss of reflexes

With loss of or diminution of reflexes on the same side, the examiner might suspect corticospinal lesions.

Loss of sensation from a segment (dermatome) coupled with loss of reflexes suggests lesions in the sensory arc. Tabes dorsalis (neurosyphilis) produces this form of disorder.

■ Indications of disease
Early indications of interruptions of the corticospinal tract

The examiner may elicit the *pronation sign* by asking the client to extend his arms at the level of

Table 20-8. Reflexes commonly tested in the physical examination

Reflexes	Segmental level
Deep tendon	
Jaw	Pons
Biceps	Cervical 5, 6
Triceps	Cervical 6, 7, 8
Brachioradialis	Cervical 5, 6
Patellar	Lumbar 3, 4
Achilles	Sacral 2
Superficial	
Corneal	Pons
Palatal	Medulla
Pharyngeal	Medulla
Abdominal (upper)	Thoracic 7, 8, 9
Abdominal (lower)	Thoracic 12, lumbar 1
Cremasteric	Lumbar 1, 2, 3
Gluteal	Lumbar 4, 5

the shoulders with the palms upward (Fig. 20-43). The arm on the affected side will drift downward and pronate.

The examiner may elicit *Barré's sign* by asking the client to flex his knees 90° while in the prone position (Fig. 20-44). The affected leg will move downward.

Fine movements of the hands, such as picking up coins or pencils, are done slowly when there are lesions of the corticospinal tract. The ability to touch the thumb to the fingers is performed less rapidly.

Cortical lesions

Disturbance in the ability to discriminate objects or symbols by means of the senses, assuming the individual previously had this skill, is termed *agnosia. Visual agnosia*, caused by lesions of the

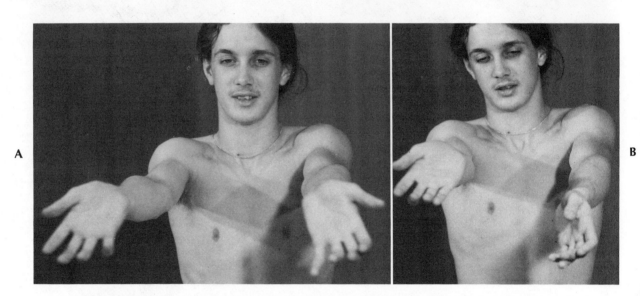

Fig. 20-43. Elicitation of the pronation sign. **A,** The client is asked to extend his arms at shoulder height with the palms upward. **B,** Frequently in disease of the corticospinal tract, the affected arm will drift downward and pronate.

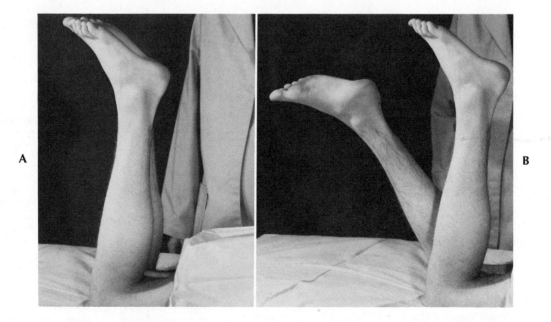

Fig. 20-44. Elicitation of Barré's sign. **A,** The client is asked to lie on his abdomen, flexing the legs at a 90° angle. **B,** Frequently in disease of the corticospinal tract, the affected leg will drift downward.

occipital cortex, is the inability to recognize objects. *Auditory agnosia,* caused by lesions below the sylvian fissure, is the inability to recognize familiar sounds. *Tactile agnosia,* caused by lesions of the parietal lobe, is the inability to recognize objects by feeling them.

A disturbance in the recognition of body parts is termed autotopagnosia.

Lack of insight of an individual to his disease is termed anosognosia.

Lesions of the cerebral hemisphere dominant for language

Aphasia, the inability to comprehend or use language symbols, is caused by a disorder of the cortical areas necessary to speech or by neural connections in the cerebral hemisphere dominant for speech; aphasia encompasses dysarthria and dysphonia. *Nonfluent aphasia* is the inability to produce words in either spoken or written form. The client with *fluent aphasia* has the ability to produce words but frequently chooses inappropriate words *(paraphasia)* or makes errors in content, occasionally creating words.

Lesions of the cerebral hemisphere not dominant for language

A disturbance in the ability to perform a purposeful act when comprehension is intact is termed apraxia. For example, given a fork, the client may be unable to use it to eat; the client may be unable to dress or button his shirt. *Constructional apraxia* is the inability to draw or construct forms of two or three dimensions.

Signs of meningeal irritation

Meningeal irritation is most commonly due to infection or to intracranial hemorrhages. The following signs are indications for laboratory work to confirm the diagnosis.

Nuchal rigidity (stiff neck) is a common sign of meningitis and may be demonstrated through the use of cervical flexing.

Brudzinski's sign (Fig. 20-45) is elicited with the client supine. The head is lifted toward the sternum. The individual with meningeal irritation will resist the movement and may flex the hips and knees. The movement is commonly accompanied by pain.

Kernig's sign is the inability to extend the lower leg when that leg is flexed at the hip, or there may be resistance or pain during the process. Knee extension is usually possible to approximately 135°.

Lasègue's sign (straight leg) is elicited by lifting the leg, supporting it under the heel, in order to maintain extension. A positive sign is pain, resistance, or a decreased angle of flexion of the hip.

Neurological "soft" signs

Signs of possible neurological significance but of unknown cause are called neurological "soft" signs. The following signs are recorded when observed: short attention span; minimal lack of coordination; clumsiness; frequent falling; hyperkinesis, both voluntary and involuntary; uneven perceptual development; incomplete laterality, for example, left handed but right footed, no side

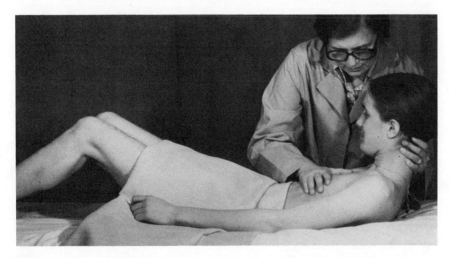

Fig. 20-45. Elicitation of Brudzinski's sign. With meningeal irritation, pain is elicited when the head is flexed.

clearly dominant; language disturbances; articulation disorders; dyslexia; motor outflow (motor movements involving more muscles than intended), and mirroring movements of the extremities, for example, when one hand performs a function, the other is also in motion.

BIBLIOGRAPHY

Alpers, B. J., and Mancall, E. L.: Essentials of the neurological examination, Philadelphia, 1971, F. A. Davis Co.

Caplan, G.: Support systems and community mental health, New York, 1974, Behavioral Publications, Inc.

DeMyer, W.: Technique of the neurologic examination, ed. 2, New York, 1974, McGraw-Hill Book Co.

Dreikurs, R.: Psychodynamics, psychotherapy and counseling, Chicago, 1967, Alfred Adler Institute.

Fieve, R. R., and Dunner, D. L.: Unipolar and bipolar affective states. In Flach, F. F., and Draghi, S. C., editors: The nature and treatment of depression, New York, 1975, John Wiley & Sons, Inc.

Haymaker, W.: Bing's local diagnosis in neurological diseases, ed. 15, St. Louis, 1969, The C. V. Mosby Co.

Kolb, L. C.: Modern clinical psychiatry, ed. 8, Philadelphia, 1976, W. B. Saunders Co.

Mayo Clinic: Clinical examinations in neurology, ed. 3, Philadelphia, 1971, W. B. Saunders Co.

Simpson, J. F., and Magee, K. R.: Clinical evaluation of the nervous system, Boston, 1973, Little, Brown and Co.

Strahl, M. O., and Lewis, N. D., editors: Differential diagnosis in clinical psychiatry, New York, 1972, Science House.

Wartenberg, R.: The examination of reflexes; a simplification, Chicago, 1945, Yearbook Medical Publishers, Inc.

Woodruff, R. A., Goodwin, D. W., and Guze, S. B.: Psychiatric diagnosis, Oxford, 1974, Oxford University Press.

21 Assessment of the pediatric client

Pediatric care is, to a large extent, health care aimed at promoting the health of the child and preventing illness and disability through early identification of problems.

The examination of the child is ideally carried out over an extended period of time in a planned sequential pattern. The dynamic changes that occur in the normal growth and development of the child require the practitioner to carefully assess the increments in growth; the changes in physiological function; and the development of cognitive, social, and motor skills of the child during each examination.

It is by comparing the individual child's current growth achievements and parameters of health with that found in previous examinations and with other normal healthy children that the health of the child is determined. The child should be seen more frequently during infancy, when the growth changes are most rapid and dramatic, and then at less frequent intervals throughout the childhood years.

The examination of the child also gives consideration to the environment in which the child lives and to the parental concerns in child rearing. The adults responsible for the child's care often have concerns about the development of the child and about their own ability to manage. They need respect, support, and guidance that encourages them to express the concerns they may have and to discuss their needs and the needs of the child. The mother is usually the person most familiar with the child and his care and is the one most likely to detect changes, both normal and abnormal, that go unnoticed by others, including the health practitioner. The practitioner should also be alert to any signs of stress between the mother and child. A mother who is concerned, anxious, or angry about a child's behavior or physical condition is showing evidence of stress that may interfere with the mother-child relationship and ultimately with the development of the child. Therefore, consideration is given to the needs of the mother or other adults caring for the child as well as to those of the child himself.

The attitude of the practitioner should always demonstrate respect for both the child and the parent, a willingness to listen to the problems, and a concerned interest in finding adequate solutions. Both the child and the parent will be sensitive to the attitudes of the practitioner and will respond according to the impressions they receive.

In essence, the examiner needs to be sensitive to the child as a growing, developing human being who is ever changing.

This chapter includes a discussion of the approaches to the child and the parent and some of the techniques used in obtaining health information and in assessing the health of the child. In addition, some of the physical differences between the child and the adult are discussed.

It is not possible to include a survey of all the components of child development that are assessed. The reader is referred to standard pediatric texts for assistance in understanding the parameters of health in children.

THE PEDIATRIC HISTORY

The pediatric history provides the opportunity to interview both the child and the parent in order to gather information about the child's health, development, relationships with others, and care. It also provides the opportunity for the child to become acquainted with the practitioner before he is examined. The pediatric history is an adaptation of the model used for an adult history.

It also incorporates areas uniquely pertinent to the child, such as the history of the mother's health during the pregnancy and the history of birth and the neonatal period.

The informant for the history may be a parent, a relative, a caretaker, or the child himself. The interviewer should identify the informant and indicate the reliability of the information obtained. It is common for the child, even the young child, to participate in the interview and to volunteer useful information. The information gained from the child should be indicated in the history.

■ Chief complaint

The chief complaint (CC) statement gives the reason for making the visit and should be in the words of the informant. Children are seen most frequently for health care, and the CC statement may indicate a visit for routine health care rather than for the treatment of a health problem. An example would be "It is time for his checkup."

■ Present illness

The present illness (PI) section incorporates the same categories of information obtained in the adult health history and includes a statement about the usual health, a description of the chronological story, any relevant family history, negative information, and a disability assessment. The following is an example of a history of the present illness of a child brought to the examiner for health care:

This 7-year-old, white female, who is a student in the second grade of the Urban Elementary School, was brought to the clinic by her mother for an annual physical examination. She has been in good health except for occasional colds, approximately four colds, since her visit 1 year ago in July. The child, Debbie, stated that she enjoys school but thinks her teacher "is too hard sometimes." Her mother indicated that all school reports are good and that Debbie has many friends in school and the neighborhood and has recently started "sleeping over" with one or two of her girl friends. The only problem that the mother expressed was in regard to dental care. Debbie has two small cavities, which were found on her first visit to the dentist 2 months ago and the mother is questioning the value of having "baby teeth filled." Debbie has complained of a toothache on only one occasion, just prior to the visit to the dentist. The pain was relieved by giving aspirin, 5 grains.

The PI description in this example is that of a child in good health who is functioning well. The negative information concerning the dental caries gives information that the dental caries are not interfering with the child's ability to function but

that further consideration is necessary to prevent a more serious problem for the child. An attempt should be made to learn the reason for deciding not to continue dental care. The mother may be seeking assurance that she is right in not making a plan for dental care or she may be seeking information that the experience will not be difficult for the child and should be planned. Whatever the outcome, information and support need to be given to help the child and the parent reach a more appropriate decision.

■ Past history

The past history of infants, young children, and any child with a possible developmental deficiency should include the following information:

1. The health of the mother during the pregnancy with this child, including the mother's feelings about the pregnancy, the amount of prenatal care, and any history of complications (excessive weight gain, hypertension, vaginal bleeding, nausea and vomiting, urinary problems, infections such as rubella or venereal disease), and any medications or drugs prescribed or used

2. The birth history, including the date, the hospital where the child was born, the duration of the pregnancy, the parity of the mother, the birth weight, the nature and duration of the labor, the type of delivery, the use of any sedation or anesthesia, the state of the infant at birth, and the use of any special procedures

3. The postnatal history, including information about color, bleeding, seizures, fever, congenital anomalies or birth injuries, difficulty in sucking, rashes, or poor weight gain during the first days and weeks after birth

4. A developmental history, including the age at which the child attained specific developmental achievements (holding the head erect, rolling over, sitting alone, pulling up, walking with help, walking alone, saying first words, using sentences, urinary continence during the day, urinary continence during the night, control of feces), a comparison of this child's development with that of siblings, any periods of decreased or increased growth, the school grade attained, and the quality of school work

5. A history of hospitalizations, serious illnesses, or injuries and dates of occurrence

6. A history of communicable diseases (measles, mumps, pertussis, chickenpox, rheumatic fever), the age at which the disease

occurred, the severity, and any complications

7. A history of immunizations, including booster inoculations and dates
8. A history of allergies to food and drugs and any history of hay fever, asthma, or eczema

Family history

The family history of the child includes questions about familial illnesses or anomalies; the health and age of the grandparents, as well as that of the parents; the age, sex, and health of siblings; and the age at death and the cause of death of immediate members of the family, including a history of stillbirths, miscarriages, and abortions.

Nutritional history

Information about the following items is obtained in the nutritional history:

1. Breast or formula feeding, including the type (if formula), amount, and duration; major changes at the time of weening; and any difficulties
2. Vitamin supplements, including the type, when they were started, the amount, and the duration of time they have been used
3. Solid foods given, including when they were started, how they are given (by spoon or in the bottle), and the types and amount of food
4. The child's appetite, food likes and dislikes, and reaction to eating

Habits and care

The history of habits and care includes a description of the following items:

1. Eating patterns
2. Sleeping habits, including the number of hours and any disturbances, restlessness, or nightmares
3. Play interests and the amount of exercise
4. Urinary and bowel continence and the care given to the child in developing independence and control
5. Medications and drugs given to the child
6. Parental concerns and management of any specific behavior, such as masturbation, thumb-sucking, temper tantrums, or bed-wetting

Social history

The social history gives information about the child's pattern of health care; his place of birth; his placement and progress in school; his relationships with family members, peers, and the important people outside the home; the socioeconomic status of the family; and the marital status of the parents.

Review of systems

The review of systems is essentially the same as that carried out in the adult history.

PHYSICAL EXAMINATION

The physical examination of the infant or child varies according to the age, development, and behavior of the child. The organization is changed to accommodate the individual child. If consideration is not given to the child's age and development, it is likely that the examination will be incomplete.

Approach to the child

When carrying out a pediatric examination, the examiner should keep in mind that each visit for health care is a learning experience for the child. The child's experience may result in increased confidence in himself and others, or the child may experience feelings of failure and distrust in the people who care for him. Thus, it is most productive to provide opportunities for the child to develop positive relationships during the visits for routine health care. It is also important to remember that any separation from the parent may be anxiety provoking and may increase the child's level of fear and distrust. It is therefore important to encourage the parent to participate in the examination in order to support the child. The older child may be able to participate more freely without the parent present. Most parents will recognize the child's developing independence and encourage him to participate by himself. Finally, it is important to prepare the child and parent for any new or painful procedure. This requires the examiner to have a special kind of appreciation for the feelings of children and parents and will result in greater cooperation on the part of the child and parent.

Little difficulty is encountered in the performance of the physical examination of the infant in the first 6 months of life, since the infant has little fear of strangers. The infant often enjoys having his clothing removed and is easily distracted by the parent or the examiner with repetitive vocal sounds and smiles. However, the examination of the ears and mouth may cause distress and should be done as the last part of the examination. It is wise to take advantage of the opportunities that are offered. If the infant is quiet or sleepy, it is best to start with the auscultation of the chest; if the infant is playful and active, it is easier to start with the extremities and wait for a quieter moment to examine the chest.

During the last half of the first year of life, the infant experiences an increasing fear of strangers; thus, it is often profitable to conduct the entire examination while the infant is held on the parent's lap. Even under the best of circumstances, it may not be possible to create a situation that is ideal; the infant may remain resistant throughout the examination. This requires the examiner to be efficient in carrying out the examination in the least amount of time and with the use of minimal restraint of the infant. The parent often experiences discomfort or embarrassment because of the infant's behavior and needs reassurance that the infant is behaving normally. The situation is ideal for helping the parent understand normal development and the needs of the infant at this age.

The child from 1 to 4 years of age is a challenge to even the most experienced examiner. The child is learning to use his body and to manipulate and experiment with all aspects of the environment. Any restraint in the pursuit of his desired activities may be seen by the child as an interference, resulting in unhappiness or frustration for the child. The child at this age is getting lots of pleasure from recently acquired skills such as walking and talking and enjoys his new ability to manipulate objects such as doors and wastebaskets. At the same time, he is still unsure of strangers and needs the parent's presence in order to feel safe. The 2- or 3-year-old child may be charming and cooperative, or difficult to examine; whichever the case, the examiner is required to make many modifications in the organization of the exam. The child may be examined in a standing position or on the parent's lap. He usually does not like to have all of his clothing removed at one time but will often cooperate if only one article of clothing is removed at a time as the examination is carried out. The child also needs the opportunity to handle and use the examining instruments. He may enjoy doing this but may also reject the offer if it is too fear provoking. Despite the difficulties in examining the child of this age, the ability of the child to relate more positively at each subsequent visit can be rewarding and profitable for the examiner.

The child at 4 or 5 years of age is usually able to understand and cooperate during the examination. He is anxious to please and is usually a delightful participant. He has better control of his feelings and his behavior than the younger child but may still lose control if his fear is great. He should receive recognition for his efforts to par-

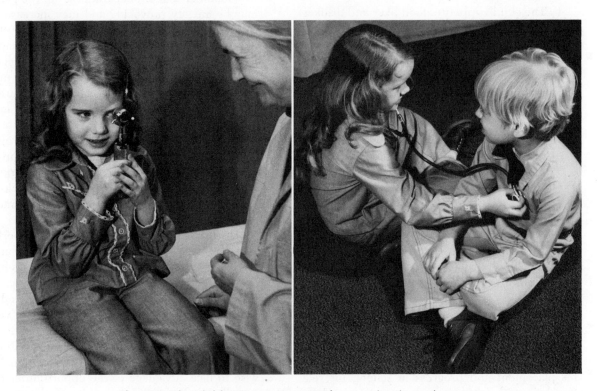

Fig. 21-1. The child enjoys trying out the examiner's equipment.

ticipate, so that his self-image is enhanced. This child especially enjoys trying out the examiner's equipment and will very likely demonstrate his new learning in future play activities; this is a way to incorporate the role of the examiner and master his fears (Fig. 21-1).

The school age child may be approached in much the same way as the adult. However, he may be extremely shy and modest. If the child is distressed about removing clothing, this modesty should be respected, as with the adult, and attempts made to conduct the examination with as little exposure as possible.

■ Measurements

The measurements of the temperature, pulse rate, respiratory rate, blood pressure, and height and weight are part of the physical examination of the child. In addition, the measurements of the head circumference and chest circumference are noted for the child under 2 years of age. The comparison of the physical measurements of a child with those of other healthy children over a period of time make it possible to determine if the child is progressing within the normal parameters of health or if there are significant deviations.

Temperature. Temperature is usually obtained rectally until the age of 6 years or even older, since it is difficult to obtain an accurate oral temperature until the child understands what is expected of him.

Temperature regulation is less exact in children than in adults. The rectal temperature is normally higher in infants and young children, and the average temperature is above 99° F (37.2° C) until the age of 3 years. The increase in temperature from infection is greater in infants and young children than in adults, except in very young infants, who may have no fever with a severe infection.

Pulse and respiratory rates. The pulse and respiratory rates are more rapid in infants and young children and change with age. The average heart rate of the child is 130 to 150 per minute at birth, 110 to 120 per minute at 1 year of age, and 90 to 110 per minute at 2 years of age. The average range of normal respirations is 30 to 80 per minute in the newborn period as compared to 20 to 40 per minute at 1 year of age and 20 to 30 per minute at 2 to 3 years of age. Pulse and respiratory rates are labile measurements in children and are more responsive to illness and activity than in adults.

The pulse rate may be obtained in infants and young children by palpation of the carotid artery or by auscultation of the heart. The respiratory rate may be obtained by inspection or auscultation. These measurements should be obtained while the child is relatively quiet or sleeping.

Blood pressure. The measurement of the blood pressure is often neglected in children because of a lack of proper equipment. There are pediatric cuffs available in several sizes; the proper cuff size is one with a width no less than one half and no more than two thirds of the length of the upper arm or thigh.

The blood pressure is best obtained before the examination of the ears and throat. The child at 3 years of age is usually able to understand and cooperate with the examiner, but it may be necessary to use the flush method with younger children and infants. In this method, the blood pressure cuff is applied; then the hand, wrist, and forearm are elevated and tightly wrapped to exclude blood, up to the point where the cuff is applied. The cuff is then inflated to a level above the suspected blood pressure, and the wrappings are removed. The pressure of the cuff is reduced slowly until flushing is noticed in the hand; the pressure at this point is close to the systolic pressure.

The levels of systolic blood pressure gradually increase during childhood; the average systolic pressure is 96 at 1 year of age, 99 at 2 years of age, and 100 at 6 years of age.

Height and weight. The height and weight measurements provide a good estimate of the overall growth of the child. The height and weight also provide a measurement that can be compared with earlier measurements of the child and with other children of a similar age. Both measurements are done at each visit and are recorded on a standardized growth chart. There will be wide variations in the patterns of growth among children, but the use of the growth chart enables the examiner to determine the pattern of growth of the individual child as compared with that of other children.

Height is most accurately measured when the child is able to stand alone. It is difficult to measure the infant's length, but a crude measurement can be obtained with the infant lying flat in the supine position with the legs extended. A tape measure is used to determine the length from the heel to the top of the head.

Failure to grow or to gain weight is sometimes the first indication of a serious problem. The weight of the child, which is more easily obtained, is usually a better index of health than is length. Weight loss indicates illness, malnutrition, or dehydration. Rapid weight gain may indicate overfeeding or the presence of edema. Plateaus in weight gain should also be noted and may deserve further investigation.

Head and chest circumferences. The head and chest circumferences are measured during each examination until the child reaches 2 years of age. The head circumference is an important measurement in the examination of the young child because it is related to intracranial volume and allows an estimation of the rate of growth of the brain. Sequential measurements should be carried out and plotted on a growth chart. Any discrepancy or deviation may result from conditions such as microcephaly and hydrocephaly. The average head circumference at birth is 35 cm (14 inches), and the chest is about 2 cm less. The head is usually about the same circumference as the chest until the child is 2 years old; then the chest circumference continues to grow rapidly while the head circumference increases slightly.

The head circumference is measured by passing a tape measure over the most prominent part of the occiput and just above the supraorbital ridges. The chest is measured at the level of the nipple when the child is supine.

Areas of assessment
Skin

The examination of the skin provides valuable information about the general health of the child as well as evidence of specific skin problems. The skin of the entire body should be noted at each examination. The normal condition of the skin changes with age, and it is helpful to become familiar with those changes seen in children.

The skin of the newborn is soft, smooth, and appears almost transparent. The superficial vessels are prominent, giving the skin its red color. A mild degree of jaundice is present after the second or third day in normal infants; if the jaundice is severe or occurrs in the first 24 hours, however, the examiner should consider the presence of a serious problem. Small papular patches, called nevus flammeus, may be present over the occiput, forehead, and upper eyelids in the newborn period and usually disappear by the end of the first year of life. The nose and cheeks are frequently covered by small white papules, caused by plugging of the sebaceous glands during the neonatal period. Both sweat and sebaceous glands are present in the newborn but do not function until the second month of life. Some desquamation is common during the first weeks and varies in individual babies. Mongolian spots,

which are blue, irregularly shaped flat areas, are found in the sacral and buttocks area of some infants, usually those who have more darkly pigmented skin. These usually disappear by the end of the first or second year but occasionally persist for a longer time. There is a considerable amount of fine hair, called lanugo, over the body of the newborn, which is lost during the first weeks of life. The nails of the full-term newborn are well formed and firm in contrast to those of the premature infant, which are imperfectly formed.

During the first year of life there is a continuing increase in the proportion of subcutaneous fat, and raw areas resulting from skin rubbing against skin are more prevalent in young, obese infants. This is called intertrigo. During the second year of life there is a decrease in the proportion of subcutaneous fat, and intertrigo is less common.

After the first year of life the normal child shows little changes in the skin until the onset of puberty, when there is considerable development of both sweat and sebaceous glands. Associated with the development of the sebaceous glands is acne vulgaris, which is so common in its mildest forms that it is sometimes considered as a normal physiological change. Early evidence of acne is the occasional comedo or blackhead on the nose and chin. At age 13 or 14, papules and small pustules may begin to appear, and by age 16 many children will have recovered completely. There are also changes in the amount and distribution of hair. Hair growth becomes heavier; the appearance of pubic, axillary, and most of the more prominent body hair is influenced by sexual development during adolescence.

Lymph nodes

Lymph nodes in children have the same distribution as that found in adults, but the nodes are usually more prominent until the time of puberty. The amount of lymphoid tissue is considerable at birth and increases steadily until after puberty. It is common to find shotlike, small, bean-sized nodules in the normal, healthy child. Lymph nodes are examined during the examination of each part of the body.

Head and neck

The shape of the newborn infant's head is often asymmetrical as a result of the molding that occurs during the passage through the birth canal, and it may be a few days or weeks before the normal shape is restored. The newborn has a skull that molds easily because the bones are soft and pliable. Trauma may result in caput succedaneum or cephalohematoma. *Caput succedaneum* is an edematous swelling of the superficial tissues of the scalp that is manifested by a generalized soft swelling not bounded by suture lines. *Cephalohematoma* occurs as a result of bleeding into the periosteum and results in swelling that does not cross the suture line. These problems are temporary and are usually resolved in a matter of days or weeks. Flattening of the head is often seen in normal children but can also be indicative of problems such as mental retardation or rickets.

The sutures of the skull are palpated and can usually be felt as ridges until the age of 6 months. The fontanels are palpated during each examination of the infant and young child to determine the size, shape, and presence of any tenseness or bulging. Normally, the posterior fontanel closes by 2 months of age and the anterior fontanel closes by the end of the second year (Fig. 21-2).

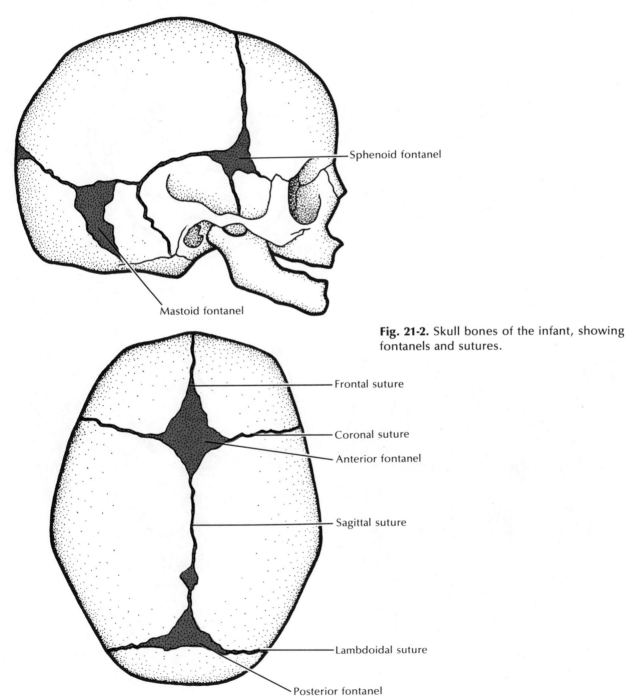

Sphenoid fontanel

Mastoid fontanel

Fig. 21-2. Skull bones of the infant, showing fontanels and sutures.

Frontal suture

Coronal suture

Anterior fontanel

Sagittal suture

Lambdoidal suture

Posterior fontanel

Tenseness or bulging of the fontanels is most easily detected when the child is in a sitting position and should be assessed when the child is quiet. Bulging of the fontanels is evidence of intracranial pressure. The fontanels may be depressed when the infant is dehydrated or malnourished. Early closure or delayed closure of the fontanels should be noted. Early closure may result from microcephaly, and delayed closure from prolonged intracranial pressure.

The importance of measuring the head circum-ference of the child up to 2 years of age has already been discussed.

Transillumination of the skull is a useful procedure in the initial examination of the infant and for any infant with an abnormal head size. Transillumination is carried out in a completely darkened room with an ordinary flashlight equipped with a rubber adaptor. The light is placed against the infant's head. If the cerebrum is absent or greatly thinned, as from increased intracranial pressure, the entire cranium lights up. Often, de-

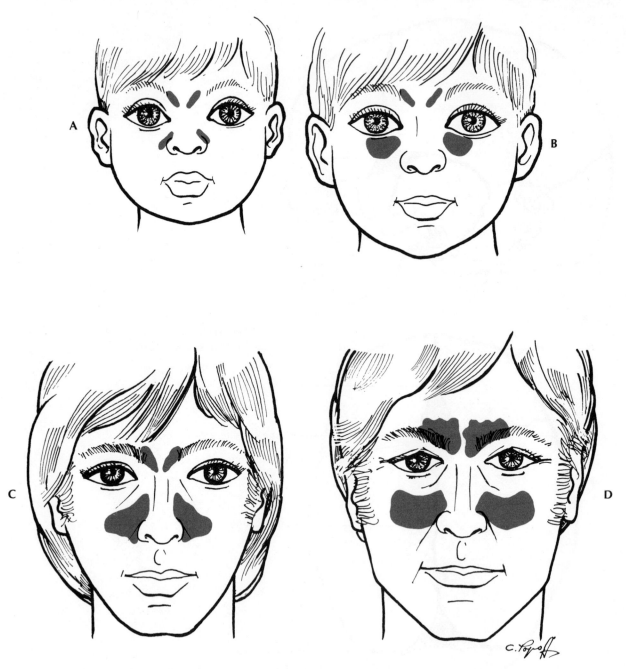

Fig. 21-3. Development of the frontal and maxillary sinuses. **A,** Early infancy. **B,** Early childhood. **C,** Adolescence. **D,** Adulthood.

fects transilluminate in a more limited way. Auscultation of the skull may reveal bruits, which are commonly found in normal children up to 4 years of age. After the age of 4, bruits are evidence of problems such as aneurysms or increased intracranial pressure.

The young infant's scalp is inspected for evidence of crusting, which often results from a seborrheic dermatitis.

The shape of the face is inspected. A facial paralysis is most easily observed when the child cries or smiles and the asymmetry is increased. An abnormal or unusual facies may indicate a chromosomal abnormality such as Down's syndrome.

The frontal and maxillary sinuses should be percussed by the direct method and palpated in the child over 2 or 3 years of age. Until that age the sinuses are too small and poorly developed for percussion or palpation (Fig. 21-3).

The submaxillary and sublingual glands are palpated in the same way as in the adult examination. Local swelling of the parotid gland is most easily determined by observing the child in the sitting position with the head raised and the neck extended and by noting any swelling below the angle of the jaw. The swollen parotid gland may be felt by palpating downward from the zygomatic arch. Unilateral or bilateral swelling of the parotid gland is usually indicative of mumps.

The neck is examined with the child lying flat on his back. The size of the neck is noted. The neck of the infant normally is short; it lengthens at about 3 or 4 years of age. The lymph nodes are palpated, as are the thyroid gland and trachea. The sternocleidomastoid muscle is carefully palpated. A mass on the lower third of the muscle may indicate a congenital torticollis. Finally, the mobility of the neck is determined by lifting the child's head and turning it from side to side. Any resistance to flexion may be indicative of meningeal irritation.

Eyes

The examination of the eyes is most easily accomplished when the child is able to cooperate. The school age child is able to participate, and the examination is carried out as described in Chapter 10, on Assessment of the eyes. The infant and young child are much more of a challenge to the examiner.

Visual function at birth is limited but improves as the structures develop. Vision may be grossly tested in the very young infant by noting the pupillary response to light; this is one of the most primitive visual functions and is normally found in the newborn infant. The blink reflex is also present in normal newborns and young infants. The infant will blink his eyes when a bright light is introduced. At 5 or 6 weeks of age the child should be able to fixate and give some evidence of following a bright toy or light. At 3 or 4 months of age the infant begins to reach for objects at different distances. For children 3 to 6 years of age

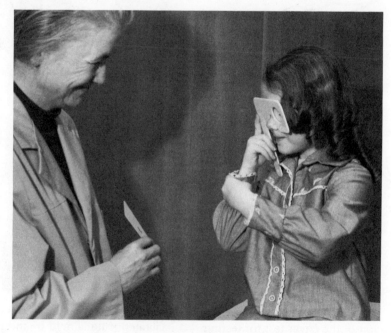

Fig. 21-4. Preparing the child for participation in testing of visual acuity.

Snellen's *E* chart can be used. The child is asked to hold his fingers in the same direction as the fingers of the *E* (Fig. 21-4). The young child is normally far sighted and does not achieve visual acuity of 20/20 until the age of 7 years.

Tests for strabismus should be carried out. Transient strabismus is frequently seen during the first months of life; if it persists beyond 6 months of age, however, or becomes fixed at an earlier age, the child should be referred to an ophthalmologist. Early recognition is essential for restoration of binocular vision. An easy method for detecting strabismus is the observation of the pupillary light reflex. The reflection of the light should come from approximately the same part of each pupil, and any deviation should be noted. Another test is the cover test (Fig. 21-5). The child's attention is attracted by a light or toy, and the examiner's hand is placed on top of the child's head with the thumb extended to cover one eye while the other eye is observed. The thumb is then removed, and both eyes are observed. If one or both eyes move, a strabismus is present. The test is repeated for the other eye.

Extraocular movements can be tested during the first weeks of life, as soon as the child is able to demonstrate following movement. The visual fields can also be at least partially examined in infants and young children by having the child sit on the parent's lap with the head in the midline and one eye covered. As the light or bright object is brought into the visual field, the child will look at it or reach for it.

Inspection of the outermost structures of the eyes is done in the same way as in the adult exam. The ophthalmoscopic examination of the eyes is dependent on the ability of the child to cooperate and on the examiner's efficiency in observing as much as possible in a limited period of time. Attempts to restrain the child and force the eyes to remain open often prove unsuccessful. If possible, the child's attention should be directed toward an object or light while the examiner approaches without touching the child. The appearance of the red reflex alone is important information for ruling out opacities of the cornea and lens, and cataracts.

Ears

Examination of the ears is often difficult but is important because the immature structure of the young child's ears makes them more prone to infection.

The external ear and the posterior mastoid areas are inspected and palpated for any obvious deformities. The position and size of the ears are

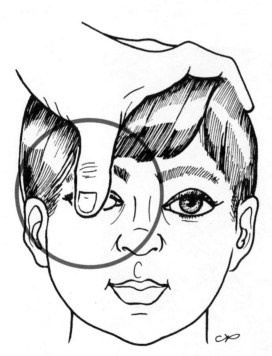

Fig. 21-5. Modification of the cover test for testing young children for strabismus.

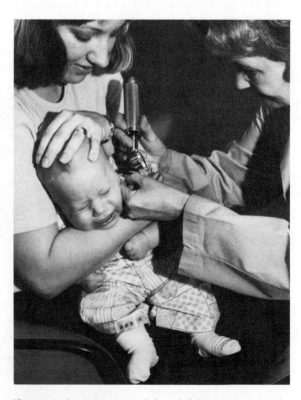

Fig. 21-6. Examination of the child's ear may be facilitated if he is held by the parent. Note that the pinna is pulled downward.

noted. Normally the top of the ear is on a horizontal line with the inner and outer canthus of the eye.

Next, the otoscope is used. This examination becomes more difficult as the child grows older, and it is usually helpful to spend some time preparing the child by letting him see the light and by inserting the speculum gently for only a few seconds and then removing it to assure him that discomfort will be minimal. When it is necessary to use restraint, the child should be held firmly by the parent. Before the otoscope is inserted, the meatus is inspected for evidence of a foreign body. In infancy and early childhood the auditory canal is directed upward, and the pinna should be pulled downward to aid in visualization. The otoscope is held so that the hand holding it rests firmly on the head, and the top of the speculum is inserted only ¼ or ½ inch into the canal to avoid any unnecessary discomfort (Fig. 21-6). Before the drum is examined, the canal should be carefully examined for evidence of furuncles or redness.

If the canal is filled with cerumen, it may occasionally be necessary to irrigate the ear. The wax should first be softened with a detergent, and the ear is then gently irrigated with lukewarm water. The procedure is unpleasant and may cause vomiting; it is not done unless necessary. It is never done if a perforation is suspected. It is inadvisable to clean the wax out with a curette unless the examiner is very skillful. This procedure causes pain and will result in crying, which only increases the redness of the tympanic membrane. It is important to avoid discomfort so that the child will not become conditioned to expect pain with future ear examinations.

The hearing is estimated. In the infant it can be tested by asking an assistant to stand behind the child and make a noise, such as a hand slap, several inches away from the ear while the examiner observes the child for an eye blink. In the young child, hearing can be grossly tested with the whispered voice. The examiner stands behind the child and whispers the child's name. The child will usually turn if he hears his name.

Nose

Any unusual shape of the nose is noted, as well as flaring of the nostrils and the character and amount of discharge.

Examination of the septum, turbinates, and vestibule is accomplished by pushing the tip of the nose upward with the thumb of the left hand and shining a light into the naris. A speculum is

usually not necessary; it might cause the child to be apprehensive.

Mouth and oropharynx

This area is usually examined last, since this examination is often the most fear provoking to the child. However, it is helpful to some children to do this examination first. The child who is anticipating discomfort may be relieved to have it accomplished and can then cooperate with the rest of the examination. This approach requires the examiner to have knowledge about the individual child's behavior and responses.

The procedures are the same as in the adult examination; however, there are differences from adults in the findings. The number of deciduous and permanent teeth and the pattern of eruption are determined by the age and development of the child. There are 20 deciduous teeth, and their eruption is completed by the age of 2½ years. The first permanent molar and lower incisor erupt at 6 years of age. The tonsils are normally larger in children than in adults and usually extend beyond the palatine arch until the age of 11 or 12 years.

Chest

The examination of the chest begins with an inspection of the general shape and circumference. In infancy the chest is almost round; the anteroposterior diameter is as great as the transverse diameter. The circumference is normally the same as or slightly less than the head circumference until the age of 2 years, as discussed earlier in this chapter. Respiratory activity is abdominal and does not become primarily thoracic until the age of 7 years. Little intercostal motion is seen in infants and young children. Therefore, if intercostal motion is seen in the young child, lung disease may be suspected.

Palpation may be carried out and tactile fremitus evaluated, while the child is crying.

Percussion of the chest may be done directly or by the indirect method; the chest is normally more resonant than in the adult.

Auscultation with the bell stethoscope is most satisfactory, because of the small size of the child's chest (Fig. 21-7). Breath sounds will seem much louder because of the thinness of the chest wall and are almost all bonchovesicular.

Heart

The examination of the cardiovascular system as described in Chapter 14 (Cardiovascular assessment: the heart and the neck vessels) applies to the examination of the child. However, there are some cardiac findings of normal children that are not considered normal in adults.

The pulse rate found in children of different ages is discussed earlier in this chapter. The palpation of pulses in all the extremities is a part of the cardiovascular examination; and the pulses in the lower extremities, especially the femoral pulses, are of special importance in children. Their absence or diminution may indicate coarctation of the aorta.

During infancy the heart is more nearly horizontal and has a larger diameter in comparison with the total diameter of the chest than it does in the adult (Fig. 21-8). The apex is one or two intercostal spaces above that considered normal for the adult. Therefore, the apical impulse in young children is normally felt in the fourth intercostal space just to the left of the midclavicular line. This location changes gradually and by 7 years of age the apical impulse is normally found in the fifth intercostal space at the midclavicular line.

Sinus arrhythmia is a normal finding in infants and children. The degree of arrhythmia is less in the young infant and greatest in the adolescent.

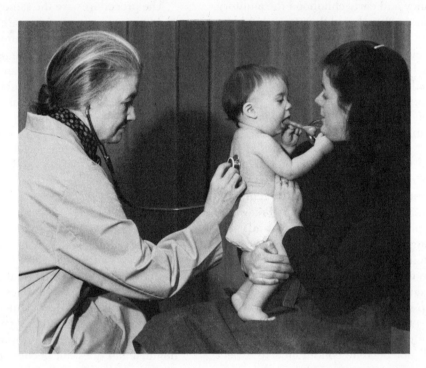

Fig. 21-7. Auscultation of breath sounds is most easily accomplished when the child is comfortable.

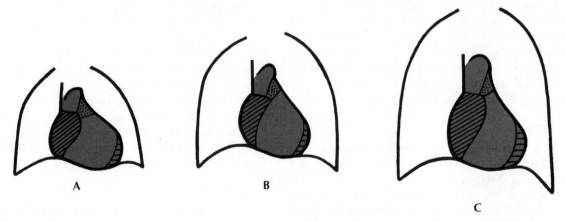

Fig. 21-8. Position of the heart at different ages. **A,** Early infancy. **B,** Early childhood. **C,** Adulthood.

The heart sounds are louder because of the thinness of the chest wall. They are also of a higher pitch and shorter duration than those of the normal adult. A splitting of the second heart sound can be heard in the second left intercostal space in most infants and children. The split normally widens with inspiration. A third heart sound is present in about one third of all children and is best heard at the apex.

Many children have murmurs without heart disease, and the significance of a murmur may be difficult to determine. Innocent murmurs are characteristically systolic in timing, are grade 1 or 2 in intensity, and are not transmitted to other areas. They are loudest in the recumbent position and disappear when the child sits up or exercises. It is not always possible to determine whether the murmur is innocent or pathological by auscultation alone, although murmurs of grade 3 or louder are usually indicative of heart disease. A venous hum is commonly found in children. It is heard either above or below the clavicles and is accentuated in the upright position.

Abdomen

The examination of the abdomen may be done first, since it requires few instruments and may be less frightening to the child. However, if the child is upset, it may be done later. When the child is relaxed, the abdomen is somewhat easier to examine than in the adult, because of the less well developed abdominal wall. To win the child's cooperation, several approaches may be helpful: a bottle may be offered to the infant; the young

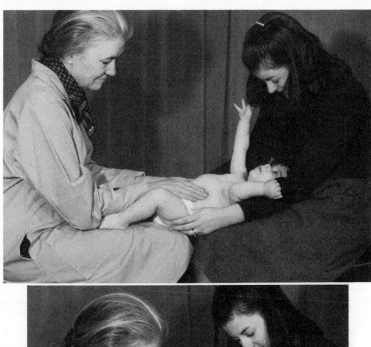

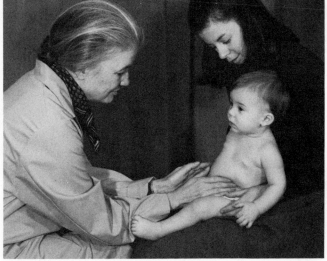

Fig. 21-9. Modifications in approach to the examination of the abdomen of the young child.

child may be more comfortable and relaxed if examined while sitting on the parent's lap. Each examiner will find the approaches that are most productive for him (Fig. 21-9).

The order of the abdominal examination procedures for the young child may be changed to avoid introducing the stethoscope and using percussion until after the child has experienced procedures that appear less threatening. First, the abdomen is inspected. The abdomen is larger than the chest in children under 4 years of age and appears "pot bellied" in both supine and sitting positions. The child up to 13 years of age will have a "pot belly" in the standing position. This normal shape needs to be differentiated from the real distention that is caused by enlargement of organs or the presence of tumors, cysts, or ascites. A depressed abdomen may result from dehydration or malnutrition. Respirations are largely abdominal in children up to 7 years of age. Any splinting or loss of movement may be indicative of peritonitis, appendicitis, or other acute problems. The umbilicus is normally closed, but umbilical hernias are common in white children up to 2 years of age and for longer periods in black children. The abdomen is also observed for peristaltic waves and dilated veins.

Palpation is carried out in the same way as in the examination of the adult except for the modifications in approach and in the positions of the child. Light palpation enables the examiner to determine the tenseness of the abdominal muscles, the presence of superficial masses, and the presence of tenderness. The child is often not able to pinpoint the area of tenderness, and only by watching the facial expressions can the examiner determine the point of maximal tenderness. The liver is generally palpable 1 to 2 cm below the right costal margin during the first year of life. If it extends more than 2 cm below the costal margin, further investigation is warranted. The spleen is normally palpable 1 to 2 cm below the left costal margin in the first weeks of life. Any increase in size should be noted, and any evidence of tenderness may be an indication of serious blood dyscrasias or other problems. Tissue turgor is also determined by grasping a few inches of skin and subcutaneous tissue over the abdomen, pulling it up, and then quickly releasing it. If the creases formed do not disappear immediately, dehydration is present. Deep palpation is done in all four quadrants by single-handed or bimanual methods. The inguinal and femoral regions are palpated for hernias, lymph nodes, and femoral pulses.

Auscultation of the abdomen is carried out in the same manner as described in the examination of the adult.

Finally, percussion may be useful in obtaining the boundaries of the liver, spleen, and any tumors.

Genitalia

The examination of the genitalia of both male and female children is usually carried out by inspection and palpation.

Male genitalia. In the male child there are two primary areas to be examined: the penis and the

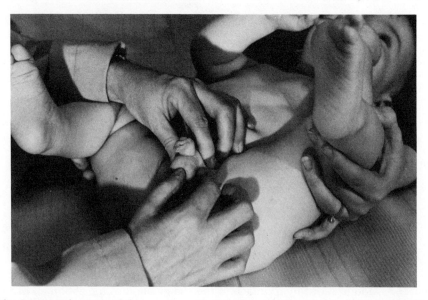

Fig. 21-10. Palpation of the scrotum to determine if the testes are descended.

scrotum. The foreskin of the penis is examined first. The foreskin of the uncircumcised infant is normally tight for the first 2 or 3 months of life and does not retract easily. If the tightness persists beyond this period, it is called a phimosis and should be observed to determine if there is any interference with urination. Any retraction of the foreskin should be done carefully, since the delicate membranes attached to the foreskin may be easily torn and result in adhesions. Next, the meatus is examined to determine its position and the presence of any ulceration. The meatus is normally located at the tip of the shaft. An abnormal location of the meatus on the ventral surface is called a hypospadias; an abnormal location on the dorsal surface is called an epispadias.

The scrotum is inspected for evidence of enlargement. An enlarged scrotum may be indicative of a hernia or hydrocele. The scrotum is also palpated to determine if the testes are descended (Fig. 21-10). The examiner's index finger is used to block the inguinal canal and is gently pushed toward the scrotum. The finger and thumb of the opposite hand are used to palpate the scrotum

and grasp the testes as it is pushed downward into the scrotum. The testes are felt as a soft mass about 1 cm in diameter and are normally descended if they can be palpated in the scrotum even if retraction into the inguinal canal occurs immediately.

Female genitalia. The genitalia of the female child is always inspected. A bloody discharge is normal, but not common, during the first weeks of life. Vaginal bleeding in children less than 8 years of age is considered abnormal and should be examined further. Purulent or mucoid discharges are indications of infection. The labia or clitoris are inspected for any abnormality in size or for evidence of adhesion or infection. The vaginal area is inspected but not usually palpated. An imperforate hymen may be noted if there is fluid retention behind it.

Musculoskeletal system

Much of the examination is done while watching the child or while playing with the child. An older child will be able to follow directions, and a routine musculoskeletal examination can be com-

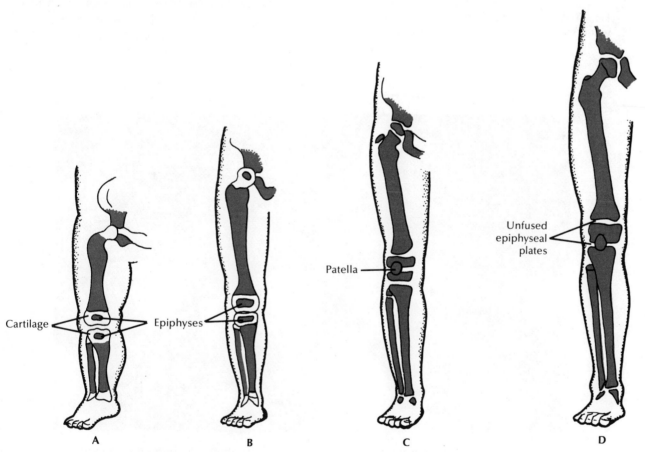

Fig. 21-11. Skeletal development of the leg. **A,** Early infancy. **B,** Early childhood. **C,** Late childhood. **D,** Adolescence.

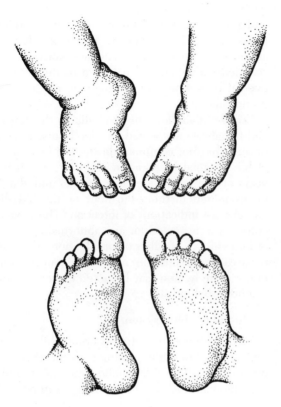

Fig. 21-12. The infant's feet may appear deformed when retained in the in utero position.

pleted. The younger child or infant is not able to understand directions, and much of the examination is done by helping the child passively go through range-of-motion movements.

The skeleton of the infant and young child is made up largely of cartilaginous tissues, which accounts for the relative softness and malleability of the bones (Fig. 21-11). It is also the reason that many defects identified early in life can be corrected with more ease than in later years.

The spine is inspected for evidence of abnormal curvatures, such as scoliosis, while the range of motion is evaluated. It is also inspected and palpated for evidence of a meningocele or a pilonidal cyst.

The extremities are inspected for symmetry, increased or decreased mobility, and anatomical defects. The newborn at rest assumes the position maintained in utero, and the feet are rarely straight. They are usually held in the varus or valgus position and simulate the clubfoot (Fig. 21-12). To determine whether this is a true abnormality or a transient position, the examiner can scratch the outside border and then the inside border of the foot. The normal foot will usually assume a right-angle position with the leg.

The hips should be routinely investigated in in-

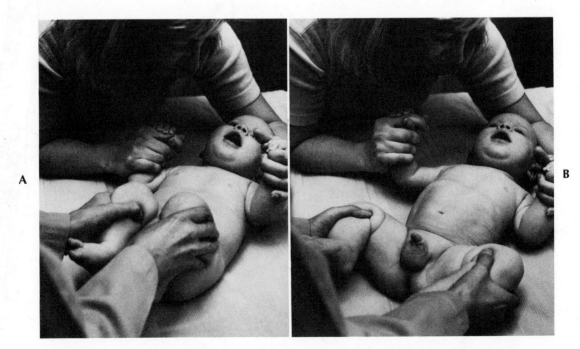

Fig. 21-13. Examination of the hips for evidence of dislocation. The hips and knees are flexed at right angles **(A)** and then abducted until the lateral aspects of the knees touch the examining table **(B).**

fants for congenital dislocation. With the infant on his back, the legs are flexed at the knees and internal and external rotation are attempted (Fig. 21-13). A determination is made as to whether the rotation is equal bilaterally. Unequal rotation is indicative of decreased mobility of one joint.

Neural system

Children of 2 years of age or older can be examined with many of the methods used in the adult neurological examination. The neurological examination of the infant or child less than 2 years of age is an assessment of the neurological development associated with the increasing myelinization and maturation of the neural system. The degree of maturation can be estimated by assessing (1) the reflex pattern, (2) motor skills, and (3) the behavior of the child.

The automatic infant reflexes that are normal at birth and disappear around 4 months of age, as voluntary control begins to develop, include the Moro reflex, the palmar grasp reflex, and the rooting reflex. Absence of these reflexes may indicate a severe problem of the central nervous system. Persistence of these reflexes may be equally serious. The *Moro reflex* is elicited by placing the infant in a supine position and surprising him with a loud noise or by allowing the head to suddenly drop a few inches. The infant will respond with an overall grasping movement; the arms extend and then flex, and the knees and hips flex. The *palmar grasp reflex* is obtained by the examiner's placing one of his fingers in contact with the palmar surface of the infant's fingers. The infant will automatically grasp the fingers tightly. The *rooting reflex* is obtained by touching the infant's cheeks. The infant will turn his head toward the stimulus as if searching for it.

The tonic neck reflex appears at 1 month of age and disappears at 5 to 7 months of age. It is elicited by placing the infant in the supine position and turning the head to the left or right. The arm on the side toward which the head is turned will extend, and the other arm will flex.

Babinski's reflex is normally present in the newborn and disappears by the age of 12 to 24 months.

The overall development of motor skills, communication skills, and behavior is evaluated by obtaining a developmental history and by observing the child's behavior. Comparison of the child's development with the expected development for his age may be accomplished by utilizing developmental charts that provide information about the range of ages in which specific developmental abilities are expected to occur.

BIBLIOGRAPHY

Barness, L. A.: Manual of pediatric physical diagnosis, ed. 4, Chicago, 1972, Yearbook Medical Publishers, Inc.

Barnett, H. L., and Einhorn, A. H.: Pediatrics, ed. 15, New York, 1972, Appleton-Century-Crofts Educational Div., Meredith Corp.

Gamstrop, I.: Pediatric neurology, New York, 1970, Appleton-Century-Crofts Educational Div., Meredith Corp.

Lowrey, G. H.: Growth and development of children, ed. 6, Chicago, 1973, Yearbook Medical Publishers, Inc.

Vaughn, V. C., McKay, R. J., and Nelson, W. E.: Nelson textbook of pediatrics, ed. 10, Philadelphia, 1975, W. B. Saunders Co.

22 Assessment of the aging client

THE INTERVIEW AND HEALTH HISTORY

The social use of the age 65 as the demarcation point between middle age and old age had its origin in Bismarck's laws. This is the time designated for retirement from work and for the eligibility for funds and services designated for the aged. Gerontologists have classified old age into two groups:

1. *Early old age or later maturity:* 65 to 74.
2. *Advanced old age:* 75 and older.

Although the use of specific years has been useful for governmental and social agency purposes, it has served to prejudice the public as well as health personnel, so that all the changes attributable to the aged, both ill and well, are expected to be present in each aged client.

The life expectancy has not changed significantly in the United States over the past 20 years. The following figures reflect the life expectancy of children born in 1970:

Race	Men	Women
White	67.5	74.9
Black	60.1	67.5

Both black and white women outlive their respective male counterparts, so that women make up more than 55% of the elderly population. The total number of elderly persons in the United States was estimated to be 20 million in 1970; this figure represents 10% of the total population. It has been said that at least 60% of all hospitalized people are elderly.

Two general thoughts should be borne in mind by the practitioner in examining the older individual. On the one hand, advancing years are not necessarily equated with disease. Thus, the practitioner should not expect all older clients to be ill. On the other hand, when one problem is identified, others must be suspected, since multiple disease is the primary characteristic of health problems in the elderly. In addition, the differentiation of the client's major problem may be complicated by decreases of acuity in the sensory processes, so that clearly defined symptoms cannot be reported.

Although a representative of the U.S. Census Bureau has declared that the bulk of the elderly in this country are poor, uneducated, and generally unemployed, it is important to remember that many clients are gainfully employed. The usual age for retirement in the United States is 62 years (and even younger in dangerous occupations), but it has been shown that 42% of individuals between 70 and 74 years of age and 19% of those between 75 and 79 years of age are still working for pay. Often, however, forced retirement means retirement from a valued job to a less satisfying form of work, such as caretaker or watchman, which this society values little and therefore allots to the elderly.

For those not working, retirement may be fraught with financial worries, particularly if the client has been living to the limit of his income during his working years or for other reasons has been unable to establish any savings. Thus, one of the problems of the elderly in this country is that of earning money to meet the costs of living without jeopardizing their qualifications for Social Security benefits. Most of the cost-of-living estimates indicate that governmental support to the elderly is not sufficient for total support. Few states have enacted legislation that will allow the elderly the option of seeking work without risking the loss of Social Security payments.

Although the more affluent may not experience the problems related to the curtailment of monetary supply, they may well participate in an even more universal feeling. This is the feeling of loss or demoralization associated with aging. This society has devalued the elderly by making them ineligible for many highly valued activities that are reserved for younger members. The aging person is considered appropriate for menial, boring, and low-paying jobs. In addition, the elderly are frequently rejected in a real or imagined sense by younger relatives and acquaintances.

The presence of emotional illness has been estimated to be as high as 20% in the otherwise well population over 65 years of age and 40% in those with physical illness. Thus particularly in assessment of the elderly, consideration must be given to both the psychological and social, as well as the physical, aspects of the client's development. One must also bear in mind that a problem associated with one of these functional areas may well lead to a disturbance in one or both of the other two.

■ Taking the health history

Although the objective of obtaining as much relevant information about the client and his problems as possible is valid for the elderly as well as for other age groups, techniques for obtaining more information may need to be adapted to compensate for aging changes. In addition, in interpreting the relationship to problems, the examiner may need to weigh the information regarding symptoms uniquely for these clients. For instance, it has been shown that the elderly complain less of pain than do younger adults with similar disease. For example, some aging clients may sense biliary colic as a dull ache. The aged complain less of pain in general. The complaint of pain may thus be less characteristic of a symptom complex.

It may be necessary to devote a good deal more time and patience in order to get an adequate history from the aging client. Difficulties in obtaining information may relate to sensory loss, since sensory losses in both reception and perception are particularly prevalent in the aging client.

The loss of auditory acuity is the most common sensory loss among aging individuals, and loss of hearing may seriously impede the progress with questions and answers during history taking. It has been reported that nearly one third of the population that is 65 years of age or older has substantial bilateral hearing loss. This loss is often associated with personality changes that may further complicate the history-taking process. Hearing loss has been shown to be associated with

suspiciousness and irritability. Communication techniques that are used with the partially deaf client should include a commonly accepted vocabulary and simple, direct questions. The examiner should give a full-face view to the client so that the client can clearly see the lips and eyes. In cases of extreme hearing loss, electronic amplifying equipment or even an old-fashioned speaking tube may be used. Since shouting obscures the consonants and only amplifies vowels, this process should be avoided with the client who has hearing loss. In instances where the client is totally deaf, it may be necessary to communicate entirely in writing. When the interview has to be conducted in writing, only the most pertinent questions should be asked, since this process is quite exhausting for the majority of such clients. It may be wiser to identify only that a symptom exists at the first interview and to establish other clues, such as how long and how much, at a subsequent interview.

Vision perception diminishes from the middle years onward. One of the changes that can be seen during the interview is a change in pupil size. The reduction in pupil size limits the amount of light that reaches the retina. The client may appear to have slow adaptation and a degree of blindness. These changes may be compensated for by increasing the illumination without glare and by utilizing color contrast. The client's ability to follow directions may be markedly increased by using color contrast in the furniture and walls of the room. "Sit on the yellow chair" may be an easier task than "Sit on the middle chair." If written interview forms are utilized, a high-wattage lamp, placed so that the light is reflected onto the page and not the client's eyes, may improve the responses that the client can make. Since light-dark adaptation occurs more slowly, the level of general illumination in examining rooms should be the same level of brightness. Differences in intensity of lighting should be avoided. Floor and table lamps should not be used; these frequently appear as spots of bright light surrounded by dark or dim spaces and are confusing to the individual with this visual impairment.

As previously mentioned, a sensory loss that makes the history taking of the elderly client difficult is the apparent decrease in the perception of pain. In the laboratory cutaneous and visual pain-producing stimuli are perceived and responded to by the aging client to a lesser degree than by the healthy young adult. That is, a more intense stimulus is required to evoke a response in the older client. Further evidence of sensory loss with aging is that the evidence of hypersensitivity reactions is less in this age group. Thus, the aging client may not report symptoms that are attested to in the early stages of some illnesses by younger individuals.

Laboratory testing has shown that there is a loss of tactile perception that accompanies aging. Thus, "I don't know why I fell" may mean that the client did not feel the object under the sole of his foot that caused him to trip. Furthermore, his loss of visual acuity may have made the object difficult to see.

One of the common fallacies of thinking that must be avoided by the examiner of aging clients is that general intelligence declines as function of advancing years. Although some of the older correlation studies would seem to support this conclusion, more recent, controlled studies deny this phenomenon. Studies performed on individuals at various time intervals in their lives (using them as their own controls) have shown an increase in intelligence test scores that continued to 55 or 60 years of age. Furthermore, there is little evidence to support the fact that a decline of intelligence occurs even after age 60 unless systemic or neurological disorders are superimposed. Impaired oxygen delivery to central nervous system (CNS) structures, such as that which accompanies decreased cerebral blood perfusion, is cited as the major cause of intellectual deterioration. Thus, the examiner should interact with the aging client with respect for both the intelligence and experience the client's years have granted him.

Although the general intelligence has been shown to remain intact, there may be an uneven decline in some of those intellectual skills thought to comprise intelligence. It has been shown that problem-solving skills involving numerical manipulation, analogies, block design, and number series suffer loss starting in early adult years. However, this may be a disuse phenomenon; if so, it should be less likely to be found in individuals using these skills in their careers, such as engineers, who would constantly challenge their mathematical skills. Vocabulary skills and inventories of available information show little change from early adulthood through the aging years. For some aged clients memory appears to be less efficient for recent events than for those of the distant past. This failure to relate events in the immediate past has also been correlated with the physical health of the client; the older person in good health has much less of a deficit.

As with any individual, learning that involves the unlearning of previously held information is the most difficult type of learning for the older client. Since it seems logical that more learning has taken place just by benefit of the client's greater number of years, it would seem that there might be a good deal to unlearn during the acquisition of most new information. Thus, difficulties for the aging person in learning new tasks may be understood.

When disorders of memory or learning ability are apparent, the examiner should be alert to the necessity of repeating questions, instructions, and explanations. Directions should be given in simple phrases and in words that would be familiar to the older client.

Should the client be confused or intellectually impaired, it may be necessary to obtain the history from a relative or an individual who has spent a good deal of time with the client. The testimony of persons who have been with the client at home may be particularly valuable in answering questions concerning changes in behavior or symptoms that the client may have identified prior to this assessment. Such a question might be "Has he complained of 'stomach' pain to you?"

Previous medical records should be sought to provide evidence concerning the duration of current symptoms and signs since particularly recent symptoms may not be remembered.

Although the family history is important, the hereditary diseases deserve less attention in the elderly client since genetic diseases are usually diagnosed at an earlier age. An exception to this might be diabetes mellitus. One of the major values of the family history is that it may yield clues as to the financial aid relatives of the client may be prepared to give.

■ Pharmaceutical history

It is particularly important to assess the medicines that may have been prescribed for the older client or that he is ingesting at his own discretion and that may be acquired without a prescription. In addition to a careful drug history taken at the initial interview, a periodic review of drug intake is important to the care of the elderly client.

Many of the drugs frequently prescribed for common medical problems pose a greater danger to the aged client than they do to the younger adult. Mucosal irritation and bleeding of the gastrointestinal tract caused by aspirin, digitalis intoxication, bizarre or hypersensitive reactions to barbiturates, bleeding phenomena due to heparin, potassium depletion due to diuretics, and extrapyramidal symptoms due to phenothiazine and phenylbutazone toxicity are known to have a higher incidence in older adults. The changes in reaction to drugs have been suggested to be caused by altered metabolism, diminished CNS function, and a reduction in elimination of drugs as a result of the functional decline of both the liver and the kidney.

Frequently, iatrogenic illness is not identified, because practitioners do not recognize symptoms as drug induced since they are a part of the stereotype of old age: slowed reaction time, confusion, disorientation, loss of memory, tremors, loss of appetite, noncompliant behavior, or anxiety.

Chronic laxative abuse is frequently seen in the elderly and may explain symptoms of potassium deficiency or general malnourishment. Tranquilizers and sleeping medications are also recognized as being frequently used by the elderly.

Just as important as the drugs that are being used are those that have been ordered by a physician and not taken. Some clients do not fill prescriptions. Others stop taking medicine because they feel better. The examiner may ask to see the containers of all drugs that are currently being taken and advise the client to bring all of his medicine with him on future visits so that the examiner may see them firsthand. This will allow the practitioner to count the pills remaining and to calculate whether they are being taken as prescribed. This may also obviate confusion from descriptions such as "It is a little yellow one with a mark in the middle."

PHYSICAL APPRAISAL

The approach to the physical examination in the elderly is essentially identical to that performed on a client of any age. The client should be allowed to establish his own pace. The examiner may need to allow more time for response to requests such as a change of position. The examiner should note evidence of muscle weakness or lack of coordination in order to give assistance to the client when he needs help in moving or turning.

Patience is the most helpful asset in dealing with the elderly. Valuable information may be lost because the practitioner did not wait to see the full range of response to a test. A hurried and annoyed manner of dealing with the elderly client may cause him to retreat or make minimal attempts to comply with procedures.

The following review of examinations includes only those parameters that may differ in the aged client as compared to the younger adult.

■ General inspection

The elderly client may measure ½ inch shorter than when he was young. This change is attributed to the thinning of cartilages between bones.

Longitudinal studies have shown a steady loss in weight in men past age 65. However, the majority of women show a tendency toward progressive weight gain.

Because cartilage continues to be laid down in old age, the ears and nose of the elderly client may be larger and appear more prominent in relation to the face.

Wrinkling and relaxation (sagging) of the skin are recognized as signs of the aging process, as is the loss of pigmentation of the hair.

■ Areas of assessment
Metabolism

The physiology of the healthy aged individual is essentially the same as that of the younger adult. However, the response to stressful stimuli occurs at a slower rate in the older person. An example of this is the slower return of normal pH seen in the person challenged with an oral dose of sodium bicarbonate.

The metabolic rate has been shown to decline with age. The thyroid gland has been shown to undergo a reduction in cell size and function with aging. The rate of thyroxin metabolism also declines with age. Glucose clearance time, the insulin secretion in response to stimulation of the beta cells, is lengthened in the aged. One estimate is that one half of the elderly population has at least minimal diabetes; that is, the response to glucose stimulation of the beta cells to produce insulin is impaired. It has been suggested that impaired glucose clearance may be related to elevated levels of insulin antagonists in the elderly client.

Eyes

The lacrimal glands decrease in tear production with aging, so that the eyes may appear dry and lusterless. Other changes associated with aging that may be observed on inspection of the eyes are arcus senilis, scleral discolorations, and diminution of pupil size. Arcus senilis is the accumulation of a lipid substance on the cornea. The deposition may be seen as a dotlike accumulation as early as the 20s or 30s. As more of the lipid is laid down, the cornea may be completely infiltrated, thickened, and even raised in appearance. Arcus senilis characteristically appears as a grayish arc or complete circle almost at the edge of the cornea. The iris may frequently have pale brown discolorations.

Loss of elasticity of the lens causes vision changes, so that many normal individuals who are aging wear corrective lenses. Normal changes in the eye may predicate changes in the eyeglasses every 3 to 5 years. The examiner should assess the visual acuity of the client with his glasses in place and determine how long the client has had them.

Peripheral vision is diminished in the aged. The elderly are also less able to perceive purple colors. Glaucoma and cataracts are other problems frequently associated with aging. Surgical removal of the cataract followed by ocular correction will obviate the loss of vision.

Ears

Hearing loss in the elderly is most frequently due to presbycusis or otosclerosis. *Presbycusis* is the name given to the loss in perception of auditory stimuli that accompanies degenerative changes of the neural structures of the inner ear or the auditory nerve, or both. The first symptom is the loss of high-frequency tones.

A common condition of the otic capsule in which abnormally excessive bone cells are laid down is called *otosclerosis*. This generally results in fixation of the footplate of the stapes in the oval window; occasionally, however, the otosclerotic process may affect the cochlea, resulting in a neural deafness.

Mouth

Atrophy of the papillae of the lateral edges of the tongue is common in persons past age 45. One of the indications of loss of taste perception is that the elderly need to be exposed to three times the concentration of sugar needed by younger clients to sense sweetness.

Most clients of age 65 or greater are edentulous. If teeth are still present, they are generally diseased.

Breasts

The amount of fat in the breasts increases in most women, whereas glandular tissues atrophy. As a rule, the general size remains the same. However, the breasts change in consistency and shape and are often described as pendulous (elongated) or flaccid. Because of the diminution of connective tissue, the presence of breast lesions is detected earlier than in the younger adult. The detection of a lump in the elderly woman is of greater significance since cystic mastitis is not common past the menopausal years.

Respiratory system

Maximum breathing capacity, forced vital capacity, vital capacity, and inspiratory reserve volume are known to decline with age. The breaths taken by the elderly client are not as deep as those taken by the younger client, and the older client may complain of discomfort if asked to breathe more deeply. Furthermore, there is a loss of diffusion capacity, the passage of oxygen from the environment into the pulmonary capillaries and of carbon dioxide from the pulmonary capillaries to the external side of the alveolus. For identical pulmonary blood flow rates, the client of 80 years of age gets one third as much oxygen into his cardiovascular system as a 20-year-old.

As with the younger adult, nocturnal dyspnea and orthopnea may point to a cardiovascular origin. The elderly client with cardiac disease more frequently presents a chief complaint of fatigue than of shortness of breath. The elderly client with known respiratory disease who has marked fatigue that has been present for only a short time is frequently found to be suffering an acute respiratory system infectious process. Cough is the most frequent symptom of pulmonary congestion.

The elderly client's complaints of chest pain may sound less severe than that described by the younger individual for both pleural and cardiac problems.

Tracheal deviation in the elderly may be due to upper dorsal scoliosis. Changes in calcium metabolism may result in an increase in the anteroposterior diameter of the chest. Bony changes responsible for this restructuring of the chest are degenerative changes in the vertebra accompanied by kyphosis and calcification of costal cartilages.

Cardiovascular system

The resting heart rate declines in the elderly, as does the cardiac output. The heart also becomes less distensible. The effective strength of blood vessels is decreased as connective tissue replaces smooth muscle cells. Elasticity is decreased as elastic fibers are replaced by fibroconnective tissue. The proximal arteries tend to thin and dilate as aging progresses, whereas the peripheral arterial walls become thicker. Baroreceptor sensitivity is known to be blunted with age.

The older individual's response to maximal exercise is not as great as that of the younger adult for either cardiac output or heart rate. The older person develops a greater increase in systolic blood pressure than does a younger adult performing the same amount of physical work.

Kyphoscoliosis, frequently seen in the aging individual, may cause a dislocation of the cardiac apex, so that its location loses diagnostic significance.

Dizziness, blackouts, or syncope seen in the elderly may be the result of marked aortic stenosis but may also result from impairment of carotid flow. Fainting also occurs when cardiac output is not increased in response to exertion and also with marked vasodilation of skeletal muscle beds.

Many elderly clients have ectopic heartbeats, which may be innocuous, but there is a need to identify those that are not.

Data from phonocardiographic studies show that murmurs are present in 60% or more of aging clients. The most common is a soft systolic ejection murmur heard at the base of the heart due to sclerotic changes at the bases of the cusps of the aortic valve.

Whereas in the younger individual there are often typical symptoms related to heart attack, that is, heavy, squeezing pressure on the sternum radiating to the neck, back, or arm, the descriptions given by the elderly client may be indefinite. This may be due to changes in perception or to the fact that the sensory nerve endings and fibers are altered in such a way that the intensity of signals reaching the brain is diminished. This decrease in pain sensation has a higher incidence in the client with diabetes mellitus. These individuals frequently report no experience of pain at the time of myocardial infarction.

Although there is an overall increase in incidence of heart disease with advancing age, there are no heart diseases that are peculiar to old age.

Tricuspid stenosis is generally found in marked rheumatic heart disease and therefore is seldom seen in the elderly, since the victims generally succumb in middle age. Thus, the practitioner need devote less attention to ruling out this phenomenon.

Pulses. The artery is felt more readily in the elderly because of a loss of adjacent connective tissue and because of increased hardness of the arteries due to arteriosclerosis and atherosclerosis. The vessels may be more tortuous as well, because vessels become longer with age; since the vessels are anchored at fixed points, lengthening results in folding or kinking. The increased rigidity is due to a deposit of fatty material (arteriosclerotic plaque) in the intima part of the artery and to calcification of the middle layer.

Abdomen

Examination of the abdominal structures may be accomplished more easily in the nonobese client than in the fat or heavily muscled client. Since there is a general loss of fibroconnective tissue as well as muscle wasting in the elderly, the abdominal wall of the elderly client will be slacker and thinner, making palpation simpler and more accurate than in the younger client.

Abdominal wall rigidity is not as common a sign of peritoneal irritation in the elderly client as it is in the younger individual.

In an acute abdominal emergency, the elderly client generally complains less of discomfort than would the younger person with a similar condition.

Gastrointestinal function. Salivation and gastric acid secretion have been shown to decline with advancing age. Decreases in the production of both hydrochloric acid and pepsin as well as in digestive enzymes of the pancreas (amylase, lipase, trypsin) have been measured and may explain the elderly client's complaints of anorexia and difficulty in digesting meals.

Constipation is also a frequent complaint. However, although a decline in the motility of the gastrointestinal tract has been proved to occur with advancing years, it has been shown that 90% of individuals over 60 years of age have at least one bowel movement a day.

Genitourinary system

Because of the decreased cardiac output, blood flow to the kidney is markedly diminished in the aged, leading to a loss of kidney function.

The two most common signs of genitourinary dysfunction in the elderly are nocturnal frequency of micturition and incontinence of urine.

In addition to the frequency of urination, the volume passed during each episode should be investigated. Small amounts of urine passed frequently may be due to a mucosal irritation caused by inflammation or trauma. Large volumes of urine passed frequently may be due to chronic renal failure or poorly regulated diabetes mellitus. The client should be questioned as to the exact amount of fluid he ingests. In addition, he should be asked if he is taking a diuretic and, if so, the time he takes it.

In the elderly male client frequency of micturition accompanied by problems in initiating and ending the stream is generally the result of prostatic enlargement with urinary retention.

Relaxation of the perineal muscles in the elderly female client leads to stress incontinence.

Reproductive status

Female client. Since the cells of the reproductive tract and the breasts are estrogen dependent both for growth and function, the decline of estrogen production starting at menopause is responsible for many changes observed in these tissues in elderly female clients.

The uterus is diminished in size because of a loss of myometrial fibers; the uterine mucosa is normally thin and atrophic and is rarely secretory. The cervix is also decreased in size, and the cervical mucus is less than during the reproductive years. When the mucus is examined, it is seen to be thick and cellular. The fern test is negative. The vagina of the elderly client is observed to be narrower and shorter due to an increase in the amount of the submucosal connective tissue. The vaginal epithelium atrophies, and the surface appears thin and pale. Because of the fragility of the mucosa, special attention should be devoted to observing for erosion, ulcerations, and adhesions. Furthermore, as estrogen deficiency becomes marked, the glycogen content and acidity of the vaginal mucus decline, allowing pathogenic organisms to replace the normally protective Döderlein's bacilli. Thus, the examiner should be alert to the presence of vaginitis. Dyspareunia is a common symptom of the loss of vaginal epithelium and associated changes in mucus.

Because some physicians routinely administer estrogen to postmenopausal women to prevent the atrophic and functional changes of the reproductive tissues, the practitioner must assess the client who is medicated with estrogen to determine the effect of the hormone and the presence of side effects. Thus, the examiner should assess this client for the presence of uterine bleeding, mastalgia, weight gain, fluid retention, hypertension, and neoplasm, all of which have been implicated in long-term estrogen therapy.

Male client. Although the decline of testosterone production in the male client occurs at a later time in life than that of estrogen in the female client, clinically observable signs and symptoms do accompany the decline in production of this reproductive hormone.

The client may report a decline in sexual en-

Table 22-1. Changes noted in the four phases of intercourse in the aging male client

Phase	Alteration
1. Excitement	Slower increment in excitement; sex flush less in duration and intensity; involuntary spasms diminished; longer time required to obtain erection; less testicular elevation and scrotal sac vasocongestion in erection
2. Plateau	Longer duration; increase in penile diameter since less preejaculatory fluid emission
3. Orgasmic	Shorter duration; fewer contractions in expulsion of semen bolus
4. Resolution (refractory)	Lasts 12 to 24 hours as compared to 2 minutes in the youthful client; loss of erection (return of penis to flaccid state) may take a few seconds as compared to minutes or hours in the youthful client

ergy. During the act of intercourse, physiological reactions are less intense and reactions are slowed.

There is a gradual decline in strength of the muscles associated with the act of intercourse. The testes decrease in size and are less firm on palpation. Histologically, there is an increase in connective tissue in the tubules, so that they are thickened. The result of this degenerative change is a decrease in production of spermatozoa. The prostate gland is increased in size, and secretion is impaired. The seminal fluid is reduced in amount and viscosity.

These changes do not necessarily mean a decrease in libido or a loss in the sense of satisfaction from the sex act. A frequency of intercourse of one to two times per week in most men over 60 has been reported.

Musculoskeletal system

Although muscle mass is known to decline progressively with age, loss of strength is not necessarily the result. The practitioner may use the opportunity afforded by the examination session to determine if the aging client is exercising all of his muscles. The client is queried concerning his planned exercise or calisthenics, movements during recreation, and the amount of activity experienced through his work. If the client is a housewife, it is important to find out just how much physical activity is actually involved in her particular housecleaning; the number of rooms in her home and the number of floors in her home (determining the extent of stair climbing), plus the thoroughness with which cleaning is done provide a wide range of exercise commitment. Remedial exercise may be advised if deficits are identified.

Osteoarthritic changes in the joints are almost universally observed in the elderly. The changes are of such a general nature that some roentgenologists claim to be able to estimate the age of individuals past 40 years of age through examination of roentgenograms of the cervical spine. Proliferative changes in the spine cause protrusion and lipping of the vertebrae. These bony overgrowths are called osteophytes. Osteoarthritic bony overgrowths involving the distal finger joints are termed Heberden's nodes. Bouchard's nodes are overgrowths involving the proximal joints.

A nodular thickening of the palmar fascia may be associated with the contraction deformity of the lateral fingers, so that full extension is impossible. A higher incidence of this contraction, called Depuytren's contraction, is observed in diabetic clients than in the nondiabetic. The overall occurrence in the aging population is 10%.

Kyphosis in the elderly client may be the first indication of osteoporosis, a type of pathophysiological condition characterized by increased mobilization of calcium from the bones. The client may complain of aches and pains along the vertebrae; this may also signal the presence of osteoporosis.

Skin

A decrease in connective tissue, which becomes more marked with aging, is evident in examination of the skin. The skin appears thinner, particularly over the backs of the hands. Because of the loss of elastic fibers, the skin, when pinched between the examiner's thumb and finger, takes a good deal longer to return to its natural shape. Sebaceous and sweat glands are less active. Thus, the client may complain of "dry skin," particularly over the extremities where circulation is less effective. In addition, hair growth often becomes scanty or absent as the peripheral circulation is compromised. This is particularly evident over the dorsum of the feet and lower legs. Along with the general thinning of the hair that is characteristic of the aging phenomenon, the elderly suffer a loss of scalp hair. In women the hairs appear finer or sparser, or both. There is also a general thinning of pubic and axillary hair. The female client may report that she no longer shaves under the arms.

In examination of the skin, the examiner should be particularly alert to the presence of ecchymoses, since the presence of a bruise may indicate a recent injury. The client may have forgotten the injury or may have been unaware of it because of the decrease in sensory perception.

Small, scarlet growths scattered over the skin, called senile telangiectasia, are noted to increase in number from the middle years onward.

Pigment may be deposited as melanotic freckles (lentigines), although overall the skin may be paler. Vitiligo, areas of skin lacking pigment (melanocytes), may be localized or generalized in distribution; there is some tendency for this hypopigmentation to increase with age.

The presence of warts or hyperkeratosis consisting of raised pale, brown, or black epidermal overgrowth may be noted. These senile warts are generally located with their long axis following those of the client's skin creases. These are normal overgrowths and are not removed unless the client desires them excised for cosmetic reasons.

Cutaneous tags called acrochordons are a common skin change seen in the elderly. The lesions are soft, flesh colored, and pedunculated and vary in size from a pinhead to a pea. They are most commonly noted on the vertical and lateral surfaces of the neck and in the axillary area. The lesions have no clinical significance and can be ignored unless the client frequently injures them with clothing or jewelry, or if they are disturbing from a cosmetic point of view.

Neural system

After age 50, brain cells decrease in number at a rate of about 1% per year. However, because of the immense number of reserve cells involved, no clinical signs may be observed.

Autopsies of individuals who were assessed as having normal behavior have shown extensive disease of neural structures. This finding has led to the conclusion that compensation to neurological disease is possible. It has been postulated that alternate tissues may be available for many functions. Thus, physical diagnostic procedures may not be sufficient to unmask all of the pathology that exists.

Conduction velocity in some nerves is known to decline with age. The startle response takes twice as long in some aged clients.

The sense of smell is markedly diminished in the older adult because of a decrease of olfactory nerve fibers and atrophy of the remaining fibers.

443

Position sense is impaired in many elderly clients. Since the tactile sense is known to be blunted, more intense clues may be used to test this sensory modality. The assessment of these sensory abilities is particularly important in effectively advising modifications of the client's living quarters to increase sensory input and to avoid serious accidents. Some suggestions to the client that may be helpful are (1) the use of very marked textural differences and (2) the use of color contrasts.

The aged need stronger signals (greater amplitude) to detect vibration; this is probably due to decline of CNS function.

Although the response to deep tendon reflex testing is decreased or absent in some elderly clients, all of these reflexes may be elicited in the healthy elderly adult.

BIBLIOGRAPHY

Agate, J. N.: The practice of geriatric medicine, ed. 2, London, 1970, William Heinemann Medical Books Ltd.

Brocklehurst, J. C.: Textbook of geriatric medicine and gerontology, Edinburgh, 1973, Churchill Livingstone.

Buckley, E. C. III, and Dorsey, F. C.: The effect of aging on serum immunoglobulin concentrations, J. Immunol. **105:**964, 1970.

Busse, E. W., and Pfeiffer, E., editors: Behavior and adaptation in late life, Boston, 1969, Little, Brown and Co.

Butler, R. N., and Lewis, M.: Aging and mental health, St. Louis, 1973, The C. V. Mosby Co.

Caird, F. I., and Judge, T. G.: Assessment of the elderly patient, London, 1974, Pitman Publishing Ltd.

Cowdry, E. V., and Steinberg, F. U.: The care of the geriatric patient, ed. 4, St. Louis, 1971, The C. V. Mosby Co.

Hershey, D.: Life span and factors affecting it, Springfield, Ill., 1974, Charles C Thomas, Publisher.

Jones, H. E.: Trends in mental abilities, 1958, Institute of Child Welfare, University of California.

Owens, W. J.: Age and mental abilities; a second adult follow-up, J. Educ. Psychol. **67:**311, 1966.

Post, F.: The clinical psychiatry of late life, Oxford, 1965, Pergamon Press Ltd.

Shanas, E.: Health status of older people, Am. J. Public Health **64:**261, 1974.

23 Integration of the physical assessment

This chapter contains a discussion of two issues relating to the complete physical assessment: the performance of an integrated, screening physical examination and the recording of the physical examination.

PERFORMANCE OF THE SCREENING PHYSICAL EXAMINATION

After practicing and acquiring proficiency in the performance of regional examinations, it is recommended that the student develop a procedure for the performance of an integrated physical examination. In actual practice, the examiner will need to perform complete regional examinations, for example, in acute care settings, as well as complete screening examinations, such as in health maintenance or screening situations.

In developing a personal routine for a complete examination, the student should consider factors of efficiency and client comfort. If procedures are performed systematically and efficiently, time is conserved and the examiner is less likely to forget a procedure or a part of the body than if the examination were performed in a haphazard fashion.

Clients who are ill or debilitated lose energy quickly. Developing a system of examination that requires the fewest number of position changes of clients will enhance acceptability and decrease the number of examinations that need to be deferred because of client intolerance.

The manner in which the examiner conducts the physical examination can enhance or destroy rapport developed during the interview for history taking. A disorganized examiner who leaves the room to obtain missing equipment, who runs around the bed several times in a short period of time, or who has the client changing positions frequently may lose the client's confidence.

The outline presented here is a suggested procedure for the performance of the physical examination. It is intended to be a guide for the beginning practitioner and is intended for use in practice sessions. In actual client care situations this outline may require adaption because of the client's age or disability or because of the examination protocols and priorities of the care agency.

The suggested procedure is organized in such a way as to avoid excessive movement of the client or examiner. Examination of body systems is integrated into the examination of body regions.

■ Outline for examination

I. *Client* is sitting on the bed or examination table, head and shoulders uncovered. *Practitioner* is facing client (Fig. 23-1).
   A. Observe generally.
   B. Observe and palpate upper extremities.
      1. Examine skin (color, temperature, vascularity, lesions, hydration, turgor, texture, edema, masses), muscle mass, and skeletal configuration.
      2. Examine nails (color and condition).
   C. Assess pulses (apical and brachial).
   D. Measure blood pressure (both arms).
   E. Measure respiration.
   F. Examine head.
      1. Ask about deformities.
      2. Observe scalp and face.
      3. Palpate head and face.
      4. Palpate sinus area.
   G. Examine eyes.
      1. Measure visual acuity (cranial nerve [CN] II).
      2. Assess visual fields (CN II).
      3. Determine alignment of eyes (perform cover test and light reflex).

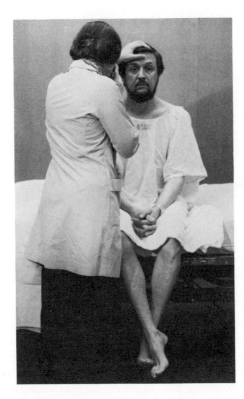

Fig. 23-1. Client seated, examiner facing client.

4. Test extraocular movements (CN III, CN IV, CN VI).
5. Observe eyebrows, eyelids, conjunctiva, cornea, sclera, iris, and lens.
6. Palpate lacrimal organs.
7. Inspect pupillary responses.
8. Perform ophthalmoscopic examination of lens, media, and retina (CN II).

H. Examine ears.
1. Inspect auricle.
2. Palpate auricle.
3. Perform otoscopic examination.
4. Determine auditory acuity (CN VIII).
5. Perform Weber and Rinne tests.

I. Examine nose.
1. Determine patency of each nostril.
2. Test for olfaction (CN I).
3. Determine position of septum.
4. Inspect mucosa, septum, and turbinates with nasal speculum.

J. Examine mouth and pharynx.
1. Inspect lips, total buccal mucosa, teeth, gums, tongue, sublingual area, roof of the mouth, tonsillar area, and pharynx.
2. Test glossopharyngeal nerve (CN IX) and vagus nerve (CN X) ("ah" and gag reflex).
3. Test hypoglossal nerve (CN XII) (tongue movement).
4. Test taste (CN VII).

K. Complete examination of cranial nerves and face.

1. Test trigeminal nerve (CN V) (jaw clenching, lateral jaw movements, corneal reflex, pain, and light touch to face).
2. Test facial nerve (CN VII) (client raises eyebrows, shows teeth, puffs cheeks, keeps eyes closed against resistance).
3. Test spinal accessory nerve (CN XII) (trapezius and sternocleidomastoid muscles).

L. Palpate temporomandibular joint.
M. Observe range of motion of the head and neck.
N. Palpate nodes (preauricular, posterior auricular, occipital, tonsillar, submaxillary, submental, anterior cervical, posterior cervical, supraclavicular, and infraclavicular nodes).
O. Palpate carotid arteries.
P. Palpate thyroid gland.
Q. Palpate for position of trachea.
R. Auscultate carotid arteries and thyroid gland.

II. *Client* is sitting on the bed or examining table, total chest uncovered if male, breasts covered if female (Fig. 23-2). *Practitioner* is standing behind client.

A. Examine back.
1. Inspect spine.
2. Palpate spine.
3. Inspect skin and thoracic configuration.
4. Palpate muscles and bones.
5. Palpate costovertebral area, asking client about tenderness.

B. Examine lungs (apices and lateral and posterior areas). *Note:* Apical, posterior, and lateral lung regions can usually be examined from a position behind client.
1. Observe respiration and total thorax.
2. Palpate for thoracic expansion and tactile fremitus.
3. Percuss systematically.
4. Determine diaphragmatic excursion.
5. Auscultate systematically.
6. Auscultate for vocal fremitus.

III. *Client* is sitting on the bed or examining table, uncovered to the waist. *Practitioner* is facing client (Fig. 23-3).

A. Examine breasts.
1. Observe breasts with client's arms and hands at the side; above the head; and pressed into the hips, eliciting pectoral contraction.
2. Observe breasts with client leaning forward.
3. Ask client about lesions; if present, palpate them.
4. If large breasts, perform a bimanual examination.

B. Palpate axillary nodes.
C. Examine lungs (anterior areas).
1. Inspect configuration and skin.
2. Palpate for tactile fremitus.

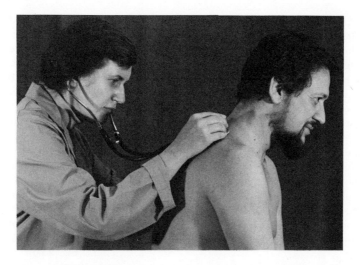

Fig. 23-2. Client seated, examiner behind client.

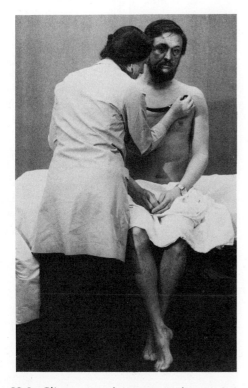

Fig. 23-3. Client seated (uncovered to waist), examiner facing client.

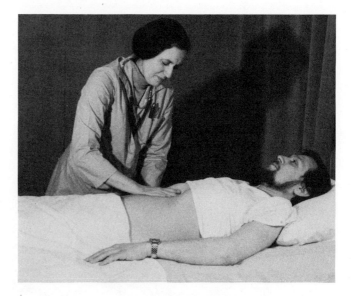

Fig. 23-4. Client lying on back, examiner at client's right side.

3. Percuss lungs systematically.
4. Auscultate lungs systematically.
D. Examine heart.
   1. Inspect precordium.
   2. Palpate precordium.
   3. Auscultate precordium.
   4. Observe external jugular vein and internal jugular pulsations.
IV. *Client* is supine. *Practitioner* is at the right side of client (Fig. 23-4).
  A. Examine breasts.

1. Palpate breasts systematically.
2. Attempt to express secretion from the nipples.
B. Examine heart.
   1. Inspect precordium.
   2. Palpate precordium.
   3. Auscultate precordium.
   4. Observe jugular venous pulses and pressures.
C. Measure blood pressure (both arms).
D. Examine abdomen.
   1. Inspect abdomen.
   2. Auscultate bowel sounds, aorta, renal arteries, and femoral arteries.
   3. Percuss liver and spleen systematically.
   4. Palpate liver, spleen, inguinal and femoral

447

node and hernia areas, and femoral pulses systematically.

5. Test abdominal reflexes.

E. Examine genitalia of male client.
1. Inspect penis, uretheral opening, and scrotum.
2. Palpate scrotal contents.

F. Examine lower extremities.
1. Inspect skin, hair distribution, muscle mass, and skeletal configuration.
2. Palpate for temperature, texture, edema, popliteal pulses, posterior tibial pulses, and dorsal pedal pulses.
3. Test range of motion.
4. Test strength.
5. Test sensation (pain, light touch, and vibration).
6. Test position sense.

V. *Client* is sitting on the bed or examining table. *Practitioner* is standing in front of client (Fig. 23-5).

A. Assess neural system.
1. Elicit deep tendon reflexes (biceps, triceps, brachioradialis, patellar, and Achilles reflexes).
2. Test for Babinski's reflex.

3. Test for coordination of upper and lower extremities.

B. Test upper extremities for strength, range of motion sensation, vibration, and position.

VI. *Female client* is in lithotomy position, genital area uncovered. *Practitioner* is sitting, facing the genital area.

A. Examine genitalia.
1. Inspect genitalia.
2. Palpate external genital area.
3. Perform speculum examination.
4. Take smears and cultures.
5. Perform bimanual vaginal examination.

B. Examine rectum: perform bimanual rectovaginal examination.

VII. *Client* is standing. *Practitioner* is standing next to client (Fig. 23-6).

A. Examine spine.
1. Observe with client bending over.
2. Test for range of motion.

B. Assess neural system.
1. Observe gait.
2. Perform Romberg test.
3. Observe heel and toe walks.

C. Test for inguinal and femoral hernias.

D. Examine male rectum: palpate rectum.

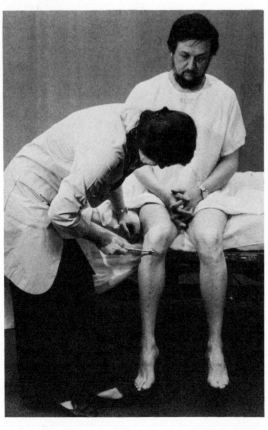

Fig. 23-5. Client seated, examiner facing client.

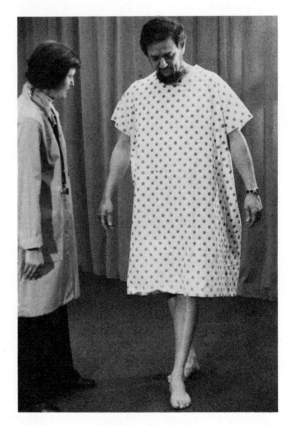

Fig. 23-6. Client standing, examiner standing next to client.

RECORDING THE PHYSICAL EXAMINATION

In recording the physical examination, the practitioner is continuously attempting to achieve a balance between the principles of conciseness and comprehensiveness. The record should describe what was seen, heard, palpated, and percussed. Whenever appropriate, the exact description is written; evaluations such as "normal," "good," or "poor" are avoided or used judiciously. Too frequently, a major system, such as the cardiovascular system, is described in one word, "normal." This description does not indicate what components of that system were assessed or the examiner's parameters of normal.

Conciseness is achieved through the use of outlines, phrases, and abbreviations. Grammar is sacrificed, and only essential words are written. Often it is helpful to use a form for recording the physical examination. A form provides an outline into which data can be entered. Forms serve as reminders for completeness; they save time; and, if they are used by all of the members of a health care system, they are useful as indices for rapid information identification. An example of a worksheet for recording a physical examination is included at the end of this chapter.

As recommended in the recording of the history (see Chapter 3 on The health history), the beginning practitioner should overrecord. The beginner should record all findings from the examination. With increased skill and discrimination regarding the significance of findings, the practitioner will be able to weed out the irrelevant information and consolidate the significant data.

Table 23-1 is a guideline that is designed to be of assistance to the beginning recorder. The first column indicates the body systems or regions that are examined. The second column contains a list of the areas of recording. These areas should be described for all clients. The third column is a partial list of areas to be recorded if abnormalities are identified in the examination of that system. The fourth column contains examples of recording for each body system or area. The examples of recording do not relate to one client; they should not be read as an example of the composite physical examination of one client.

Table 23-1. Areas and examples of recording for the physical examination

Area of examination	Descriptions usually recorded	Descriptions recorded in detail if abnormalities are present (partial listing only)	Examples of recording

Vital signs	Temperature: oral or rectal
	Pulse
	Respiration
	Blood pressure: both arms in at least two positions (lying and sitting recommended)
	Weight: indicate if client is clothed or unclothed
	Height: without shoes
		Blood pressure in standing position and in both thighs	T: 98.6° F (oral)
			P: 76/min—strong and regular; R: 16/min
			BP:
			    Lying: R, 110/70; L, 112/68
			    Sitting: R, 116/74; L, 120/76
			Wt: 130 lb unclothed
			Ht: 5 ft 3 in

General health	Appearance as relative to chronological age Apparent state of health Awareness Personal appearance Emotional status Nutritional status Affect Response Cooperation	Handshake Speech Respiratory difficulties Gross deformity Movements Unusual behavior	Slightly obese, alert, white male who looks younger than his stated age of 45 years. Moves without difficulty; no gross abnormalities apparent. Appears healthy and in no acute distress; is neatly dressed, responsive, and cooperative. Responds appropriately; smiles frequently.
Skin and mucous membranes	Color Edema Moisture Temperature Texture Turgor	Discharge Drainage Lesions: distribution, type, configuration Superficial vascularity Mobility Thickness	*Skin:* Uniformly brown in color; soft, warm, moist, elastic, of normal thickness. No edema or lesions. *Mucous membranes:* Pink, moist, slightly pale.

Continued.

Table 23-1. Areas and examples of recording for the physical examination—cont'd

Area of examination	Descriptions usually recorded	Descriptions recorded in detail if abnormalities are present (partial listing only)	Examples of recording
Nails	Color of beds Texture	Lesions Abnormalities in size or shape Presence of clubbing	Nail beds pink, texture hard, no clubbing.
Hair and scalp	Quantity Distribution Color Texture	Lesions Parasites	*Hair:* Normal male distribution; thick, curly; black color with graying at temples. *Scalp:* Clean, no lesions.
Cranium	Contour Tenderness	Lesions	Normocephalic, no tenderness.
Face	Symmetry Movements Sinuses CN V CN VII	Tenderness Edema Lesions Parotid gland	Symmetrical at rest and with movement. Jaw strong, no crepitations in temporomandibular joint. Sinus areas not tender. Sensory: pain and light touch intact.
Eyes	Visual acuity Visual fields Alignment of eyes Alignment of eyelids Movement of eyelids Conjunctiva Sclera Cornea Anterior chamber Iris Pupils: size, shape, symmetry, reflexes (PERRLA may be used for "Pupils, equally round, react to light and accommodation") Lens Lacrimal apparatus Ophthalmological examination (media, disc, vessels, retina, macular areas)	Eyebrows Tonometry Lesions Exophthalmia	Vision (with glasses): R, 20/40; L, 20/30; can read newspaper at 18 inches. Visual fields full. Alignment: no deviation with cover test; light reflex equal; palpebral fissure normal. Extraocular movements: bilaterally intact; no nystagmus, ptosis, lidlag. Conjunctiva: clear, slightly injected around area of R inner canthus. Sclera: white. Cornea: clear, arcus senilis, R eye. Anterior chamber: not narrowed. Iris: blue, round. Pupils: PERRLA. Lens: clear. Fundoscopic examination: normal veins and arteries; disc round, margins well defined, color yellowish pink; macular areas normal; no arteriolovenous nicking, hemorrhages, exudates. Lacrimal system: no swelling or discharge. Corneal reflex: present.
Ears	Auricle Canal Otoscopic examination (color, presence of landmarks) Rinne and Weber tests	Discharge Pathological alterations present on otoscopic examination Lesions Mastoid tenderness General tenderness	Auricle: no lesions, canal clean. Otoscopic examination: drum intact, color gray, landmarks present. Hearing: finger rub heard in both ears at 3 ft. Rinne and Weber tests: normal, AC > BC.
Nose	Patency of each nostril Olfaction Turbinates and mucous membranes	External nose Vestibule Transillumination of sinuses	Nostrils patent, odors identified. Septum: slightly deviated to R. Turbinates and membranes: pink, moist, no discharge.
Oral cavity	Buccal mucosa Gums Teeth (decayed, missing, filled) Floor of mouth Hard and soft palate Tonsillar areas Posterior pharyngeal wall	Breath Lips Lesions Laryngoscopic examination Palpation of mouth Parotid duct	Membrane: pink and moist, no lesions. Gums: no edema. Teeth: 3D, 1M, 10F (approximately). Palate: intact, moves symmetrically with phonation, gag reflex present. Tonsils: present, not enlarged. Pharynx: pink and clean. Tongue: strong, moves symmetrically.

Table 23-1. Areas and examples of recording for the physical examination—cont'd

Area of examination	Descriptions usually recorded	Descriptions recorded in detail if abnormalities are present (partial listing only)	Examples of recording
Oral cavity —cont'd	Taste Tongue		Taste: able to differentiate sweet and sour.
Neck	Movements: rotation and lateral bend Symmetry Thyroid gland Tracheal position Glands and nodes	Postural alignment Tenderness Tone of muscles Lesions Masses	Full ROM, strong symmetrically, thyroid not palpable, trachea midline, no enlargement of head and neck regional nodes.
Breasts	Axillary nodes Supraclavicular nodes Infraclavicular nodes Breasts: observation and palpation Nipples Discharge Masses	Retraction Dimpling	No nodes palpable—axillary, infraclavicular, or supraclavicular; no masses, retraction, or discharge; L breast slightly larger than R breast, otherwise symmetrical at rest and with movement.
Chest and respiratory system	Shape of thorax Symmetry of thorax Respiratory movements Respiratory excursion Palpation: tactile fremitus, tenderness, masses Percussion notes Diaphragmatic excursion and level Auscultation: breath sounds, adventitious sounds	Adventitious sounds Deformity Use of accessory muscles of respiration Vocal fremitus Egophony, bronchophony, whispered pectoriloquy	Thorax oval, A.P. diameter < lateral diameter; symmetrical at rest and with movements; excursion normal; tactile fremitus equal bilaterally; no masses or tenderness; percussion tones resonant, diaphragmatic excursion 5 cm bilaterally between T10 and T12; vesicular breath sounds bilaterally; no adventitious sounds.
Central cardiovascular system	Position in which the heart was examined: lying, sitting, left lateral, recumbent Inspection: bulging depression, pulsation (precordial and juxtaprecordial) Palpation: thrusts, heaves, thrills, friction rubs Point of PMI Auscultation: rate and rhythm, character of S_1, character of S_2, comparison of S_1 in aortic and pulmonic areas, comparison of S_1 and S_2 in major auscultary areas, presence or absence of extra sounds—if present, description	Murmur or extra sound: whether systolic or diastolic; intensity; pitch; quality; site of maximal transmission; effect of position, respiration, and exercise; radiation	Examined in sitting and lying positions; no abnormal pulsations or lifts observed; PMI in the 5th ICS, slightly medial to the LMCL; no abnormal pulsations palpated. Apical pulse: 72, regular; S_1 single sound; S_2 splits with inspiration; A_2 is louder than P_2, S_1 heard loudest at apex, S_2 heard loudest at base; no murmurs or other sounds.
Arterial pulses	Radial pulse: rate, rhythm; consistency and tenderness of arterial wall Amplitude and character of peripheral pulses: superficial temporal, brachial, femoral, popliteal, posterior tibial, dorsal pedal	Any abnormality: analysis of type	Radial pulse: bilaterally equal, regular, strong; no tenderness or thickening of vessels; 76/min. Peripheral pulses:

	Temporal	Brachial	Femoral
R	as above	as above	as above
L	as above	as above	as above

	Popliteal	Posterior tibial	Dorsal pedal
R	not felt	as above	as above
L	not felt	as above	as above

Continued.

451

Table 23-1. Areas and examples of recording for the physical examination—cont'd

Area of examination	Descriptions usually recorded	Descriptions recorded in detail if abnormalities are present (partial listing only)	Examples of recording
Arterial pulses —cont'd	Carotid pulses: equality, amplitude, thrills, bruits		Carotid pulses: equal, strong, no bruits.
Venous pulses and pressures	Jugular venous pulsations, presence of waves a, c, and v Venous pressure: distention present at 45°	Hepatojugular reflex Analysis of jugular venous waves	Jugular venous pressure, 5 cm with client at 45°; venous a and v waves present, a wave strongest.
Abdomen	Inspection: scars, size, shape, symmetry, muscular development, bulging, movements Auscultation: peristaltic sounds—present or absent; vascular bruits—present or absent Palpation Masses Tenderness (local, referred, rebound), tone of musculature Liver: size, contour, character of edge, consistency, tenderness Kidney (indicate if palpable or not) Costovertebral area: tenderness Percussion: liver size at MCL, spleen, masses	Diastasis Distension Mass or bulging: specific description Palpable spleen: indication of size, surface contour, splenic notch, consistency, tenderness, mobility Palpable kidney: indication of location, size, shape, consistency Distention of urinary bladder Fluid wave Flank dullness Shifting dullness Aorta Gallbladder	Healed scar RLQ (appendectomy); slightly obese, protuberant; symmetrical, no bulging; normal bowel sounds, no bruits; no abnormal movements, symmetrical; no masses; no tenderness; liver 11 cm in RMCL; no CVA tenderness; no organs palpated; muscle tones lax. Area of midline diastasis: 6 cm × 2 cm inferior and superior to the umbilicus.
Neural system	Orientation Intellectual performance Emotional status Insight Memory Cranial nerves Coordination Sensory: touch, pain, position, vibration Babinski's sign Romberg's sign	Thought content Speech Sensory: hot, cold, two-point discrimination Stereognosis Involuntary movements	Alert, oriented ×3; mood appropriate and stable; remote and recent memory intact; several calculations by 6 accurate; insight normal; cranial nerves all intact, examined and recorded in head and neck regions; all movements coordinated; able to perform rapid coordinated movements with upper and lower extremities.

Reflexes (0-4+)
0 = absent
+ (or 1+) = decreased
++ (or 2+) = normal
+++ (or 3+) = hyperactive
++++ (or 4+) = clonus

Sensory: light touch, pain, and vibration to face, trunk, and extremities normal and symmetrical; walks with coordination, able to maintain standing position with eyes closed.

Table 23-1. Areas and examples of recording for the physical examination—cont'd

Area of examination	Descriptions usually recorded	Descriptions recorded in detail if abnormalities are present (partial listing only)	Examples of recording
Extremities and musculo-skeletal system	Both upper and lower extremities: general assessments—size, shape, mass, symmetry, hair distribution, color; temperature; edema; varicosities; tenderness; epitrochlear lymph nodes Bones and joints: range of motion, tenderness, gait Muscles: size, symmetry, strength, tone, tenderness, consistency Back: posture, tenderness; movement—extension, lateral bend, rotation	Lesions Deformities Color and temperature changes on elevation and dependency Homans' sign Redness Heat Swelling Deformity Crepitations Contractures Muscle spasms Tenderness Atrophy Hypertrophy	Muscular development and mass normal for age; arms and legs symmetrical; skin warm, soft, neither moist nor dry; normal male hair growth on arms, legs, and feet; no edema, varicosities, or tenderness; no nodes palpated; joints nontender, not swollen; normal ROM; muscle tone and strength normal bilaterally; back—full ROM; no tenderness or deformities.
Rectal area	Anal area Skin Hemorrhoids Sphincter tone Rectum Tumors Stool color Occult blood	Lesions Fissures Pilonidal sinus Condition of perineal body Tenderness Proctoscopic examination	Skin clean, no lesions; sphincter tone good; no hemorrhoids or masses noted; stools brown, guiac negative.
Inguinal area	Hernia: inguinal, femoral Nodes	Size, shape, consistency, tenderness, reducibility of hernia or nodes	Hernias not present; no enlargement of nodes noted.
Male genitalia	Penis: condition of prepuce, skin Scrotum: size, skin, testes, epididymides, spermatic cords Prostate gland: size, shape, symmetry, consistency, tenderness Seminal vesicles: size, shape, consistency	Scars Lesions Structural alterations Masses Swelling Nodules	Penis: circumsized, clean, no lesions. Scrotum and contents: normal size, no masses or tumors noted. Prostate and inferior portions of seminal vesicles: palpated. Prostate: not enlarged, rubbery, not tender. Seminal vesicles: soft, not nodular.
Female genitalia	External: hair distribution; labia; Bartholin's glands, urethral meatus, Skene's glands (BUS); hymen; introitus Vaginal observation: presence or absence of rectocele, urethrocele, cystocele; tissue; discharge (smears or cultures taken); cervix Bimanual examination: cervix, uterus, adnexa Rectovaginal examination; uterus, cul-de-sac, septum	Lesions Tumors Prolapses	Normal female hair distribution; no lesions or masses. BUS: no tenderness, redness, or discharge. Hymen: present in caruncles. Labia: approximate, intact. Introital tone: good; no prolapses; no scars, perineum thick. Vagina: pink; discharge—small amount, thin, clean, nonodorous. Cervix: pink, nulliparous, firm, not tender, movable, midline. Uterus: pear shaped, movable, normal size, firm, no masses. Tubes: not palpable. Ovaries: palpable, movable, not tender; approximately 2 × 3 × 2 cm; smooth surface, no lesions, firm consistency. Rectovaginal septum: thick and firm; no masses palpated in rectum or cul-de-sac.

WORKSHEET FOR RECORDING A PHYSICAL EXAMINATION

Vital signs

Temperature _____ Respiration _____ BP   (L)   Arm   (R)

_____ Supine _____

_____ Sitting _____

_____ Standing _____

Height _____ Weight _____ (Stripped or clothed)

General

Skin, hair, nails, mucous membranes

Head

Scalp _____

Face _____

(CNs V, VII) _____

_____

Sinus areas _____

Nodes _____

Cranium _____

Eyes

Visual acuity _____

Visual fields _____

Ocular movements (CNs III, IV, VI) _____

Corneal light reflex _____

Lids, lacrimal organs _____

Conjunctiva, sclera _____

Cornea (CN V) _____

Lens and media _____

Pupils: Pupillary reflexes (CN III) _____

Light, direct and consensual _____

Near point _____

Fundi (CN II) _____

Intraocular pressure _____

Ears

External structures _____

Canal _____

Tympanic membranes _____

Hearing (CN VIII) _____

2

Nose

Septum _____

Mucous membranes _____

Patency _____

Olfactory sense (CN I) _____

Oral cavity

Lips _____

Mucous membranes _____

Gums _____

Teeth _____

Palates and uvula (CNs IX and X) _____

Tonsillar areas _____

Tongue (CN XII) _____

Floor _____

Voice _____

Breath _____

Neck

General structure _____

Trachea _____

Thyroid _____

Nodes _____

Muscles (CN XI) _____

Breasts and area nodes

_____

_____

_____

Chest, respiratory system

Chest shape _____

Type of respiration _____

Expansion _____

Fremitus _____

General palpation _____

Percussion _____

_____ Diaphragmatic excursion: (R) _____ cm (L) _____ cm

Breath sounds _____

_____

_____

_____

Adventitious sounds _____

_____

Continued.

WORSHEET FOR RECORDING A PHYSICAL EXAMINATION—cont'd

3

Cardiovascular system

Rate and rhythm: Radial (palpation) _____

Apical (auscultation) _____

Precordium: Inspection _____

Palpation _____

Auscultation _____

S_1 _____

S_2 _____

S_3 _____

S_4 _____

Extra sounds _____

Murmur(s): Systolic _____

Diastolic _____

Carotids _____

Jugular venus pulse and pressure _____

Description of peripheral pulses

	Brachial	Radial	Femoral	Popliteal	Dorsal pedal	Post. tibial
R						
L						

Abdomen and inguinal areas

Contour, tone _____

Scars, marks _____

Auscultation _____

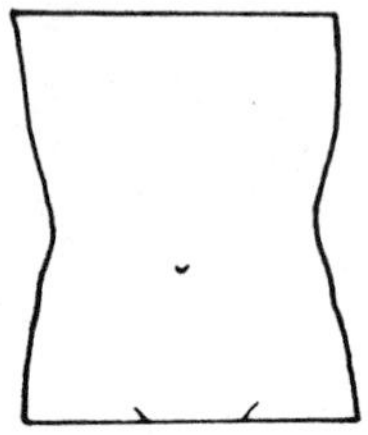

Liver _____ Span _____ cm at RMCL

Spleen _____

Kidneys _____ CVA tenderness _____

Bladder _____

Hernias _____

Masses _____

Palpation _____

Percussion _____

Genitalia and area nodes

_____
_____
_____
_____

Rectal examination

4

Musculoskeletal system

Gait _____

Deformities _____

Joint evaluation _____

_____

Muscle strength _____

_____

Muscle mass _____

Range of motion _____

Spine

Contour _____

Position _____

Motion _____

_____

Nervous system

Mental status _____

Language _____

Cranial nerves (summarize) _____

Motor: Coordination: Upper extremities _____

Lower extremities _____

Involuntary movements _____

Deep tendon reflexes:

Note: +s denote finger jerks, brachioradialis, biceps, triceps, reflexes, 4-quadrant abdominal scratch reflexes, patellar Achilles reflexes, and plantar reflexes. Abdominal reflexes are recorded as 0 or +. Scale: 0-4 (++++); normal = 2 (++).

Sensory

Light touch _____

Pain (pinprick) _____

Vibration _____

Position _____

24 Clinical laboratory procedures

The information obtained through the physical examination is augmented and in many cases verified through the judicious use of laboratory diagnostic procedures to provide a biochemical data base for use in the analysis of the client's state of health.

The tests most frequently included in a screening workup include a blood chemistry profile, hematology, a serological test for syphilis, urinalysis, a chest roentgenogram, the Papanicolaou (Pap) cytological examination for cancer diagnosis, hormonal evaluation of ovarian function in women from puberty onward, a proctoscopic examination, and an electrocardiogram (ECG) for all persons older than 40 years of age.

Blood chemistry profiles characteristically include determinations of sodium, potassium, chloride, calcium, phosphorus, glucose, bilirubin, blood urea nitrogen (BUN), uric acid, total proteins, albumin, cholesterol, serum glutamic-oxaloacetic transaminase (SGOT), lactic dehydrogenase (LDH), and alkaline phosphatase.

The hematology screening examination includes a study of the red blood cell (RBC) count, hematocrit, hemoglobin, mean corpuscular volume, and mean corpuscular hemoglobin concentration. In addition, the total white blood cell (WBC) count and a differential count based on morphological types are included.

Urinalysis is performed for analysis of specific gravity, pH, and the presence of glucose, protein, acetone, blood, and microscopic formed elements.

The procedure for the Pap smear is described in Chapter 17 on Assessment of the female genitalia and procedures for smears and cultures.

The tables of normal ranges found in textbooks of clinical pathology are to be considered as relative guidelines. The values are often those of a group of medical or nursing student volunteers and laboratory technicians and thus are not specific as to sex and age.

Furthermore, values vary from one clinical laboratory to another even though the same procedure may be used in each laboratory.

There may be real differences in values observed in geographically separated population groups, as well as seasonal changes; for example, generally higher cholesterol values are observed in sample populations in San Francisco. Uric acid levels are observed to be greater in winter than in other seasons.

When abnormal values are observed in test results, the examiner should review the interview data to determine if any circumstances in the client's life-style, environment, drug use, or state of nutrition or hydration may have influenced the value. For instance, an elevated protein-bound iodine (PBI) level and low resin-uptake value (tri-iodothyronine [T_3]) may indicate that the client has been taking oral contraceptives.

Posture is known to affect laboratory values. Blood albumin, total protein, hemoglobin, cholesterol and calcium values are known to be higher in the client who has been standing for a long period of time.

Diet and alcohol may also alter laboratory values. Bilirubin and SGOT values have been shown to be elevated during fasting. High fat content in the diet will produce hyperlipemia. High-protein meals may produce an increased BUN level. Most professionals are aware of the possibility of increased blood glucose values incurred as a result of a "carbohydrate binge." Alcohol consumption or alcoholic liver damage has been shown to result in increased levels of uric acid, glucose, calcium, phosphorus, LDH, SGOT, creatine phosphokinase (CPK), alkaline phosphatase, and triglycerides, accompanied by a low PBI level and albumin-globulin (A/G) ratio.

The blood specimens collected from a dehydrated individual will show the values to be consistent with the more concentrated fluid. These include increased levels of sodium, potassium, chloride, calcium, phosphorus, glucose, BUN, uric acid, cholesterol, total protein, globulin, LDH, SGOT, and creatinine.

The overhydrated client might be expected to have decreased concentrations of sodium, potassium, chloride, calcium, phosphorus, BUN, uric acid, albumin, total proteins, and cholesterol in the blood.

Improper handling of specimens may also result in erroneous test results. Test tubes that have been washed with detergent and poorly rinsed may cause spuriously elevated calcium, sodium, and potassium levels.

Possible applications of results of laboratory procedures include:

1. Provision of health assessment parameters of both a morphological and biochemical nature that are unavailable through the health history and physical examination.
2. Confirmation of a biochemical state of health when physical examination findings are negative.
3. Provision of further information in the differential diagnosis of disease. For example, the client with easy fatigability, shortness of breath on exertion, dizziness on exercise, and pale buccal mucosa may have a diagnosis of anemia confirmed through the results of screening hematological studies.
4. Provision of a gauge of the severity of disease. The degree of anemia that is disclosed may determine the therapeutic regimen for the client. The milder form of iron deficiency anemia may well be ameliorated in time through diet and rest, allowing the client's blood-forming organs to make up the deficit. Medication may be necessary for more severe involvement, and blood replacement by transfusion may be necessary for marked reduction in hemoglobin and RBCs.
5. Provision of biochemical clues that will indicate appropriate dosages of medication. A serum iron determination may be done for the client who is suspected of having iron deficiency anemia to substantiate the physical examination findings. The serum iron levels may be used to monitor the efficiency of the treatment regimen.

BLOOD CHEMISTRY PROFILE

Automated machines are available in many pathology laboratories for the purpose of performing chemistry tests. These machines commonly perform 6 to 24 determinations, using a single small sample of blood. Two types of machines are utilized. The first type is a discrete sample analyzer (DSA), which separates the sample into as many chambers as there are tests to be performed. Translated into the language of technician-performed testing, this means the sample is separated into an individual test tube for each ordered test. The second type is a continuous flow analyzer (CFA), which separates the sample within a single tubing into discrete sections through the use of bubbles. These sections pass through the tubing, stopping at specific sites for analysis. Some caution must be used with these machines to be certain that the tubing is thoroughly cleaned between samples.

Table 24-1 lists some of the machines used in the performance of blood chemistry profiles.

Most of these machines provide a printout sheet that records the client's data against a range of normal for the particular instrument. Graphs provided with the SMA 12/60 and SMA 6 are seen in Fig. 24-1 and 24-2.

Blood chemistry tests are performed on venous samples that are obtained following a period of fasting (usually at least 6 hours).

Some of these machines provide test results at a rate of greater than 3,000 per minute and thus provide significantly more data at less cost to the consumer.

In general, the machines are carefully self-calibrated and are more accurate than the results produced when humans do the testing.

Table 24-1. Machines used in the performance of blood chemistry profiles

Instrument	Type	Size of sample required (ml)	Number of tests possible	Choice of test or machine runs all possible tests
SMA 12/60	CFA	1.0	12	All
SMA C	CFA	0.5	20	All
AcuChem	DSA	0.5	17	Choice
Coulter Chemistry	DSA	3.0	21	Choice
Hycel 17, Super 17	DSA	1.2	17	Choice

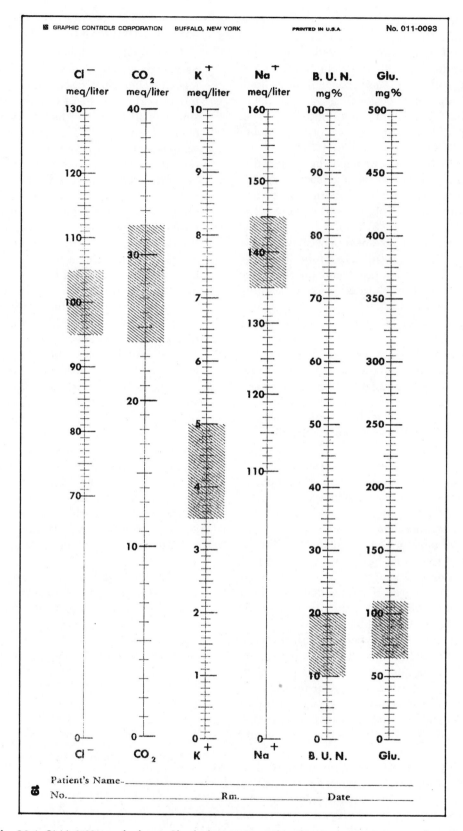

Fig. 24-1. SMA 6/60 graph sheet. Shaded areas in each column represent normal ranges. The machine draws a line representing the values of the specimen. Thus, deviation from the normal range is prominently displayed. (Courtesy Graphics Controls Corp., Buffalo, N.Y.)

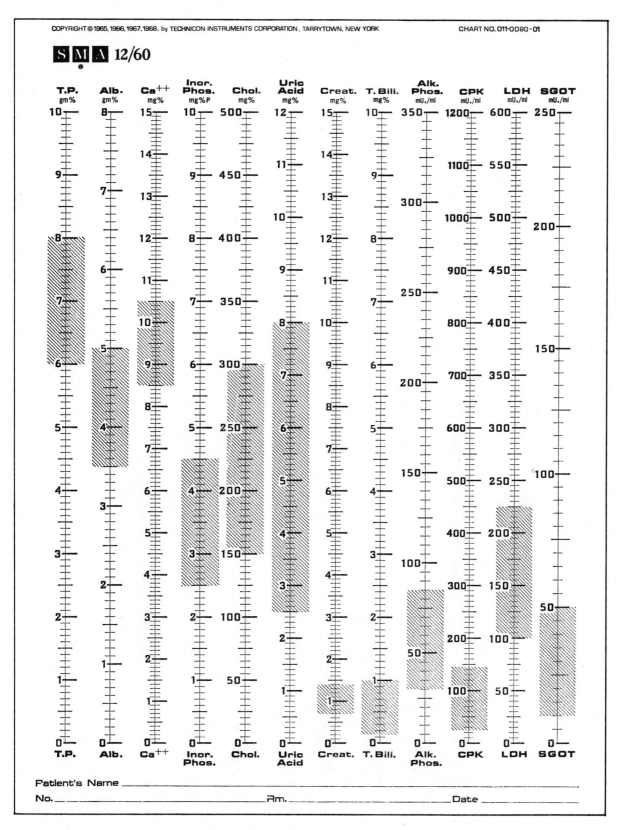

CHART NO. 011-0080-01

SMA 12/60

Fig. 24-2. Chart paper for Technicon™ SMA™ 12/60 multichannel analyzer. (Courtesy Technicon Instruments Corp., Tarrytown, N.Y.)

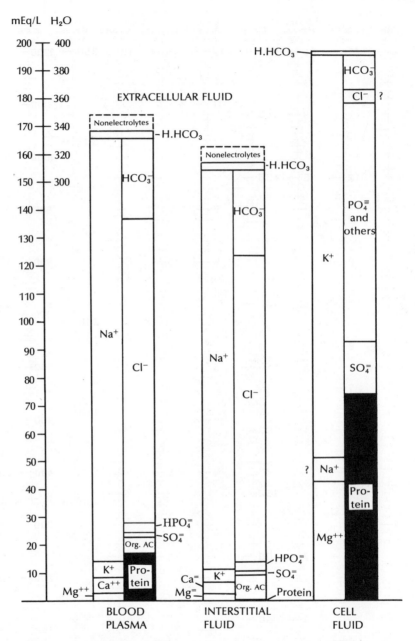

Fig. 24-3. Electrolyte distribution in the fluid compartment of the body. The column of figures on the left (200, 190, 180, and so on) indicates amounts of cations or anions; the figures on the right (400, 380, 360, and so on) indicate the sum of cations and anions. Note that chloride and sodium values in cell fluid are questioned. It is probable that at least muscle intracellular fluid contains some sodium but no chloride. (From Anthony, C. P., and Kolthoff, N. J.: Textbook of anatomy and physiology, ed. 9, St. Louis, 1975, The C. V. Mosby Co. Adapted from Mountcastle, V. B., editor: Medical physiology, vol. 2, ed. 13, St. Louis, 1974, The C. V. Mosby Co.; after Gamble, J. L.: Harvey Lect. **42:**247, 1946-1947.)

One disadvantage to the practitioner and the client is that more data may be generated than is actually necessary to assess the client's health status.

■ Electrolytes

Some electrolytes that are routinely analyzed in a screening examination include sodium (Na^+), potassium (K^+), chloride (Cl^-), and carbon dioxide CO_2 combining power.

Plasma is an aqueous solution (90% water) that contains approximately 1% electrolytes.

The distribution of electrolytes in the normal individual is represented by the following values:

Na^+	136 to 142 mEq/L		Cl^-	95 to 103 mEq/L
K^+	3.8 to 5 mEq/L		PO_4^{3-}	1.8 to 2.6 mEq/L
Ca^{2+}	4.5 to 5.3 mEq/L		SO_4^{2-}	0.2 to 1.3 mEq/L
Mg^{2+}	1.5 to 2.5 mEq/L		HCO_3^-	21 to 28 mEq/L
			Protein	$\cong$ 17 mEq/L

The distribution of these ions in the plasma is compared with those of the interstitial and cellular fluids in Fig. 24-3.

Electrolytes are carefully controlled through a variety of physical and chemical mechanisms, so that the range of normal for each of these compartments is quite narrow.

Sodium

Sodium is the major cation of the body. It is the most abundant extracellular ion and as such plays a prominent role in the osmolality of the extracellular fluid. The ion is necessary to the resting potential of excitable cells. The intake of sodium in the average adult diet is 10 to 12 gm, but the amount is variable.

The kidney plays the principal role in homeostasis of sodium in the body fluids. Aldosterone is secreted by the adrenal cortex due to activation of the renin angiotensin system when the whole blood sodium concentration or blood volume are decreased or when the potassium concentration is increased. ACTH directly stimulates the cells of the adrenal cortex. Thus, aldosterone is also secreted in times of stress. Aldosterone facilitates the reabsorption of sodium in the distal tubule of the kidney.

The concentration of the ions is necessarily dependent on the water content of the blood. Although the whole blood sodium content might stay constant, the concentration of the sodium ions will be greater when water stores are less in quantity.

Osmotic diuretic agents, such as mannitol and glucose, are known to carry out sodium with

Serum sodium: normal values and deviations

Normal values: 136 to 142 mEq/L
Normal osmolality of the blood: 280 to 295 mOsm/L

Deviations	Etiology
Hyponatremia	Dehydration with loss of electrolytes
	Sweating
	Diarrhea
	Burns
	Nasogastric tube
	Addison's disease
	Diuretics
	Mercurial
	Chlorothiazide
	Chronic renal insufficiency
	Starvation
	Diabetic acidosis
	Water retention or dilution
	Cirrhosis
	Congestive heart failure
	Renal insufficiency
	Excessive ingestion of water
	Overhydration with intravenous therapy
Hypernatremia	Deficient water intake
	Excessive water loss—lack of antidiuretic hormone (ADH)
	Cushing's disease
	Primary hyperaldosteronism

them. In some cases of acidemia, the concentration of SO_4^{2-}, Cl^-, PO_4^{3-}, and organic acids overwhelms the kidney's capacity to secrete H^+ and NH_3 while exchanging Na^+. Thus, the ions are excreted in the urine with fixed base, which is sodium for the most part.

Potassium

Potassium is the most abundant intracellular cation; since the majority of potassium is found within the cells, the total body content of the ion cannot be measured readily. Furthermore, the relationship between intracellular potassium and serum potassium is a highly dynamic one. For instance, intracellular potassium readily leaves the cell in the event of serum potassium deficiency. Potassium ions compete with hydrogen ions for excretion by the kidney. Dietary intake of potassium is excreted largely by these two mechanisms, though some may be lost in sweat and gastrointestinal secretions.

The importance of homeokinetic control of extracellular potassium ions relates to the function of potassium in neuromuscular excitability. The resting membrane potential of the cells of these

463

Serum potassium: normal values and deviations

Normal values: 3.8 to 5 mEq/L

Deviations	Etiology	Possible effects

Hyperkalemia	Excretion of K^+
	   Kidney disease
	   Intestinal obstruction
	Addison's disease
	Iatrogenic K^+ replacement therapy
	Trauma
	Burns
		Changes in ECG
		   >8 mEq/L widened
		   p wave
		Widened QRS complex
		Depressed ST segment
		   >11 mEq/L
		Symmetrical peaking of
		   T wave
		Ventricular fibrillation
		Heart block in
		   diastole
		Neuromuscular changes
		Numbness
		Tingling
		Flaccidity
		Muscle paralysis

Hypokalemia	↓ Ingestion of K^+
	Excretion of K^+
	   Prolonged gastrointestinal suctioning
	   Vomiting
	   Diuretics
	Excessive administration of bicarbonate (K^+ enters the cells)
	Cirrhosis
	Cushing's disease
	Treatment with steroids
	Aldosteronism
	Intravenous infusion of K^+ free fluids
		Changes in ECG
		Prolonged Q-T interval
		Prolonged T wave
		Malaise
		Apathy
		Nausea and vomiting
		↓ Reflexes
		↓ Smooth muscle tone
		   Distention
		   Paralytic ileus
		↓ Diastolic blood
		   pressure

Serum chloride: normal values and deviations

Normal values: 95 to 103 mEq/L

Deviations	Etiology	Possible effects
Hypochloremia	Hypokalemic alkalosis Ingestion of potassium compounds that do not contain chloride Potassium-sparing diuretics Excessive loss of gastric secretions Vomiting Nasogastric tube	Associated with ↓ K^+, ↑ CO_2 combining power
Hyperchloremia	Renal tubular acidosis	

tissues is directly related to the ratio of intracellular to extracellular potassium concentrations.

Chloride

Chloride is the major anion of the body and in general is found to behave in concert with sodium. More precisely, the chloride passively follows sodium in its transport through membranes. Chloride plays a prominent role in acid-base balance. In acidemia, Cl^- concentration is increased and thus more Cl^- is associated with sodium. In alkalemia, more bicarbonate (HCO_3^-) is associated with sodium. Chloride deficit leads to increased reabsorption of bicarbonate in the distal tubules of the kidney and thereby to alkalemia. Since chloride is necessary to the synthesis of hydrochloric acid in the stomach, excessive loss of gastric secretions leads to alkalemia.

Calcium

Plasma calcium (Ca^{2+}) occurs in three forms. About half of the calcium is bound to protein. Calcium in this form does not diffuse through the capillary wall. A second, nonionized, nondiffusable group of calcium compounds makes up approximately 5% of the plasma calcium. Somewhat less than half (45%) of the plasma calcium is ionized. This third form of calcium diffuses through the capillary membrane and is physiologically active.

The effect of calcium on skeletal and cardiac muscle, nerve tissue, and bone are due to the ionized calcium. The ionized calcium of the plasma is maintained within a fairly narrow range (±5%) due to the influence of parathyroid hormone (PTH) and thyrocalcitonin (TCT). PTH increases plasma ionized calcium by increasing absorption of calcium from the intestinal tract and reabsorption of calcium from the renal tubules of the kidney and by absorbing calcium salts from the bones through its action of osteoclasts. TCT lowers serum ionized calcium by increasing depositions of calcium in the bones through its influence on the osteoblasts.

A metabolite of vitamin D increases the absorption of calcium from the intestine through the stimulation of a calcium-binding protein.

Phosphorus

The serum level of phosphate (PO_4^{3-}) generally bears a combination relationship with serum calcium concentration. Parathyroid hormone increases the amount of phosphate absorbed in the intestinal tract since phosphate is absorbed when calcium is absorbed. The excretion of phosphate

Serum calcium: normal values and deviations

Normal values
Adults
Ionized: 4.2 to 5.2 mg/100 ml
2.1 to 2.6 mEq/L
Total: 9 to 10.6 mg/100 ml
4.5 to 5.3 mEq/L
Infants 11 to 13 mg/100 ml

Etiology	*Possible effects*
Deviations	
Hypercalcemia	
↑ PTH	↓ Neuromuscular excitability
↓ TCT	Skeletal muscle
↑ Vitamin D	(↓ tone, weakness)
↑ Ingestion of Ca^{2+}	Smooth muscle (observed in such
Acidosis	signs as constipation)
Paget's disease	Heart muscle
Destructive bone lesions	Shortening of Q-T interval of ECG
	↓ Plasma phosphate
	Renal calculi due to precipitation of calcium phosphate ($Ca_3 [PO_4]_2$)
	Associated with ↑ alkaline phosphatase
Hypocalcemia	
↑ TCT	↑ Neuromuscular excitability (tetany)
↓ PTH	Prolongation of the S-T segment of the ECG
↓ Absorption of Ca^{2+} from the gastrointestinal tract	Osteomalacia in adults
Steatorrhea	Rickets in children
Sprue	
Celiac disease	
↓ Vitamin D (hypovitaminosis)	
Hypoalbuminemia	
Pregnancy	
Diuretic ingestion	
Hypomagnesemia	
Starvation	

Serum phosphorus: normal values and deviations

Normal values
Adults: 3 to 4.5 mg/100 ml
1.8 to 2.6 mEq/L
Children: 4 to 7 mg/100 ml
2.3 to 4.1 mEq/L

Deviations	*Etiology*	*Possible effects*
Hyperphosphatemia	↑ TCT	Associated with ↑ BUN, creatinine
	↑ Growth hormone	Symptoms of hypocalcemia
	↑ Ingestion of PO_4^{3-}	Associated with ↑ gamma globulin
	Chronic glomerulonephritis	
	Sarcoidosis	
Hypophosphatemia	↑ PTH	↓ ATP
	↓ Ingestion of PO_4^{3-}	Symptoms of hypercalcemia
	Hyperinsulinism	Associated with indications of hypoglycemia

Serum magnesium: normal values and deviations

Normal values: 1.5 to 2.5 mEq/L
1.8 to 3 mg/100 ml

Deviations	*Etiology*	*Possible effects*
Hypermagnesemia	↑ Ingestion of Mg^{2+} (milk of magnesia)	↓ Neuromuscular excitation
		↓ Muscle tone
Hypomagnesemia	Malabsorption syndrome	↑ Neuromuscular excitation (tetany)
	Acute pancreatitis	Peripheral vasodilation
		Arrhythmias

Magnesium

Magnesium (Mg^{2+}) influences muscular activity in much the same direction as does calcium. The ion appears to be necessary for the coenzyme activity in the metabolism of carbohydrate and protein.

■ Gases and pH

The blood gases are not usually tested in the screening examination but may be indicated as necessary tests by clinical signs such as cyanosis or hyperventilation.

Oxygen

Tests for blood oxygen analysis are generally performed on arterial blood. The blood may be tested for oxygen content, hemoglobin satura-

is accomplished largely by the kidney and is determined by the fact that phosphate is a threshold substance. Thus, the kidney regulates the serum phosphate level by secreting phosphate when the serum level exceeds 1 millimol/L and retaining phosphate when the serum concentration is less.

Blood oxygen: normal values and deviations

Normal values

	ARTERIAL BLOOD	MIXED VENOUS BLOOD
Content:	15 to 23 vol%	
Saturation:	94% to 100%	70% to 75%
Tension:	95 to 100 mm Hg	35 to 40 mm Hg

Deviations	*Etiology*	*Possible effects*
Anoxic hypoxia	Inadequate environmental O_2 supply, such as occurs in high altitude (acute) Impaired respiratory exchange	Low PaO_2 Inadequate saturation of the arterial blood with oxygen Cyanosis ↑ Respiratory rate
Chronic hypoxia	Living at high altitude	↑ O_2 carrying capacity as RBCs increase
Anemic hypoxia	↓ Hemoglobin Competition for hemoglobin-binding sites (carbon monoxide poisoning)	↓ Saturation of hemoglobin possible
Stagnant hypoxia	↓ Circulatory function (failure to deliver O_2 to tissues) 　Cardiac failure 　Shock 　Peripheral impairment of flow (embolism)	Blood O_2 values may be normal
Histotoxic hypoxia	↓ Ability of cells to take up or utilize O_2, such as in poisoning	
Hyperoxia	Pure O_2 delivered at 1 atmosphere (766 mm Hg)	Bronchitis in 12 to 24 hours Fall in vital capacity in 60 hours Retrolental fibroplasia

tion, and the gas tension (PaO_2, arterial blood; PvO_2, venous blood). The oxygen content of the blood reflects the hemoglobin concentration. At standard temperature and pressure 1.34 ml of oxygen combines with 1 gm of hemoglobin at full saturation. The oxygen saturation of hemoglobin is a comparison of the percentage of oxygen that is bound to hemoglobin with the total amount that it is possible for the hemoglobin to carry. The erythrocyte carries 98.5% of the oxygen in the blood bound to hemoglobin. Since the normal hemoglobin content of the adult male is 15 gm/100 ml, the oxygen-carrying capacity is approximately 20 ml/100 ml of blood, or 20 vol%.

At standard conditions arterial blood contains 0.3 ml of oxygen dissolved in 100 ml of plasma;

this exerts a pressure of 100 mm Hg. The amount of oxygen combined with hemoglobin is decreased with an increase in temperature, acidity, and carbon dioxide tension ($PaCO_2$, arterial blood; $PvCO_2$, venous blood).

Carbon dioxide

Carbon dioxide in the blood occurs in three forms: as bicarbonate, combined with protein (carbamino), and in simple solution. Carbon dioxide in an aqueous solution is in potential equilibrium with carbonic acid. The enzyme carbonic anhydrase is necessary to the catalysis of the equilibrium:

$$CO_2 + H_2O \rightleftharpoons H_2CO_3$$

The only test for carbon dioxide that is generally performed as part of the screening battery is the carbon dioxide–combining power, which measures the buffering capacity of the blood. The sample is collected, and the serum is removed after clotting and centrifugation. The carbon dioxide tension of the serum is equilibrated to normal alveolar tensions of 40 mm Hg. The bicarbonate is converted to carbon dioxide by hydrolysis, and the gas that is given up is measured. Subtraction of the known amount of dissolved carbon dioxide in the blood gives a value that is essentially that of bicarbonate alone.

Normal $PaCO_2$: 35 to 45 mm Hg
Normal $PvCO_2$: 41 to 55 mm Hg
Normal arterial whole blood HCO_3^-: 22 to 26 mEq/L
Normal venous whole blood HCO_3^-: 22 to 26 mEq/L

The base excess (BE) is a measure of alkaline substances in the blood. This includes bicarbonate and other bases in the blood.

Normal arterial BE: −2 to +2
Normal venous BE: −2 to +2

pH

Hydrogen ion concentration of the blood is reflected in the pH value. The degree of alkalinity or acidity of the body is important in that many enzymes are active only within narrow pH ranges. Furthermore, many other physiological processes are pH dependent, notably respiration. Acidosis is the process whereby an individual develops acidemia, the accumulation of excess hydrogen ions in the blood—or decreased pH. The affected person is described as acidotic.

Alkalosis, on the other hand, is the process whereby alkalemia is incurred. Alkalemia may be defined as decreased hydrogen ion concentration in the blood—or increased pH—and the individual may be described as alkalotic.

The Henderson-Hasselbalch equation describes pH relationships:

$$pH = pK + \log \frac{base}{acid}$$

pK is the dissociation constant (the ability to release hydrogen ions of the acid described). In the human being the bicarbonate ion is the most important buffering system, since the ion is present in large quantities. Thus, the equation may be written:

$$pH = 6.1 + \log \frac{HCO_3^-}{H_2CO_3}$$

The ratio $\dfrac{HCO_3^-}{H_2CO_3} = \dfrac{20}{1}$ in the normal person.

The bicarbonate ion is controlled by the lungs through the expiration of carbon dioxide and the kidneys, which control excretion of bicarbonate and hydrogen ions.

Whole blood pH: normal values and deviations

Normal values
Arterial: 7.38 to 7.44 (7.40)
Venous: 7.30 to 7.41 (7.36)

Deviations
Acidemia (acidosis): <pH 7.35
Alkalemia (alkalosis): >pH 7.45

Glucose

Sucrose, lactose, and starches make up the majority of the carbohydrates ingested by man. Slight amounts of alcohol, lactic acid, pyruvic acid, pectins, and dextrins are also consumed. These carbohydrates are hydrolyzed in the intestinal tract, so that they are broken down to the monosaccharides: glucose (80%), fructose (10%), and galactose (10%) in which form they are absorbed into the bloodstream.

Glucose is the principal form of fuel for cellular function; and the liver can convert fructose and galactose to glucose, so that all of the absorbed sugars can be utilized. Fats and proteins may also be converted to glucose during fasting states or in times of increased glucose utilization, as in exercise. Glucose in excess of energy needs is converted to storage forms. The body is capable of storing about 100 gm of glucose as glycogen. The majority of the remainder of glucose is converted to fat, but some is converted to amino acids.

The pancreatic hormones, insulin and glucagon, play a prominent role in glucose metabolism, as well as in the metabolism of protein and lipid. Insulin is produced by the beta cells of the pancreas, and its secretion is primarily deter-

Blood glucose: normal values and deviations

Normal values
Serum or plasma: 70 to 110 mg/100 ml (Folin-Wu)
65 to 90 mg/100 ml (Somogyi-Nelson)
65 to 90 mg/100 ml (Glucose oxidase)

Deviations	Etiology	Possible effects
Hyperglycemia	Diabetes mellitus (most common cause)	Ketoacidosis
	Pancreatic insufficiency	$\downarrow CO_2$ combining power
	Cushing's disease	
	Treatment with steroids	
	$\uparrow$ Catecholamines	
	Pheochromocytoma	
	Pancreatic neoplasm	
	Hyperthyroidism (look for hypocholesterolemia)	
	Thiazide diuretics	
Hypoglycemia	Beta cell neoplasm (hyperinsulinism)	
	Addison's disease	
	Hypothyroidism	
	Hepatocellular disease	
	Starvation (late)	
	Glycogen storage diseases	

mined by the concentration of blood glucose. The secretion of insulin is increased by an increase from basal of blood glucose; it is decreased as the concentration of blood glucose becomes less than normal. Blood insulin values in excess of normal produce the following major changes in glucose metabolism: (1) the rate of glucose metabolism is increased by facilitating the transport of glucose into the cells via facilitated diffusion, (2) the process of glycogen storage is enhanced, and (3) the process of glucose entry into fat cells is enhanced and fat storage increased.

On the other hand, a decrease of blood insulin is accompanied by (1) glycogenolysis, or a breakdown of glycogen to glucose, and (2) gluconeogenesis, the manufacture of glucose by the liver from amino acids derived from protein stores and from glycerol derived from fat stores.

Thus, blood glucose concentration in the fasting state is maintained within reasonably narrow limits. Blood glucose determination at any one time will provide data concerning the state of the body's metabolism for that specific point in the individual's daily cycle. However, the practitioner must bear in mind that the metabolic processes are determined by the state of nutrition and the energy expenditure. The normal individual, in dynamic equilibrium, will show remarkable variation throughout the day; the picture is even more complex in disease.

Care of specimens for blood glucose determination deserves special attention; glucose values for whole blood decrease 10 mg/100 ml per hour (at room temperature) unless a satisfactory preservative is employed. Fluoride is currently recognized as the most effective preservative.

Glucose analysis is accomplished by reducing and enzymatic methods. In both cases a protein-free filtrate of the blood sample is tested. The reducing methods include the Folin-Wu and Somogyi-Nelson tests, both of which consist of color changes that occur in copper solutions. The enzymatic (glucose oxidase) tests measure hydrogen peroxide that is released during the enzymatic conversion of glucose to gluconic acid.

Blood glucose values are 120 to 130 mg/100 ml in mild hyperglycemia, and >500 mg/100 ml in marked hyperglycemia.

Serum bilirubin: normal values and deviations

Normal values
Total: 0.1 to 1.2 mg/100 ml
Newborn: 1 to 12 mg/100 ml

Deviations	Etiology	Possible effects
Hyperbili-rubinemia	Destruction of red cells Hemolytic diseases Hemorrhage Hematoma Hepatic dysfunction	Jaundice
↑ Unconjugated bilirubin	Autoimmune disease Transfusion-initiated hemolysis Hemolytic diseases Sickle cell anemia Pernicious anemia Glucuronyl transferase deficiency (hemolytic disease of the newborn) Hemorrhage (bleeding into body cavities) Hematoma Impaired hepatic uptake of bile (infectious or toxic hepatitis)	Brain damage (22 mg/100 ml or more)
↑ Conjugated bilirubin	Impaired glucuronide excretion Hepatocellular disease (infectious, toxic, or autoimmune hepatitis) Cirrhosis Obstruction of biliary ducts Calculi Tumor Extrinsic pressure Cholangiolitis	"Regurgitation" of conjugated bilirubin back into the blood

A rising blood glucose concentration stimulates excessive insulin secretion in some individuals. Some amino acids (leucine) may also stimulate excessive beta cell secretion. Thus, glucose levels may be depleted as the insulin effects are manifested.

Two-hour postprandial glucose test. The 2-hour postprandial glucose test consists of the serial collection of samples for blood glucose determination following a 100-gm carbohydrate meal given to a client who has fasted for 12 hours. The following represent hyperglycemic results:

Time	Blood glucose determination
1 hour after meal	>170 mg/100 ml
2 hours after meal	>120 mg/100 ml

Glucose tolerance test. The glucose tolerance test is performed in the fasting individual following the ingestion of 100 gm of glucose; the blood glucose level rises 30 to 60 mg/100 ml above the fasting level by 30 minutes. By the end of an hour the blood glucose level begins to decline (20 to 50 mg/100 ml), and after 2 to 3 hours returns to the fasting level. Urine specimens are collected. Glucose does not appear in the urine of the normal individual during the course of the glucose tolerance test. The glucose tolerance test shows elevated values in the period following myocardial infarction.

■ Bilirubin

Bilirubin is a pigment most of which is derived from the breakdown of heme in the hemoglobin of RBCs in Kupffer's cells of the reticuloendothelial system. The pigment has a golden hue and is the major pigment found in bile. Plasma containing the pigment enters the hepatic parenchymal cells and is enzymatically conjugated with glucuronic acid in preparation for excretion. The conjugated bilirubin is soluble in an aqueous medium and is actively excreted into the bile. A small amount of the conjugated bilirubin is returned to the blood and accounts for the direct-reacting bilirubin found in the plasma of normal subjects. Because it passes through membranes, it may be detected in the urine.

Intestinal bacteria act on bilirubin to form urobilinogen. Since urobilinogen is highly soluble, it is readily reabsorbed through the intestinal mucosa into the blood and is for the most part recycled in the liver back to the intestine; some, however, is excreted in the urine.

Bilirubin is analyzed through its reaction (color change) with diazo reagents; this is the basis of van den Bergh's test. The conjugated form reacts expediently with the diazo reagents in aqueous solution and is called direct reacting. The unconjugated form must be treated with methyl alcohol for the reaction to occur and is called indirect reacting.

Bilirubin is called unconjugated, free, or indirect reacting before it is combined with glucuronic acid in the liver cell. It does not cross the membranes of the capillary or of the glomerular capsule. After combination with glucuronic acid in the hepatic cells, bilirubin is referred to as conjugated, glucuronide, or direct reacting.

The occurrence of jaundice (yellowish tint of the skin) represents the failure to remove or excrete the bilirubin. The skin may appear jaundiced when serum bilirubin levels are about three times the normal value. In most individuals pigmentation of the tissues is visible when serum bilirubin levels exceed 1.5 mg/100 ml.

■ Blood urea nitrogen

Urea is the end product of protein metabolism and is formed through deamination of amino acids in the liver. Urea is excreted by the kidneys.

Ingestion of protein does not cause a significant change in the BUN level. However, in the interest of accuracy this test is done in the fasting individual.

The severity of uremia is an indicator of the seriousness of renal involvement.

BUN: normal values and deviations

Normal values
8 to 18 mg/100 ml
Normal values tend to be higher in male subjects than in female subjects.

Deviations	Etiology
Increased BUN level (uremia)	High protein intake
	Dehydration
	Protein catabolism
	Burns
	Intestinal obstruction
	Gastrointestinal hemorrhage
	Renal disease
	Glomerulonephritis
	Pyelonephritis
	Prostate hypertrophy
Decreased BUN level	↓ Protein ingestion
	Starvation
	Liver dysfunction
	Cirrhosis (loss of 80% to 85% hepatic function)

■ Creatinine

The metabolism of creatinine phosphate, a high-energy compound produced in skeletal muscle, results in the production of creatinine. The serum creatinine level does not vary markedly with diet or exercise and may be regarded as an indicator of total muscle mass.

Creatinine clearance by the kidney has been used as a measure of renal function. In addition to the fact that the serum creatinine level is fairly constant, using creatinine clearance as a measure offers another advantage to the client in that an intravenous injection of the substance used in the clearance study is not needed. Renal plasma clearance of creatinine (C) is equal to the rate of creatinine excretion (UV) divided by the plasma concentration of creatinine (P):

$$C = \frac{UV}{P}$$

Since endogenous creatinine is fully filtered in the glomerulus and not reabsorbed by the tubules, its clearance is a useful clinical tool for estimation of the glomerular filtration rate (GFR). Thus, the removal of creatinine from the blood is a measure of renal efficiency. As renal function declines, the creatinine level rises.

■ Uric acid

Uric acid production is the final step in purine metabolism. Uric acid is not in stable solution at a normal human blood pH of 7.4. Uric acid is continuously produced in the human being and is excreted by the kidney. The quantity of uric acid found in the urine is about 10% of that which is filtered. Thus, it is obvious that uric acid is reabsorbed in the proximal tubules. It has been further shown that uric acid is secreted in the proximal tubules.

However, reabsorption overrides this process, and the plasma uric acid represents the

Serum creatinine: normal values and deviation

Normal values
0.6 to 1.2 mg/100 ml
Normal values for male subjects are slightly higher than for female subjects.

Deviation	Etiology	Possible effects
Hypercreatinemia	Renal disease (75% of nephrons are nonfunctional)	Signs of renal failure
	Chronic glomerulonephritis	
	Nephrosis	
	Pyelonephritis	

Serum uric acid: normal values and deviation

Normal values
Females: 2 to 6.4 mg/100 ml
Males: 2.1 to 7.8 mg/100 ml

Deviation	Etiology	Possible effects
Hyperuricemia (gout)	↑ Destruction of nucleic acid and purine products Chronic lymphocytic and granulocytic leukemia Multiple myeloma Chronic renal failure Fasting ↑ Ingestion of protein ↓ Excretion of uric acid Gout Toxemia of pregnancy Glomerulonephritis Thiazide diuretics Alpha-lipoprotein deficiency (Tangier disease) Hypoparathyroidism ↑ Salicylate ingestion Ethanol ingestion	Monosodium urate precipitate in joints (tophi) Often associated with hyperlipidemia, atheromatosis Impaired clearance of uric acid

balance of uric acid production and excretion.

Monosodium urate deposits may occur in the presence of a normal serum uric acid value.

Hypouricemia is seldom observed unless the client is being treated with allopurinol, which depresses uric acid production.

■ Total proteins

Plasma proteins make up approximately 7% of the plasma volume. Albumin and globulin in the free state as well as in combination with lipid and carbohydrate substances are the major plasma proteins. Through the application of zone electrophoresis and ultracentrifugation, the plasma proteins have been defined as albumin, the globulins (alpha-1, alpha-2, beta-1, beta-2, and gamma), lipoproteins, and fibrinogen. Separation through centrifugation is possible because the sedimentation rate at high speeds is determined by molecular size and shape. Electrophoresis is the process of migration of charged particles in an electrolyte solution through which an electrical current is passed. The proteins move at various rates depending on size, shape, and electrical charge. Immunoelectrophoresis separates the immune globulin fractions through a combination of electrophoresis and immunodiffusion.

The plasma proteins are large molecules that do not readily diffuse through the capillary membrane. The small amount of protein that does pass through the capillary wall is taken up by the lymphatic system and returned to the blood. It has been demonstrated that the plasma protein concentration exceeds that of the interstitial space nearly four times. Since the plasma proteins are the only dissolved substances in the plasma that do not pass through the capillary membrane, they are responsible for plasma oncotic pressure. Thus, proteins help to regulate intravascular volume. The plasma proteins also serve as buffers in acid-base balance and as binding and transporting agents for lipids, triglycerides, hormones, vitamins, calcium, and copper. In addition, they participate in blood coagulation. Furthermore, in the event that body tissues become depleted of protein, plasma proteins may be used for replenishment. The liver synthesizes nearly all of the plasma albumin and fibrinogen and about one half of the globulins.

The rate of synthesis is dependent on the availability of amino acids in the plasma.

Normal plasma protein values
Total: 6 to 7.8 gm/100 ml
Albumin: 3.2 to 4.5 gm/100 ml
Globulins: 2.3 to 3.5 gm/100 ml

Alpha-1 globulin	0.2 to 0.4 gm/100 ml
Alpha-2 globulin	0.5 to 0.9 gm/100 ml
Beta globulin	0.5 to 1.0 gm/100 ml
Gamma globulin	1.0 to 2.0 gm/100 ml

Fibrinogen: 0.2 to 0.4 gm/100 ml

Albumin

Normal plasma albumin, essentially all of which is synthesized in the liver, makes up 52% to 68% of the blood and is responsible for 80% of the oncotic pressure. Thyroxin, bilirubin, fatty acids, salicylates, barbiturates, and other drugs are bound and transported by albumin. Since the albumin molecule is small in comparison to other blood proteins, it is the plasma protein most frequently detected in the urine in the event of renal damage.

Deviation	Etiology
Hypoalbuminemia (2.5 gm or less)	Chronic liver disease Protein malnutrition Malabsorption syndrome, especially of protein Nephrotic syndrome Chronic infection Acute stress

Serum albumin elevation is seldom encountered.

The normal pregnant woman has decreased albumin levels that are progressive through delivery and do not return to normal until 8 weeks postpartum.

Globulins

The five globulin fractions serve as transport media or antibodies. Approximately 50% of the globulins are manufactured by the liver; the remainder are synthesized in the lymphatic tissue and other reticuloendothelial cells.

Alpha-1 globulins bind carriers for cortisol (transcortin), thyroxine (thyroxine-binding globulin), fats, lipids, and fat soluble vitamins.

Alpha-2 globulins contain copper (ceruloplasmin), hemoglobin (haptoglobulin), lipids, triglycerides, erythropoietin, glycoprotein, mucoprotein, prothrombin, angiotensinogen, enzymes such as cholinesterase, lactic acid dehydrogenase, and alkaline phosphatase.

Beta globulins bind and transport heme (hemopexin) and iron (transferrin) and include lipid soluble vitamins, hormones, glycerides, phospholipids, lipoprotein, cholesterol, fibrinogen, profibrinolysin, and complement components.

The gamma globulin fraction includes the immunoglobulins, or antibodies, and the cryoglobulins, or cold agglutinins.

Deviations	Etiology
Hyperglobulinemia	Hypergammaglobinemia
	Hodgkin's disease
	Leukemia
	Myeloproliferative diseases
	(multiple myeloma)
	Chronic granulomatous infectious diseases (tuberculosis)
	Chronic hepatitis
	Collagen disease
	Sarcoidosis
Alteration in globulin fractions	
Absence of alpha-1 globulins	Alpha-1 (antitrypsin deficiency)
↓ Alpha-1 globulins	Nephrotic syndrome
↑ Alpha-2 globulins	Stress situations
	Infection
	Injury
	Surgery
	Tissue necrosis
	Myocardial infarction
	Nephrotic syndrome
↑ Beta globulins	Pregnancy (third trimester)
	Associated with serum cholesterol
	Hypothyroidism
	Biliary cirrhosis

Deviations—cont'd	Etiology—cont'd
	Nephrosis
	Obstructive jaundice
	Hepatitis
↓ Gamma globulins	Hypogammaglobulinemia
	Nephrotic syndrome
	Lymphosarcoma
	Lymphocytic leukemia
	Multiple myeloma
↑ Gamma globulins	Infections
	Collagen diseases
	Hypersensitivity diseases
	Hodgkin's disease
	Malignant lymphoma
	Chronic lymphocytic leukemia
	Multiple myeloma
	Liver disease
	Hepatitis
	Cirrhosis
	Obstructive jaundice

Albumin-globulin ratio

In the normal client, the albumin is about double that of globulin.

Normal A/G ratio: 1.5:2.5

An A/G ratio of 2.5:3 is strongly suggestive of chronic liver disease.

The levels of each of the globulins obtained from the electrophoretic zone patterns are more valuable data than the A/G ratio.

Fibrinogen

The bulk of fibrinogen is produced in the liver. Fibrinogen is the precursor of fibrin.

Deviation	Etiology	Possible effects
Hypofibrinogenemia	Hepatic dysfunction	Disseminated intravascular coagulation

■ Lipids

Several lipid elements are present in the normal plasma. These lipids are bound to specific proteins and phospholipids that render them soluble in the aqueous media of the blood. The lipids that are transported in the blood are comprised of exogenous triglycerides, (glycerol esterified with fatty acids from ingested foods, endogenous triglycerides (manufactured by the liver), cholesterol, phospholipids, and free fatty acids. All of the serum lipoproteins contain these same substances and vary only in the amount of each substance and in the size of the molecule.

Exogenous triglycerides

Exogenous triglycerides are the major constituent of chylomicrons, the largest lipids; these lipids contain a lesser quantity of cholesterol (10%), phospholipids (7%), and protein (24%). The high triglyceride content results in a density less than water. Thus, the chylomicrons may rise to the top of the blood left standing. The large size of the molecule results in light scattering, resulting in a turbid appearance of the plasma. The disappearance of chylomicrons from the blood is dependent on the presence of the enzyme lipoprotein lipase. The chylomicrons should return to basal levels within 6 hours following a fat-containing test meal.

Since the chylomicron (and thus, triglyceride) level varies with dietary intake of fats, the most valuable data are obtained from testing done in the fasting state.

Endogenous triglycerides

Endogenous triglycerides are manufactured by the liver. Hepatic triglyceride synthesis appears to be independent of the sudden increase in dietary intake of fats but shows a relationship to the total ingestion of foodstuffs, particularly in regard to caloric value.

Endogenous triglycerides are transported in molecules that are less dense than chylomicrons;

these molecules are called very low density lipoproteins (VLDLs). Endogenous triglycerides are the major constituent (55%) of these molecules; protein contributes a lesser amount (2% to 15%), and the remainder is made up of free and esterified cholesterol and phospholipids.

Cholesterol

Exogenous cholesterol is absorbed from the small intestine into the lymph. Endogenous cholesterol is formed by all the cells of the body. Most of the endogenous cholesterol in the plasma is formed by the liver from acetate. It is the endogenous cholesterol that is measured in blood chemistry profiles. A control mechanism exists for these two processes, since endogenous cholesterol production is inhibited when cholesterol ingestion is increased. Cholesterol is present in the plasma primarily as low-density (beta) lipoproteins (LDLs). Analyses of high-density (alpha) and very low density (prebeta) lipoproteins also reveal the presence of cholesterol. Cholesterol testing was the forerunner of serum lipid analysis and has served as a valuable tool for the prediction of coronary artery disease due to atheromatous or arteriosclerotic artery disease.

Because the liver esterifies cholesterol, the ratio of esterified to unesterified cholesterol may be considered an indication of liver function. The normal serum esterified cholesterol value ranges from 20% to 30%.

Obstruction of the biliary ducts is typified by an increased cholesterol level with a decrease in the amount of esterified cholesterol.

High-density lipoproteins. High-density lipoproteins (HDLs) have been suggested to be carriers of cholesterol from the tissues for metabolism and excretion and repositories for lipolytic enzyme activators. Observations provide an inverse correlation between HDLs and coronary artery disease potential.

Phospholipids

Lecithin and sphingomyelin are the major serum phospholipids. Phospholipids are constituents of both alpha (high-density) and beta (low-density) lipoproteins.

Normal serum phospholipid values: 150 to 375 mg/100 ml

Free fatty acids

Free fatty acids are transported in the blood in combination with albumin. At this point little diagnostic information is gained by measuring these

---

Serum cholesterol: normal values and deviations

Normal values: 150 to 250 mg/100 ml

Deviations	Etiology	Possible effects
Hypercholesterolemia (marked: 400 mg/100 ml)	Liver disease Nephrotic stage of glomerulonephritis Familial hypercholesterolemia Hypothyroidism Pancreatic dysfunction Diabetes mellitus	Associated with ↑ alkaline phosphatase, ↑ bilirubin, ↑ BUN, ↑ creatinine
Hypocholesterolemia (significant: 150 mg/100 ml)	↓ Ingestion of cholesterol Malnutrition Fasting Liver disease Megaloblastic or hypochromic anemia ↑ Estrogen ↑ Thyroid hormone Hypermetabolic states Fever Exercise	

acids, and they are not included in clinical lipid evaluation.

Hyperlipemias are clinically important when values exceed 100 mg/100 ml.

■ Enzymes

Enzymes are individual or aggregates of protein molecules occurring in globular form. Enzymes act as catalysts to biochemical reactions. In the event of cellular destruction of an organ or tissue, the cytoplasmic enzymes are released into the plasma from the diseased cells. Enzymes are categorized by their functional effect. These groupings are called isoenzymes. Isoenzymes are enzymes with the same functional effect but with variations in configuration and physical characteristics. The isoenzyme content of many tissues and structures has been determined. There is sufficient variation in the enzyme content of the various organs that changes in the enzyme concentration in the blood may serve as an indicator of the site of disease. Electrophoresis may be used to separate these proteins. Serum enzyme determination results are also used to assess tissue rejection following transplantation procedures.

SGOT, serum LDH, and serum alkaline phosphatase determinations are included in most screening laboratory examinations. Enzyme determinations currently and commonly encountered in clinical practice are described in this section.

Serum glutamic-oxaloacetic transaminase

SGOT is found in many tissues. The transaminase enzymes catalyze the conversion of an amino acid to keto acid while another keto acid is converted to an amino acid in the glycolytic cycle. This enzyme catalyzes conversions of glutamic and oxaloacetic acids. High tissue concentrations of SGOT have been demonstrated for the heart and liver, but appreciable amounts are found in RBCs, muscle, and kidney.

Colorimetric and spectrophotometric techniques are used in determining the serum concentration of these enzymes. Elevated levels of the enzyme may be identified 8 hours after tissue damage occurs. In the case of a single injury (such as myocardial infarction) that is not followed by further damage, the enzyme reaches a peak level in 24 to 36 hours and declines to basal levels in about 4 to 6 days.

The SGOT concentration is directly related to the degree of cellular damage.

Total serum lipids: normal values and deviations

Normal values: 350 to 800 mg/100 ml (adult)

Deviations	Etiology	Predominant lipoprotein
Cholesterol: marked elevation; triglyceride: no change or elevation	↑ Ingestion of cholesterol	LDL (Type IIa)
Cholesterol: elevation; triglyceride: no change or elevation	↑ Cholesterol manufacture by liver Obesity Hereditary ↓ LDL catabolism Hypothyroidism Hereditary ↓ Remnant removal Hypothyroidism Hereditary	LDL (Type IIa) or LDL and VLDL (Type IIb) LDL (Type IIa) Remnants (Type III) or VLDL and chylomicrons)
Cholesterol: no change or elevation; triglyceride: elevation	↑ Triglyceride snythesis Dietary intake (caloric) Alcohol Hyperinsulinism Obesity Corticosteroids Estrogen Hereditary ↓ Triglyceride clearance Insulin (diabetes) Hypothyroidism Renal failure Hereditary	VLDL (Type IV) or VLDL and chylomicrons VLDL (Type IV) or VLDL and chylomicrons (Type V)

SGOT: normal values and deviation

Normal values: 8 to 33 U/100 ml (Reitman-Frankel)
10 to 40 mU/ml (SMA 12/60)

Deviation	Etiology

Elevation of SGOT values
  Elevation greater than 1,000 U/ml (or more than 10 times normal
 	
  Elevation to 40 to 100 U/ml
	Myocardial infarction
	Hepatocellular disease
	  Infectious or toxic hepatitis
	  Liver necrosis
	Skeletal muscle damage
	Tachyarrhythmias
	Congestive heart failure
	Pericarditis
	Pulmonary infarction
	Cirrhosis
	Cholangitis
	Pancreatitis
	Metastatic liver disease
	Generalized infection (infectious mononucleosis)
	Trauma
	Muscle disease
	  Muscular dystrophy
	  Dermatomyositis

Serum glutamic-pyruvic transaminase

Serum glutamic-pyruvic transaminase (SGPT) catalyzes conversions between glutamic and pyruvic acid in the glycolytic pathway. The liver contains the highest concentration of SGPT, but the enzyme is prominent in kidney, heart, and skeletal muscle. The pattern of release of SGPT is similar to SGOT in the face of cellular damage, though more damage than that necessary to produce an elevation of SGOT is generally present when SGPT levels are increased.

Lactic dehydrogenase

The tissue concentrations of LDH mimic those of SGOT. Furthermore, elevations in serum LDH levels correlate with the same conditions underlying increases in SGOT concentrations. LDH catalyzes the conversions between pyruvate and lactate in the glycolytic cycle. Following myocardial infarction, serum LDH levels increase five to six times in the first 48 hours and may remain elevated for as long as 6 to 10 days. LDH has been separated into five isoenzymes, making it a sharper diagnostic tool. These isoenzymes may be separated by electrophoresis.

A variety of colorimetric tests are available for assessment of this serum enzyme concentration.

A hemolyzed blood specimen may give spuriously high values for LDH concentration in the serum since the damaged RBCs give up LDH; this will be reflected in the concentration of the enzyme in the sample.

Alkaline phosphatase

Determinations of serum alkaline phosphatase levels are frequently used to determine the presence of liver and bone cell disease, since the enzyme has its greatest content in these two tissues. However, it is also found in significant concentrations in intestine, kidney, and placenta. The enzyme is thought to catalyze reactions in the process of bone matrix formation, because increased

SGPT: normal values and deviation

Normal values: 5 to 35 U/ml (Reitman-Frankel)

Deviation	Etiology
Elevation of SGPT values	
Marked elevation	Infectious or toxic hepatitis
	Infectious mononucleosis
Moderate elevation	Obstructive jaundice
	Postnecrotic cirrhosis
Slight elevation	Cirrhosis
	Myocardial infarction

Serum LDH: normal values and deviation

Normal values: 200 to 400 U/ml (Wroblewski)
100 to 225 mU/ml (SMA 12/60)

Deviation	Etiology
Evaluation of LDH values	
Elevation greater than 1,400 Wroblewski units	Hemolytic disorders (marked hemolysis)
	Pernicious anemia
	Myocardial infarction
Elevation of 500 to 700 Wroblewski units	Chronic viral hepatitis
	Malignant neoplasms
	Liver
	Kidney
	Brain
	Skeletal muscle
	Heart
	Destruction of lung tissue
	Pulmonary emboli
	Pneumonia
	Destruction of renal tissue
	Infarction
	Infection

Serum alkaline phosphatase: normal values and deviation

Normal values
Adults: 1.5 to 4.5 U/100 ml (Bodansky)
4 to 13 U/100 ml (King-Armstrong)
0.8 to 2.3 U/ml (Bessey-Lowry)
30 to 100 mU/ml (SMA 12/60)
Children: 5 to 14 U/100 ml (Bodansky)
3.4 to 9 U/ml (Bessey-Lowry)
15 to 30 U/100 ml (King-Armstrong)
(The level in children is about three times that of the adult.)

Deviation	Etiology
Elevation of alkaline phosphatase values	
Marked elevation (15 U/ 100 ml or more— Bodansky)	Liver disease
	Obstructive disease
	Neoplasm
	Bone disease:
	Paget's disease
	Sarcoma
	Metastatic carcinoma
Slight to moderate elevation (8 to 10 U/100 ml— Bodansky)	Liver disease
	Cholangitis
	Cirrhosis
	Hyperparathyroidism
	Osteomalacia
	Renal infarction, tissue rejection

serum alkaline phosphatase levels correlate with osteoblastic activity. The isoenzymes from the liver, bone, intestine, kidney, and placenta can be separated by electrophoresis; thus, the source of the enzyme can be determined. Synthesis of alkaline phosphatase is thought to be small in the normal hepatic cell. The serum alkaline phosphatase level reflects placental function and may be used to monitor the progress of pregnancy.

A low alkaline phosphatase level may be associated with hypophosphatemia, hypothyroidism, or vitamin C deficiency.

Acid phosphatase

Acid phosphatase occurs in greatest amount in prostatic tissue. In the normal individual the enzyme is excreted in prostatic fluids. However, in prostatic metastatic carcinoma, the serum acid phosphatase level rises and thus becomes a tool in differential diagnosis.

Normal serum acid phosphatase values: 1 to 4 U/100 ml (King-Armstrong)

Creatine phosphokinase

Creatine phosphokinase (CPK) catalyzes the phosphorylation of creatine by adenosine triphosphate (ATP). The greatest tissue content of CPK is found in skeletal and cardiac muscle although significant amounts occur in the brain. The serum CPK level may be elevated as a result of intramuscular injection or following surgery and returns to basal levels in 24 to 48 hours. Since CPK is not produced by the liver, elevated serum

Serum CPK: normal values and deviation

Normal values: 0 to 200 units (Sigma)
Males: 5 to 50 mU/ml (Oliver-Rosalki)
Females: 5 to 30 mU/ml (Oliver-Rosalki)

Deviation	Etiology

Elevation of serum CPK values	Muscle disease
	   Duchenne's muscular dystrophy (early)
	   Dermatomyositis
	   Polymyositis
	   Trauma
	Myocardial infarction
	Encephalitis
	Bacterial meningitis
	Cerebrovascular accident
	Hepatic coma
	Uremic coma
	Strenuous exercise
	Ingestion of salicylates

values of this enzyme may help eliminate liver disease in differential diagnosis.

Aldolase

Aldolase catalyzes the splitting of fructose 1,6-diphosphate into glyceraldehyde phosphate and dihydroxyacetone phosphate. Aldolase occurs in greatest concentration in skeletal and heart muscle, but the liver contains a moderate amount, and all tissues contain some of the enzyme.

Amylase

Pancreatic amylase is synthesized in the pancreatic cells and secreted into the pancreatic ducts for transport to the duodenum, where it catalyzes the hydrolysis of starch and glycogen. Elevated serum amylase levels may be used to monitor damage to pancreatic cells. Although the salivary glands produce amylase, diseases of these cells do not affect the serum lipase level.

Lipase

Lipase is synthesized by the pancreatic cells and secreted into the pancreatic ducts for transport to the duodenum, where it catalyzes the

Serum aldolase: normal values and deviation

Normal values: 3 to 8 U/100 ml (Sibley-Lehninger)

Deviation	Etiology

Elevation of serum aldolase values	Muscle disease
	   Progressive muscular dystrophy
	   Dermatomyositis
	   Trichinosis
	Myocardial infarction
	Viral hepatitis
	Hepatic cellular necrosis
	Granulocytic leukemia
	Carcinomatosis

Serum amylase: normal values and deviation

Normal values: 60 to 150 U/100 ml (Somogyi)

Deviation	Etiology
Elevation of serum amylase values	Acute pancreatitis

Serum lipase: normal values and deviation

Normal values: 0 to 1.5 U/ml (Cherry-Crandall)

Deviation	Etiology
Elevation of serum lipase values (lipasemia)	Acute pancreatitis

hydrolysis of triglycerides to fatty acids. Elevation of serum lipase concentrations indicates damage to pancreatic cells. Serum lipase levels remain elevated longer following acute pancreatitis than do amylase levels.

Cholinesterase

Cholinesterase (ChE) catalyzes the hydrolysis of acetylcholine and other cholinesters and has been classified as "true" cholinesterase or as pseudocholinesterase. "True" cholinesterase, or acetylcholinesterase, is more rapid in its action on acetylcholine and is found in greatest concentration in the brain and in RBCs. Pseudocholinesterase is found in plasma but not in the erythrocytes and is thought to be manufactured by the liver. Both of these enzymes are inactivated by organophosphates. Testing of acetylcholinesterase provides an indication of toxicity from insecticides containing these compounds.

Normal ChE (RBC) values: 0.65 to 1.00 pH units
Pseudocholinesterase (plasma): 0.5 to 1.3 pH units

Red blood cells: normal counts and deviations

Normal counts
Males: 4.6 to 6.2 × 10⁶/μl
Females: 4.2 to 5.4 × 10⁶/μl

Deviations	Etiology	Possible effects
Elevated RBC count (polycythemia)	Bone marrow hyperplasia (polycythemia vera)	Hyperviscosity of blood Tendency toward thrombosis Sluggish blood flow to tissues (tissue hypoxia) Hypervolemia Headache Tinnitus Dizziness Ruddy cyanosis
Decreased RBC count (anemia)	RBC production deficiency states Protein Iron Vitamin B₁₂ Folic acid Toxicity (depressed bone marrow) Metabolites (urea, creatinine) Drugs (chloramphenicol) Ionizing radiation Hypothyroidism Hereditary (thalassemia)	

SCREENING HEMATOLOGICAL EXAMINATIONS

The hemogram, or complete blood cell count (CBC), includes the following determinations: RBC count, hematocrit (HCT), hemoglobin (Hgb), white blood cell (WBC) count, and differential WBC count. Other commonly performed hematological examinations are determinations of the mean corpuscular volume (MCV), mean corpuscular hemoglobin (MCH), and mean corpuscular hemoglobin concentration (MCHC).

■ Red blood cells
RBC count

Erythropoiesis, the manufacture of RBCs, occurs in the bone marrow. Erythropoietin, a hormone produced by the kidney exposed to hypoxia, plays a prominent role in the control of erythropoiesis.

Electronic counting devices (such as the Coulter device) are faster and produce more accurate blood cell determinations than those of a technician counting the smear under a microscope.

Both anemias and polycythemias are classified as relative if they result from changes in plasma volume.

Hematocrit

The hematocrit examination is used to determine the volume packed (centrifuged) RBCs in 100 ml of blood.

Normal hematocrit values
Males: 40% to 54%
Females: 38% to 47%

Hemoglobin

Hemoglobin consists of heme, a pigmented compound containing iron and globin, a colorless protein. Hemoglobin binds with oxygen as well as with carbon dioxide. The hemoglobin molecule binds oxygen and transports it to the periphery; it binds carbon dioxide as it is transported to the lung.

Normal hemoglobin values
Males: 13.5 to 18 gm/100 ml
Females: 12.0 to 16 gm/100 ml

Mean corpuscular volume

The MCV test measures RBCs in terms of individual cell size. The value can be calculated through the use of the following formula:

$$MCV = \frac{HCT}{RBC}$$

The result is expressed in microcubic millimeters per blood cell.

Normal MCV: 80 to 94 μmm^3

This test is used to classify anemias as microcytic (RBC size smaller than normal), normocytic, or macrocytic (larger than normal).

Deviations	Etiology
Microcytic anemia	Hypochromic
	Iron deficiency
	Thalassemia
	Chronic infections
	Chronic renal disease
	Malignancy
Normocytic anemia	Hypochromic
	Lead poisoning
	Chronic infection
	Chronic renal disease
	Malignancy
	Normochromic
	Hemorrhage
	Hemolytic anemia
	Bone marrow hypoplasia
	Splenomegaly
Macrocytic anemia	Normochromic
	Pernicious anemia
	Folic acid deficiency
	Hypothyroidism
	Hepatocellular disease

Mean corpuscular hemoglobin

The MCH examination measures the hemoglobin concentration of the individual RBCs. Expressed in picograms (micromicrograms), it can be calculated by dividing the hemoglobin in grams by the RBCs:

$$MCH = \frac{Hgb}{RBC}$$

The test allows the classification of anemia as hypochromic or normochromic.

Normal MCH values: 27 to 31 pg

Mean corpuscular hemoglobin concentration

The MCHC test measures the concentration of hemoglobin in grams per 100 ml of RBCs. Expressed in percentages, it can be calculated using the following formula:

$$MCHC = \frac{Hgb\ in\ grams}{HCT}$$

Normal mean cell hemoglobin concentration: 32% to 36%

An elevation of MCHC is seen only in hereditary spherocytosis.

Sedimentation rate

The erythrocyte sedimentation rate (ESR) is the speed with which RBCs settle in unclotted blood. The speed with which the RBCs settle is dependent on the concentration of the various plasma protein fractions and on the concentration of the RBCs. The cells settle out more rapidly when the plasma concentration is high and the RBC count is low. Increased concentration of fibrinogen or of the globulins speeds up the rate of sedimentation. The rate of settling is accelerated in many inflammatory conditions, in pregnancy, and in multiple myeloma. The sedimentation rate is decreased in sickle cell anemia; this may be due to the abnormal shape and stickiness of the RBCs.

Normal ESR rate (Westergren)
    Men under 50: <15 mm/hr
    Men over 50: <20 mm/hr
    Women under 50: <20 mm/hr
    Women over 50: <30 mm/hr

Microscopic RBC examination

A stained smear of whole blood is examined microscopically to assess the morphological characteristics of the RBCs.

Normal RBC: Nonnucleated, biconcave disc, 7μ to 8μ in diameter; contains 95% hemoglobin (Fig. 24-4)

Nucleated RBCs may be observed in periods of marked erythropoiesis as a result of marrow stimulation. These immature cells are released from the marrow and are found in the circulating blood.

Reticulocytes. A reticulocyte is a cell that is larger than the normal RBC and that stains more with basic dye. The center does not appear pale, as does the normal RBC. In the normal individual 0.5% to 1.5% reticulocytes are present in the circulating blood. During periods of accelerated erythropoiesis the number of reticulocytes in the general circulation increases. The reticulocyte count is generally elevated as a result of hemorrhage or hemolysis.

Nuclear fragments. Structures that represent the degenerated nucleus of the erythroblast are seen as coarse dots, blue lines, and imperfect rings in the smear.

Basophilic stippling. The term basophilic stip-

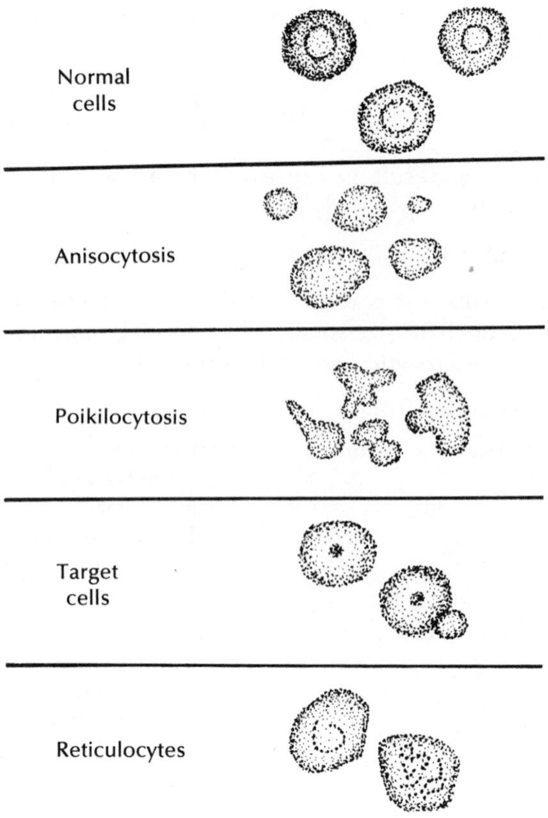

Fig. 24-4. The average red blood cell is 7μ in diameter and is slightly indented in the center. This produces a gradual lessening of color toward the center of the cell. In evaluation of shape, only cells that do not touch neighboring cells are considered. Irregularity in size is referred to as anisocytosis. Irregularity in shape is referred to as poikilocytosis. Increased basophilia is seen in younger cells, such as reticulocytes. (From Fowkes, W. C., Jr., and Hunn, V. K.: Clinical Assessment for the nurse practitioner, ed. 1, St. Louis, 1973, The C. V. Mosby Co.)

pling refers to the presence of homogenous blue dots observed in RBCs treated with Wright stain. This stippling may indicate thalassemia or toxic manifestations resulting in abnormal hemoglobin production.

Siderotic granules. Granules of iron-containing substances in addition to hemoglobin may be seen in some cells of smears of RBCs treated with Prussian blue dye. The cells are termed siderocytes and are increased in number following splenectomy and during the course of hemolytic anemias.

Heinz bodies. The RBCs of the individual with glucose-6-phosphate dehydrogenase deficiency may contain inclusion bodies containing denatured hemoglobin called Heinz bodies.

Poikilocytosis. A poikilocyte is an RBC of abnormal shape. Poikilocytosis is the term used to designate the presence of abnormally shaped RBCs in the blood. Leptocytes (target, or "Mexican hat," erythrocytes) are characterized by a central pigment bulls-eye area surrounded by a clear area, which is ringed by a hemoglobinated peripheral border. This type of erythrocyte is seen in the blood of individuals with hemoglobin C or A, or a combination of C and S. They are frequently seen in thalassemia. Liver disease has

Platelets: normal count and deviations

Normal count: 300,000/μl

Deviations	Etiology
Thrombocytopenia	Bone marrow depression
Thrombocytosis	Polycythemia Splenectomy

been shown to be present in some individuals with demonstrated poikilocytosis. The sickle cell disease is characterized by long, crescent-shaped cells.

Anisocytosis. Anisocytosis is the term used for blood containing erythrocytes with excessive variations in size.

Platelets (thrombocytes). Platelets may be seen in the microscopic examination of whole blood smears. The platelets are granular fragments of cytoplasm of megakaryocytes in the bone marrow. The platelets are largely phospholipids and polysaccharides. They are carriers for a variety of enzymes as well as for clotting factors and serotonin. Thus, platelets play a major role in blood coagulation.

Thrombocytopathy is a term for platelet cells of unusual size or shape.

White blood cells: normal counts and deviations

Normal counts: 4,500 to 11,000/μl whole blood

Deviations	Etiology
Elevated WBC count (leucocytosis)	Leukemia
	Bacterial infection
	Polycythemia (due to bone marrow stimulation)
Decreased WBC count (leucopenia)	Bone marrow depression
	Ionizing radiation
	Chloramphenicol
	Phenothiazines
	Sulfonamides
	Phenylbutazone
	Agranulocytosis
	Acute viral infection
	Acute alcohol ingestion

■ White blood cells

WBC count

The WBC count is the assessment of the number of WBCs (leucocytes) in 1μl of whole blood. The WBCs function to protect the body against infectious disease. Neutrophils and monocytes destroy microorganisms by phagocytosis. Lymphocytes and plasma cells are thought to produce antibodies. Eosinophils play a role in allergy. Granulocytes, monocytes, and some lymphocytes are produced in the bone marrow; lymphocytes and plasma cells are produced in the lymph nodes and thymic tissue. Disease processes may result in changes within individual leucocyte groups, which may include morphological and functional changes as well as variations in total numbers. These alterations may provide valuable clues that can be used in differential diagnosis.

Differential WBC count

Six different types of WBCs have been identified in the blood: polymorphonuclear neutrophils (PMNs) polymorphonuclear eosinophils (PMEs), polymorphonuclear basophils (PMBs), monocytes, lymphocytes, and plasma cells. Platelets (thrombocytes) are particles of megakaryocytes.

Increased granulation of leucocytes may indicate toxicity reactions.

A shift to the left means that increased numbers of immature neutrophils are present in the specimen and that they are band forms rather than lobulations. Acute stress to the bone marrow and severe bacterial infection may cause the release of early granulocytes. Increased lobulation (3 to 6) or segmentation of neutrophils is often ob-

Differential WBC count: normal percentages and deviations

Normal differential count

TYPE OF CELL	PERCENTAGE OF TOTAL WBC COUNT	RANGE
Neutrophils (PMNs)	56%	50% to 70%
Eosinophils (PMEs)	2.7%	5% to 6%
Basophils (PMBs)	0.3%	0 to 1%
Lymphocytes	34%	20% to 40%
Monocytes		0 to 7%

Deviations	Etiology
Neutrophilic leucocytosis	Bacterial infections
	Pneumonia
	Systemic infections
	Inflammatory disease
	Rheumatic fever
	Rheumatoid arthritis
	Pancreatitis
	Thyroiditis
	Carcinoma
	Trauma (tissue destruction)
	Burns
	Crush injury
	Stress
	Cold
	Heat
	Exercise
	Electroshock therapy
	Panic, fear, anxiety
	Increased catecholamines
	Increased corticosteroids
	Cushing's disease
	Acute gout
	Diabetes mellitus
	Lead poisoning
	Acute hemorrhage
	Hemolytic anemia
Neutrophilopenia	Acute viral infections
	Bone marrow damage
	Nutritional deficiency
	Vitamin B_{12}
	Folic acid
Basophilic leucocytosis	Myeloproliferative diseases
	Myelofibrosis
	Polycythemia vera
Basophilopenia	Anaphylactic reaction
Eosinophilic leucocytosis	Allergic manifestations
	Asthma
	Hay fever
	Parasitic infestations
	Roundworm
	Flukes

Continued.

Differential WBC count: normal percentages and deviations—cont'd

Normal differential count

	Malignancy (Hodgkin's disease)
	Colitis
	Eosinophilic granulomatosis
	Eosinophilic leukemia
Lymphocytosis	Leukemia (80% to 90% of total WBCs)
	Infectious diseases
	Infectious mononucleosis
	Pertussis
	Viral infections with exanthema
	Measles
	Rubella
	Roseola
	Chickenpox
	Thyrotoxicosis
	Cushing's disease
Monocytosis	Typhoid fever
	Tuberculosis
	Subacute bacterial endocarditis
	Malaria

served in association with vitamin B_{12} deficiency.

Mild to moderate leucocytosis associated with mild to moderate lymphocytosis is characteristic of chronic infections such as tuberculosis. Relative lymphocytosis is the condition in which the total number of circulating lymphocytes remains constant but the WBC count is low because of neutropenia. Relative lymphocytosis is normal between 4 months and 4 years of age.

Monocytosis may occur even though there is no increase in WBCs.

Abnormal white blood cells of diagnostic importance

Plasma cells. Plasma cells are not normally found in the circulating blood. The presence of plasma cells in the blood predicates the necessity to differentiate multiple myeloma, infectious mononucleosis, serum sickness, and rubella.

Downey cells. Downey cells are abnormal lymphocytes that differ from the normal cells in size, cytoplasmic structures (vacuolated, foamy), and immature chromatin pattern. These cells are observed in individuals with infectious mononucleosis, viral diseases (hepatitis), and allergic states.

LE cell. The LE cell is a polymorphonuclear leucocyte, generally a neutrophil that contains an inclusion body. The inclusion body has been shown to be denatured nuclear protein that is being phagocytosed by the neutrophil. The LE cell, which can be induced in the laboratory in the presence of LE factor, is present in the blood of many individuals who have lupus erythematosis.

DETECTION OF SYPHILIS (LUES)

Syphilis is the disease caused by the spirochete *Treponema pallidum.* The disease is described in terms of its early or late manifestations or in terms of primary, secondary, and tertiary stages. The disease is transmitted by intimate mucous membrane contact or in utero. The destructiveness of the organism is attributed to its invasiveness and the elaboration of a weak endotoxin. Immunity is established by a single infection. One to 4 months after contraction of syphilis, two distinct antibodies appear in the serum. The complement fixation and flocculation diagnostic tests are based on one of these, syphilitic reagin, which combines with certain tissue lipids. *T. pallidum* is sensitive to penicillin. Thus, detection of the infection provides an opportunity for curative intervention.

■ Immunological tests for syphilis

The first serological test for syphilis (STS) was devised by Wassermann and, like Kolmer's modification, which superseded it, was a complement fixation test. Wassermann used extract from a syphilitic liver that had as its reactive ingredient cardiolipin, which is found in many tissues and is not actually specific for syphilis. Thus, it was fortuitous that the syphilitic reagin reacted with it. A lipoidal substance is found in spirochetes that is thought to be similar to the cardiolipin lipoprotein complex, which would explain the reaction.

The procedure for the complement fixation test involves first mixing the sample serum with cardiolipin reagent. The antigen-antibody reaction serves to bind the complement, removing it from the reaction. Sheep blood indicator is then added to the mixture. Hemolysis of the blood cells indicates the presence of free complement. If the cells do not hemolyze, complement is absent because of an earlier antigen-antibody reaction. False positive results may occur if the serum contains anticomplement activity.

The flocculation tests include the Venereal Disease Research Laboratory (VDRL), rapid plasma reagin (RPR), Kahn, Hinton, Kline, and Mazzini tests. These tests are performed by adding a suspension of cardiolipin antigen particles to the sample serum. If the syphilitic reagin (antibody) is present, it produces clumping, or flocculation. The reaction is quantitated by the degree of flocculation.

T. pallidum immobilization test

Nichols strain of pathogenic spirochetes can be cultured in rabbits. These spirochetes are incubated with the suspected serum for the *T. pallidum* immobilization (TPI) test. If the specific antibody is present, the spirochetes are immobilized. This reaction can be observed under the microscope. Other treponema spirochetes are known to give positive reactions to this test.

Reiter protein complement fixation test

The nonpathological Reiter strain of spirochetes can be cultured in artificial media for the Reiter protein complement fixation (RPCF) test. Antigen has been prepared from this strain and used in a complement fixation technique.

Fluorescent treponemal antibody absorption test

In the fluorescent treponemal antibody absorption (FTA-ABS) test, nonspecific cross-reacting antibodies are absorbed from the suspected serum through the use of the Reiter treponema antigen. The remaining serum is incubated on a smear of killed Nichols spirochetes. Following this, a solution containing fluorescent antibodies produced against human globulins is exposed to the sample.

Accuracy of test results

The STS tests are reported to produce as many as 25% to 45% biological false positive (BPF) results. That is, many positive tests have been reported for individuals who definitely have not been exposed to or do not have syphilis. Further investigation has shown these individuals to have acute viral or bacterial infections, hypersensitivity reactions, or a recent vaccination; in some cases such individuals have been found to have chronic systemic illness, such as collagen disease, malaria, or tuberculosis.

Positive tests results obtained from nonspecific methods may be confirmed with the FTA-ABS tests, which yields positive results midway through or at the end of the primary stage. Thus, in screening procedures a flocculation STS test is done initially and is followed up with the more specific FTA-ABS test.

All tests for syphilis give positive results in the secondary stage.

Antibiotic therapy may cause tests for syphilis to be negative.

■ Darkfield examination

Serous fluid exudate may be removed from a syphilitic lesion by pipet. *T. pallidum*, if present, may then be identified by darkfield microscopy. This provides positive identification of the spirochete and may be the earliest method of identification, since antibodies are not apparent until late in the primary stage.

URINALYSIS

The urine that is examined for screening purposes is generally a voided specimen collected without regard to circadian variation of the components; that is, it is voided at any time during the 24-hour period. More accuracy can be expected in electrolyte determination and less likelihood of bacterial contamination can be expected if a midstream or clean-catch specimen is employed. Ideally, the urine is collected on the client's arising following a period of 12 hours in which no fluids were taken. The urine should be tested within 2 hours following its collection; spurious results may be obtained if urine is allowed to stand for long periods at room temperature; the urine pH is greater, bacteria multiply, and leucocytes and casts are known to deteriorate.

The standard urinalysis includes description of appearance, determination of specific gravity, pH, glucose, protein ketones, and microscopic examination of urinary sediment.

■ Appearance

The normal color of urine is pale golden yellow. Diluted urine is even more pale in hue. The color is only reported in the event of abnormality. Orange, red, and brown hues of the urine may be associated with porphyria, hemoglobinuria, urobilinuria, or bilirubinemia. Porphyria may be indicated by urine that becomes burgundy red on exposure to light.

Deviations	Etiology
Orange hue	Bile
	Ingestion of Pyridium
Red hue	Blood
	Porphyria
	Urates
	Ingestion of Dorbane
Brown hue	Blood
	(Melanin may turn black on standing)

■ Specific gravity

The specific gravity of the urine provides an indicator of the ability of the kidney to concentrate urine. The test is reported as the ratio of the weight of the urine tested to the weight of water.

Normal specific gravity of the urine
  1.016 to 1.022 (in states of euhydration)
  1.001 to 1.035 (range of normal without reference to hydration)

Low values suggest renal tubular dysfunction. Concentrated urine is observed in ADH deficiency.

■ **pH**

pH of urine: normal pH and deviation

Normal pH: Freshly voided urine is generally acidic with a pH of 4.6 to 8.

Deviation	Etiology
Alkaline urine	Metabolic alkalemia (except hypokalemic chloremia)
	Proteus infections
	Aged specimen

■ **Glucose**

The presence of glucose is not a normal finding for urine. Although glucose is freely filtered by the renal glomerulus it is fully reabsorbed by the tubules. Only when the blood glucose levels reach the tubular maximum (T_m) of glucose (320 mg/min) or plasma threshold of 160 to 190 mg/100 ml is the kidney unable to completely reabsorb it. Glycosuria may indicate that the individual has a low renal threshold for glucose. The most common cause, however, is the presence of diabetes mellitus. Occasionally after high carbohydrate intake the blood glucose level may be high enough to allow spilling of glucose into the urine. Both reducing and enzymatic tests may be used to identify urinary glucose.

The practitioner may measure both blood and urinary glucose concentrations through the means of dipsticks, chemically treated papers that change color on exposure to glucose. Color charts provided with the testing materials allow standard comparison and, thereby, identification of the degree of glucose concentration of the tested body fluid.

Deviation	Etiology
Glucosuria	Diabetes mellitus
	Increased intracranial pressure
	Cushing's disease
	Pheochromocytoma
	Pregnancy

■ **Protein**

Tests for the protein content in urine are dependent on the principle that protein precipi-

tates in the presence of heat in acidic urine. Sulphosalicylic acid is the acid most frequently used for this purpose. An estimate of the protein content is made from the density of the precipitate as noted below:

Precipitate description	Value	Percent protein
Faintly cloudy	1+	
Cloudy but transparent	2+	0.1
Opaque with clumping	3+	0.2 to 0.3
Dense, solid gel	4+	0.5

Normally, very small amounts of protein appear in urine that are not detectable by routine methods. Even trace quantities are an indication that follow-up should be done. A 24-hour quantitation of the protein excreted by the kidneys may be done. In addition, an electrophoretic determination of the type of protein that is in the urine may be done. Albumin is the most frequently encountered protein, since its molecular size is smaller than that of the globulins or fibrinogen.

The urine specimen may be contaminated with vaginal secretions. This should be borne in mind for the female client. In many agencies it has become routine to use a clean-catch urine collection technique for this determination in order to obviate this protein contamination.

Bence Jones protein is an abnormal protein that appears in the urine of individuals with multiple myeloma.

■ **Acetone and diacetic acid (ketone bodies)**

Ketones are products of fat metabolism and are increased in the blood during periods when increased fats are being used as fuel, such as in starvation, after glycogen stores have been depleted. In diabetes mellitus, the lack of insulin makes

Urinary protein: normal excretion and deviation

Normal excretion: 0.1 gm/24 hr

Deviation	Etiology
Proteinuria	Pregnancy
	Strenuous physical exercise
	Orthostatism
	Fever
	Kidney disease
	Glomerulonephritis
	Nephrotic syndrome
	Neoplasm
	Infarction
	Postrenal infection

glucose relatively unavailable to the cells, so that fats are again metabolized in greater quantity. The blood ketones are increased more rapidly than they can be metabolized and are excreted in the urine. Acetone determinations are indicated whenever the urinary glucose test is positive or blood glucose is elevated.

The acetone level of urine may be tested with a chemically treated dipstick that changes color in the presence of ketone bodies. This is read against a standard scale provided with the test papers.

▪ Microscopic examination of urinary sediment

The normal urinary sediment may contain one or two RBCs as well as WBCs and an occasional cast. All other substances are considered pathological.

Red blood cells. Since RBCs are too large to filter through the glomerulus, the presence of blood in the urine indicates bleeding within the genitourinary tract. Common causes are calculi, cystitis, neoplasm, tuberculosis, and glomerulonephritis.

White blood cells. WBCs may indicate infection in any part of the genitourinary tract. Glomerulonephritis is typified by the presence of WBCs, casts, and bacteria. As a rule, pyuria from the kidney is associated with proteinuria, whereas only very small amounts of protein are present in the urine of the individual with an infection of the lower urinary tract.

Casts. Gelled protein and cellular debris precipitated in the renal tubules and molded to the tubular lumen are called casts. Portions of these casts may break off and are found in the urine. The casts are hyaline, granular, or cellular in nature. Epithelial casts are made up of columnar renal epithelium or round cells. The hyaline casts are almost transparent and consist of homogenous protein. The granular casts are dark colored and a degenerated form of the hyaline casts. The tubular shape of the casts has led to the use of the term cylinduria.

Casts consisting of WBCs are typical of pyelonephritis and the exudative stage of acute glomerulonephritis. Casts containing RBCs may appear clear or yellow.

The deposition of amyloid substance in urinary casts gives them a waxy appearance.

Urine that contains hyaline casts and protein may indicate a nephrotic syndrome.

Crystals. The acidity or alkalinity of the urine determines the type of crystals that may be identified in it. A urine with low pH is characterized by calcium oxalate, cystine, uric acid, and urate crystals. Alkaline urine is most frequently associated with carbonate crystals and amorphous phosphates.

EXAMINATION OF THE STOOL

In most cases a stool specimen is obtained by asking the individual to defecate, but digital removal of feces from the rectum can be done to facilitate collection when time constraints so dictate. Frequently a laxative is recommended to soften the stool, particularly if the individial has given a history of constipation. Because chemical analyses are calculated on the basis of daily output, the entire stool is sent to the laboratory. The feces are analyzed for size, shape, consistency, and color.

The normal individual excretes 100 to 200 gm of feces daily. The volume is dependent on the fluid content of the bowel. About 500 to 1,000 ml of chyme (liquid stool) are delivered to the colon each day, but most of the water and electrolytes are reabsorbed, primarily in the proximal colon. Sodium is absorbed, and chloride follows passively. The gradient established results in absorption of water. In addition, bicarbonate ions are secreted by the colon and an equal amount of chloride is absorbed. About one fourth of the stool is solid material which consists of the undigested residue of food, intestinal mucus and epithelium, bacteria, fat, and waste materials from the blood.

The rapid passage of stool through the colon in diarrhea results in larger stools (by volume) containing more liquid. Diarrhea is generally caused by inflammation of the colon but may also result from malabsorption syndromes.

A fecalith or stercolith is a dried, hardened fecal mass.

▪ Color

The normal color of the stool is brown as a result of food pigments as well as the breakdown products of bilirubin. Bilirubin is converted to biliverdin (green bile) by intestinal bacteria and then to stercobilin (a brown substance). Increased motility of the stool in diarrhea may result in green stools due to the presence of biliverdin that was allowed insufficient time for bacterial conversion in the colon.

Melena is the name given to a black stool caused by gastrointestinal bleeding (more than 100 ml) high enough in the tract that it is partially digested. Bleeding of the lower gastrointestinal tract is observed as bright-to-dark red blood in the stool. The guiac test for occult blood is described in Chapter 15 on Assessment of the abdomen and rectosigmoid region.

Deviation	Etiology
Melena	Esophagitis
	Esophageal varices
	Hiatus hernia
	Gastritis
	Peptic ulcer
	Carcinoma
Presence of bright-to-dark red blood	Polyps of the colon
	Carcinoma of the colon
	Diverticulitis
	Colitis
	Hemorrhoids

Ingestion of iron or bismuth compounds may cause the stool to be green to black. Green vegetables ingested in excessive amounts may also turn the stool green. A dietary intake that contains a good deal of milk but is low in protein may result in a light-colored stool.

■ Odor

The odor of feces and flatus are the result of bacterial action and are dependent on the colonic bacterial flora and the type of food ingested.

The normal stool is 10% to 20% fat. Excessive amounts of fat in the stool is termed steatorrhea. The stool may appear grossly oily. Steatorrhea may be the result of pancreatic or small bowel malabsorption problems or liver disease. Sudan stain is an iodine compound that colors fat droplets, rendering them visible under the microscope. Excessive fat loss in the stool may also be associated with deficiency of the fat soluble, vitamin D.

Quantitative evaluation of fecal fat content is sometimes performed. In the performance of this test the amount of dietary fat is usually controlled at 100 gm of fat per day. A 3-day stool collection containing more than 5 gm of fat for each day is considered pathological.

■ Microscopic examination

The stool may be examined under the microscope in order to identify ova and parasites. At least three separate specimens are examined, since one negative examination is not sufficient to rule out the infestation.

The presence of WBCs in the stool is indicative of an inflammation in the gastrointestinal tract.

BIBLIOGRAPHY

Bauer, J. D., Ackermann, P. G., and Toro, G.: Clinical laboratory methods, St. Louis, 1974, The C. V. Mosby Co.

Cromwell, L., Arditti, M., Weibell, F. J., and others: Medical instrumentation for health care, Englewood Cliffs, N.J. 1976, Prentice-Hall, Inc.

Davidsohn, I., and Henry, J. B., editors: Todd-Sanford's clinical diagnosis by laboratory methods, ed. 15, Philadelphia, 1974, W. B. Saunders Co.

Eastham, R. D.: Clinical hematology, ed. 4, Baltimore, 1974, The Williams & Wilkins Co.

French, R. M.: Guide to diagnostic procedures, ed. 4, New York, 1975, McGraw Hill Book Co.

Ravel, R.: Clinical laboratory medicine, ed. 2, Chicago, 1973, Yearbook Medical Publishers, Inc.

Skydell, B., and Crowder, A. S.: Diagnostic procedures; a reference for health practitioners and a guide to patient counseling, Boston, 1975, Little, Brown and Co.

Tilkian, S. M., and Conover, M. H.: Clinical implication of laboratory tests, St. Louis, 1975, The C. V. Mosby Co.

Wallach, J.: Interpretation of diagnostic tests, a handbook synopsis of laboratory medicine, ed. 2, Boston, 1974, Little, Brown and Co.

Widmann, F. K.: Goodale's clinical interpretation of laboratory tests, ed. 7, Philadelphia, 1973, F. A. Davis Co.

Tables of normal values

Many of the normal values are based on the experience in the Department of Pathology, Mount Sinai Hospital, Chicago, Illinois, and the Division of Clinical Pathology, State University Hospital, State University of New York, Syracuse, New York. Actual values may vary with different techniques or in different laboratories.

ABBREVIATIONS USED IN TABLES

<	= less than
>	= greater than
dl	= 100 ml
gm	= gram
IU	= International Unit
kg	= kilogram
mEq	= milliequivalent
mg	= milligram
ml	= milliliter
mM	= millimole
mm Hg	= millimeters of mercury
mIU	= milliInternational Unit
mOsm	= milliosmole
$m\mu$	= millimicron
ng	= nanogram
pg	= picogram
μEq	= microequivalent
μg	= microgram
μIU	= microInternational Unit
μl	= microliter
μU	= microunit

Reproduced with permission from Davidsohn, I., and Henry, J. B., editors: Todd-Sanford's clinical diagnosis by laboratory methods, ed. 15, Philadelphia, 1974, W. B. Saunders Co.

Table A-1. Whole blood, serum, and plasma (chemistry)

Test	Material	Normal value	Special instructions
Acetoacetic acid			
Qualitative	Serum	Negative	
Quantitative	Serum	0.2-1.0 mg/dl	
Acetone			
Qualitative	Serum	Negative	
Quantitative	Serum	0.3-2.0 mg/dl	
Albumin, quantitative	Serum	3.2-4.5 gm/dl (salt fractionation)	
		3.2-5.6 gm/dl by electrophoresis	
		3.8-5.0 gm/dl by dye binding	
Alcohol	Serum or whole blood	Negative	
Aldolase	Serum	Adults: 3-8 Sibley/Lehninger U/dl at 37° C	
		Children: Approximately 2 times adult levels	
		Newborn: Approximately 4 times adult levels	
Alpha-amino acid nitrogen	Serum	3-6 mg/dl	
δ-Aminolevulinic acid	Serum	0.01-0.03 mg/dl	
Ammonia	Plasma	20μg-150μg/dl (diffusion)	Collect with sodium heparinate; specimen must be analyzed immediately
		40μg-80μg/dl (enzymatic method)	
		12μg-48μg/dl (resin method)	
Amylase	Serum	60-160 Somogyi units/dl	
Argininosuccinic lyase	Serum	0-4 U/dl	
Arsenic	Whole blood	<3μg/dl	
Ascorbic acid (vitamin C)	Plasma	0.6-1.6 mg/dl	Analyze immediately
	Whole blood	0.7-2.0 mg/dl	
Barbiturates	Serum, plasma, or whole blood	Negative	
Base excess	Whole blood	Male: −3.3 to +1.2	
		Female: −2.4 to +2.3	
Base, total	Serum	145-160 mEq/L	
Bicarbonate	Plasma	21-28 mM/L	
Bile acids	Serum	0.3-3.0 mg/dl	
Bilirubin	Serum	Up to 0.3 mg/dl (direct or conjugated)	
		0.1-1.0 mg/dl (indirect or unconjugated)	
		Total: 0.1-1.2 mg/dl	
		Newborns total: 1-12 mg/dl	
Blood gases			
pH		7.38-7.44 arterial	
		7.36-7.41 venous	
Pco_2		35-40 mm Hg arterial	
		40-45 mm Hg venous	
Po_2		95-100 mm Hg arterial	
Bromide	Serum	0-5 mg/dl	
BSP (bromsulfonphthalein) (5 mg/kg)	Serum	<6% retention after 45 min	
Calcium	Serum	Ionized: 4.2-5.2 mg/dl	
		2.1-2.6 mEq/L or	
		50%-58% of total	
		Total: 9.0-10.6 mg/dl	
		4.5-5.3 mEq/L	
		Infants: 11-13 mg/dl	

Table A-1. Whole blood, serum, and plasma (chemistry)—cont'd

Test	Material	Normal value	Special instructions
Carbon dioxide (CO₂ content)	Whole blood, arterial	19-24 mM/L	
	Plasma or serum, arterial	21-28 mM/L	
	Whole blood, venous	22-26 mM/L	
	Plasma or serum, venous	24-30 mM/L	
CO₂ combining power	Plasma or serum, venous	24-30 mM/L	
CO₂ partial pressure (PCO₂)	Whole blood, arterial	35-40 mm Hg	
	Whole blood, venous	40-45 mm Hg	
Carbonic acid	Whole blood, arterial	1.05-1.45 mM/L	
	Whole blood, venous	1.15-1.50 mM/L	
	Plasma, venous	1.02-1.38 mM/L	
Carboxyhemoglobin (carbon monoxide hemoglobin)	Whole blood	Suburban nonsmokers: <1.5% saturation of hemoglobin	
		Smokers: 1.5%-5.0% saturation	
		Heavy smokers: 5.0%-9.0% saturation	
Carotene, beta	Serum	40μg-200μg/dl	
Cephalin cholesterol flocculation	Serum	Negative to 1+ after 24 hours; 2+ or less after 48 hours	
Ceruloplasmin	Serum	23-50 mg/dl	
Chloride	Serum	95-103 mEq/L	
Cholesterol, total	Serum	150-250 mg/dl (varies with diet and age)	
Cholesterol, esters	Serum	65%-75% of total cholesterol	
Cholinesterase	Erythrocytes	0.65-1.00 pH units	
Pseudocholinesterase	Plasma	0.5-1.3 pH units	
		8-18 IU/L at 37° C	
Citric acid	Serum or plasma	1.7-3.0 mg/dl	
Congo red test	Serum or plasma	>60% after 1 hour	Severe reactions may occur if dye is injected twice; check patient's record
Copper	Serum or plasma	Male: 70μg-140μg/dl	
		Female: 85μg-155μg/dl	
Cortisol	Plasma	8 AM-10 AM: 5μg-25μg/dl	
		4 PM-6 PM: 2μg-18μg/dl	
Creatine	Serum or plasma	Males: 0.2-0.6 mg/dl	
		Females: 0.6-1.0 mg/dl	
Creatine phosphokinase (CPK)	Serum	Males: 55-170 U/L at 37° C	
		Females: 30-135 U/L at 37° C	
Creatinine	Serum or plasma	0.6-1.2 mg/dl	
Creatinine clearance (endogenous)	Serum or plasma and urine	Male: 123 ± 16 ml/min	
		Female: 97 ± 10 ml/min	
Cryoglobulins	Serum	Negative	Keep specimen at 37° C

Test	Material		*Percent*	*Gm/dl*	Special instructions
Electrophoresis, protein	Serum	Albumin	52-65	3.2-5.6	
		Alpha-1	2.5-5.0	0.1-0.4	
		Alpha-2	7.0-13.0	0.4-1.2	
		Beta	8.0-14.0	0.5-1.1	
		Gamma	12.0-22.0	0.5-1.6	

Test	Material	Normal value	Special instructions
Fats, neutral	Serum or plasma	0-200 mg/dl	
Fatty acids			
Total	Serum	9-15 mM/L	
Free	Plasma	300μEq-480μEq/L	
Fibrinogen	Plasma	200-400 mg/dl	

Continued.

Table A-1. Whole blood, serum, and plasma (chemistry)—cont'd

Test	Material	Normal value	Special instructions
Fluoride	Whole blood	<0.05 mg/dl	
Folate	Serum	5-25 ng/ml (bioassay)	
	Erythrocytes	166-640 ng/ml (bioassay)	
Galactose	Whole blood	Adults: None	
		Children: <20 mg/dl	
Gamma globulin	Serum	0.5-1.6 gm/dl	
Globulins, total	Serum	2.3-3.5 gm/dl	
Glucose, fasting	Serum or plasma	70-110 mg/dl	Collect with heparin-fluoride mixture
	Whole blood	60-100 mg/dl	
Glucose tolerance, oral	Serum or plasma	Fasting: 70-100 mg/dl	Collect with heparin-fluoride mixture
		30 min: 30-60 mg/dl above fasting	
		60 min: 20-50 mg/dl above fasting	
		120 min: 5-15 mg/dl above fasting	
		180 min: fasting level or below	
Glucose tolerance, IV	Serum or plasma	Fasting: 70-110 mg/dl	Collect with heparin-fluoride mixture
		5 min: Maximum of 250 mg/dl	
		60 min: Significant decrease	
		120 min: Below 120 mg/dl	
		180 min: Fasting level	
Glucose-6-phosphate dehydrogenase (G-6-PD)	Erythrocytes	250-500 units/10^9 cells	
		1,200-2,000 mIU/ml of packed erythrocytes	
γ-Glutamyl transpeptidase	Serum	2-39 U/L	
Glutathione	Whole blood	24-37 mg/dl	
Growth hormone	Serum	<10 ng/ml	
Guanase	Serum	<3 nM/ml/min	
Haptoglobin	Serum	100-200 mg/dl as hemoglobin binding capacity	
Hemoglobin	Serum or plasma	Qualitative: Negative	
		Quantitative: 0.5-5.0 mg/dl	
	Whole blood	Female: 12.0-16.0 gm/dl	
		Male: 13.5-18.0 gm/dl	
Hemoglobin A$_2$	Whole blood	1.5%-3.5% of total hemoglobin	
α-Hydroxybutyric dehydrogenase	Serum	140-350 U/ml	
17-Hydroxycorticosteroids	Plasma	Male: 7μg-19μg/dl	Perform test immediately or freeze plasma
		Female: 9μg-21μg/dl	
		After 25 USP units of ACTH IM: 35μg-55μg/dl	
Immunoglobulins	Serum		
IgC		800-1,600 mg/dl	
IgA		50-250 mg/dl	
IgM		40-120 mg/dl	
IgD		0.5-3.0 mg/dl	
IgE		0.01-0.04 mg/dl	
Insulin	Plasma	11μIU-240μIU/ml (bioassay)	
		4μU-24μU/ml (radioimmunoassay)	
Insulin tolerance	Serum	Fasting: Glucose of 70-110 mg/dl	Collect with heparin-fluoride mixture
		30 min: Fall of 50% of fasting level	
		90 min: Fasting level	

Table A-1. Whole blood, serum, and plasma (chemistry)—cont'd

Test	Material	Normal value	Special instructions
Iodine			Test not reliable if iodine-containing drugs or radiographic contrast media were given prior to test
Butanol extraction (BEI)	Serum	$3.5\mu g$-$6.5\mu g$/dl	
Protein bound (PBI)	Serum	$4.0\mu g$-$8.0\mu g$/dl	
Iron, total	Serum	$50\mu g$-$150\mu g$/dl	Hemolysis must be avoided
Iron-binding capacity	Serum	$250\mu g$-$450\mu g$/dl	
Iron saturation, percent	Serum	20%-55%	
Isocitric dehydrogenase	Serum	50-250 U/ml	
Ketone bodies	Serum	Negative	
17-Ketosteroids	Plasma	$25\mu g$-$125\mu g$/dl	
Lactic acid	Whole blood, venous	5-20 mg/dl	Draw without stasis
	Whole blood, arterial	3-7 mg/dl	
Lactate dehydrogenase (LHD)	Serum	80-120 Wacker units 150-450 Wroblewski units 71-207 IU/L	
Lactate dehydrogenase isoenzymes	Serum	Anode: LDH_1 17%-27% LDH_2 27%-37% LDH_3 18%-25% LDH_4 3%-8% Cathode: LDH_5 0%-5%	
Lactate dehydrogenase (heat stable)	Serum	30%-60% of total	
Lactose tolerance	Serum	Serum glucose changes are similar to those seen in a glucose tolerance test	
Lead	Whole blood	0-$50\mu g$/dl	
Leucine aminopeptidase (LAP)	Serum	Male: 80-200 Goldbarg-Rutenburg units/ml Female: 75-185 Goldbarg-Rutenburg units/ml	
Lipase	Serum	0-1.5 Cherry-Crandall U/ml 14-280 mIU/ml	
Lipids	Serum		
Total		400-800 mg/dl	
Cholesterol		150-250 mg/dl	
Triglycerides		10-190 mg/dl	
Phospholipids		150-380 mg/dl	
Fatty acids		9.0-15.0 mM/L	
Neutral fat		0-200 mg/dl	
Phospholipid phosphorous		8.0-11.0 mg/dl	
Lithium	Serum	Negative Therapeutic level: 0.5-1.5 mEq/L	
Long-acting thyroid-stimulating hormone (LATS)	Serum	None	
Luteinizing hormone (LH)	Plasma	Male: <11 mIU/ml Female: Midcycle peak >3 times baseline value Premenopausal: <25 mIU/ml Postmenopausal: >25 mIU/ml	

Continued.

Table A-1. Whole blood, serum, and plasma (chemistry)—cont'd

Test	Material	Normal value	Special instructions
Macroglobulins, total	Serum	70-430 mg/dl	
Magnesium	Serum	1.5-2.5 mEq/L	
		1.8-3.0 mg/dl	
Methemoglobin	Whole blood	0-0.24 gm/dl	
		0.4%-1.5% of total hemoglobin	
Mucoprotein	Serum	80-200 mg/dl	
Nonprotein nitrogen (NPN)	Serum or plasma	20-35 mg/dl	
	Whole blood	25-50 mg/dl	
5′ Nucleotidase	Serum	0-1.6 units	
Ornithine carbamyl transferase (OCT)	Serum	8-20 mIU/ml	
Osmolality	Serum	280-295 mOsm/L	
Oxygen			
Pressure (PO_2)	Whole blood, arterial	95-100 mm Hg	
Content	Whole blood, arterial	15-23 vol%	
Saturation	Whole blood, arterial	94%-100%	
pH	Whole blood, arterial	7.38-7.44	
	Whole blood, venous	7.36-7.41	
	Serum or plasma, venous	7.35-7.45	
Phenylalanine	Serum	Adults: <3.0 mg/dl	
		Newborns (term): 1.2-3.5 mg/dl	
Phosphatase, acid, total	Serum	0-1.1 U/ml (Bodansky)	Hemolysis must be avoided; perform test without delay or freeze specimen
		1-4 U/ml (King-Armstrong)	
		0.13-0.63 U/ml (Bessey-Lowry)	
		1.4-5.5 U/ml (Gutman-Gutman)	
		0-0.56 U/ml (Roy)	
		0-6.0 U/ml (Schinowara-Jones-Reinhart)	
Phosphatase, alkaline, total	Serum	Adults: 1.5-4.5 U/dl (Bodansky)	
		4-13 U/dl (King-Armstrong)	
		0.8-2.3 U/ml (Bessey-Lowry)	
		15-35 U/ml (Shinowara-Jones-Reinhart)	
		Children: 5.0-14.0 U/dl (Bodansky)	
		3.4-9.0 U/ml (Bessey-Lowry)	
		15-30 U/dl (King-Armstrong	
Phospholipid phosphorus	Serum	8-11 mg/dl	
Phospholipids	Serum	150-380 mg/dl	
Phosphorus, inorganic	Serum	Adults: 1.8-2.6 mEq/L	Separate cells from serum promptly
		3.0-4.5 mg/dl	
		Children: 2.3-4.1 mEq/L	
		4.0-7.0 mg/dl	
Potassium	Plasma	3.8-5.0 mEq/L	
Proteins	Serum		
Total		6.0-7.8 gm/dl	
Albumin		3.2-4.5 gm/dl	
Globulin		2.3-3.5 gm/dl	
Protein fractionation	Serum		
Protoporphyrin	Erythrocytes	15μg-50μg/dl	

Table A-1. Whole blood, serum, and plasma (chemistry)—cont'd

Test	Material	Normal value	Special instructions
Pyruvate	Whole blood	0.3-0.9 mg/dl	
Salicylates	Serum	Negative	
		Therapeutic level: 20-25 mg/dl	
Sodium	Plasma	136-142 mEq/L	
Sulfate, inorganic	Serum	0.2-1.3 mEq/L	Hemolysis must be
		0.9-6.0 mg/dl as SO_4	avoided
Sulfhemoglobin	Whole blood	Negative	
Sulfonamides	Serum or whole blood	Negative	
Testosterone	Serum or plasma	Male: 400-1,200 ng/dl	
		Female: 30-120 ng/dl	
Thiocyanate	Serum	Negative	
Thymol flocculation	Serum	0-5 units	

Test	Material	Normal value		Special instructions
Thyroid hormone tests	Serum	*Expressed as thyroxine*	*Expressed as iodine*	
T_4 (by column)		5.0µg-11.0µg/dl	3.2µg-7.2µg/dl	
T_4 (by competitive binding Murphy-Pattee)		6.0µg-11.8µg/dl	3.9µg-7.7µg/dl	
Free T_4		0.9-2.3 ng/dl	0.6-1.5 ng/dl	
T_3 (resin uptake)		25-38 relative % uptake		
Thyroxine-binding globulin (TBG)		10µg-26µg/dl (expressed as T_4 uptake)		

Test	Material	Normal value	Special instructions
Transaminases			
GOT	Serum	8-33 U/ml	
GPT	Serum	1-36 U/ml	
Triglycerides	Serum	10-190 mg/dl	
Urea nitrogen	Serum	8-18 mg/dl	
Urea clearance	Serum and urine	Maximum clearance: 64-99 ml/min	
		Standard clearance: 41-65 ml/min or more than 75% of normal clearance	
Uric acid	Serum	Male: 2.1-7.8 mg/dl	
		Female: 2.0-6.4 mg/dl	
Vitamin A	Serum	15µg-60µg/dl	
Vitamin A tolerance	Serum	Fasting: 15µg-60µg/dl	Administer 5,000
		3 hr or 6 hr after 5,000 units vitamin A/kg: 200µg-600µg/dl	units vitamin A in oil per kg body
		24 hr: Fasting values or slightly above	weight
Vitamin B_{12}	Serum	Male: 200-800 pg/ml	
		Female: 100-650 pg/ml	
Unsaturated vitamin B_{12} binding capacity	Serum	1,000-2,000 pg/ml	
Vitamin C	Plasma	0.6-1.6 mg/dl	Collect with oxalate and analyze within 20 minutes
Xylose absorption	Serum	25-40 mg/dl between 1 and 2 hr; in malabsorption, maximum approximately 10 mg/dl	For children administer 10 ml of a 5% solution of
		Dose	D-xylose per kg
		Adult: 25 gm D-xylose	of body weight
		Children: 0.5 gm/kg D-xylose	
Zinc	Serum	50µg-150µg/dl	
Zinc sulfate turbidity	Serum	<12 units	

Table A-2. Urine

Test	Type of specimen	Normal value	Special instructions
Acetoacetic acid	Random	Negative	
Acetone	Random	Negative	
Addis count	12-hr collection	WBC and epithelial cells: 1,800,000/12 hr RBC: 500,000/12 hr Hyaline casts: 0-5,000/12 hr	Rinse bottle with some neutral formalin; discard excess
Albumin			
Qualitative	Random	Negative	
Quantitative	24 hr	10-100 mg/24 hr	
Aldosterone	24 hr	$2\mu g$-$26\mu g$/24 hr	Keep refrigerated
Alkapton bodies	Random	Negative	
Alpha-amino acid nitrogen	24 hr	100-290 mg/24 hr	
δ-Aminolevulinic acid	Random	Adult: 0.1-0.6 mg/dl Children: <0.5 mg/dl	
	24 hr	1.5-7.5 mg/24 hr	
Ammonia nitrogen	24 hr	20-70 mEq/24 hr 500-1,200 mg/24 hr	Keep refrigerated
Amylase	2 hr	35-260 Somogyi units per hour	
Arsenic	24 hr	$<50\mu g$/L	
Ascorbid acid	Random	1-7 mg/dl	
	24 hr	>50 mg/24 hr	
Bence Jones protein	Random	Negative	
Beryllium	24 hr	$<0.05\mu g$/24 hr	
Bilirubin, qualitative	Random	Negative	
Blood, occult	Random	Negative	
Borate	24 hr	<2 mg/L	
Calcium			
Qualitative (Sulkowitch)	Random	1+ turbidity	Compare with standard
Quantitative	24 hr	Average diet: 100-250 mg/24 hr Low calcium diet: <150 mg/24 hr High calcium diet: 250-300 mg/24 hr	
Catecholamines	Random	0-$14\mu g$/dl	
	24 hr	$<100\mu g$/24 hr (varies with activity)	
Chloride	24 hr	110-250 mEq/24 hr	
Concentration test (Fishberg)	Random after fluid restriction	Specific gravity: >1.025 Osmolality: >850 mOsm/L	
Copper	24 hr	0-$3\mu g$/24 hr	
Coproporphyrin	Random	Adult: 3-$20\mu g$/dl	Use fresh specimen and do not expose to direct light; preserve 24-hr urine with 5 gm Na_2CO_3
	24 hr	$50\mu g$-$160\mu g$/24 hr Children: 0-$80\mu g$/24 hr	
Creatine	24 hr	Male: 0-40 mg/24 hr Female: 0-100 mg/24 hr Higher in children and during pregnancy	
Creatinine	24 hr	Male: 20-26 mg/kg/24 hr 1.0-2.0 gm/24 hr Female: 14-22 mg/kg/24 hr 0.8-1.8 gm/24 hr	
Cystine, qualitative	Random	Negative	
Cystine and cysteine	24 hr	10-100 mg/24 hr	
Diacetic acid	Random	Negative	
Epinephrine	24 hr	0-$20\mu g$/24 hr	

Table A-2. Urine—cont'd

Test	Type of specimen	Normal value	Special instructions
Estrogens, total	24 hr	Male: 5µg-18µg/24 hr Female Ovulation: 28µg-100µg/24 hr Luteal peak: 22µg-105µg/24 hr At menses: 4µg-25µg/24 hr Pregnancy: Up to 45,000µg/24 hr Postmenopausal: 14µg-20µg/24 hr	Keep refrigerated
Estrogens, Fractionated	24 hr	Non-pregnant, mid-cycle	
Estrone (E1)		2µg-25µg/24 hr	
Estradiol (E2)		0-10µg/24 hr	
Estriol (E3)		2µg-30µg/24 hr	
Fat, qualitative	Random	Negative	
FIGLU (N-formi-minoglutamic acid)	24 hr	<3 mg/24 hr After 15 gm of L-histidine: 4 mg/8 hr	
Fluoride	24 hr	<1 mg/24 hr	
Follicle-stimulating hormone (FSH)	24 hr	Adult: 6-50 mouse uterine units/24 hr Prepubertal: <MUU/24 hr Post-menopausal: >MUU/24 hr	
Fructose	24 hr	30-65 mg/24 hr	
Glucose			
Qualitative	Random	Negative	
Quantitative	24 hr		
Copper-reducing substances		0.5-1.5 gm/24 hr	
Total sugars		Average: 250 mg/24 hr	
Glucose		Average: 130 mg/24 hr	
Gonadotropins, pituitary (FSH and LH)	24 hr	10-50 MUU/24 hr	
Hemoglobin	Random	Negative	
Homogentisic acid	Random	Negative	
Homovanillic acid (HVA)	24 hr	<15 mg/24 hr	
17-Hydroxycorticosteroids	24 hr	Male: 5.5-14.5 mg/24 hr Female: 4.9-12.9 mg/24 hr Lower in children After 25 USP units ACTH, IM: a 2- to 4-fold increase	Keep refrigerated
5-Hydroxyindoleacetic acid, qualitative	Random	Negative	Some muscle relaxants and tranquilizers interfere with test
5-HIAA, quantitative	24 hr	<9 mg/24 hr	
Indican	24 hr	10-20 mg/24 hr	
Ketone bodies	Random	Negative	Fresh, keep cool
17-Ketosteroids	24 hr	Male: 8-15 mg/24 hr Female: 6-11.5 mg/24 hr Children: 12-15 yr, 5-12 mg/24 hr; <12 yr, <5 mg/24 hr After 25 USP units ACTH, IM: 50%-100% increase	Keep refrigerated
Androsterone		Male: 2.0-5.0 mg/24 hr Female: 0.8-3.0 mg/24 hr	
Etiocholanolone		Male: 1.4-5.0 mg/24 hr Female: 0.8-4.0 mg/24 hr	
Dehydroepiandrosterone		Male: 0.2-2.0 mg/24 hr Female: 0.2-1.8 mg/24 hr	

Continued.

Table A-2. Urine—cont'd

Test	Type of specimen	Normal value	Special instructions
11-Ketoandrosterone		Male: 0.2-1.0 mg/24 hr	
		Female: 0.2-0.8 mg/24 hr	
11-Ketoetiocholanolone		Male: 0.2-1.0 mg/24 hr	
		Female: 0.2-0.8 mg/24 hr	
11-Hydroxyandrosterone		Male: 0.1-0.8 mg/24 hr	
		Female: 0.0-0.5 mg/24 hr	
11-Hydroxyetiochol-anolone		Male: 0.2-0.6 mg/24 hr	
		Female: 0.1-1.1 mg/24 hr	
Lactose	24 hr	12-40 mg/24 hr	
Lead	24 hr	<100μg/24 hr	
Magnesium	24 hr	6.0-8.5 mEq/24 hr	
Melanin, qualitative	Random	Negative	
3-Methoxy-4-hydroxy-mandelic acid (VMA)	24 hr	1.5-7.5 mg/24 hr (adults) 83μg/kg/24 hr (infants)	No coffee or fruit 2 days prior to test
Mucin	24 hr	100-150 mg/24 hr	
Myoglobin			
Qualitative	Random	Negative	
Quantitative	24 hr	<1.5 mg/L	
Osmolality	Random	500-800 mOsm/L	May be lower or higher, depending on state of hydration
Pentoses	24 hr	2-5 mg/kg/24 hr	
pH	Random	4.6-8.0	
Phenolsulfonphthalein (PSP)	Urine, timed after 6 mg PSP IV		
	15 min	20%-50% dye excreted	
	30 min	16%-24% dye excreted	
	60 min	9%-17% dye excreted	
	120 min	3%-10% dye excreted	
Phenylpyruvic acid, qualitative	Random	Negative	
Phosphorus	Random	0.9-1.3 gm/24 hr	Varies with intake
Porphobilinogen			
Qualitative	Random	Negative	
Quantitative	24 hr	0-2.0 mg/24 hr	
Potassium	24 hr	40-80 mEq/24 hr	Varies with diet
Pregnancy tests	Concentrated morning specimen	Positive in normal pregnancies or with tumors producing chorionic gonadotropin	
Pregnanediol	24 hr	Male: 0-1 mg/24 hr	Keep refrigerated
		Female: 1-8 mg/24 hr	
		Peak: 1 week after ovulation	
		Pregnancy: 60-100 mg/24 hr	
		Children: Negative	
Pregnanetroil	24 hr	Male: 1.0-2.0 mg/24 hr	Keep refrigerated
		Female: 0.5-2.0 mg/24 hr	
		Children: <0.5 mg/24 hr	
Protein			
Qualitative	Random	Negative	
Quantitative	24 hr	10-100 mg/24 hr	
Reducing substances, total	24 hr	0.5-1.5 mg/24 hr	
Sodium	24 hr	80-180 mEq/24 hr	Varies with dietary ingestion of salt
Solids, total	24 hr	55-70 gm/24 hr Decreases with age to 30 gm/24 hr	

Table A-2. Urine—cont'd

Test	Type of specimen	Normal value	Special instruction
Specific gravity	Random	1.016-1.022 (normal fluid intake) 1.001-1.035 (range)	
Sugars (excluding glucose)	Random	Negative	
Titrable acidity	24 hr	20-50 mEq/24 hr	Collect with toluene
Urea nitrogen	24 hr	6-17 gm/24 hr	
Uric acid	24 hr	250-750 mg/24 hr	Varies with diet
Urobilinogen	2 hr	0.3-1.0 Ehrlich units	
	24 hr	0.05-2.5 mg/24 hr or 0.5-4.0 Ehrlich units/24 hr	
Uropepsin	Random	15-45 units/hr	
	24 hr	1,500-5,000 units/24 hr	
Uroporphyrins			
Qualitative	Random	Negative	
Quantitative	24 hr	$10\mu g$-$30\mu g$/24 hr	
Vanillylmandelic acid (VMA)	24 hr	1.5-7.5 mg/24 hr	
Volume, total	24 hr	600-1,600 ml/24 hr	
Zinc	24 hr	0.15-1.2 mg/24 hr	

Table A-3. Gastric fluid

Test	Normal value
Fasting residual volume	20-100 ml
pH	<2.0
Basal acid output (BAO)	0-6 mEq/hr
Maximal acid output (MAO) after histamine stimulation	5-40 mEq/hr
BAO/MAO ratio	<0.4

Table A-4. Hematology

Test	Normal value		
Hemoglobin A_2	1.5%-3.5%		
Hemoglobin F	<2%		
	% NaCl	*% Lysis (fresh)*	*% Lysis (after 24-hr incubation at 37° C)*
Osmotic fragility	0.20	97-100	95-100
	0.30	90-99	85-100
	0.35	50-95	75-100
	0.40	5-45	65-100
	0.45	0-6	55-95
	0.50	0	40-85
	0.55		15-70
	0.60		0-40
	0.65		0-10
	0.70		0-5
	0.75		0

Continued. **495**

Table A-4. Hematology—cont'd

Test	Normal value	
Platelet count	150,000-400,000/μl	
Reticulocyte count	0.5%-1.5%	
	25,000-75,000 cells/μl	
Sedimentation rate (ESR)	Men under 50 yr: <15 mm/hr	
(Westergren)	Men over 50 yr: <20 mm/hr	
	Women under 50 yr: <20 mm/hr	
	Women over 50 yr: <30 mm/hr	
Viscosity	1.4-1.8 times water	
Complete blood count (CBC)		
Hematocrit	Male: 40%-54%	
	Female: 38%-47%	
Hemoglobin	Male: 13.5-18.0 gm/dl	
	Female: 12.0-16.0 gm/dl	
Red cell count	Male: 4.6-6.2 $\times$ 10^6/μl	
	Female: 4.2-5.4 $\times$ 10^6/μl	
White cell count	4,500-11,000/μl	
Erythrocyte indices		
Mean corpuscular volume (MCV)	82-98 cu microns (fl)	
Mean corpuscular hemoglobin (MCH)	27-31 pg	
Mean corpuscular hemoglobin concentration (MCHC)	32%-36%	
White blood cell differential (adult)	*Mean percent*	*Range of absolute counts*
Segmented neutrophils	56%	1,800-7,000/μl
Bands	3%	0-700/μl
Eosinophils	2.7%	0-450/μl
Basophils	0.3%	0-200/μl
Lymphocytes	34%	1,000-4,800/μl
Monocytes	4%	0-800/μl
Blood volume	Male: 69 ml/kg	
	Female: 65 ml/kg	
Plasma volume	Male: 39 ml/kg	
	Female: 40 ml/kg	
Coagulation tests		
Bleeding time (Ivy)	1-6 min	
Bleeding time (Duke)	1-3 min	
Clot retraction	½ the original mass in 2 hr	
Dilute blood clot lysis time	Clot lyses between 6 and 10 hr at 37° C	
Euglobin clot lysis time	Clot lyses between 2 and 6 hr at 37° C	
Partial thromboplastin time (PTT)	60-70 sec	
Kaolin activated	35-50 sec	
Prothrombin time	12-14 sec	
Venous clotting time		
3 tubes	5-15 min	
2 tubes	5-8 min	
Whole blood clot lysis time	None in 24 hr	

Table A-5. Miscellaneous

Test	Specimen	Normal value
Bile, qualitative	Random stool	Negative in adults; positive in children
Chloride	Sweat	4-60 mEq/L
Clearances	Serum and timed urine	
Creatinine, endogenous		115 ± 20 ml/min
Diodrast		600-720 ml/min
Inulin		100-150 ml/min
PAH		600-750 ml/min
Diagnex blue (tubeless gastric analysis)	Urine	Free acid present
Fat	Stool, 72 hr	Total fat: <5 gm/24 hr and 10%-25% of dry matter
		Neutral fat: 1%-5% of dry matter
		Free fatty acids: 5%-13% of dry matter
		Combined fatty acids: 5%-15% of dry matter
Nitrogen, total	Stool, 24 hr	10% of intake or 1-2 gm/24 hr
Sodium	Sweat	10-80 mEq/L
Trypsin activity	Random, fresh stool	Positive (2+ to 4+)
Thyroid ^{131}I uptake		7.5%-25% in 6 hr
Urobilinogen		
Qualitative	Random stool	Positive
Quantitative	Stool, 24 hr	40-200 mg/24 hr
		30-280 Ehrlich units/24 hr

Table A-6. Serology

Test	Normal value
Antibovine milk antibodies	Negative
Antideoxyribonuclease (ADNAase)	<1:20
Antinuclear antibodies (ANA)	<1:10
Antistreptococcal hyaluronidase (ASH)	<1:256
Antistreptolysin-O (ASLO)	<160 Todd units
Australia antigen	See hepatitis-associated antigen
Brucella agglutinins	<1:80
Coccidioidomycosis antibodies	Negative
Cold agglutinins	<1:32
Complement, C′3	100-170 mg/dl
C-reactive protein (CRP)	0
Fluorescent treponemal antibodies (FTA)	Nonreactive
Hepatitis-associated antigen (HAA or HBAg)	Negative
Heterophile antibodies	<1:56
Histoplasma agglutinins	<1:8
Latex fixation	Negative
Leptospira agglutinins	Negative
Ox cell hemolysin	<1:480
Rheumatoid factor	
Sensitized sheep cell	<1:160
Latex fixation	<1:80
Bentonite particles	<1:32
Streptococcal MG agglutinins	<1:20
Thyroid antibodies	
Antithyroglobulin	<1:32
Antithyroid microsomal	<1:56

Continued.

Table A-6. Serology—cont'd

Test	Normal value
Toxoplasma antibodies	<1:4
Trichina agglutinins	0
Tularemia agglutinins	<1:80
Typhoid agglutinins	
O	<1:80
H	<1:80
VDRL	Nonreactive
Weil-Felix (Proteus OX-2, OX-K, and OX-19 agglutinins)	Fourfold rise in titer between acute and convalescent sera

Table A-7. Cerebrospinal fluid

Test or constituent	Normal value	Special instructions
Albumin	10-30 mg/dl	
Albumin/globulin ratio	1.6-2.2	
Calcium	2.1-2.9 mEq/L	
Cell count	0-8 cells/μl	
Chloride	Adult: 118-132 mEq/L	These values are invalidated by admixture of blood
	Children: 120-128 mEq/L	
Colloidal gold curve	0001111000	
Globulins		
Qualitative (Pandy)	Negative	
Quantitative	6-16 mg/dl	
Glucose	45-75 mg/dl	
Lactate dehydrogenase (LDH)	Approximately $1/10$ of serum level	
Protein		
Total CSF	15-45 mg/dl	
Ventricular fluid	8-15 mg/dl	
Protein electrophoresis		
Pre-albumin	4.1 ± 1.2%	
Albumin	62.4 ± 5.6%	
Alpha-1 globulin	5.3 ± 1.2%	
Alpha-2 globulin	8.2 ± 2.0%	
Beta globulin	12.8 ± 2.0%	
Gamma globulin	7.2 ± 1.1%	
Xanthochromia	Negative	

Glossary

abduction Movement away from the axial line (for a limb) or the median plane (for the digits).

abscess Localized collection of pus.

achalasia Failure of smooth muscle of the gastrointestinal tract to relax; particularly significant for sphincters, such as the esophagogastric sphincters.

achondroplasia Disturbance in cartilage development.

acromegaly Chronic disease due to hypersecretion of the pituitary gland; characterized by overgrowth of the small parts.

acute Experience of short duration and marked severity.

adduction Movement toward the axial line (for a limb) or the median plane (for the digits).

adenoid Resembling a gland.

adenoma Tumor consisting of glandular cells.

adiposis Excessive accumulation of adipose (lipoid) tissue; obesity or corpulence; fatty infiltration of an organ or tissue.

afferent Carrying to the center from the periphery.

agnosia Inability to discriminate sensory stimuli. *Acoustic or auditory agnosia:* impaired ability to recognize familiar sounds. *Tactile agnosia:* impaired ability to recognize familiar objects by touch or feel. *Visual agnosia:* impaired ability to recognize familiar objects by sight. *Autotopagnosia:* disturbance in recognition of body parts.

amaurosis Blindness without perceptible disease of the visual structures.

amyotonia Lack of tone of the musculature of the body.

amyotrophy Wasting or atrophy of muscle tissue.

analgesia Loss of sensation; used particularly to denote relief of pain without loss of consciousness.

anarthria Loss of articulation.

anesthesia Loss of sensation.

aneurysm Dilated artery or vein of the heart.

angina pectoris Pain—substernal or radiating to the left arm, neck, or jaw; frequently correlated with myocardial ischemia.

anorexia Loss of appetite.

anosmia Inability to smell.

anosognosia Lack of insight of an individual to his disease.

antrum Cavity or chamber.

anuria Absence of secretion of urine.

aphasia Dysfunction or loss of the ability to express thoughts by speech, writing, symbols, or signs. *Fluent aphasia:* ability to produce words but with frequent errors in the appropriate choice of words or in the creation of words. *Nonfluent aphasia:* inability to produce words, either in spoken or written form.

aphonia Inability to produce laryngeal voice sounds.

aplastic Impairment in blood formation.

apraxia Impairment of the ability to carry out purposeful movement, draw, or construct forms of two or three dimensions.

aqueous humor Fluid secreted in the ciliary body and found in the anterior and posterior chambers of the eye.

arcus senilis Gray to white opaque ring surrounding the cornea, generally seen in individuals older than 50 years of age, due to lipoid position.

arrhythmia Any deviation from the normal pace of the heart.

arteriosclerosis Hardening (sclerosis) and thickening of the walls of arterioles.

arthritis Inflammation of a joint.

arthropathy General term for disease in a joint.

ascites Effusion and collection of fluid within the peritoneal cavity.

asthenia Weakness; loss of strength or energy.

asthma Paroxysmal dyspnea (wheezing) due to obstruction of the bronchi or to spasm of smooth muscle.

ataxia Impairment of coordination of muscular activity.

atelectasis Incomplete expansion of a lung that had never expanded completely; collapse of the adult lung.

atherosclerosis Type of arteriosclerosis characterized by deposits (atheromas) of cholesterol, lipoid material, and lipophages in the walls of large arteries and arterioles.

athetosis Involuntary writhing movements, particularly in the hands.

atrophy Wasting; decrease in the size of a cell, tissue, organ, or body part.

aura Premonitory sensation, generally applied to sensations preceding epileptiform convulsions.

auscultation Examination made by listening, usually through the stethoscope.

AV block Impairment of impulse conduction from the atria to the ventricles.

basophilia An abnormal increase in the basophilic leucocytosis.

borborygmus Audible bowel sound, generally due to gas propulsion through the intestine.

bradycardia Slower than normal heart rate (<50 beats per minute).

bronchiectasis Chronic disease characterized by dilatation of the bronchi. Signs include expectoration of mucopurulent material, paroxysmal coughing, and a foul-smelling breath.

bronchitis Acute or chronic bronchial inflammation.

bronchophony Sound resembling normal voice sounds over the bronchus, heard through the stethoscope; this increased vocal resonance may indicate pulmonary consolidation.

bruit Murmur (blowing sound) heard over peripheral vessels.

buccal Pertaining to the cheek.

bullous Characterized by vesicles (blisters) usually 2 cm or more in diameter.

cachexia Marked malnutrition.

chorda tympani Nerve running across the middle ear.

chorea Involuntary movements that may appear well coordinated.

chronic obstructive pulmonary disease (COPD) General term for disease involving airway obstruction, such as chronic bronchitis, emphysema, or asthma.

clonus Alternate contraction and relaxation of a muscle, induced by stretching the muscle.

clubbing Proliferation of soft tissue of terminal phalanges, generally associated with relative hypoxia of peripherial tissues, loss of the angle between the skin and nail base, and sponginess of the nail base.

colic Acute abdominal pain associated with smooth muscle contraction of the gastrointestinal tract.

colitis Inflammation of the colon.

coma Deep unconsciousness from which the individual cannot be aroused, even by painful stimuli. *Comatose:* the condition of being affected by coma.

confabulation Psychiatric term for conversation by an individual wherein the truth is little regarded. Synonym: fabrication.

consensual Reflex reaction in one pupil mimicking that occurring in the other, which is being stimulated.

consolidation Process of liquid or solid replacement of lung parenchyma as exudate from an inflammatory condition is amassed.

constipation Infrequent or difficult evacuation of feces; often associated with drying and hardening of the stool.

contralateral On the opposite side.

convulsion Series of involuntary muscle contractions.

cor pulmonale Disease of the heart secondary to pulmonary disease.

crepitus Grating, cracking noise heard in (1) beginning solidification of the lung, (2) joints from rubbing dry synovial surfaces together, or (3) the skin due to the presence of air.

cretinism Disease due to congenital lack of thyroid hormone; characterized by retarded physical and mental development

crisis Sudden change in the course of a disease.

cyanosis Dusky blue color imparted to skin when the hemoglobin saturation is less than 75% to 85% or Pa_{O_2} is less than 50 mm Hg.

cyst Collection of fluid surrounded by a membrane.

dermographia Abnormal skin sensitivity, so that firm stroking with a dull instrument or light scratching results in a wheal surrounded by a red flare; may be due to allergy.

desquamation Scaling, shedding of epithelial tissue.

diarrhea Increased frequency and liquid content of fecal evacuation.

dicrotic pulse Presence of two sphygmographic elevations to one beat of the pulse.

diopter Refractive power of a lens with a focal distance of 1 meter; a unit of measure of refractive power.

diplopia Double vision; perception of two images for a single item.

disease Cluster of symptoms or signs with a more or less predictable course.

diverticulum Pouch or sac created by herniation of mucosal lining of a hollow organ (bladder or gastrointestinal tract) through a defect in the muscular wall.

dysarthria Difficulty in articulating single sounds or phonemes of speech. Individual letters: *f, r, g;* labials—sounds produced with the lips: *b, m, v* (cranial nerve [CN] VII); gutterals—sounds produced in the throat (CN X); linguals—sounds produced with the tongue: *l, t, n* (CN XII).

dyschezia Difficulty in passing stool; pain associated with defecation.

dysdiadochokinesia Impairment in the ability to stop a movement and to institute the opposite movement, such as pronation to supination.

dysesthesia Impairment of any sensation, particularly of touch.

dysgeusia Impairment or perversion of the sense of taste.

dyslexia Disturbance in understanding the written word; difficulty in reading.

dyspepsia Impairment of the ability to digest food; especially, discomfort after eating a meal.

dysphasia Disturbance in understanding or expressing words.

dysphonia puberum Difficulty in controlling laryngeal speech sounds that occur as the larynx enlarges in puberty.

dysphoria Restlessness, agitation.

dysplasia Disorder in the size, shape, or organization of adult cells.

dyspnea Difficult or labored respiration.

dysprosody Difficulty in speech wherein inflection, pronunciation, pitch, and rhythm are impaired.

dysuria Difficulty in or painful micturition.

ectopic Abnormally located.

eczema Superficial inflammatory process of the epidermis associated with redness, itching, weeping, and crusting; of multiple etiology.

edema Abnormal increase in the quantity of interstitial fluid.

efferent Carrying from the center to the periphery.

egophony Voice sound of a nasal (telephonelike or bleating) quality, heard through the stethoscope; often defined by asking the client to say "ee," which sounds like "ay" through the stethoscope.

embolism Sudden obstruction of an artery by a clot or other foreign substance.

emphysema Collection of pus in a body cavity, generally the pleural cavity.

encephalitis Inflammation of the brain.

enteritis Inflammation of the small intestine.

enuresis Involuntary urination during sleep.

epilepsy Paroxysmal disturbances in brain function characterized by loss of consciousness, motor or sensory impairment, and disturbance of emotions or thought process.

epispadias Congenital anomaly wherein the urethra opens on the dorsum of the penis.

eructation Act of belching or bringing up gas (air) from the stomach.

erythema Enlargement of capillaries resulting in redness of the skin.

exanthem General eruption of the skin accompanied by fever.

exophthalmos Greater than normal protrusion of the eye.

festination Involuntary tendency to accelerate the speed of walking; occurs in paralysis agitans.

fever Pyrexia; elevation of the body temperature above normal for a given individual.

fiberoptics Transmission of an image along flexible bundles of coated glass or plastic fiber having special optical properties.

fibrillation Quivering or local, involuntary contraction of muscle fibers; visible through the skin.

flaccid Relaxed, without tone, flabby.

flatulence Excessive amount of gas in the gastrointestinal tract.

fremitus Palpable vibration.

friction rub Sound of a crackling or grating quality, heard through the stethoscope over inflamed pleural surfaces.

fusiform Spindle or cigar shaped.

gallop rhythm Heart rate characterized by three sounds in the presence of tachycardia.

gastritis Inflammation of the stomach.

goiter Increase in size of the thyroid gland.

gout Disease caused by deposition of crystals of monosodium urate; characterized by a disorder in purine metabolism and associated with exacerbations of arthritis of a single joint.

gumma Neoplasm composed of soft, gummy tissue resembling granulation tissue; may occur in tertiary syphilis or in tuberculosis.

gynecomastia Hypertrophy of breast tissue in a male subject.

hallucination Psychiatric term for perception of a sensory experience for which no phenomenon or object can be discerned by others.

hematemesis Vomitus containing blood that is more or less entrapped in an organ, tissue, or space.

hematoma Localized collection of blood due to rupture of a blood vessel.

hematuria Presence of blood in the urine.

hemolytic Pertaining to the release of hemoglobin from red blood cells.

hemophilia Genetic predisposition to bleed more than normal due to a deficiency of the clotting factors.

hemoptysis Expectoration containing blood.

hernia Abnormal protrusion of an organ or tissue through an opening. *Incarcerated hernia:* protrusion of abdominal contents through a weakness in the abdominal wall, so that the contents cannot be returned to the abdominal cavity. *Inguinal hernia: direct*—protrusion of abdominal contents through a weakness in the abdominal musculature, region of Hesselbach's triangle; *indirect*—protrusion through an internal inguinal ring hernia descending beside the spermatic cord. *Scrotal hernia:* protrusion (generally indirect) of abdominal contents into the scrotal sac.

herpes Virus disorder of the skin characterized by numerous small vesicles in clusters.

hyaline Glasslike, as of casts in the urine.

hydrocele Circumscribed collection of fluid, particularly in the scrotum.

hyperesthesia Abnormally increased sensitivity of the skin or another sense organ.

hyperplasia Increase in the size of a tissue or organ due to an increase in the number of cells.

hyperpnea Increased rate and depth of respiration.

hyperpyrexia Marked elevation of temperature, usually above 105.8° F (41° C).

hypertension Persistent elevation of blood pressure.

hypertrophy Abnormally enlarged tissue or structure.

hypochondriasis Abnormal concern with one's state of health, frequently accompanied by symptoms that cannot be explained pathophysiologically.

hypochromic Abnormally decreased color; used to describe anemias wherein the amount of hemoglobin in red blood cells is deficient.

hypoesthesia Abnormally decreased sensitivity of the skin or another sense organ.

hypoglossal Below the tongue.

icteric Jaundiced.

infarction Obstruction of circulation followed by ischemic necrosis.

inflammation Localized protective condition associated with vascular dilatation, exudation of plasma, and leucocytes. Clinical signs include redness, swelling, pain, heat, and limitation of function.

ipsilateral On the same side.

keratitis Inflammation of the cornea.

koilonychia Spoon-shaped nail surface, frequently associated with iron deficiency anemia.

kyphosis Increased posterior convexity of the spine (humpback).

lamella Small sheet or leaf.

leucopenia Abnormal diminution of leucocytes.

lordosis Anterior concavity of the lumbar spine (swayback, saddleback).

lysis Gradual return to normal following a disease; generally refers to a fever.

macula Small spot on the skin that differs in color from the surrounding tissue and is not elevated above the surrounding skin.

malignant Disease that is severe in nature—life threatening.

mastitis Inflammation of breast tissue.

melena Dark-colored stools (may be black or tarry) due to the presence of partially digested blood.

migraine Paroxysmal headache, frequently unilateral.

miosis Pupillary constriction.

mumps Viral infection involving the parotid gland.

murmur Blowing sound due to turbulence of blood flow, heard over the heart or the great vessels.

mydriasis Dilatation of the pupils.

myopathy Disease of the muscles.

nausea Feeling that emesis is impending.

neuralgia Pain associated with the course of a nerve.

neurosis Psychiatric term for an emotional problem thought to be related to unresolved conflict; differs from a psychosis in that hallucinations, delusions, and illusions generally do not occur.

nevus Well-demarcated malformation of the skin, such as an area of pigmentation or a mole.

nuchal Pertaining to the nape of the neck.

nystagmus Involuntary oscillation of the eyeballs; may be horizontal, vertical, or rotary.

obstipation Severe constipation.

oliguria Abnormally decreased urine secretion (<400 ml/24 hours).

onychia Inflammation of the matrix of the nail.

opisthotonos Abnormal arching of the back due to muscle spasm.

orthopnea Dyspnea relieved by sitting upright.

orthostatic Pertaining to the upright or standing position or caused by the erect position.

Paget's disease Condition characterized by excoriating or scaling lesion of the nipple overlying a malignancy.

palpate Examination conducted by feeling or touching the object to be evaluated.

palpebra Eyelid.

palpitation Awareness of the pulsations of the heart and arteries.

papilledema Edema of the optic papilla.

paraesthesia Altered or perverted sensation, such as itching, burning, or "pins and needles."

paresis Slight or incomplete paralysis; weakness.

percussion Examination conducted by listening to reverberation of tissue after striking the surface with short, sharp blows.

peristalsis Wave of contraction moving along a muscular tube, particularly the gastrointestinal tract.

petechia Small area of extravasation of blood into the skin.

-plegia Complete paralysis. *Diplegia:* paralysis of both upper or lower limbs. *Hemiplegia:* paralysis of one side of the body. *Paraplegia:* paralysis of both legs and the lower part of the body. *Quadraplegia:* paralysis of all four limbs.

plethora Pertaining to a red, florid complexion.

pleural effusion Fluid of any kind in the pleural cavity.

pleurisy Pain accompanying pleural inflammation.

polycythemia Abnormal increase in the number of red blood cells.

polydipsia Increased sensation of thirst.

polyuria Increased urinary excretion.

prepuce Foreskin.

priapism Prolonged erection of the penis.

proctoscopy Examination of the rectum with a short cylindrical instrument called a proctoscope.

prognathism Protrusion of the jaw.

proprioceptive sensation Muscle and joint sensation.

psoriasis Papulosquamous dermatosis; characteristic lesion is bright red macule, papule, or plaque covered with silver scales.

psychosis Psychiatric term for a mental disorder associated with thought disorders, pathological perception (delusions, hallucinations), or extremes of affect.

ptosis Flaccid drooping tissue, usually the sagging of an eyelid.

pulse Palpable rhythmic expansion of the artery.

pyemia Septicemia.

pyorrhea purulent Inflammation of the gums.

pyrexia Fever; elevation of the body temperature above normal for a given individual.

pyuria Presence of pus in the urine.

rale Discrete, noncontinuous sound resembling fine crackling, radio static, or hairs being rubbed together, heard through the stethoscope; generally produced by air bubbling through an exudate.

regurgitation Reversal of the flow of a substance through a vessel, such as blood flow in the wrong direction or the return of food to the mouth without vomiting.

rhonchus Wheezing or snoring sound produced by airflow across a partially constricted air passage. *Sibi-*

lant rhonchus: wheeze produced in a small air passage. *Sonorous rhonchus:* wheeze produced in a large air passage.

rigor Common term for shivering accompanying a chill or for muscle rigidity accompanying depletion of adenosine triphosphate, as in death (rigor mortis).

scoliosis Lateral deviation of the spine.

scotoma Blind or partially blind area in the visual field.

sign Objective evidence of disease that is perceptible to the examiner.

somatic Pertaining to the body.

sordes Materia alba, undigested food bacteria encrusting the lips and teeth.

spastic Rigid; characterized by muscle spasm.

steatorrhea Abnormal increase of fat in the feces.

stereognosis Discrimination of objects by the sense of touch.

sthenic Sturdy or strong; active.

stomatitis Inflammation of the mouth.

strabismus Deviation of the eye (heterotropia, squint, manifest deviation); visual axes not aligned to produce a single image of the object viewed.

strangulated hernia Hernia for which the blood supply to the protruded tissue is obstructed.

stress incontinence Involuntary urination incurred on straining, coughing, or lifting.

stridor Harsh, high-pitched respiratory sound heard in respiratory obstruction.

stupor Decreased responsiveness; partial unconsciousness.

succussion Procedure involving shaking an individual to demonstrate fluid in a hollow cavity.

symptom Subjective perception of a client of an alteration of bodily or mental function from basal conditions; change perceived by the individual.

syncope Fainting; temporary unconsciousness.

syndrome Consistent group of symptoms and signs that are produced by a similar pathological change in different individuals.

tachycardia Rapid heart rate (>100 beats per minute). *Atrial flutter:* rapid, regular, uniform atrial contraction due to AV block; ventricular rhythm varies with the degree of AV block. *Atrial tachycardia:* arrhythmia due to the atria; rapid, regular beat of all the heart. *Ventricular tachycardia:* arrhythmia due to the ventricles; rapid, relatively regular heartbeat.

tachypnea Rapid respiratory rate.

telangiectasis Localized group of dilated capillaries.

tenesmus Uncomfortable straining; particularly, unsuccessful attempts at stool or urination.

thrill Palpable murmur; vibration accompanying turbulence in the heart or the great vessels.

tic Muscle twitch, spasmodic movement.

tophus Deposits of monosodium urate, seen in gout.

tympany Drumlike note produced by percussion, generally over a gas-filled region.

undulant Wavelike variations, particularly as in fever, diurnal circadian variations.

urticaria Rash characterized by wheals.

valgus Angulation of an extremity toward the midline. *Genu valgus:* a knock-kneed person.

varicocele Distention of the veins of the spermatic cord.

varicose Dilated, particularly a vein.

varus Angulation of an extremity away from the midline. *Genu varus:* a bow-legged person.

vertigo Illusion that the environment is moving, whirling around the individual affected; frequently seen in disease of the inner ear or vestibular apparatus.

vitiligo Skin affliction characterized by patches of depigmented skin due to destruction of melanophores.

whispered pectoriloquy Increased resonance of the whispered voice as heard through the stethoscope.

xerostomia Dryness of the mouth.

Index